KA

MASTER THE BOARDS
PEDIATRICS

SECOND EDITION

THE HIGHEST-YIELD REVIEW FOR THE ABP EXAM

William G. Cvetnic, MD, FAAP

Printed in the United States of America

10 9 8 7 6 5 4 3 2 1

ISBN-13: 978-1-60978-879-7

Kaplan Publishing books are available at special quantity discounts to use for sales promotions, employee premiums, or educational purposes. For more information or to purchase books, please call the Simon & Schuster special sales department at 866-506-1949.

About the Author

William G. Cvetnic, MD, FAAP, is a board-certified pediatrician and neonatologist. He has an extensive clinical and academic background, and has taught in medical school classrooms, in clinical settings, and as an invited lecturer and consultant. He received his BS in molecular biology from Johns Hopkins and his MD and MBA from the University of Pittsburgh. He completed his pediatrics residency at the University of California, San Diego, and a fellowship in neonatal-perinatal medicine at the University of California, Irvine. Dr. Cvetnic has served on the pediatrics faculties in neonatal-perinatal medicine of the University of California, Irvine, and the University of Pittsburgh; was the medical director of the Neonatal Intensive Care Unit at Magee-Women's Hospital, University of Pittsburgh; and also had an appointment at Children's Hospital of Pittsburgh. Besides academic neonatology, he has practiced inpatient and PICU hospital medicine, outpatient acute care, neonatal follow-up, developmental pediatrics, pediatric pulmonology, and office general pediatrics. In addition, he was the vice president and medical director of a private medical company, teaching family-centered, developmentally supportive care to the staffs of NICUs around the country. Dr. Cvetnic has been teaching and preparing educational materials for Kaplan since 2004. He resides in Jacksonville, Florida.

KAPLAN MEDICAL ADVISORY PANEL

JACK SILLS, MD, is Clinical Professor of Pediatrics at the University of California, Irvine. Dr. Sills graduated from Northwestern University's Feinberg School of Medicine in 1979 and completed training in pediatrics at the University of California, Irvine, in 1982, and a perinatal-neonatal fellowship at the University of California, San Diego, in 1984. His expertise is in bedside teaching and clinical research in the areas of risk management, evidence-based outcomes, pulmonary disease processes, and neonatal nutrition and pharmacology.

CHRISTINE E. KOERNER, MD, is Associate Professor of Emergency Medicine and Chief, Division of Pediatric Emergency Medicine, at the University of Texas Health Science Center at Houston.

TABLE OF CONTENTS

For Test Changes or Late-Breaking Developments

kaptest.com/publishing

The material in this book is up-to-date at the time of publication. However, the American Board of Pediatrics (ABP) may have instituted changes in the test after this book was published. Be sure to carefully read the materials you receive when you register for the test. If there are any important late-breaking developments—or any changes or corrections to the Kaplan test preparation materials in this book—we will post that information online at *kaptest.com/publishing*.

INTRODUCTION

If you are preparing to take the general pediatrics exam for the first time, it may feel like a daunting task to go back and review the entire field. After all, most of you will not have seen or taken care of patients with every condition about which you are expected to know. Even though learning through direct patient experience always leads to the best understanding and retention of disease processes, you have also been exposed to many other types of indirect learning since medical school—classroom lectures, journal clubs, clinical discussions, noon conferences, and your own reading. You have most of the material that you need for this exam somewhere in your cerebral cortex; it just needs to be brought to the foreground, organized, and solidified. Again, this may be a daunting task, but it is easier if you have been keeping up with your reading through your residency and afterward, into subspecialty training or practice. Hopefully, that is the situation, so that what you really need is just a review of the most important concepts in order to take an exam and perform well. You need not restudy absolutely everything that has anything to do with pediatrics. Most of the exam questions are based on clinically relevant issues related to managing wellness in children, preventing disease, and diagnosing and treating disease. While there may be questions on some basic science issues, these also tend to have a clinical relevance, rather than simply testing about an isolated, perhaps obscure, basic science fact. The highest percentage of questions is related to the more common issues; however, you also need to know about many less common illnesses that many (maybe most) of you have never seen.

HOW TO USE THIS BOOK

Master the Boards: Pediatrics is not a textbook—it is a review book: a review of the information that you need to know for this exam, as presented in the exam content outline of the American Board of Pediatrics (ABP). The ABP basically tells you what you need to know, and if you study that material, and study it well, you have the potential to score high.

This book is organized in a similar manner to that of the content outline for the exam. There is more detail given for those topics that represent a higher percentage of exam content. For example, the topics representing about 35 percent of the exam are growth and development; nutrition and nutritional disorders; preventive pediatrics; infectious disease; respiratory disorders; ear, nose, and throat disorders; adolescent medicine and gynecology; and behavioral and mental health issues. These topics are covered in greater detail than some of the less represented exam topics, such as metabolic disorders and ethics for primary care physicians. Nonetheless, all aspects of the content outline contain the information that you need. The only topics that are beyond the scope of this book from the content outline are pharmacokinetics, research and statistics, and patient safety and quality improvement. These three areas represent about 5 percent of the exam, and you should go back and review the basics of these topics.

The layout is primarily presented as an outline, mostly with the use of short phrases either in paragraph form or bulleted lists. Comparative material is presented in tables, basic figures, and flow diagrams. In each section, the emphasis is on the etiology of a disease process; key words in making a diagnosis; major associations with the disease; choosing the best initial test, the most accurate test, and the best initial therapy; and the most effective therapy and outcome. In addition to illnesses, all aspects of well-child care and development through adolescence are discussed. The most important words and concepts are in bold for you to particularly focus on, and perhaps to allow for a briefer, final review prior to taking your exam.

ABOUT THE GENERAL PEDIATRICS CERTIFYING EXAM

The General Pediatrics Certifying Exam is given once a year in the fall throughout the United States. In order to sit for the exam, a candidate must be a graduate of an accepted medical school (the Liaison Committee on Medical Education in the United States, the Royal College of Physicians and Surgeons of Canada, or the American Osteopathic Association); otherwise, if the medical school is listed by the World Health Organization, a standard certificate from either the Educational Commission for Foreign Medical Graduates (ECFMG) of the Medical Council of Canada is required. In addition, candidates must have a valid, unrestricted license to practice medicine in one of the United States or a province of Canada, or unrestricted privileges to practice in the U.S. Armed Forces. Candidates must complete three years of pediatric training in programs accredited by the Accreditation Council for Graduate Medical Education (ACGME) or in accredited Canadian programs. Program directors must verify satisfactory completion of training and evaluate the acceptability of the applicant. The information in this section was current at time of publication, but it's a good idea to check in at ABP: gpcert@abp.org.

EXAM BLUEPRINT

The exam is taken in a single day, and there are four sections, each 1 hour and 45 minutes long, for a total testing time of 7 hours. However, you can expect to spend around 9 hours at the testing center, accounting for the required arrival time (30 minutes before your test appointment), introduction and honor code (5 minutes), optional 10-minute tutorial, two optional 15-minute breaks, a 45-minute lunch break after Section Two, and closing examinee survey.

This computer-based test consists of 330–350 questions. Question formats include multiple-choice and single best answer, and most reflect patient-based clinical scenarios. An unanswered question automatically counts as an incorrect answer, so be sure to answer every question even if you must guess.

REGISTRATION

The registration process varies depending on your situation. For the most accurate, up-to-date information about registration and test day procedures, go to abp.org. At the time of publication, the registration fee is $2,225. (There is a $340 late fee.)

SCORING
Pass Rates

The most recent pass rate, from 2012, was 86.0 percent (and has generally been increasing since 2005, when it was 76.6 percent), according to the ABP.

Score Reporting

Results of the exam are reported to the candidate online within 90 days of having taken the exam. Passing the exam gives the examinee initial board certification in Pediatrics.

ABOUT THE MAINTENANCE CERTIFYING EXAM (MOC)

The ABP offers a Maintenance of Certification Program that is a continuous process of self-assessment and maintenance of skills, and a secure exam every 10 years.

ON THE DAY OF THE EXAM

1. Arrive at the test center at least 30 minutes before your scheduled testing time to allow for check-in. If you arrive late, you may not be permitted to take the exam.

2. You must bring your scheduling permit and an acceptable, unexpired form of identification with a recent (within the last 10 years) photograph. Acceptable forms of identification include a driver's license or a U.S. passport. Check any questions or concerns with the test maker before your scheduled exam.

Others, besides those taking the general pediatric exam for the first time, may find this book helpful. While the material goes beyond that needed for the USMLE, all of the pediatric knowledge for that exam is presented (and reflective of the types of questions typically asked). Physicians who need to recertify in pediatrics may find that a reading of this book is a useful way to prepare. It may also be used as a quick office reference guide, although there are no specifics in terms of dosing of drugs or the use of precise treatment protocols.

So whatever your goal, you should find this review book useful in terms of strengthening your pediatric knowledge. You might even learn something that you previously did not know. Remember that one major key to succeeding on standardized tests is overlearning. Study all parts thoroughly and never assume that because something is uncommon, you will not see a question on it. If you take that attitude, you may end up not studying for 15 percent of the exam (the lowest percentage of questions regarding less common material). So study everything well, and good luck.

THE NEONATE

DELIVERY ROOM RESUSCITATION

Apgar Score

Definition: The Apgar score is a tool used for immediate assessment of the newborn that helps identify infants requiring resuscitation.

✓ State of the infant by scoring at 1 and 5 minutes (and every 5 minutes as long as resuscitation continues)

✓ **1 minute:** need for immediate resuscitation, but DO NOT WAIT; begin resuscitation as soon as it is evident that ventilation is inadequate to sustain an adequate heart rate irrespective of the score.

✓ **5 minutes** and beyond: probability of successful resuscitation (The score itself does **not** determine when to resuscitate.)

✓ Does **not** predict long-term neurological outcome (is normal in most patients with cerebral palsy), but an Apgar score of ≤3 beyond 10 minutes is predictive of a worse outcome. Scores ≥ 7 are generally considered to be good.

✓ BUT a 5-minute score of 0–3 PLUS an umbilical artery pH of ≤7.0 significantly increases relative risk of neonatal mortality

Scoring:			
	0	**1**	**2**
Heart rate	0	<100	≥100
Respiration	None	Slow, irregular	Good cry
Muscle tone	Flaccid	Some flexion	Active
Reflex irritability	None	Grimace	Cry
Color	Pale, blue	Peripheral cyanosis	Pink

The newborn establishes regular respirations by 1 minute of age. The following resuscitation schema applies if: there is presence of meconium, there is decreased breathing or crying effort, the infant is not pink, there is decreased tone, or gestational age is less than term:

Initial steps in neonatal resuscitation

- **Radiant warmer** (prone to heat loss due to high surface area-to-body mass ratio)
- Suction trachea (if **thick, particulate meconium** is present in a **non-vigorous** infant → intubate, visualize cords, then **suction** through endotracheal tube)
- Dry (heat loss in delivery room reduced with radiant warmer and drying)
- Position head → suction mouth, then nose
- Decreased responsiveness → tactile stimulation
- EVALUATE **respirations, heart rate, and color**

Next if there are decreased (or no) respirations and/or if the heart rate is <100

Positive pressure ventilation with 100% oxygen through bag and mask for 15–30 seconds. **If no response after 30 seconds,** perform intubation and ventilation with 100% oxygen with a bag through the endotracheal tube (ETT). **If the heart rate remains <100,** continue ventilation.

If heart rate is <60 despite effective positive pressure ventilation and 100% oxygen for at least 30 seconds, initiate **chest compressions** at 120/minute (compression:ventilation = 3:1; lower third of sternum with two fingers perpendicular to sternum or with thumbs with fingers encircling the chest).

If the heart rate is <60 despite effective ventilation and compressions, give **epinephrine** (umbilical vein or ETT) 0.1–0.3 mL/kg of 1:10,000 solution. May repeat every 3–5 minutes.

If there is evidence of significant volume depletion (e.g., secondary to placental abruption), give 10–20 mL/kg IV or an isotonic crystalloid solution or colloid (albumin, filtered cord blood, or O-negative red blood cells, if acute hemorrhage).

If the infant has respiratory depression and the mother has been given an analgesic drug within 4 hours of delivery, give 0.1 mg/kg of **naloxone hydrochloride** either IV or via the ETT.

If there is a prolonged resuscitation and metabolic acidosis has been documented → give 2 mEq/kg (0.5 mEq/mL of a 4.2% solution) **sodium bicarbonate** slowly AND ONLY after you have effective ventilation.

After resuscitation, if the infant has poor perfusion (weak pulses, low blood pressure, low urine output), start a continuous infusion of **dopamine or dobutamine** at 5–20 µg/kg/min along with maintenance IV fluids. If still no response, consider **epinephrine** at 0.1–1.0 µg/kg/min (severe shock).

BIRTH TRAUMA

Table 1.1: Major Birth Injuries

Trauma	Key Diagnostic Words	First Diagnostic Step in Management	Treatment	Prognosis
Caput succedaneum	Presenting scalp (most parietal, occipital), fluctuant edema (most serous) above periosteum; crosses suture lines	None	If hemorrhagic (less common) and patient is jaundiced, follow bilirubin	Resolves completely within days
Cephalohematoma	Subperiosteal blood; does not cross suture line; possible underlying linear skull fracture	Most important is to follow the bilirubin; skull radiographs only if severe and concern for significant fracture	May need phototherapy	Most resolve in 2 weeks to 3 months; may have calcium deposition for up to 1–5 years
Subcutaneous fat necrosis	Difficult deliveries and with maternal cocaine use; at sites of trauma → well-defined, hard, irregular lesions of skin; necrosis at 6–10 days of life	None unless anorexia, vomiting, irritability and increased sleep → obtain serum calcium	May need to treat significant hypercalcemia with IV fluids, furosemide and hydrocortisone	Becomes soft within 2 months and then regresses
Skull fracture	Most linear and with cephalohematoma; usually not recognized; depressed—mostly secondary to forceps delivery	None unless depressed → x-ray, possibly CT if suspect underlying brain trauma	Usually none, unless large, depressed → immediate surgery	Most heal within months without problems
Facial nerve paralysis	Most with forceps delivery; smooth forehead, open eye, no nasolabial fold, corner of mouth droops on ipsilateral side; tongue not affected so feeding is fine	None	None	Most resolve within days to weeks (months in most severe, uncommon)
Subconjunctival hemorrhage	Red patch in bulbar conjunctiva; common with any delivery	None	None	Absorbed in 1–2 weeks

(continued on next page)

Table 1.1: Major Birth Injuries (cont.)

Trauma	Key Diagnostic Words	First Diagnostic Step in Management	Treatment	Prognosis
Clavicular fracture	Most frequent neonatal fracture; difficult delivery of shoulder in vertex or extended arms in breech; if complete → at birth with irritability (pain), decreased arm movement, discoloration, deformation at clavicle, no Moro on ipsilateral side	Plain radiograph	Control pain → immobilize arm/shoulder	Bone contour normal after several months
Brachial palsy	*Duchenne-Erb:* prolonged and difficult delivery; C5–C6; most common; arm adducted and internally rotated with extension at elbow, pronation of forearm; no reflexes *Klumpke:* rare; C8-T1 (Horner syndrome); hand and wrist paralyzed	Possible plain radiographs of shoulder including lower cervical spine, clavicle, and upper humerus to exclude other bone/soft tissue injuries	Physical therapy and monthly evaluations; if no correction by 3–9 months → explore brachial plexus for surgery	Most resolve completely; others may have improvement with early surgery
Phrenic nerve injury	Most unilateral with ipsilateral brachial palsy; hemi-diaphragmatic paralysis; recurrent cyanosis, difficult respirations and no diaphragmatic movement; decreased breath sounds	Plain radiograph → elevated diaphragm, shift of mediastinum to opposite side and atelectasis bilaterally; best test: real-time ultrasound	Position with involved side down, oxygen as needed, IV fluids; may need ventilation; if no resolution within 2 months → surgical plication of diaphragm	Most recover spontaneously
Sternocleidomastoid injury	Muscular torticollis; hyperextension in difficult breech or head delivery or in-utero constraint; hematoma → scarring → muscle shortening; may see at birth or 10–14 days after birth; head forward to the involved side and chin to opposite shoulder	Plain radiographic studies to exclude other pathology	Daily stretching exercises, stimulate infant to look in involved direction; place on affected side during sleep; try for 6 months → if no improvement, then surgery	Most recover within 2–3 months; if not corrected by 3–4 years, skull becomes foreshortened and may have lower cervical and upper thoracic scoliosis

HIGH-RISK INFANTS

Premature, Low Birth Weight, Post-Term, and Large for Gestational Age

Estimate of gestational age (appropriate-AGA, small-SGA, large-LGA) based on physical and neurological criteria made at birth with the modified **Ballard scoring** system provides estimation of gestational age with physical and neurological exam features. It is accurate within ±2 weeks.

Premature or preterm delivery: **<37 weeks** from first day of last menstrual period, due to many causes (fetal, placental, uterine, and maternal). Significant cause is in-utero infection → **chorioamnionitis.**

Low birth weight (LBW): birth weight **<2,500 g**. Due to premature birth, intrauterine growth retardation (IUGR; SGA), or both. Result in a significant part of neonatal morbidity and mortality (through the first 28 days).

Very low birth weight (VLBW): birth weight **<1,500 g**. Most are preterm. **Most accurate predictor** of neonatal mortality rate.

Intrauterine growth retardation (IUGR): Higher neonatal mortality rate than appropriate-for-gestational-age (AGA) infants; more prone to fasting hypoglycemia, temperature instability, polycythemia, and perinatal asphyxia.

1. <u>Early-onset or symmetric:</u> Decreased cell number; problems early in gestation. Weight, length, and head circumference (i.e., brain size) are decreased to relatively same extent. Major causes: chromosomal, malformation syndromes, teratogenic, intrauterine infections. Main complications are directly related to underlying cause.
2. <u>Late-onset, asymmetric, or head-sparing:</u> Decreased size beginning in third trimester. Head circumference (and hence brain size) is normal, but weight and length are decreased. Major causes: poor maternal nutrition, placental vascular disease (preeclampsia, toxemia), maternal illnesses (e.g., chronic hypertension, renal disease, anemia). Main complications related to degree of placental-fetal perfusion and may result in perinatal asphyxia, hypoglycemia, and polycythemia-hyperviscosity, or fetal death.

Post-term infants: Delivery after 42 weeks from last menstrual period. May have placental insufficiency → hypoxia and meconium staining (more than term). Significant increase in mortality if delivery is delayed **more than 3 weeks after term**. Increased birth weight, no lanugo, decreased or absent vernix, loose skin, long nails, lots of scalp hair, and white, desquamating skin.

Large for gestational age: Infants weighing above the 90th percentile for gestational age. Neonatal mortality rates increase at >4,000 g. Most significant factors are **maternal obesity and diabetes**; higher incidence of birth injuries, congenital anomalies, and mental/developmental retardation.

NEONATAL INFECTIONS

Bacterial Sepsis

- Newborn is at particular risk for infection due to immunologic deficiencies
- Exposure to many organisms from the mother and postpartum environment
- May look very much like other systemic problems.
- Infection evaluations performed and antibiotics started until evidence of no infection (i.e., negative final cultures).

Early-onset neonatal sepsis

- Infection **before or during delivery**, usually manifesting in the first week of life. Vast majority seen in the first 24 hours.
- Acquired from **colonized maternal genitourinary tract**. Results from either transplacental or ascending infection.
- Most occur with **prolonged rupture of membranes** (PROM **>18 hours** of ruptured membranes).
- **Chorioamnionitis**: maternal fever, foul-smelling amniotic fluid, uterine tenderness, maternal leukocytosis, and fetal tachycardia
- Intrapartum complications and a higher rate of infection in premature infants
- Most are multisystem (**pneumonia, sepsis** common)
- Most common organisms: **Group B *Streptococcus*** (GBS), enteric organisms (primarily *Escherichia coli*), and *Listeria monocytogenes*
- Prevention: All pregnant women should receive **vaginal and rectal screening cultures** at 35–37 weeks gestation; high-risk patients (premature delivery, PROM, fever, previous infant with GBS disease) receive **intrapartum antibiotic prophylaxis**. This has decreased the incidence of early-onset neonatal GBS disease.

Late-onset neonatal sepsis

- Infection from the **caregiving environment** (nursery, NICU, home) from indwelling catheters, intravenous and arterial lines, caregivers
- Occurs from **7 days to 90 days after birth**
- Usually no intrapartum complications; focal infections more common (meningitis)
- Most common organisms: **coagulase-negative staphylococci**, *Staphylococcus aureus*, *Candida*, Gram-negatives, anaerobes, and GBS

Diagnostic key words—temperature instability (decreased temperature more common), poor feeding, vomiting, diarrhea, abdominal distension, jaundice, liver dysfunction, petechiae, bleeding, apnea, respiratory distress, cyanosis, pallor, tachycardia, bradycardia, hypotension, decreased urine output, irritability, lethargy, hypotonia

Next step in management
- Full **infection evaluation**
- Prompt **institution of broad-spectrum antibiotics**
- After stabilization, a complete review of the maternal history, prenatal course, labor and delivery records, and postpartum course should be performed, along with a thorough physical exam.

Laboratory studies
- CBC, differential and platelet count
  - **Neutropenia** is more common than neutrophilia,
  - Thrombocytopenia is nonspecific,
  - Suggestive of infection: **immature: total neutrophil count >0.2**
- Must document a **positive blood culture**.
- **Urine culture** collected by suprapubic aspiration or sterile catheterization
- Chest radiograph
- Not every infant requires a lumbar puncture. It should be done if the infant is symptomatic or if the blood culture is positive

Prophylactic antibiotics
- Early-onset disease: **ampicillin plus an aminoglycoside** (gentamicin, commonly)
- For presumptive meningitis: meningitic doses of ampicillin **plus third-generation cephalosporin** (cefotaxime), as most parenteral aminoglycosides do not achieve high levels in the cerebrospinal fluid (CSF). Do not use a cephalosporin alone (**L. monocytogenes and enterococcus are resistant**).
- Late-onset infections: must cover for **coagulase-negative staphylococci** so substitute vancomycin for the ampicillin.
- Once organism is identified and sensitivities determined, switch to the most appropriate drug or combination of drugs.
- Most treatment should be at least 7–10 days or 5–7 days after clinical improvement. Repeat the blood culture at 24–48 hours after initiation of treatment to demonstrate sterility.

INTRAUTERINE INFECTIONS (TORCH)
- Maternal illness during pregnancy (mild or even asymptomatic) → organism circulated in the blood
- May cause a **transplacental infection**, affecting the fetus
- Severity of fetal infection correlates to the gestational age when maternal infection is acquired

Toxoplasmosis (T)

Organism: *Toxoplasma gondii* (protozoan)

Acquisition: Maternal ingestion of contaminated undercooked or raw meat, or exposure to cat feces

Severity: If mother is affected in first trimester

Most signs and symptoms: Chorioretinitis, hydrocephalus, intracranial calcifications, hepatosplenomegaly, prematurity, IUGR

Diagnosis: **Most accurate test:** If evidence of acute infection in mother → polymerase chain reaction (PCR) amplification of B1 gene for *T. gondii* in amniotic fluid. Then serial ultrasounds to look for fetal organ damage (early). **Best initial test for infant** is IgM enzyme-linked immunosorbent assay (ELISA) or IgM immunosorbent agglutination assay.

Treatment: Mother: **spiramycin** to prevent fetal infection. If ultrasound shows evidence of fetal infection, change to **pyrimethamine plus sulfadiazine (with folinic acid** to block marrow suppressive effects of these two drugs).

Outcome: Poor outcome with delay in diagnosis and treatment. Chorioretinitis → to **visual problems, including blindness**; intracranial calcifications → to seizures and/or intellectual and developmental delay, including mental retardation. Cognitive defects may be significant.

Other (O)

Syphilis

Organism: *Treponema pallidum*

Acquisition: 100% vertical transmission to fetus from mother who has most likely first- or second-stage syphilis during pregnancy; newborn considered to have **second-stage** syphilis.

Severity: Correlated with diagnosis and appropriate maternal treatment. Without treatment, many fetal or neonatal deaths occur.

Most signs and symptoms: **Early** (<2 years old): IUGR, hepatosplenomegaly, jaundice, **snuffles** (persistent nasal discharge), **chorioretinitis, nephrotic syndrome, periosteitis, osteochondritis, mucocutaneous lesions (may involve palms and soles and may desquamate).**

Late: (untreated) Rhagades (linear scars radiating from anus, nares, mouth), saddle nose deformity, saber shins (anterior tibial bowing), Clutton joints (painless synovitis), mulberry molars (multiple small cusps), Hutchinson teeth (notched, peg-shaped upper central incisors).

Diagnosis: **Best initial test**: First, screen with nontreponemal test (Venereal Disease Research Laboratory [VDRL] or rapid plasma reagin [RPR]); quantitative results correlate with disease activity so can follow titers for response to therapy. Will become negative in a few months. **Then,** confirm with a treponemal test (*T. pallidum* immobilization test [TPI], fluorescent treponemal antibody absorption test [FTA-ABS], or microhemagglutination assays [MHA-TP]). Will remain positive. **Most accurate test**: finding organisms with dark-field microscopy or direct immunofluorescence on tissue (placental, umbilicus, skin, nasal discharge, amniotic fluid).

Treatment:

- A nontreponemal test at least 4 times greater than the mother's
- Physical, laboratory, and radiographic evidence of disease in the infant
- Positive VDRL in cerebrospinal fluid (CSF) or elevated CSF protein or WBC count
- Placental or umbilical cord positive with direct immunofluorescence

---

Rx: If positive, perform lumbar puncture and radiography. First week of life: **penicillin G** 100,000–150,000 U/kg/24 hours divided q 12 hrs (q 8 hrs after week 1) for 10 days OR **procaine penicillin** 50,000 U/kg/day IM for 10 days. Follow nontreponemal test until negative. Adequate Rx of mother (penicillin at least **4 weeks prior to delivery**) does not require treatment of infant.

Outcome: Nontreponemal tests should decrease by 3 months and become negative by 6 months. Re-treat if still reactive. For neurosyphilis, repeat CSF q 6 months. Re-treat if still reactive at 6 months. Infants symptomatic at birth CAN develop late congenital syphilis despite appropriate treatment.

Varicella zoster

Organism: Varicella zoster virus (VZV)

Acquisition: Varicella infection (chickenpox) in susceptible mother early in pregnancy leads to **congenital varicella syndrome**, whereas transplacental infection at delivery → **neonatal varicella**. (Shingles during pregnancy causes neither).

Severity: Greatest fetal risk at 6–12 weeks (development of limb buds) and 16–20 weeks (maturation of eye and brain).

Most signs and symptoms: **Cicatricial skin lesions (scarred primary lesions), limb hypoplasia and atrophy**, club foot, microcephaly, **IUGR, mental deficiency**.

Diagnosis: Maternal history and fetal ultrasound/newborn exam; VZV-specific IgM and IgG in cord blood

Treatment: Once maternal infection is present, varicella-zoster immunoglobulin (VZIG) will not protect the fetus; acyclovir to mother with severe disease, but is of no value to infant after birth because the virus does not actively replicate.

Outcome: Up to half die in early infancy. Wide spectrum of severity for mental deficiency and seizures.

Parvovirus B19

Organism: Parvovirus B19 (small, single-stranded DNA virus). Humans are the only host.

Acquisition: Primary infection from respiratory route

Severity: Greatest fetal risk prior to 20 weeks—virus causes **lysis of RBC precursors → transient RBC aplasia**

Most signs and symptoms: Most are normal newborns. **Nonimmune hydrops fetalis (from severe fetal anemia).**

Diagnosis: **Best initial test**: specific IgM or rise in titer of specific IgG. **Most accurate test**: PCR for viral DNA in amniotic fluid, fetal blood, or fetal tissue.

Treatment: Serial ultrasounds and alpha-fetoprotein with possible intrauterine transfusion for severe hydrops. Exchange transfusions after birth for hydrops.

Outcome: Varies per study; most do not have hydrops and do well.

Human immunodeficiency virus (HIV)

Organism: Human immunodeficiency virus type 1 (HIV-1)

Acquisition: HIV-infected mother by transplacental infection, **exposure to blood during labor and delivery**, or contaminated human milk

Maternal illness: HIV-positive or AIDS

Severity: **Highest perinatal transmission correlates to maternal HIV RNA viral load at delivery.**

Most signs and symptoms: Usually **asymptomatic** at birth; may have lymphadenopathy, hepatosplenomegaly, failure to thrive, pneumonia, oral candidiasis

Diagnosis: **PCR for HIV DNA** at birth, 1 and 4 months (two samples positive → infant has HIV). All infants will be seropositive (transplacental passage of antibodies) until 18 months (can use ELISA and Western blot thereafter).

Treatment: Primary treatment is prevention. Elective C-section prior to rupture of membranes (ROM). **No breast milk** (in United States, where there is safe formula); treat mother with oral **zidovudine** (ZDV, AZT) prenatally and with IV ZDV intrapartum. Begin infant on ZDV immediately after birth for at least 6 weeks or when disease absence is established. **Significantly reduces the transmission.**

Outcome: **Best outcome correlates with decrease in maternal viral load during labor and delivery with appropriate use of combination antiretrovirals**

Rubella (R)

Organism: Rubella virus (RNA virus in Togavirus family)

Acquisition: Respiratory tract spread from infected person; then viremia and intrauterine transmission

Severity: Worse in first trimester.

Most signs and symptoms: Majority show no problem at birth, but do so years later; IUGR with postnatal growth failure, **blueberry-muffin spots** on head, neck, and trunk (dermal extramedullary hematopoiesis), sensorineural **deafness**, **congenital heart disease** (with infection in first 8 weeks), **patent ductus arteriosus (PDA)**, **cataracts**, microcephaly, mental retardation

Diagnosis: **Prenatal:** documented seroconversion in mother at start of pregnancy; rubella-specific IgM in mother 7–14 days after a rash illness. **Infant: best initial test:** detection of rubella-specific IgM in cord blood or increasing titers of IgG over time; **most accurate test:** isolate virus from newborn's blood, nasopharynx, CSF, or urine by PCR for viral RNA.

Treatment: Congenitally affected children are contagious for **up to a year** unless repeated cultures are negative. No treatment.

Outcome: More than 25% of patients may have some degree of mental retardation, with smaller numbers showing behavioral and neurological problems and autism.

Cytomegalovirus (CMV) (C)

Organism: CMV is a member of the Herpesvirus family

Acquisition: Close contact with infected secretions; viral excretion is more prolonged after primary rather than reactivation infection; **vertical transmission:** transplacental, intrapartum, breast milk; **horizontal transmission:** contact with contaminated saliva, urine, blood

Severity: Higher with primary infection in first half of pregnancy; classic cytomegalic inclusion disease if infected around time of conception; worse outcomes with intracranial calcifications, chorioretinitis, and profound sensorineural hearing loss

Most signs and symptoms: Majority are **asymptomatic** at birth, but still at risk for late sequelae; IUGR, prematurity, **hepatosplenomegaly**, jaundice (direct hyperbilirubinemia), petechiae and purpura **(thrombocytopenia)**, **microcephaly, periventricular calcifications, sensorineural hearing loss**; hydrocephalus, chorioretinitis

Diagnosis: **Best initial test:** isolation of virus from infant in first 2–3 weeks of life (urine most commonly; typically, three separate specimens; improved yield with PCR); CMV-specific IgM or a 4-fold rise in IgG titers.

Treatment: Approved controlled trials use of **ganciclovir** for severely affected infants. Most effective for retinitis and hearing loss.

Outcome: Few normal survivors. **Profound bilateral, progressive sensorineural hearing loss.** Intellectual impairment; chorioretinitis may result in optic atrophy and severe visual defects; other neurological defects, including seizure disorder.

Herpes Simplex (H)

Organism: Herpes simplex virus 1 and 2 (HSV-1, HSV-2)

Acquisition: Viral acquisition during delivery **(intrapartum transmission)** but also by ascending infection and crossing of intact membranes. Postnatal spread (mostly HSV-1). Primary genital infection (more commonly with HSV-2); **may have asymptomatic shed of virus during labor (from recent infection).**

Severity: Higher with **maternal primary herpes**; higher if infection in third trimester and at birth with ROM >4–6 hours. Higher with **fetal scalp monitors**.

Most signs and symptoms: <u>Neonatal:</u> Prematurity, most with lesions (**vesicles** mostly over presenting parts and appearing as clusters) on skin and mucous membranes; **CNS involvement** with or without mucocutaneous involvement, **disseminated** with or without CNS involvement; encephalitis: irritability, poor feeding, seizures, lethargy. Disseminated disease highest in: **liver, adrenal glands, lungs**; usually present in first or second week of life with signs of shock, then disseminated intravascular coagulation (DIC), pneumonitis, hepatitis.

Diagnosis: **Best initial and most accurate test:** PCR identification of virus isolated from vesicles, CSF, urine, stool, nasopharynx, or conjunctivae.

Treatment: **C-section** within 4–6 hours of ROM; immediate isolation, and culture at infant age 24 and 48 hours; no circumcision until discharge and negative cultures; breastfeeding contraindicated *only* if lesions present on breast; **acyclovir** for symptomatic infants (or presence of vesicles).

Outcome: Mortality greatest with **disseminated infection**, then with CNS and least with focal mucocutaneous lesions; sequelae more common with HSV-2 and with encephalitis, disseminated disease, or seizures (mental retardation, seizure disorders, visual and hearing defects, chronic liver dysfunction)

NEONATAL GLUCOSE PROBLEMS
Hypoglycemia
- **Blood glucose ≤35 mg/dL at 2–3 hours after birth**, regardless of gestational age
- Glucose is lowest at 30–90 minutes after birth, then increases gradually in full-term infants to 40–80 mg/dL.
- Levels are lower in preterm and SGA infants.
- **If initial documented hypoglycemia in the first 2 hours after birth → Continue to** check the glucose every 10–15 minutes until recovery occurs. If hypoglycemia is persistent and/or the infant is symptomatic, then treatment is needed (see below).
- **Key diagnostic words:** Irritability, jitteriness, hypotonia, tachycardia, sweating, tachypnea, apnea, hypothermia, hypotonia, lethargy, feeding difficulties, cyanotic spells, seizures
- **Major causes of neonatal transient hypoglycemia**
  - **Maternal:** intrapartum glucose administration, maternal diabetes and drugs (mechanisms result in fetal insulin release): beta-sympathomimetic tocolytic drugs (e.g., ritodrine, terbutaline), propranolol, thiazide diuretics, salicylates, oral hypoglycemics
  - **Neonatal:** IUGR, asphyxia, infections, polycythemia-hyperviscosity, hypothermia, erythroblastosis fetalis
- **Major causes of neonatal persistent hypoglycemia**
  - **Hyperinsulinism:** Beckwith-Wiedemann syndrome, beta-cell hyperplasia
  - **Endocrine:** pituitary, adrenal problems (see Chapter 16)

- **Inborn errors of metabolism:** disorders of carbohydrates, fatty acids, and amino acids (see Chapter 2)
- **Treatment: With symptoms** (not seizures), give 2 mL/kg of 10% glucose (4 mL/kg with seizures) followed by an infusion at 8 mg/kg/min. **If still hypoglycemic**, or **if hypoglycemia is recurrent**, gradually increase the glucose to 15–20%. If still hypoglycemic, consider hyperinsulinemia (see below). Follow the serum glucose every hour until levels are at least 40 mg/dL, and then every 4–6 hours. Gradually withdraw supplemental glucose (other than normal feedings) over 24–48 hours.

Other Most Common Metabolic Problems and Anomalies

Either from hyperinsulinism or teratogenic effect of hyperglycemia:

- **Caudal regression** syndrome (agenesis or hypoplasia of pelvis and femurs and agenesis of lower vertebrae and sacrum)
- Cardiomegaly with heart failure; obstructive **asymmetric septal hypertrophy** (spontaneously resolves within 6 months
- Congenital heart disease: **ventricular septal defect (VSD)**, atrial septal defect (ASD), **transposition**, truncus arteriosus
- **Small left colon** (abdominal distension due to transient delay in development of descending colon)
- **Renal vein thrombosis** (flank mass, hematuria, and thrombocytopenia, usually with polycythemia)
- **Hypocalcemia** (decreased parathyroid hormone [PTH] production and persistently elevated calcitonin) and hypomagnesemia (unknown etiology)

Transient Neonatal Hypoglycemia

Table 1.2: Infants of Diabetic Mothers (IODM)

Maternal Diabetes		Fetus		Neonate
Lack of good control with repeated bouts of hyperglycemia and high HbA1c levels	→	Fetal hyperinsulinemia	→	Macrosomia, visceromegaly, increased adipose tissue, hypoglycemia
Fetal hyperinsulinemia and hyperglycemia	→	Decreased surfactant production and maturity	→	Respiratory distress syndrome (even in a term infant)
Increased fetal substrate uptake → increased metabolic rate and oxygen consumption	→	Relative hypoxemia	→	Increased erythropoietin → polycythemia, hyperviscosity and hyperbilirubinemia

Best preventive treatment

Good control of glucose during pregnancy to maintain normal rates of glucose production and basal metabolism with decreased incidence of macrosomia and anomalies.

Most important management after the birth

- Check the blood glucose within an hour and then hourly for 6–8 hours in the asymptomatic infant.
- Symptomatic infants may need more frequent checks.
- Start feeds as soon as possible (as long as the patient is stable and there are no contraindications), every 3 hours.
- Treat persistent hypoglycemia with frequent feeds (every 2–3 hours or continuous nasogastric feeds) and intravenous glucose infusion to maintain a glucose delivery of at least **6–8 mg/kg/min**.
- Avoid hypertonic boluses of glucose, as that will lead to cycles of hyperinsulinemia and hypoglycemia.

Persistent Hypoglycemia

Hyperinsulinemia

<u>Nesidioblastosis-adenoma spectrum</u> **(persistent neonatal hyperinsulinemic hypoglycemia):** Hyperinsulinemia from focal pancreatic adenomatous beta-cell hyperplasia or diffuse beta-cell hyperplasia (nesidioblastosis). Most cases are sporadic, but some are familial.

Key diagnostic words: large-for-gestational-age (LGA) infant; severe signs of **hypoglycemia** soon after birth requires high concentrations of glucose infusions.

Best initial test: Check concomitant serum glucose with serum insulin. **Insulin will be high** or normal.

Most accurate test: Pathologic exam of pancreas with immunocytologic and electron microscopic studies

Treatment: Initial treatment for hypoglycemia described above. If still hypoglycemic despite 20% glucose solution (14 mg/kg/min), start **diazoxide**. If still hypoglycemic, start **octreotide** (a long-acting somatostatin analogue). Hydrocortisone and glucagon may also be helpful. Most patients require a **subtotal (85% removal) or total (95–98% removal) pancreatectomy**.

Outcome: Some with spontaneous remission; may have diabetes and exocrine pancreatic insufficiency; high incidence of neurological damage secondary to persistent hypoglycemia.

<u>Beckwith-Wiedemann syndrome</u> **(congenital overgrowth syndrome):** Caused by altered imprinting on 11p15.5 chromosome; found as sporadic and familial cases and with chromosomal abnormalities.

Most common findings are:

- **Macrosomia** with large muscle mass (length remains >95% through adolescence and weight at 75–95%)
- **Macroglossia** (may partially occlude the respiratory tract, leading to breathing and feeding problems; partial glossectomy may be needed)
- Pancreatic beta-cell hyperplasia (**hypoglycemia**, responsive to hydrocortisone and usually required for first 4 months)
- **Hemihypertrophy** (differences in size of right vs. left side)
- Abdominal wall defect (**omphalocele**, umbilical hernia, diastasis recti)
- Cardiac defects
- Mild to moderate mental deficiency
- Tumors (**Wilms**, adrenocortical carcinoma, hepatoblastoma; appears to be related to presence of hemihypertrophy)

Hyperglycemia
- Presents less often than hypoglycemia
- More readily adapt to increases in glucose because of ability to decrease glucose production and increase glucose uptake
- Serum glucose levels above 180–200 mg/dL.

PULMONARY PROBLEMS
Normal arterial blood gas values after birth are: paO_2 60–90 mm Hg, pCO_2 35–45 mm Hg.

Transient Tachypnea of the Newborn (TTN)
- Caused by decreased absorption of fetal lung fluid at birth and leads to a decrease in lung compliance; if not monitored carefully, hypoxemia may lead to **pulmonary artery hypertension**
- **Tachypnea** is the primary problem and lasts from hours to days
- **Key diagnostic words:** term infant (most) after C-section (occurs with vaginal deliveries as well) with tachypnea (may have respiratory distress) with or without oxygen desaturation
- **Best test:** Chest radiograph (**hyperinflation**, increased vascular markings and **fluid** in the fissures)
- **Next step in management:** Monitor **oxygen saturation** with pulse oximetry, and monitor heart rate and respirations
- **Treatment: Oxygen** as needed; intravenous maintenance fluids if oral feeding contraindicated due to respiratory distress; wean oxygen as tolerated; when respirations have normalized, start feedings

Meconium Aspiration Syndrome

- Passage of meconium in utero and at birth into amniotic fluid usually indicates **fetal hypoxemia**
- May aspirate from **in-utero gasping** or postpartum aspiration of meconium in airway
- Proximal airway obstruction, peripheral airway obstruction, and pneumonitis from inflammatory mediators → severe ventilation-perfusion mismatching with hypoxemia, hypercarbia, and acidosis
- **Air-trapping** may lead to pneumothorax and severe hypoxemia to pulmonary vascular remodeling **(pulmonary artery hypertension)**.
- **Initial step in management: Immediate intubation and suctioning** of the airway for all depressed infants born with early passage of meconium (no routine intubation of all infants); careful observation of infants with meconium suctioned from below vocal cords and any infant who is symptomatic.
- **Key diagnostic words:** If meconium has been aspirated: tachypnea, signs of **respiratory distress**, **oxygen desaturation**, cyanosis, poor perfusion
- **Best initial test:** Chest radiograph: if there is an aspiration, → **patchy infiltrates**, increased lung inflation with flattening of the diaphragm, variable aeration with areas of atelectasis and areas of over-expansion (**air-trapping**); may have pneumothorax.
- **Treatment of infant with aspiration: Gentle positive-pressure ventilation** (avoid air leak, barotrauma) with 100% oxygen and early administration of **exogenous surfactant** (as there is surfactant inactivation); depending on presence of pulmonary artery hypertension, ancillary therapies may be required (high-frequency ventilation, inhaled nitric oxide, or extracorporeal membrane oxygenation [ECMO]).

Congenital Diaphragmatic Hernia (CDH)

- Malformation resulting in communication between abdominal cavity and hemithorax, usually with abdominal contents in thorax; primarily refers to the **Bochdalek type** (posterolateral, the vast majority; most on left side); small numbers are **Morgagni type** (anterolateral, retrosternal, more on right side; most are asymptomatic and diagnosed later than neonatal period). Survival is dependent upon degree of **pulmonary hypoplasia** (may be bilateral) and degree of pulmonary vascular remodeling resulting in **pulmonary artery hypertension**. About one-third of the cases have associated anomalies (CNS, cardiovascular, omphalocele, esophageal atresia) and may be associated with chromosomal abnormalities (XO, trisomy 21, trisomies 13 and 18, and others).
- **Key diagnostic words:** Severe respiratory distress in delivery room or shortly after birth (most within first 48 hours) **scaphoid abdomen** and increased chest wall diameter; bowel sounds may be heard in hemithorax, breath sounds are decreased, and cardiac point of maximal intensity (PMI) may be displaced.
- **Diagnostic steps:** Prenatal diagnosis can be made with **ultrasonography between 16 and 24 weeks**; then need high-speed MRI for further definition. After delivery, obtain chest radiograph and, if needed for further study, CT scan.
- **Initial steps in management: Intubate** a suspected or known patient with CDH; **gentle** positive-pressure ventilation with 100% oxygen to allow for **permissive hypercarbia**

(pH ≥7.3). Nasogastric tube; sedation, intravenous fluids, frequent arterial blood gases (via umbilical artery catheter); measure pulmonary and systemic pressures and cardiac function with echocardiography.

- **Further management:** Most will have significant **pulmonary artery hypertension** and require high-frequency oscillatory ventilation, inhaled nitric oxide, and/or **ECMO** prior to surgery. Wait until infant has stable oxygenation and ventilation, decreasing pulmonary artery pressure.
- **Outcome:** Overall survival close to 70%, but many with neurological and cognitive defects, gastroesophageal reflux disease, and chronic lung disease

Apnea

- Mostly occurs in the preterm infant because of **idiopathic apnea of prematurity** (AOP) and/or due to a specific problem
- **Periodic breathing** is also common: breathing pauses of 5–10 seconds, followed by 10–15 seconds of rapid breathing at 50–60/min, and infant is usually asymptomatic.
- Both AOP and periodic breathing are inversely correlated with gestational age.
- May be obstructive (nasal obstruction, unstable pharynx, flexion of the neck), central (decreased response to hypercarbia and paradoxical response to hypoxemia in preterm infants), or mixed (most); most start on day 2–7 of life
- Serious pauses defined at >20 seconds.
- **Most common causes (other than idiopathic AOP):** Sepsis, pneumonia, meningitis, intraventricular hemorrhage, anemia, necrotizing enterocolitis, hypoxia, hypoglycemia, hypothermia, hypocalcemia, seizures
- **Diagnosis:** Observation and monitoring (sleep studies rarely required); must search for possible pathology as cause, depending on clinical presentation.
- **Management:** Gentle tactile stimulation, maintenance of good oxygenation; diagnose and treat underlying problem; for central AOP, use **caffeine** (preferred; is more potent, has fewer side effects and once-daily dosing) or theophylline; for obstructive or mixed, use continuous positive airway pressure (**CPAP**; stents upper airway) and high-flow nasal cannula oxygen.

Pulmonary Artery Hypertension (primary pulmonary artery hypertension of the newborn; persistent fetal circulation)

- Primary pulmonary hypertension of the newborn (PPHN) occurs in the term and post-term infant.
- Most cases are secondary (PAH) to causes that result in **hypoxemia, hypercarbia, acidosis, or metabolic disturbances** such as hypoglycemia and polycythemia.
- May also result from maternal medication prior to birth, especially **nonsteroidal anti-inflammatory drugs (NSAIDs) or selective serotonin reuptake inhibitors (SSRIs)**.
- Problem is continued elevation (or re-elevation) of pulmonary vascular resistance → increased pulmonary artery pressure and decreased pulmonary blood flow → right-to-left shunting across fetal channels.

- **Key diagnostic words: severe respiratory distress and cyanosis; hypoxemia resistant to 100% oxygen**, but may show initial improvement with intubation and ventilation.
- **Diagnostic studies: Best initial test:** a preductal (right radial) vs. postductal (umbilical artery). paO2 difference of >20 mm Hg is suggestive of a right-to-left shunt (or difference by pulse oximetry of at least 5%). **Most accurate test:** can visualize shunt using real-time Doppler echocardiography.
- **Management:** First, gentle positive-pressure ventilation with 100% oxygen, with **permissive hypercarbia** (excellent outcome compared to previous theory of hyperventilation and hypocapnia); sedation; may need inotropes (dopamine and dobutamine first); if minimal or no response → **inhaled nitric oxide** (endothelial-derived relaxation factor of smooth muscle) followed by inhaled or IV prostacyclin (PGI_2); ECMO is used for nonresponders (>34 weeks) with severe respiratory insufficiency.

Respiratory Distress Syndrome (RDS, surfactant deficiency)

- RDS is due to **surfactant deficiency** and immaturity.
- Incidence inversely proportional to gestational age, and is highest in white males.
- Surfactant mature and in sufficient quantity after 35 weeks' gestation (although infants past this gestational age may present with RDS).
- Conditions that lead to **stress in the fetus** decrease the incidence and severity (e.g., pregnancy-induced hypertension, antenatal steroids).
- Without the appropriate amount of mature surfactant, alveolar surface tension is increased and there is **alveoli collapse at end-expiration** → diffuse **atelectasis and decreased compliance**.
- **Increased work of breathing** as the infant needs more pressure to open collapsed alveoli.
- Alveoli are perfused but not ventilated → initial problem is hypoxemia.
- Hypercarbia with respiratory and metabolic acidosis ensues.
- May be pulmonary artery vasoconstriction with right-to-left shunting.
- **Key diagnostic words:** Premature infant presents with **tachypnea, grunting** (expiration against a partially closed glottis; increases end-expiratory pressure), **nasal flaring** and chest wall **retractions** (noncompliant lungs with overly compliant chest wall); breath sounds may be normal or decreased with fine rales at the bases; if untreated, irregular respirations and apnea develop, and then hemodynamic instability.
- **Major differential diagnosis: GBS pneumonia** (may look just like RDS radiographically and clinically and may be superimposed). **Total anomalous pulmonary venous return, obstructed type** may have a similar clinical and radiographic presentation.
- **Diagnostic tests: Best initial test**: chest x-ray (decreased lung volume, fine reticulogranular or "ground glass" pattern, and air-bronchograms). **Most accurate test**: lung profile on amniotic fluid prior to birth or tracheal aspirate after birth. **Most common: L/S ratio** (lecithin-to-sphingomyelin ratio) and **PG (phosphatidylglycerol)**; as surfactant maturity, L/S should be at ≥2 and PG should be present in more than trace amounts.

- **Prenatal management:** (1) Careful timing of induction of labor or C-section (after completion of 39th week of gestation); (2) mature amniotic fluid lung profile with induction or elective C-section; (3) **betamethasone** 48 hours prior to delivery to all mothers in preterm labor (24–34 weeks) who are likely to deliver within one week → leads to significant decrease in incidence and severity of RDS and other complications of prematurity.
- **Management:** Most important first step is to **monitor oxygenation and use oxygen** as needed for low saturations. Early **CPAP**, especially in the very low birth weight (VLBW) infant (or if cannot sustain a paO_2 >50 mm Hg on an FIO_2 >0.6).
- **Exogenous surfactants:** Synthetic (Exosurf®) or natural animal (Survanta® [bovine], Infasurf® [calf], Curosurf® [porcine]; natural surfactants seem to work better, possibly due to presence of surfactant-associated proteins (faster onset, increased survival, decreased air leak). Exogenous surfactant administration strategies:
  - (1) **Prophylactic or early rescue:** immediately after birth or in first few hours; decreases mortality and air leak but not the course of bronchopulmonary dysplasia (BPD). Can extubate to CPAP after surfactant has been given. If cannot attain PaO_2 >50 mm Hg on CPAP and FIO_2 >0.6 if apnea persists, then intubate for positive pressure ventilation, always with positive end-expiratory pressure (PEEP). Goal is for paO_2 of 50–70 mm Hg, $paCO_2$ of 45–70 mm Hg, and pH of 7.2–7.35 to minimize effects of barotrauma.
  - (2) **Rescue:** multidose surfactant beginning in first 24 hours after need for intubation and dosed every 6–12 hours for 2–4 doses.
- **Complications:** PDA (see Chapter 12), **intraventricular hemorrhage** (see below), retinopathy of prematurity, and **BPD**; BPD is a form of chronic lung disease caused by a combination of effects from **barotrauma, volutrauma, and oxygen**. Chest x-ray may show hyperinflation, atelectasis alternating with areas of air-trapping, pulmonary interstitial emphysema (**PIE**), **cysts**, edema, and **fibrosis**. Principles of therapy include good nutrition with added calories, fluid restriction with use of diuretics, oxygenation, and inhaled bronchodilators (albuterol and ipratropium), but no routine corticosteroids unless severely affected (then a tapering short course). Highest mortality if still ventilated for 6 months.

HEMATOLOGICAL PROBLEMS
Normal Newborn Hematocrit and Anemia
- Average hematocrit (Hct) at term is **51 g/dL** with 2 standard deviations below the mean at **42 g/dL**.
- Upper limit of normal is **65 g/dL**.
- Less than the expected values = anemia. Physiological anemia occurs between **8 and 12 weeks after birth in the full-term infant** with a **nadir of 9–11 g/dL** and at **6 weeks in the preterm infant** with low values of **7–10 g/dL**.
- **Etiology:** With a relatively hypoxic intrauterine environment, fetal erythropoietin (EPO) production is high and therefore infants are born with high red-cell mass;

the infant is born into a comparatively oxygen-rich environment and EPO is downregulated. The hemoglobin (Hgb) and Hct fall gradually until tissue oxygen needs can no longer be met and EPO production is increased again. Hgb spontaneously increases to normal. The vast majority of term infants have no symptoms and do not require treatment; preterm infants who are in the NICU generally require frequent transfusions.

- Neonatal anemia is usually a result of **acute or chronic blood loss**, diseases resulting in **hemolysis** and **underproduction**. Acute blood loss usually results in severe distress and shock after birth or in the first day of life vs. chronic loss, which is generally milder and presents with pallor and either mild or no distress. After the first few days, anemia due to hemolysis, hemorrhagic disease of the newborn (see below), and mucosal bleeding or bleeding into organs is seen. Underproduction problems manifest later.

- **Transplacental hemorrhage:** During labor and delivery, fetal-to-maternal transfusions of variable amounts of blood are common. If the infant is anemic, the **Kleihauer-Betke test** can be performed and may show significant fetal Hgb and red blood cells in maternal blood (resistant to denaturation by strong alkali and persists).

Diagnostic workup of neonatal anemia

After establishing via CBC that an infant is anemic, obtain:

(1) **Reticulocyte count:** A low count is suggestive of a congenital anemia congenital infections (e.g., TORCH) or rarely, congenital leukemia. If reticulocyte count is normal to high, then go to (2).

(2) **Direct Coombs test:** Positive Coombs = isoimmunization, usually due to Rh, ABO blood type, or minor blood group antibodies. If Coombs is negative, then go to (3).

(3) **Mean corpuscular volume (MCV):** Low MCV is consistent with alpha-thalassemia or chronic blood loss. If MCV is normal to high, then go to (4).

(4) **Blood smear:** Abnormalities may be seen with membrane defects, with DIC, and at times with the enzyme defects; normal smears are seen with blood loss and infection (and some other, very rare causes).

Polycythemia and Hyperviscosity

- Central Hct ≥65 mg/dL; increased viscosity present in most and accounts for symptoms
- Higher incidence in: post-term infants (vs. term), SGA (vs. AGA and LGA), delayed cord clamping, recipient of a twin-twin transfusion (monozygotic twins), IODM, asphyxia, and birth at high altitudes
- Presentation: Lethargy, irritability, tachypnea, cyanosis, respiratory distress, plethora, hyperbilirubinemia, and hypoglycemia; severe hyperviscosity: necrotizing enterocolitis, renal vein thrombosis, pulmonary artery hypertension, seizure, and stroke
- Management: Treat all symptomatic and asymptomatic infants with central Hct >70 mg/dL with a partial exchange transfusion using normal saline (volume of saline = [blood volume × (observed Hct – desired Hct)] / [observed Hct]).

Erythroblastosis Fetalis

- Transplacental passage of maternal antibodies **against paternal red-cell antigens** of the infant results in red-cell destruction.
- Most with the **D antigen** (Rh), the ABO groups, and less commonly, minor blood groups.

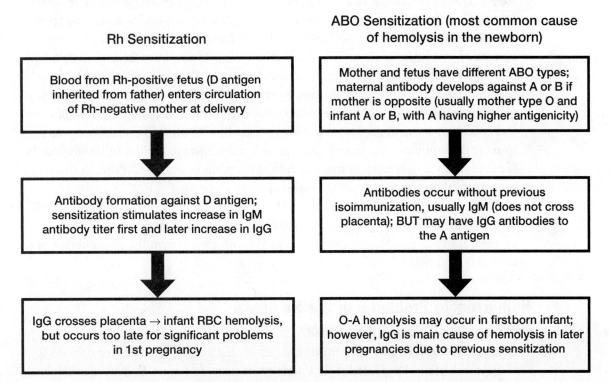

Rh Sensitization

> Blood from Rh-positive fetus (D antigen inherited from father) enters circulation of Rh-negative mother at delivery

> Antibody formation against D antigen; sensitization stimulates increase in IgM antibody titer first and later increase in IgG

> IgG crosses placenta → infant RBC hemolysis, but occurs too late for significant problems in 1st pregnancy

ABO Sensitization (most common cause of hemolysis in the newborn)

> Mother and fetus have different ABO types; maternal antibody develops against A or B if mother is opposite (usually mother type O and infant A or B, with A having higher antigenicity)

> Antibodies occur without previous isoimmunization, usually IgM (does not cross placenta); BUT may have IgG antibodies to the A antigen

> O-A hemolysis may occur in firstborn infant; however, IgG is main cause of hemolysis in later pregnancies due to previous sensitization

Figure 1.1: Pathophysiology of Rh and ABO isoimmunization

- Rh sensitization is generally significantly worse and **worsens with each pregnancy**.
- Wide severity or presentation from mild to severe anemia with **hydrops fetalis** (excessive fluid in at least two compartments, e.g., skin, peritoneal, pericardial, and pleural) → **cardiac failure and circulatory collapse**.
- **Jaundice** may be evident in the first 24 hours of life and with severe disease.
- Significant risk of developing **kernicterus**.
- With ABO sensitization there is generally mild jaundice, which may be apparent in the first day of life, no to mild anemia, and stable hemodynamics with much lower incidence of kernicterus.

Diagnostic studies and management:

- _Antenatal:_ Test parental blood types and Rh; if setup exists, follow serial maternal antibodies (IgG) to the D antigen. If there are significant titers or rapid rise, must assess fetus **noninvasively with Doppler ultrasound of the middle cerebral artery** (increased peak velocity of systolic blood flow correlates with fetal anemia and distress). Then treatment of choice is a **percutaneous umbilical blood sample (PUBS)** to assess fetal

Hgb and to **transfuse packed red cells** (umbilical vein transfusion; cross-matched blood with mother, CMV-negative, irradiated). This is repeated as needed every 3–5 weeks and delivery is planned for 35–37 weeks' gestation, when there is fetal lung maturity. Primary prevention is to administer **RhoGAM** (anti-D gammaglobulin) immediately after each pregnancy that involves an Rh-negative mother and Rh-positive infant.

- *Postnatal:* In the delivery room or immediately after birth, **expand volume and treat anemia** with small transfusion (fresh O-negative, cross-matched, irradiated, and leukoreduced). Ventilate as needed and treat metabolic acidosis (after an arterial blood gas is obtained). Obtain Hgb and Hct, reticulocyte count, ABO type and Rh, and direct Coombs test. If the Coombs is positive, then draw blood for a serum bilirubin and panel for antibodies in the mother's blood. For a significant increase in serum bilirubin and reticulocyte count, perform **a double volume (2 × 85 mL/kg) exchange transfusion** via the umbilical vein in conjunction with **phototherapy**. Follow bilirubin and Hgb/Hct every 4–6 hours and monitor rate of bilirubin rise until bilirubin decreases spontaneously in the absence of phototherapy.
- ABO sensitization is diagnosed with an ABO incompatibility, positive direct Coombs test, and increased indirect bilirubin; Hgb is usually normal or may be mildly decreased, with a reticulocyte count increased to 10–15%. Generally, phototherapy is all that is required.

Hemorrhagic Problems in the Newborn

Hemorrhagic disease of the newborn

- Occurs if **vitamin K** is not administered after birth. Lack of maternal free vitamin K and absence of newborn intestinal bacteria → decreased vitamin K–dependent factors **(II, VII, IX, X)** at birth, increases by 7–10 days of life.
- **Key diagnostic words: Early onset** of bleeding (birth to 24 hours), manifested mostly by: bleeding from the **umbilical cord**; **circumcision**; and **mucocutaneous**, intra-abdominal, gastrointestinal, intracranial, and scalp bleeding.
- **Diagnostic lab studies:** Increased prothrombin time **(PT)**, partial thromboplastin time **(PTT)**, and **blood coagulation time** with a decrease in the vitamin K–dependent factors
- **Prevention: Intramuscular injection of vitamin K immediately after birth** prevents in full-term infants but variably in preterm infants. Treatment for bleeding may be given with vitamin K, 1–5 mg, intravenously and fresh frozen plasma for significant bleeding.

Other bleeding issues

- Maternally administered drugs (interference with vitamin K function): **early bleeding** from effects of antenatal diphenylhydantoin, phenobarbital, isoniazid (INH), rifampin, warfarin
- Swallowed blood: day 2–3 of life; determine if swallowed (during delivery or from a fissured nipple while breastfeeding) vs. bleeding from gastrointestinal tract. Perform **Apt test**: fetal Hgb is alkali-resistant; mother's blood (adult Hgb) is changed to hematin after alkali is added. A difference in colors after the addition of sodium hydroxide indicates the difference.
- Malabsorption and cholestasis: **late bleeding** (>2 weeks through 6 months), e.g., biliary atresia, cystic fibrosis

NEUROLOGICAL PROBLEMS

Intracranial Hemorrhage (ICH)

- The most common reasons for ICH in the term or near-term infant are **trauma** (cephalo-pelvic disproportion) and **asphyxia**.
- More common with precipitous delivery or prolonged labor, assisted delivery, and breech presentation.
- May be secondary to congenital bleeding diatheses or vascular anomalies.
- Subdural hematomas are more common. Majority of **subdural and epidural hemorrhages** are small and resolve without problem.
- Large, acute bleeds lead to rapid deterioration and death.
- Symptomatic hemorrhages become evident with increasing head size, a bulging fontanelle, and seizures.
- **Subarachnoid hemorrhages** are rare and are secondary to tearing of bridging veins or meningeal arteries. Most are small and are either asymptomatic or present with a non-recurring **seizure** on the second day of life.
- **Diagnosis:** Patients presenting as above should have a **CT scan** of the brain.
- **Management:** Increased subdural fluid should be removed by **needle aspiration** through the anterior fontanelle. Maintain the airway, breathing, and circulation, and treat seizures (see below).

Intraventricular Hemorrhage (IVH)

- Risk of IVH is inversely proportional to gestational age, with most occurring in the LBW infant (**especially <1,000 g**).
- Origin of bleeding is the **subependymal germinal matrix** (periventricular origin of CNS neurons and glial cells)—highly vascular, and the vessels are immature and poorly supported, so are prone to hemorrhage into the lateral ventricles.
- Germinal matrix matures after 34 weeks gestational age, and IVH becomes uncommon.
- Highest incidence is in the **first 3 days** of life; less common after first week.
- **Key diagnostic words:** preterm infant, most commonly in first three days of life with onset of **apnea**, cyanosis, **pallor**, hypotonicity, twitching, and a **decreased Hct and metabolic acidosis**
- **Diagnosis:** All infants **<32 weeks of age** should have **screening ultrasounds** performed through the anterior fontanelle (**best initial test**); in first few days for the lowest birth-weight infants (<1,000 g) and at 7 days for larger infants. If an IVH is present, perform serial ultrasounds and a final ultrasound at 36–40 weeks postconceptional age to look for any findings suggestive of periventricular leukomalacia (see below).
- **Staging based on severity:**
  - **Grade I**: subependymal germinal matrix hemorrhage only
  - **Grade II**: blood in the ventricles but without ventricular dilatation
  - **Grade III**: intraventricular blood plus ventricular dilatation
  - **Grade IV**: intraventricular and parenchymal hemorrhage; now considered to be a periventricular hemorrhagic infarction (severe IVH with venous congestion)
- *Periventricular leukomalacia (PVL)*: **white-matter necrosis** in the **corticospinal tracts** → **motor** abnormalities (**cerebral palsy** [CP]). Higher incidence with smaller, more

premature, and sicker infants, often with fluctuations of blood pressure and hence (decreased cerebral perfusion and reperfusion resulting in release of toxic inflammatory mediators) → focal necrosis; with early ultrasound (at age 3–10 days), may see areas of **increased echodensity, and then cysts** (as early as 14–20 days of life).

- **Diagnosis:** Ultrasonography as above. Any evidence of periventricular pathology requires an **MRI (most accurate test)** of the brain.
- **Treatment: Ventriculoperitoneal shunt** (VP shunt); diuretics and acetazolamide are not effective. But most infants with IVH do not require a shunt. Best prevention involves expert perinatal care, antenatal corticosteroids (decreases incidence of grade III and IV IVH and PVL), and avoidance of blood-pressure swings and pneumothorax in the newborn.
- **Outcome:** Most patients with grade I–II IVH do well (but even without any evidence of IVH, up to one-third of infants <1,000 g have CP and/or cognitive dysfunction). **Poor outcome** is associated with severe IVH requiring a shunt and PVL (CP, cognitive dysfunction, death).

Hypoxic-Ischemic Encephalopathy (HIE)

- Decreased oxygen supply with decreased perfusion to the brain resulting in tissue damage.
- Most likely outcomes are CP, developmental delays, mental retardation, and death.
- Most are secondary to perinatal (not prenatal) events or after birth from any condition leading to sustained or significant hypoxia in the newborn infant (e.g., respiratory disease, cyanotic heart disease, pulmonary vascular disease, infection, shock); multisystem problem, often with severe pathological changes.
- **Key diagnostic words:** Intrapartum fetal distress based on monitoring (late decelerations, decreased variability, fetal acidosis, presence of meconium). Earliest postnatal findings are apnea, irregular respirations, bradycardia, hypotonia (and may become hypertonic), decreased or absent reflexes (i.e., stupor or coma), and seizures (often refractory).
- **Best initial test:** Head CT for possible focal hemorrhage, but **most accurate test** for cortical injury is the diffusion-weighted MRI. Also continuous EEG recording (detects subclinical seizures and provides quick information regarding those at highest risk for the worst brain injury). Also evaluate other organ systems (echocardiography, chest x-ray, electrolytes, BUN, creatinine, liver enzymes and bilirubin, complete CBC, platelets, and clotting studies).
- **Management:** Systemic hypothermia, started within the first 6 hours of life, decreases cortical injury and improves early developmental outcome. Prevent hypoxia and hypotension; treat seizures aggressively (initial drug of choice is phenobarbital, but refractory seizures may require others); supportive treatment of other organ systems.
- **Outcome:** Depends on severity of the insult, timing, duration, gestational age, and adverse effect on the cardiovascular system. The worse cases in terms of severity of neurodevelopmental outcome or death are those with low Apgar score and no spontaneous breathing at 20 minutes of age with an abnormal neurological exam at 2 weeks of age.

Neonatal Drug Withdrawal

Table 1.3: Prenatal Substance Abuse and Postnatal Effects

Drug	Early Withdrawal—Major Symptoms*	Late Effects	Long-Term Effects	Treatment
Heroin	IUGR, prematurity, hyperirritability, tremors, decreased sleep, hyperacusis, diarrhea and vomiting, high-pitched cry, apnea, seizures, tachypnea, hyperreflexia, **no increase in congenital anomalies**	Gradual decrease in symptoms with appropriate treatment	Growth deficiencies; perception, cognitive, behavioral, and neurological problems	Decrease environmental stimuli, swaddling and drugs for severe symptoms: *best is* combination of tincture of opium and phenobarbital
Methadone	More severe and prolonged withdrawal symptoms within 48–72 hours, higher birth weights than with heroin, decreased head circumference not related to SGA, higher incidence of seizures, **no increase in congenital anomalies**	Late withdrawal syndrome in some between 2 and 4 weeks of age—similar symptoms with ↑ appetite, poor weight gain, and systolic hypertension	High incidence of learning and behavior disorders, hyperactivity, and poor social adjustment	Same as heroin, but usually longer
Barbiturates (phenobarbital)	Usually born at term and AGA; symptoms begin at 2–14 days of age; brief acute stage with constant cry and irritability, decreased sleep, hiccups; subacute phase with increased appetite, spitting and gagging, irritability, abnormal sleep, sweating, and hyperacusis	Second phase symptoms may last 2–4 months	Not known	Same as for heroin
Alcohol	Withdrawal is uncommon; tremors, hyperactivity, and seizures for 72 hours, lethargy for 48 hours prior to return to normal; may develop hypoglycemia and metabolic acidosis; alcohol is a teratogen → fetal alcohol syndrome (see Chapter 2).	Fetal alcohol syndrome with chronic abuse	With chronic use: persistent growth retardation, many developmental deficits, including learning disabilities and decreased intellect	For acute withdrawal: same as for heroin

(continued)

Table 1.3: Prenatal Substance Abuse and Postnatal Effects *(cont.)*

Drug	Early Withdrawal—Major Symptoms*	Late Effects	Long-Term Effects	Treatment
Cocaine	Prematurity, IUGR (most consistent effect), decreased head circumference, placental abruption, asphyxia, association with vascular occlusive defects, CNS hemorrhagic infarcts and cysts; significant increase in incidence of sudden infant death syndrome (SIDS)	Variable reports of neurobehavioral problems	Catch-up growth by 12 months, variable long-term developmental and cognitive defects (often related to head circumference)	Symptomatic treatment; no drugs
Amphetamines/ methamphetamine	Increased perinatal morbidity and mortality; prematurity, IUGR; drowsiness, jitteriness, respiratory distress	Several months of lethargy with poor weight gain and frequent infections; CNS pathology similar to cocaine	Increased tone, hypersensitivity to sound, abnormal sleep patterns, problems with coordination	Symptomatic treatment; no drugs
Tobacco	Decreased fetal weight proportional to number of cigarettes smoked; related morbidity to IUGR (uterine vasoconstriction and fetal hypoxia from nicotine and metabolites); also carbon monoxide and cyanide binds to Hgb and decreases oxygen binding	Dependent upon initial effects related to hypoxia and growth restriction	Not known	Symptomatic treatment
Marijuana	Prolonged and arrested labor, preterm labor, increased incidence of meconium; *with chronic use:* decreased birth weight, tremors, changes in state regulation, altered visual responses, abnormal sleep	None	No physical or developmental problems through age 1 year; but with heavy smokers, later sleep disturbances, developmental delays, conduct problems	Symptomatic treatment

Note: A number of neonatal abstinence scoring systems are available, as well as evaluation with the NICU Network Neurobehavioral Scale (NNNS); testing for drugs in meconium is more accurate than in urine.

GASTROINTESTINAL AND LIVER DISEASE

Table 1.4: Abdominal Wall Defects

Umbilical Hernia	Omphalocele	Gastroschisis
• Failure of umbilical ring contracture at 8–11 weeks' gestation • Small fascial defect with (at most) small intestinal herniation • More common in black race • Most disappear by age 1 year, unless >2 cm; if >2 cm, more likely to persist • Surgery only if symptomatic or persisting after **age 4–5 years**	• Arrest of migration and fusion of cranial, caudal, and lateral folds, so there is not an intact umbilical ring at 5 weeks' gestation • Insertion of umbilical cord into central **omphalocele sac** with a surrounding fascial defect • Large defects may contain stomach, liver, spleen • Significant increase in extra-GI **malformations**: cardiac, neurologic, genitourinary, skeletal • High incidence of **genetic/chromosomal syndromes** (Beckwith-Wiedemann; trisomies 13, 18, 21)	• Smaller size abdominal wall defect **lateral to umbilicus** with normal cord attachment immediately left of the defect; **no sac** • Appears to be caused by involution of the right umbilical vein or a vascular accident involving the omphalomesenteric artery leading to rupture of the abdominal wall • Most contain small intestine and ascending colon • **Bowel ischemia, atresias** of varying length

- **Prenatal diagnosis:** In-utero diagnosis by ultrasound. If other anomalies, may do a karyotype.
- Optimal delivery by C-section.
- **First steps in management:** Prevent fluid loss, heat loss, and infection; **wrap in warm, fluid-impermeable dressing**; intravenous fluids (increased due to insensible losses) and broad-spectrum antibiotics.
- **Definitive management:** Surgery individualized based on the size and type of defect. Primary repair cannot be done if it would cause a rapid increase in intra-abdominal pressure (elevation of diaphragm and compromise of inferior vena cava). Therefore, in most (and certainly large) defects a prosthetic silo is created (mesh-reinforced silastic material) around the defect for daily reduction (may take up to 10 days) and then primary closure.

Congenital Bowel Obstruction

Esophageal atresia (EA) + tracheoesophageal fistula (TEF)

- Most common: upper esophageal blind pouch with distal TEF; half with other anomalies, mostly **VACTERL** (see Chapter 2)
- **Key diagnostic words: polyhydramnios** during pregnancy; first day of life: **frothing** at the mouth with cough, respiratory distress, and cyanosis; feeding results in **immediate regurgitation,** possibly other VACTERL findings

- **First diagnostic step:** Pass nasogastric (NG) tube (can feel immediate resistance); a plain radiograph will show the tube **coiled in the blind pouch**; a pure EA will show a **gasless abdomen**, but if there is a distal TEF, there will be a large air-distended stomach. **Best test** for TEF is either esophagram or bronchoscopy using methylene blue.
- **Management:** maintain patent airway and prevent aspiration until surgery (prone position with good suctioning); avoid intubation if possible (more air distension with TEF)

Duodenal atresia

- Failure to recanalize after solid phase of intestinal development at 4–5 weeks' gestation; most born preterm; lack of connection distal to ampulla of Vater
- **Key diagnostic words: bilious vomiting with no abdominal distension on first day of life**; higher incidence in **trisomy 21**
- **First diagnostic step:** plain radiograph → shows **"double-bubble"** (distended stomach and distended obstructed proximal duodenum) **with no distal bowel gas**
- **Management:** with any obstruction, **place NG** or orogastric (OG) tube for gastric decompression and begin IV fluids; definitive management is surgical correction.

Jejuno-ileal atresia

- Intestinal vascular accident → ischemic necrosis and resorption; extraintestinal anomalies less common
- **Key diagnostic words: abdominal distension and biliary emesis** most do not pass meconium; hyperbilirubinemia (increased enterohepatic circulation)
- **First diagnostic step:** obtain plain radiograph; shows **many air-fluid levels that are uniformly dilated. Most accurate test:** upper and lower contrast studies or ultrasound can localize the site of obstruction and differentiate atresia from meconium ileus/plug and Hirschsprung disease.
- **Management:** First, place NG tube and start IV fluids; then surgical correction.

Malrotation with midgut volvulus

- Caused when the gut fails to rotate during return to abdominal cavity by 8 weeks' gestation. Last part of duodenum, jejunum, and ileum move to the right and the colon to the left → **failure of normal fixation** to the abdominal cavity; the cecum fails to move to the right lower quadrant and **Ladd bands** (fibrous bands of tissue) may extend from the cecum to the right upper quadrant and **partially obstruct the duodenum**; **volvulus** is acute twisting on the mesenteric axis because of lack of normal fixation → partial or complete obstruction with decreased mesenteric blood supply and ischemic necrosis of bowel; most neonates present in **first week of life**; the next most common presentation is the first month.
- **Key diagnostic words:** if acute: **bilious vomiting**, then with vascular compromise ischemic bowel becomes firm and dilated → **abdominal distension and acute pain** (crying, screaming, extreme irritability); with fluid shifts, the patient may be hypotensive and acidotic → peritonitis and shock.
- **Next step in management:** If patient has an acute abdomen, immediate surgery is the next step (exploratory laparotomy); if stable, can begin with a plain radiograph—may

show a **double-bubble with some distal bowel gas** (compare to duodenal atresia) or may see an abrupt cutoff of air at a point in the distal duodenum ("bird's-beak" sign). **Most accurate test:** either ultrasound (inversion of the superior mesenteric vessels) or contrast studies (upper: malposition of ligament of Treitz; barium enema (not the preferred study): abnormal position of cecum, hepatic and splenic flexures) can be diagnostic. Surgical correction is definitive.

Meconium plugs

- Decreased water content of meconium resulting in obstruction in **lower colon or anorectal area**, or may result in mucosal ulceration and perforation; major associations: small left colon (with IODM), cystic fibrosis (less commonly than meconium ileus; see below), tocolysis with magnesium sulfate and prenatal maternal opiate use.
- **Key diagnostic words:** abdominal distension and failure to pass meconium in a child with above associations
- **First diagnostic step:** Plain x-ray shows many dilated loops of bowel with no air in lower bowel and rectum.
- **Next step in management:** Gastrografin (high osmolality) enema to relieve impacted meconium

Meconium ileus

- Highest association with **cystic fibrosis** (CF; 80–90% with meconium ileus will be diagnosed with CF, but only 10% of patients with CF present with meconium ileus) → meconium becomes viscid and impacts most commonly in **distal ileum**; may lead to a perforation → can see **peritoneal calcifications** on x-ray
- **Key diagnostic findings:** abdominal distension with vomiting and **failure to pass meconium**; on exam, may palpate masses that have a **dough-like feel**
- **First diagnostic step: plain x-ray: varying width loops of bowel** (compared to an atresia, where bowel loops tend to be more evenly gas-filled) proximal to obstruction with no distal bowel gas; may see a **bubbly** appearance where meconium is mixed with air (also called "ground-glass")

Next step in management: if diagnosis is suspected, **Gastrografin enema**, as above; if not relieved, then surgery. Patient will need to be tested for CF (see Chapter 7).

Hirschsprung disease

- Abnormal bowel innervation beginning at the **internal anal sphincter** and proceeding proximally to variable lengths; most are **rectosigmoid**; may involve the entire colon or entire bowel = **congenital aganglionic megacolon**. May be associated with other defects and syndromes (Currarino triad: anorectal malformations, sacral bone anomalies, presacral masses); aganglionic segment is non-peristaltic → proximal bowel becomes dilated and increased intraluminal pressure leads to decreased blood flow to the mucosa with mucosal deterioration. Stasis and infection lead to **enterocolitis** and possible perforation, peritonitis, sepsis, and death.

- **Key diagnostic words: full-term infant with delay in passage of meconium and abdominal distension**; digital exam may show fecal mass in left lower quadrant and no air in the rectum, which may result in release of fecal material
- **Best diagnostic tests: rectal manometry** (a balloon distends the rectum and there is failure of relaxation of the internal sphincter) followed by **definitive rectal suction biopsy** if manometry is equivocal or positive. For initial screening of less certain cases, a **barium enema** may be performed. This shows a transition zone (but may not be present in first 2 weeks of life) with proximal dilatation. A repeat study 24 hours later may show continued presence of barium.
- **Management:** Surgical removal of aganglionic segment and possible ostomy.

Necrotizing Enterocolitis (NEC)

- Most common GI emergency in the neonate; **transmural necrosis** of intestine (most in terminal ileum and proximal colon); may lead to perforation, peritonitis, sepsis, and death; **intramural gas (pneumatosis intestinalis)**; related to **prematurity (most consistent finding)** + enteral feeding + infection (*Escherichia coli, Klebsiella, Clostridium perfringens, Staphylococcus epidermidis*)
- **Key diagnostic words:** insidious or acute deterioration in preterm infant, usually on enteral feedings. Nonspecific findings: lethargy, temperature instability, hypoglycemia, apnea, acidosis with or without GI findings, e.g., **abdominal distention, rectal bleeding (or occult blood), vomiting, residual feeds in stomach.**
- **Next steps in management: stop feeding immediately**, remove umbilical catheters, start **IV fluids**, culture and start **broad-spectrum antibiotics** for Gram-positive, Gram-negative, and anaerobic organisms; obtain **plain abdominal films**: presence of **pneumatosis intestinalis, portal venous air, intraperitoneal air, abnormal bowel gas patterns**; follow electrolytes, acid-base status, respiratory status, and coagulation studies frequently; repeat frequent exams and x-rays; early surgical consult (surgery if free air, deterioration, failure of medical management).

Hyperbilirubinemia and Jaundice

Physiologic jaundice (non-pathologic)

- Umbilical cord total bilirubin 1–3 mg/dL; visible jaundice on the **second to third day of life** with peak bilirubin between **second and fourth days of life**; no abnormal direct component (i.e., **<2 mg/dL**); total bilirubin uncommonly >12 mg/dL (but may have an exaggerated physiological jaundice with higher bilirubin levels); rate of rise **<5 mg/dL/24 hours**; total decreased to <2 mg/dL **by fifth to seventh day of life**, with adult levels reached at **10–14 days of life**.
- **Increased risk (of higher and/or longer-lasting bilirubin levels) with East Asian or Native American race, male gender, prematurity**, polycythemia, IODM, extensive **bruising**, cephalohematoma, and inadequate **breastfeeding**.

Pathologic jaundice

- May be exaggerated physiologic jaundice
- Due to an excessive load of bilirubin
- Hepatocellular damage and cholestasis resulting in direct hyperbilirubinemia (see discussion of cholestasis and liver disease in Chapter 13).
- **Possible pathology if there are findings outside those for physiologic jaundice.**

Diagnostic evaluation:

Direct hyperbilirubinemia

- Possible causes: sepsis, TORCH infections, giant-cell hepatitis, biliary atresia, choledochal cyst, severe hemolysis, metabolic diseases, prolonged hyperalimentation, bile duct and bile acid abnormalities
- Workup per likely diagnoses based on history and physical

Indirect hyperbilirubinemia

1. Check Coombs

    If positive → Isoimmunization

    If negative → Check Hgb or Hct
2. If Hgb or Hct is high → causes of polycythemia
3. If Hgb or Hct is low or normal → check reticulocyte count
4. If reticulocyte count is normal
    - Poor feeding with decreased calories
    - Asphyxia
    - Increased enterohepatic circulation (intestinal obstruction)
    - Enclosed hemorrhage (cephalohematoma)
    - Prolonged jaundice: breast milk, hypothyroidism, Down syndrome, Gilbert syndrome, Crigler-Najjar syndrome
5. If reticulocyte count is elevated → check blood smear
6. Blood smear

    If RBCs appear abnormal → membrane defects

    If smear is nonspecific → enzyme defects (DIC)

Breastfeeding vs. Breast-Milk Jaundice

Table 1.5: Breastfeeding vs. Breast-Milk Jaundice

Breastfeeding Jaundice	Breast-Milk Jaundice
When: Early; first days to week	*When:* Second week of life; peaks at 2–3 weeks, then gradually decreases through 10 weeks
Why: Inadequate breastfeeding → decreased calories → decreased peristalsis → increased enterohepatic circulation	*Why:* Glucuronidase present in some breast milk
Presentation: Indirect hyperbilirubinemia and dehydration	*Presentation:* Good breastfeeding with jaundice appearing in the second week
Management: Rehydrate, lactation consultation for breastfeeding techniques; no glucose water supplementation (bilirubin increases due to decreased calories from breast-milk substitution)	*Management:* (1) Check bilirubin (can be high, requiring phototherapy or even exchange transfusion); (2) Stop breastfeeding for 2–3 days (place on formula) and then recheck bilirubin (expect significant drop); (3) Breastfeeding thereafter (rarely increases back to original level)

Kernicterus

- Bilirubin encephalopathy due to **unconjugated bilirubin** crossing the blood–brain barrier to the **basal ganglia and brain-stem nuclei**
- Rare in term infants who do not have hemolysis and whose total serum bilirubin is **<25 mg/dL.**
- Onset most often in first week of life, but could be delayed.
- **Key diagnostic words:** Poor feeding, lethargy, and absent Moro reflex (all nonspecific); then within days to weeks, decreased to absent deep tendon reflexes, bulging fontanelle, opisthotonus, respiratory distress, spasms, twitching, high-pitched cry, extensor hypertonia, and seizures. Those who survive may develop **choreoathetosis with involuntary spasms, extrapyramidal findings, high-frequency hearing loss, and dysarthric speech.**
- **To decrease the incidence of kernicterus**—AAP Revised Guidelines (2004) suggest:
  - Prior to hospital discharge, determine risk for severe jaundice: measure total serum bilirubin (TSB) and transcutaneous bilirubin (TcB), assess risk factors.
  - Schedule appropriate follow-up based on time of discharge: 2 to 5 days.
  - Advise breastfeeding (at least 8–12 times per day in the first days of life).
  - Provide parents with information regarding risks associated with jaundice.

Treatment of Jaundice

- The primary treatment of jaundice is with the use of **phototherapy**; if the bilirubin continues to rise despite maximum phototherapy, **exchange transfusion** needs to be performed. There are hour-specific graphs for levels of bilirubin with low, intermediate, and high risk zones. In general, phototherapy is started at **50–70% the maximal**

bilirubin level at which one would initiate an exchange transfusion. This decreases with gestational age, birth weight, and degree of illness present.
- Measure wattage accurately at the skin surface
- Specific blue lights for maximal phototherapy
- May use fiberoptic bilirubin under back (also for home therapy)
- Cover eyes for prevention of corneal damage
- Monitor body temperature
- Contraindicated with porphyria and with direct fraction >50% of total

- **Complications of phototherapy: overheating, dehydration, corneal damage**, erythematous macular rash, **bronze baby syndrome** (gray-brown skin, usually with direct hyperbilirubinemia and cholestasis; photo-induced modifications of porphyrins, which are often present in cholestatic disease; does not preclude use of phototherapy if needed for high indirect bilirubin)

- **Ancillary therapy:** IVIG with isoimmune disease—recommended when bilirubin approaches exchange levels despite maximum phototherapy (decreases hemolysis in Rh and ABO incompatibility and the need for exchange transfusion); tin mesoporphyrin (SnMP) is a competitive inhibitor of the rate-limiting step (heme → biliverdin); a single IM dose on the first day of life in cases with expected hyperbilirubinemia (e.g., isoimmunization) decreases the need for phototherapy and exchange transfusion. Phenobarbital can increase glucuronyltransferase activity but because of potential toxicities is used for specific, high-risk conditions.

Hereditary Nonhemolytic Hyperbilirubinemia

Unconjugated Hyperbilirubinemia

Gilbert syndrome: defective hepatic uptake of bilirubin and decreased UDPGT activity; mostly seen in adults with mild indirect hyperbilirubinemia

Crigler-Najjar syndrome type I: absence of UDPGT; autosomal recessive; severe persistent hyperbilirubinemia without hemolysis and with early signs of kernicterus; diagnosis with percutaneous liver biopsy and microassay for enzyme; enzyme is not inducible with phenobarbital; aggressive phototherapy and exchange transfusions to keep bilirubin <20 mg/dL in first weeks of life

Crigler-Najjar syndrome type II: more common than type I; early unconjugated hyperbilirubinemia but usually <20 mg/dL; kernicterus is rare; good response to oral phenobarbital

Lucey-Driscoll syndrome: familial severe unconjugated hyperbilirubinemia in first 48 hours (may develop kernicterus) due to serum inhibitor of UDPGT in neonates and mothers; inhibition gradually diminishes after delivery and normalizes by 14th day

Conjugated Hyperbilirubinemia

Dubin-Johnson and Rotor syndromes: autosomal recessive conditions resulting in defective transfer of bilirubin and other organic anions from liver to bile; usually detected in adolescence or adulthood as a chronic, mild-conjugated hyperbilirubinemia

HOSPITAL DISCHARGE

The American Academy of Pediatrics (AAP) and American College of Obstetrics-Gynecology (ACOG) have put forth the following conditions for early discharge (24–48 hours):

- Uncomplicated antepartum, intrapartum, and postpartum course
- Vaginal delivery
- Singleton delivery at 38–42 weeks
- Normal vital signs in open crib
- Exam with no abnormalities needing immediate attention
- Good urine output and at least one stool (evidence of meconium passage)
- At least two successful consecutive feedings
- No excessive bleeding 2 hours after circumcision
- No jaundice within 24 hours of birth
- Appropriate parental knowledge, abilities, and compliance
- Physician availability and follow-up
- Laboratory evaluation as needed (bilirubin, VDRL, HBsAg, Coombs test, state screening) plus first hepatitis B vaccine
- No social risks

NEONATAL SCREENING

- All 50 states have neonatal screening programs that vary from state to state; but all screen for **hypothyroidism and phenylketonuria** (PKU).
- Heelstick blood placed on filter paper and sent to the state laboratory
- Results reported back to the primary physician, and appropriate follow-up must occur for all infants
- **Expanded newborn screening programs** use tandem mass spectrometry to test for a number of inherited metabolic diseases (e.g., homocystinuria, maple syrup urine disease, propionic academia, disorders of carbohydrate and fatty acid metabolism) and other conditions such as cystic fibrosis, sickle-cell disease, and 21-hydroxylase deficiency.
- All infants need to be tested **after at least 24 hours** of normal protein and lactose feeding (formula-fed infants may not have an abnormality at <36 hours and breastfed at <48–72 hours) and by 7 days.
- The AAP recommends screening all full-term infants as close to discharge as possible.
- If the first screen is done at <24 hours of life, **rescreening should be done at 14 days** of age (some geneticists recommend a 14-day re-screen if the first was done at <48 hours of life).

Hearing Screening

- Universal newborn screening programs instituted in 32 states thus far
- AAP's policy—hearing loss should be detected in every infant by **3 months of age** and appropriate intervention instituted no later than **6 months of age.**

- Unless there is a bilateral profound loss, early detection and intervention should lead to normal language skills. Initial recommended screen is the **otoacoustic emission test (OAE).**
- There is no response if hearing is worse than detection of **30–40 dB**, regardless of the cause. Infants with an abnormal screen should then have an **auditory brain-stem evoked response test (ABR)**, which can identify the degree and type of the loss.

GENETIC AND METABOLIC DISEASE

2

PART ONE: GENETICS AND DYSMORPHOLOGY

Prenatal Diagnosis

Major reasons for prenatal testing are:

- Maternal age >35 years
- Previous child with chromosomal anomaly
- Affected parent with a microdeletion syndrome, parent with a balanced translocation
- Need to determine fetal sex for possible severe X-linked traits

Ultrasound

- Performed safely throughout pregnancy for fetal anatomical abnormalities and for fetal size and growth
- Diagnoses may be made as early as the 16th week of gestation (e.g., anencephaly, myelomeningocele, certain gastrointestinal defects, and congenital heart disease)
- Ultrasound Doppler for blood-flow velocity and vascular resistance (fetal hypoxia)

Amniocentesis

- Transabdominal needle aspiration of amniotic fluid between 15 and 18 weeks' gestation
- Risk of fetal loss. Can determine fetal lung maturity, karyotype, chromosomal abnormalities, single gene defects, and enzyme analysis

Alpha-fetoprotein

- Can be analyzed in amniotic fluid or in maternal serum
- Decreased in trisomies and aneuploidy
- Increased in fetal death, intestinal atresias, neural tube defects, multiple gestation

Chorionic villus sampling (CVS)

Allows for earlier detection (10–12 weeks' gestational age) of karyotype, DNA analysis, enzyme assay; risk of fetal loss

Examples of Etiologies of Genetic Disorders

Chromosomal maldistribution—Most result from error in cell division leading to genetic imbalance (e.g., monosomy, trisomy; increased mortality); error in first or second meiotic division is nondisjunction → abnormal chromosome number in sex cells; error later in embryonic development → mosaicism; older maternal age is a factor

Chromosomal breakage—Break in at least one chromosome with subsequent rearrangement = translocation; a balanced translocation leads to no phenotypic expression; during meiosis I, increased risk of imbalance in the germ cell (if the germ cell has the translocation chromosome and the normal one from the same parent → trisomy); therefore, in trisomies resulting from translocation, the parents must be karyotyped to look for a balanced translocation carrier state; if this is the case, the recurrence risk increases (4–5% vs. 1% for full trisomy, depending on maternal age). Breakage can also result in a deletion; a microdeletion is so small that high-resolution methods are required for detection; most are new mutations, so recurrence risk is negligible unless parents have the deletion and express the phenotype; in that case, the recurrence risk is 50%.

Genetic imprinting—Some genes assess different phenotypes depending on whether they are on the male or the female chromosome. In Prader-Willi syndrome, the inherited abnormality is from the paternal 15 chromosome, and in Angelman syndrome, the abnormal gene is inherited from the maternal 15 chromosome.

Unstable gene mutations—The human genome contains short repeat trinucleotide sequences (purpose may be unknown); increased copies of these sequences leads to instability and an abnormality in the offspring. The best example of this is fragile X syndrome.

Uniparental disomy—Both alleles are from the same parent; initial trisomy and then elimination of the extra chromosome; remaining may be from the same parent, which leads to genetic imbalance (some cases of mosaicism, imprinting effects and autosomal recessive effects).

Patterns of Inheritance

Autosomal dominant

- Presence of the trait in a single allele produces the phenotypic expression.
- Most likely pattern: one parent is heterozygous for the dominant trait and the other does not carry the trait (Aa × aa); **50% of the offspring will inherit the trait and express the phenotype** (if both parents are heterozygous carriers [Aa × Aa], then 75% will express the phenotype.
- **Variability in penetrance leads to different expression** (depending on the extent and degree of mutation).
- Significant number of **new mutations** (especially with older paternal age).

Autosomal recessive

- The phenotypic expression requires the presence of both abnormal alleles.
- Most likely pattern: both parents are **heterozygous carriers** (aA × aA); **25% of offspring of each pregnancy will be homozygous recessive and therefore will express the phenotype**; of the children who do not express the phenotype, two-thirds are carriers; but there is low risk of random marriage to another carrier so the recurrence risk is low.

X-linked dominant

- The gene is carried on the **x-chromosome** and requires only one copy for expression, which results in **phenotypic expression in females (XX) and severe or lethal effects in males (XY)**.
- Inheritance: **50% of offspring** of heterozygous XX carriers and normal males will be affected
- **50% of girls and 50% of boys** will show the phenotype (this is not a common inheritance pattern).

X-linked recessive

- One copy produces minor or no phenotypic expression.
- Except in rare instances, **only males** are affected. If the mother is a carrier, **50% of daughters are carriers and 50% of sons are affected**. Transmission, then, is through mildly affected or unaffected females.

Mitochondrial inheritance

- Mitochondria carry a circular genome (37 genes encoding 13 proteins of the subunits of the respiratory chain complex).
- Inheritance is exclusively maternal, so no males are affected. All of the daughters will show the abnormality. Effects of mutations are worse over time. There are different proportions of normal vs. abnormal mitochondria in various tissues, and a threshold must be exceeded for expression of the abnormality to occur.

Multifactorial inheritance

- Threshold of phenotypic expression based on interactions between different genes and environmental factors.
- Malformations seen at differing frequencies in different ethnic groups.
- Normal parents with one affected child, risk for first-degree relatives is approximately the risk of the square root of the risk in the population (mostly 3–5%); with two affected children, the risk increases to 10–15%.
- Significantly decreased risk in second-degree relatives.
- Recurrence risk greater with greater numbers of affected family members and increasing severity of the abnormality.
- Recurrence risk increases for relatives of the least affected sex (if there are obvious sex differences in expression).

Patterns of Abnormal Morphogenesis

Malformation—Error in morphogenesis resulting in abnormal formation of tissues (dysplasia = abnormal arrangement of cells into tissues)

Deformation—Normally formed tissues that become abnormal in form as a result of extrinsic with or without intrinsic forces; most common extrinsic force is uterine constraint (primigravida, abnormal fetal lie, large-for-gestational-age [LGA] fetus, multiple gestation, oligohydramnios, uterine fibromas, bicornate uterus, small uterus)

- Combinations of extrinsic and intrinsic factors may lead to a number of **positional limb deformations** (see Chapter 17)
- **Breech presentation** (late gestational, prolonged): head elongated with prominent occiput; asymmetric shoulder compression with asymmetry of mandible; torticollis; hip dislocation; club foot
- **Plagiocephaly-torticollis sequence:** most cases from uterine constraint; head compressed to one side in late gestation → asymmetric molding of head (often rhomboid, may progress if uncorrected) and face (plagiocephaly) → shortening of the sternocleidomastoid with possible ischemia and fibrosis; mild cases resolve spontaneously or with neck-stretching exercises; more severe cases may require an orthocephalic helmet (specifically molded)
- **Craniosynostosis:** limitation of normal growth at one or more cranial sutures due either to a primary defect in brain growth (symmetric small head and brain) or to uterine head constraint and early suture closure; growth is limited and there may be a bony ridge that forms along the synostosis; multiple synostosis may lead to abnormal brain growth and increased intracranial pressure (ICP), and these are major reasons for surgery

Disruption—Breakdown of previously normally formed tissue from extrinsic factors (see below for further discussion/example)

- **Amnion rupture sequence:** Early rupture of the amnion → small amniotic strands → encircle and constrict fetal structures → amputation, limb reductions, clefts, umbilical cord compression; diagnosis is made by finding bands of amnion on the placental membranes; majority of cases are idiopathic and sporadic

Syndrome—An error in morphogenesis leading to a recognized pattern of multiple malformations

Sequence—A single initiating event leading to a pattern of malformation, where the subsequent malformation is related to the formation of the previous malformation

- **Oligohydramnios sequence (Potter sequence):** Defect of fetal urinary output and therefore decreased to absent urine into amniotic cavity (agenesis, dysplasia, obstruction) + amniotic fluid leakage → oligohydramnios → fetal compression → breech presentation, craniofacial anomalies (Potter facies: inner canthal and infra-orbital skin folds, flat nose and ears), aberrant positioning of the hands and feet with decreased joint mobility and compression of the fetal lungs with delayed development → pulmonary insufficiency (pulmonary hypoplasia = most common cause of death)

- **Robin sequence:** Hypoplasia of the mandible → retrognathia (posterior tongue positioning) → abnormal soft palate (rounded to cleft); most important issue in first month of life is possibility of airway obstruction; most patients have catch-up of mandibular growth and long-term prognosis is good.
- **Cleft lip sequence:** failure of lip fusion → possible failure of closure of palatal shelves (i.e., cleft lip + cleft palate); may have abnormal tooth development and nares closure; may have other malformations (especially in isolated cleft palate); increased incidence of conductive hearing loss and speech problems; most follow pattern of multifactorial inheritance but there are familial patterns of autosomal dominant transmission

Association—Nonrandom pattern of malformations that have no clear interrelationship

- **VACTERL association:** sporadic occurrence of nonrandom associations of: **V,** vertebral defects; **A,** anal atresia; **C,** cardiovascular defects (most ventricular septal defects [VSDs]; single umbilical artery); **T-E,** fistula with or without esophageal atresia; **R,** renal defect; **L,** limb anomaly (most radial defect)
- **CHARGE association:** unknown cause of nonrandom associations of: **C,** coloboma (from iris to retinal); **H,** heart defect; **A,** atresia choanae; **R,** retardation (mental and growth); **G,** genital hypoplasia in males; **E,** ear anomalies with or without deafness

Table 2.1: Types of Craniosynostosis (major findings)

Sagittal	Coronal	Lambdoidal	Metopic	Sagittal + Coronal
– Most common – **Biparietal constraint** – Head long and narrow **(dolichocephalic)** with prominent forehead and occiput – **Ridge** from mid to posterior sagittal suture **(scaphocephaly)**	– Limited forward head growth **(brachycephaly)** – Short cranial base and upward growth → **high forehead and shallow orbits;** and lateral growth → **ocular hypertelorism** – **Midface hypoplasia,** narrow maxilla	– Least common – Abnormal fetal lie → constraint of **posterior head** – **Unilateral:** ipsilateral flat occiput and anterior pinna displacement; **bilateral:** brachycephaly with small posterior fossa	– Lateral constraint of the front of the head – Narrow and forward-projecting forehead with prominent metopic suture ridge – Upslanted palpebral fissures and hypertelorism	– Not common; **significant problem with brain growth and increased ICP** – Proptosis, optic atrophy, visual impairment – **Early surgery** to reduce ICP and allow brain growth and development

Abbreviations: intracranial pressure, ICP

Major Malformation Syndromes

Chromosomal

Table 2.2: Major Chromosomal Malformation Syndromes

Syndrome	Major Diagnostic Findings	Major Morbidities	Diagnostic Studies	Outcomes
Trisomy 21 (Down)	**Upslanting palpebral fissures**, mild microcephaly, **flat occiput, inner epicanthal folds** (not specific for Down), **Brushfield spots** (speckling of iris); small, abnormal ears; single palmar **crease** (not specific to Down), fifth finger brachydactyly and clinodactyly, **hypotonia**; small penis and testicles	**Mental deficiency** (variable), **hearing loss** (conductive, sensorineural, or mixed), congenital heart disease (**endocardial cushion defect** most common); gastrointestinal anomalies (**duodenal atresia**, tracheoesophageal fistula, Hirschsprung disease); **atlantoaxial instability; leukemia; thyroid disorders**	Karyotype; also of parents if translocation	Hypotonia improves with age; variation in mental and social performance; short stature; progressive gonadal deficiency; **major mortality early in life is congenital heart disease**
Trisomy 13 (Patau)	**IUGR, microcephaly, microphthalmia, cleft lip and palate**, parietal-occipital **cutis aplasia, finger flexion, polydactyly**, cryptorchidism with **abnormal scrotum**, single umbilical artery	Most with **cardiac defect** (septal defects most common); other **CNS defects** (**holoprosencephaly**); renal defects	Karyotype; also of parents if translocation	**Stillborn or death** in vast majority in first month of life; any survivors have severe mental defects and failure-to-thrive
Trisomy 18 (Edwards)	**IUGR, severe mental deficiency, microcephaly, clenched hand with index finger over the third and fifth finger over the fourth; short sternum**, omphalocele cryptorchidism, rocker-bottom feet	**Cardiac defects** (most are septal defects), renal defects, bone and joint abnormalities, omphalocele	Karyotype; also of parents if translocation	**Stillborn or death** in first week with less surviving over first year; severe mental deficiency and psychomotor retardation

(continued)

Syndrome	Major Diagnostic Findings	Major Morbidities	Diagnostic Studies	Outcomes
XO (Turner)	**Small stature** (may have IUGR) **and gonadal dysgenesis; congenital lymphedema, broad chest with widely spaced nipples; low, abnormal posterior hairline; webbed neck, loose skin at posterior neck, bone and joint abnormalities (cubitus valgus most common)**	Psychomotor and neuropsychological defects (may have some degree of mental retardation); renal defects (**horseshoe kidney**), cardiac defects (**most with bicuspid aortic valve, then coarctation of the aorta; mitral valve prolapse**), renovascular **hypertension; hypothyroidism;** rarely any functional ovarian tissue by adolescence; estrogen therapy is indicated; growth hormone allows for some growth	**Karyotype in any girl with unexplained short stature or lack of pubertal development at 13 years of age**	Some pure XO are stillborns; higher mosaicism in live-borns; adults at risk for aortic dissection
XXY (Klinefelter)	**Tall and thin** (decreased ratio of upper to lower segment due to long lower limbs); **small penis and testes, gynecomastia**	**Average IQ mildly decreased** (wide range); **learning disabilities, behavioral problems; infertility** (decreasing testosterone levels late in adolescence)	Karyotype XXY/XY mosaics have better testicular function; other karyotypes with more profound mental deficiency and behavioral problems	Most require help with learning; testosterone replacement is helpful
Fragile X syndrome	Males (carrier females less affected) with **mild to severe mental retardation; large head early and large jaw after puberty;** large ears; **macro-orchidism** (especially after puberty)	Mental retardation, inattention and hyperactivity, autism; mitral valve prolapse, aortic dilation	X chromosome region of large number of **repeat trinucleotide (CGG) → molecular analysis**	Normal life span
Aniridia-Wilms tumor association (WAGR)	**W,** Wilms tumor; **A,** aniridia (and other eye defects); **G,** genitourinary anomalies (cryptorchidism, hypospadias, others); **R,** mental retardation (moderate to severe)	More patients with full spectrum develop Wilms tumor compared to those with just aniridia or GU defect	Most new mutation of 11p13 deletion → molecular analysis	Mortality related to diagnosis and treatment of Wilms tumor

Abbreviations: central nervous system, CNS; intrauterine growth retardation, IUGR

Other syndromes

Table 2.3: Syndromes with Short Stature

Syndrome	Major Diagnostic Findings and Problems
Noonan syndrome (Turner-like)	Abnormal gene at 12q; occurs **also in boys; short stature, mild to moderate mental retardation**, dysmorphic facial features, **posterior neck findings as in Turner syndrome**; pectus deformations, small penis and cryptorchidism (normal fertility if descended testes; females are fertile), various **bleeding disorders, pulmonic valvular stenosis**
Williams syndrome	Abnormal gene on the 7th chromosome; mild IUGR and microcephaly; **mental retardation and learning disorders**; very **friendly and talkative**; facial dysmorphism, renal anomalies (and renovascular hypertension), **supravalvular aortic stenosis; hypercalcemia**

Table 2.4: Syndromes with Skeletal/Connective Tissue Dysplasias or Hamartoses

Syndrome	Major Diagnostic Findings and Problems
Achondroplasia	Abnormal **fibroblast gene** on chromosome 4; **autosomal dominant** with almost all cases as new mutations; **older paternal age; rhizomelic short stature** (shortening in proximal segments of legs) → **increased upper to lower segment ratio; large head with short base** (may have hydrocephalus if small foramen magnum), prominent forehead and midface hypoplasia; **lumbar lordosis**; abnormal vertebral bodies with short intervertebral spaces (**spinal compression**); intelligence usually normal; later obesity (*Note:* hypochondroplasia is similar but without significant craniofacial features and without severe spinal abnormalities.)
Marfan syndrome	Mutations in the **fibrillin gene** on chromosome 15; **autosomal dominant** with wide expression. Marfanoid phenotype: **tall (with decreased upper to lower segment ratio because of long legs), thin, arachnodactyly (long spider-like fingers, long arms with arm span > height)**; joint laxity → **hyperextensibility; kyphoscoliosis, pectus deformations, upward lens subluxation** (suspensory ligament defect); **dilatation of ascending aorta** (may have dissecting aneurysm) → **aortic insufficiency**, mitral valve prolapse
Ehlers-Danlos syndrome	Deficiency of **fibrillar collagen; autosomal dominant** with wide expression; six types. Classic (type I): **small stature more common, hyperextensible and fragile skin** (and ears) and blood vessels with **poor healing; hyperextensible joints**; lens dislocation; **aortic root dilatation**, mitral valve prolapse
Homocystinuria	**Autosomal recessive**; decreased cystathionine synthetase → accumulation of homocystine and methionine and decrease in cystathionine and cystine → interference with **crosslinking of collagen; Marfanoid appearance** with similar bone/joint problems; **downward lens subluxation; thromboembolism** most important morbidity due to degeneration and subsequent fibrosis of elastic arteries

Table 2.5: Syndromes with Early Overgrowth

Syndrome	Major Diagnostic Findings and Problems
Beckwith-Wiedemann syndrome (see Chapter 1)	Dosage imbalance of gene on chromosome 11; sporadic appearance; pancreatic islet cell hyperplasia → severe hypoglycemia; macrosomia, large tongue, hemihypertrophy, omphalocele, abdominal tumors (Wilms)
Sotos syndrome	**LGA** at birth with **increased growth velocity** through childhood and **advanced bone age; macrocephaly** at birth, facial dysmorphism, bone problems, variable **mental deficiency**; neurodevelopmental and behavioral problems

Abbreviations: large for gestational age, LGA

Table 2.6: Syndromes with Limb Defects

Syndrome	Major Diagnostic Findings and Problems
Poland sequence	Primary defect in development of proximal subclavian artery → unilateral decreased blood flow to **pectoral muscles and limb**; most on the **right**; majority of cases in **males**; hypoplasia to aplasia of pectoralis major and nipple with rib defects; distal arm hypoplasia, short or missing fingers; **dextrocardia** if on the left
Radial aplasia-thrombocytopenia syndrome (TAR)	**Bilateral absent radius, ulnar hypoplasia or aplasia**, abnormal humerus; **thumbs are present**; abnormal or absent megakaryocytes → severe **thrombocytopenia with hemorrhage** (cause of early death); heart and CNS defects

Abbreviations: central nervous system, CNS

Table 2.7: Syndromes with Major Facial Defects (and associated with hearing loss)

Syndrome	Major Diagnostic Findings and Problems
Treacher Collins syndrome	Autosomal dominant with wide expression, most new mutations; gene on chromosome 5; **down-slanting palpebral fissures, mandibular and malar hypoplasia**; scalp hair on lateral cheek, external ear malformations, **partial or complete absence of lower eyelids, lower lid coloboma**; may have early respiratory insufficiency because of a narrow airway; **visual and hearing loss**
Waardenburg syndrome	Autosomal dominant; gene on chromosome 2; partial **oculocutaneous albinism with white forelock, deafness (severe, bilateral), bushy eyebrows with medial flare (may meet in midline)**

Table 2.8: Syndromes with Prominent Brain/Neuromuscular Findings

Syndrome	Major Diagnostic Findings and Problems
Prader-Willi syndrome	Early-onset childhood **obesity** (large caloric intake and decreased activity; most important therapy is **dietary regulation** and exercise; secondary complications related to **morbid obesity** including **decreased life span**); **severe hypotonia** in infancy; **short stature, small hands and feet, mental retardation (most mild to moderate), learning problems, small/hypoplastic external genitalia with cryptorchidism in boys**
Angelman syndrome (Happy puppet syndrome)	**Ataxia with jerky arm movements (like a puppet);** cerebral atrophy, early seizures, severe **mental and motor retardation; very few words to absent speech** (may use sign language) with **laughter paroxysms** (brain stem defect)
Menkes kinky hair syndrome	X-linked recessive inheritance; **copper-transporting gene abnormality** (low copper and ceruloplasmin); **neurodegeneration** beginning in early infancy with **death by age 3 years; hair loses pigmentation starting at 6 weeks of age, and becomes sparse, broken, and twisted;** abnormally pigmented, thick, dry skin; vascular, skeletal, gastrointestinal and urinary tract abnormalities

Table 2.9: Teratogenic Syndromes

Syndrome	Major Diagnostic Findings and Problems
Fetal alcohol syndrome	Fetal effects are **dose-related** intake of alcohol; **IUGR and poor postnatal growth; microcephaly; midface dysmorphism; mild to severe mental retardation** with various neurological abnormalities; **irritability, hyperactivity; joint abnormalities; VSD, ASD, tetralogy of Fallot**
Fetal warfarin syndrome	Use of **coumarin** derivatives, especially in the **first trimester; IUGR with later catch-up growth;** severe **mental retardation and seizures; nasal hypoplasia, depressed nasal bridge, groove on nose;** short fingers with nail hypoplasia; may have CNS and eye malformations
Retinoic acid embryopathy	Isotretinoin (Accutane™) taken **subsequent to the 15th day after conception → mental deficiency, facial asymmetry, external ear anomalies,** small jaw, **facial paralysis;** flat, depressed nasal bridge, hypertelorism, **heart defects** (conotruncal lesions); **CNS anomalies**
Fetal hydantoin syndrome	Prenatal exposure to **phenytoin** (also similar effects from **valproate, carbamazepine, phenobarbital); IUGR and poor postnatal growth;** may have **mild mental deficiency;** facial dysmorphism, hypoplasia of distal phalanges with small nails; other findings including CNS, eye, heart, genitourinary, and gastrointestinal
Fetal valproate syndrome	Prenatal exposure to **valproic acid;** mental deficiency (less common), **midface hypoplasia, high forehead, epicanthal folds, flat nasal bridge, short nose with anteverted nostrils;** cleft lip; long, thin fingers; many types of **cardiac defects** (conotruncal, hypoplastic left heart); **meningomyelocele;** bone abnormalities

Abbreviations: atrial septal defect, ASD; central nervous system, CNS; intrauterine growth retardation, IUGR; ventral septal defect, VSD

PART TWO: INBORN ERRORS OF METABOLISM

Note: Studying the inborn errors is often quite complex, and thorough knowledge of all of the biochemistry and clinical presentations is needed only for subspecialty exams in genetics and metabolism. The following discussion is limited to the most important information and most common clinical presentations of the major metabolic diseases for diagnostic exam questions. As usual, key words to associate with each of the problems are in bold.

Most inborn errors are due to single-gene defects and are inherited as autosomal recessive disorders. Many present in the neonatal period, but may have a gradual and delayed onset. Presenting findings suggestive of a metabolic problem include: an acute, life-threatening disease in the neonatal period; coma; feeding problems with persistent vomiting and failure-to-thrive; changes in tone with other neurological abnormalities and developmental delay; hepatosplenomegaly with severe liver disease or specific metabolic abnormalities (hypoglycemia, metabolic acidosis, ketosis, hyperammonemia).

The most important initial management is to stabilize the patient: airway, breathing (oxygen, ventilation), circulation, and obtain serum glucose (see later chapters for other considerations). Other labs: complete blood count and differential, cultures (if infection is considered likely), electrolytes, BUN and creatinine, liver enzymes, prothrombin time (PT), partial thromboplastin time (PTT), serum osmolality, serum lactate, plasma ammonia, arterial blood gas, and urinalysis; depending on the results, urine and plasma amino acids and organic acids.

- More specifically, to sort out the most common etiologies of a metabolic disease, the following may be used: Obtain a plasma ammonia, blood pH, and serum electrolytes (to calculate the anion gap; see Chapter 3), *then:*
  a. **Hyperammonemia with no acidosis = urea cycle defect**
  b. **Normal to high ammonia with an increased anion gap acidosis = organic acidemia**
  c. **Normal ammonia with a normal anion gap = aminoacidemia or galactosemia**

Amino-Acid Disorders

Phenylketonuria

- Most common inborn error that may result in mental retardation; newborn screening is critical to prevent mental retardation.
- **Deficiency**—Phenylalanine (PHE) hydroxylase (PAH)
- **Biochemistry/testing**—With onset of milk feedings → gradual increase of **phenylketones in the urine**
  - Increased phenylpyruvic acid → positive **urine ferric chloride test** (urine turns green)
  - Increased phenylacetic acid → **musty or mousy urine odor**
  - Newborn screen measures increased [PHE] in blood so if there is a positive screen, a **serum [PHE]** must be drawn.

- **Clinical presentation**—Initial feeding problems with **vomiting**, weight loss, and failure-to-thrive; then **lethargy, increased muscle tone and deep tendon reflexes**, seizures, developmental delay, acquired microcephaly and mental retardation; exam may show **light complexion and eczema or seborrhea**

Treatment—Special formulas with decreased PHE; but still need PHE in diet to maintain plasma levels as close to normal as possible

Others
Most important things to know:

- **Maple syrup urine disease:** Deficiency in enzyme for metabolism of **branched chain amino acids** (leucine [leu], isoleucine [iso], and valine [val]); there is an **odor of maple syrup** from the breath, urine, and stool; in the classic form, presents in the newborn period with initial poor feeding, vomiting, and progressive lethargy; then **alternating hypotonia with hypertonia, opisthotonos, seizures, and coma**; survivors with severe motor defects and mental retardation; labs: **increased anion gap metabolic acidosis; ketonuria and increased plasma levels of leu, iso, and val.**
- **Hereditary tyrosinemia:** Deficiency in last step of tyrosine (tyr) metabolism; an increase in serum tyrosine leads to severe **liver, kidney, and peripheral nervous system** disease; **neonatal screen** detects increased tyr in blood (proportional to dietary intake); most present from 2–6 months of life with **acute liver disease**; also development of **Fanconi syndrome** (renal proximal tubular disease); high progression to **liver failure and later hepatocellular carcinoma**. **Transient tyrosinemia:** delayed maturation of enzyme activity, more common in premature infants; usually normal by 1 month of age with decreased protein intake.
- **Nonketotic hyperglycinemia:** Rare defect of **glycine** (gly) metabolism; severe acute onset of disease in newborn period: hypotonia, decreased reflexes, lethargy, seizures, and coma within the first 2 days of life; significant increase in serum and urine glycine; diagnostic is an increase in **cerebrospinal fluid (CSF) glycine** out of proportion to that in the serum (i.e., a very **large ratio of CSF: plasma gly**); increased plasma ammonia but without acidosis or ketosis; most die in the neonatal period; **transient form:** normal by 2 months of age, usually with no long-term problems.

Organic Acidemias and Disorders of Fatty-Acid Oxidation and Carnitine Metabolism
- Most from **methylmalonic and propionic acidemia**; also isovaleric acidemia and multiple carboxylase deficiency; mostly arise from defects in catabolism of branched-chain amino acids (**iso and val**), threonine, methionine, cholesterol, and **odd-chain fatty acids**.
- Hallmarks are **metabolic acidosis and encephalopathy**.
- Newborn disease: feeding problems, vomiting, lethargy, seizures with **respiratory distress** (severe metabolic acidosis) and hepatomegaly; labs: **increased anion gap metabolic acidosis, ketosis and some degree of hyperammonemia**; urine shows characteristic high amounts of specific metabolites.

Isovaleric acidemia

- Catabolism of leucine.
- Presents basically the same as described above
- Baby has a characteristic **odor of sweaty feet**; blood lab studies show the same, but again the specific increased metabolite in the urine can be identified.
- Definitive diagnosis may be made with cultured skin fibroblasts showing decreased or absent enzymatic activity, or molecular genetic testing can be performed.

Examples of disorders of fatty-acid oxidation

- Various **acyl-CoA dehydrogenase deficiencies** (short, medium, long, and very-long chain deficiencies)
- **Carnitine** transporter defect
- Carnitine palmitoyltransferase
- Acylcarnitine translocase deficiencies; also defects of **ketone** metabolism.

Abnormalities of fatty-acid oxidation

- Especially important with any etiology of **decreased caloric intake and with exercise** (skeletal muscle).
- Main clinical manifestations (**medium-chain acyl-CoA dehydrogenase deficiency** is the most common) involve **skeletal muscle, liver, and heart**.
- Presenting findings can be: acute-onset **coma and hypoglycemia** with mild **hepatomegaly** (fatty)
- **Muscle weakness** and chronic **cardiomyopathy**
- Particularly symptomatic when the child is old enough to sleep through the night (and therefore have a long **period of fasting**).
- Labs: **hypoglycemia but with low plasma and urinary ketones (hypoketotic hypoglycemia) and no metabolic acidosis**
- **Increased liver enzymes and abnormal liver function tests**. Elevation of specific urinary organic acids is seen.
- **Newborn screening** can detect abnormal acylcarnitines. Genetic testing can determine the specific mutation.

Carnitine

- Needed to **transport free fatty acids** across the inner mitochondrial membrane, where beta-oxidation occurs (i.e., in the **mitochondria**).
- Carnitine deficiency (transport defect) leads to abnormal fatty-acid oxidation.
- Most present in the first several years of life with **progressive muscle weakness and cardiomyopathy**.
- Plasma and muscle **carnitine levels are very low**.

Electron transfer defects

- Generally produce severe illness in the neonate (acidosis, hypoglycemia, cardiomyopathy, and coma)

Defects in ketone synthesis

- Generally similar to fatty-acid oxidation, i.e., fasting hypoketotic hypoglycemia, but without any skeletal or cardiac muscle impairment (with one enzymatic defect) or episodes of severe fasting ketoacidosis (with another).

For disorders of very-long chain fatty acids (the peroxisomal disorders), see Chapter 22.

Urea-Cycle Defects

- **Free ammonia**, which is toxic, is produced from **amino acid catabolism**.
- Converted to **urea** in the urea cycle with a series of **five enzymes:** carbamyl phosphate synthetase (CPS), ornithine transcarbamylase (OTC), argininosuccinate synthetase (AS), argininosuccinate lyase (AL), and arginase.
- Most present in the neonatal period within days of normal feeding: **feeding problems, hepatomegaly, tachypnea, lethargy, seizures, and coma.**
- Labs: **hyperammonemia, and no acidosis** (compare to the organic acidemias).
- **Mild, transient hyperammonemia** may be present in **very low birth weight (VLBW)** infants for the first 2 months of life; they are asymptomatic and do well.
- Some premature infants, however, may have **significant transient hyperammonemia** with very high levels of plasma ammonia, which may be life-threatening.

The specific enzyme diagnosis may be sorted out as follows:

Hyperammonemia with no acidosis

- Obtain **plasma amino acids:** A specific pattern of elevation will be diagnostic of AS, AL, and arginase deficiencies
- **Nonspecific pattern** (elevated levels of glutamine, alanine, and aspartate) is seen with OTC deficiency, CPS deficiency, and transient hyperammonemia of the newborn.

To distinguish between these:

- Obtain **urine for orotic acid. High orotic acid** concentration is characteristic of **OTC** deficiency. **Normal to low** concentration is characteristic of **either CPS or transient hyperammonemia of the newborn.**
- Obtain a **plasma citrulline** level. In **CPS, it will be low;** whereas in **transient hyperammonemia of the newborn, it will be normal or increased.**

- Treatment of acute hyperammonemia is **to prevent protein breakdown** with adequate calories (glucose, lipids, and minimal amounts of essential amino acids), **to correct dehydration and electrolyte abnormalities,** and **to remove ammonia** (sodium benzoate, sodium phenylacetate, and arginine hydrochloride). If the plasma ammonia fails to significantly correct, **dialysis** is required.

Defects in Carbohydrate Metabolism

Galactosemia

The source of galactose is **lactose** (glucose + galactose), primarily from milk and other dairy products. Galactose has a small contribution to the production of glucose (conversion of galactose-1-phosphate [Gal-1-P] to glucose-1-phosphate [Glu-1-P]).

Important in the synthesis of glycolipids, glycoproteins, and glycosaminoglycans.

There are three enzyme deficiencies that may lead to galactosemia (see Table 2.10).

Table 2.10: Comparison of the Three Enzymatic Deficiencies that Cause Galactosemia

Features	Galactose-1-Phosphate Uridyl Transferase (Classic Galactosemia)	Galactokinase	UDP-Galactose-4-Epimerase
Biochemistry	Cannot convert Gal-1-P to Glu-1-P; Gal-1-P accumulates in brain, liver, and kidney; may begin prenatally with transplacental galactose	Catalyzes initial phosphorylation of galactose; accumulation of galactose and galactitol	Converts UDP-Gal to UDP Glu; accumulation of cellular UDP-Gal
Types	Classic complete (or almost-complete) deficiency vs. partial deficiency with milder to asymptomatic presentation		Benign, asymptomatic; diagnosed with neonatal screen vs. severe—resembles transferase deficiency
Clinical presentation	Neonate with vomiting, lethargy, failure to gain birth weight; **hepatomegaly, jaundice,** liver and renal failure; **cataracts;** increased risk of *Escherichia coli* **sepsis;** if survives untreated, → cirrhosis and mental retardation	Asymptomatic except for **cataracts**	A **benign form evident only with a positive neonatal screen** (deficiency only in RBCs and WBCs); or a severe form similar to transferase deficiency and with **hypotonia and sensorineural deafness**

Abbreviations: galactose-1-phosphate, Gal-1-P; glucose-1-phosphate, Glu-1-P; red blood cells, RBCs; uridine diphosphate, UDP; white blood cells, WBCs

Diagnosis and treatment

- Urine dipstick with a Clinitest will be positive for reducing substances (glu, gal, fru) but a subsequent Clinistix (glucose oxidase for glucose) will be negative.
- Diagnosis is confirmed by assaying the enzyme in RBCs.
- Treatment is with a lactose-free diet (elimination of gal from the diet).
- With this, all of the findings will regress except for any mental/developmental delays.

Fructose deficiencies

- **Sucrose** (fructose + glucose + sorbitol) and free fructose are the dietary sources of fructose.

- Deficiency in fructokinase (conversion of fructose to fructose-1-phosphate) leads to an increased fructose content in the liver and high excretion of fructose in the urine, but this does not lead to problems (**benign fructosuria**). It usually becomes apparent with a urine analysis, where one finds a **reducing substance** present.
- Deficiency of fructose 1,6-biphosphate aldolase is called **hereditary fructose intolerance**. This enzyme hydrolyzes fructose 1,6-biphosphate and fructose-1-phosphate. There is a **toxic** accumulation of fructose-1-phosphate (when fructose or sucrose is introduced into the diet) that leads to hypoglycemia and features resembling classic galactosemia.

Glycogen storage diseases

Deficiencies result in abnormalities in **the breakdown of glycogen to glucose with accumulation of glycogen**. There are more than 12 types, and any of the 12 causes prominent **liver or muscle problems**. The most common types are discussed briefly below:

- **Von Gierke disease (Type I):** Glucose-6-phosphatase deficiency (little to no activity in liver, kidney, and intestine); problem in conversion of glucose-6-phosphate to glucose; most present in first months of life with **hypoglycemia** (may have seizures), **lactic acidosis, and hepatomegaly** (with **protuberant abdomen**); may develop cirrhosis and renal failure; characteristic features: **short stature with thin extremities** and what is described as **doll-like facies**; diagnosis with molecular genetic analysis.
- **Pompe disease (Type II):** Acid maltase deficiency leads to abnormal breakdown of glycogen in **lysosomes** (other glycogen storage diseases with glycogen accumulation in cytoplasm) with lysosomal glycogen accumulation mostly in **skeletal, smooth, and cardiac muscle**. Infantile type (with cirrhosis and cardiac failure; huge heart on x-ray) leads to early death. More common presentation: any time from childhood to adult with **progression of weakness** (more in legs) leading to wheelchair-dependence; there is no severe heart involvement. Labs: increased creatine kinase (CK), lactic acid dehydrogenase (LADH), and aspartate aminotransferase. Diagnosis is enzyme activity in skin biopsy.
- **McArdle disease (Type V):** Muscle phosphorylase deficiency which leads to glycogen accumulation and decreased production of ATP; presents later in childhood or in the adult with **exercise intolerance**, cramps, myositis, and **rhabdomyolysis**, leading to **myoglobinuria** (during exercise) with acute renal failure.

Primary lactic acidosis

Caused by defects in gluconeogenesis (e.g., phosphoenolpyruvate carboxylase deficiency) or in the **metabolism of pyruvate** (during glycolysis or the citric acid cycle). With an unexplained increased anion gap acidosis, blood should be obtained for **pyruvate, lactate, and acylcarnitine with urine for organic acids**.

Lactic acidosis from:

- **Hypoxemia or respiratory chain defects:** Serum pyruvate is normal and lactate is significantly increased, therefore there is an **increased lactate–pyruvate ratio**.
- **Pyruvate dehydrogenase or gluconeogenesis:** Serum pyruvate and lactate are increased, so the **lactate–pyruvate ratio is normal**.

Mucopolysaccharidoses (MPS)

Deficiency in enzymes in lysosomes needed to metabolize **glycosaminoglycans** (primarily heparan sulfate); these are complex carbohydrates (with neutral and amino sugars and uronic acid). They are protein-linked for the formation of **proteoglycans** (in connective tissue and cell/nuclear membranes). With a deficiency in one of the enzymes involved in the breakdown of heparan sulfate, fragments accumulate in the **lysosomes**, which then interfere with cell function.

MPS I (spectrum of Scheie to Hurler syndromes)

Alpha-L-iduronidase deficiency; depending on the type of mutation, there is variable expression of the disease from the mild Scheie disease to severe Hurler (with an intermediate form); **autosomal recessive** inheritance; *Hurler* is **severe with death** by 10 years of age (respiratory or heart failure); babies are normal at birth but may have **inguinal hernias** (clue to diagnosis); diagnosis is made thereafter in the first 2 years of life: **coarse facies with large tongue and prominent forehead; hepatosplenomegaly, corneal clouding, short stature, joint contractures, skeletal dysplasia** (called dysostosis multiplex); patients with Hurler may have **cardiomyopathy** (with valvular regurgitation and narrowing of the coronary arteries), hydrocephalus, and obstructive airway disease (with repeat infections and deteriorating pulmonary function).

MPS II (Hunter disease)

Deficiency of iduronate sulfatase; **X-linked recessive** inheritance, so essentially only in males; wide spectrum of disease; severe disease may look like Hurler, except there is **no corneal cloudiness and there is slower progression** of the disease features, with initial findings detected later than Hurler. Most Hunter patients live slightly longer than those with Hurler; may have many **Mongolian spots** at birth (clue to diagnosis).

The other forms of MPS include four types of Sanfilippo disease, two types of Morquio disease, Maroteaux-Lamy disease, Sly disease, and hyaluronidase deficiency.

Sphingolipidoses

These are **lysosomal storage diseases**, where deficiency in a hydrolyase leads to accumulation of a specific lipid substrate consisting of **ceramide**, which is the basis for the production of the **sphingolipids** (essential part of all **cell membranes**); the sphingolipids are broken down in the nervous system and in visceral organs, RBCs, and WBCs; accumulation of the **glycosphingolipids in the CNS results in neurodegenerative disease**; systemic findings are present with storage in other organ systems. There is often a broad clinical spectrum of the disease, with various ages of onset, acuity, and severity. Diagnosis is demonstrating decreased or absent enzyme activity in cultured fibroblasts and with molecular genetic testing to identify the carrier state and for prenatal diagnosis and genetic counseling. In some cases, specific therapies are of value (e.g., recombinant enzyme replacement, liver transplantation, bone marrow transplantation, gene therapy), but much of the therapy is supportive.

All of the following have **autosomal recessive** inheritance.

Tay-Sachs disease and Sandhoff disease (GM$_2$ gangliosidosis)
- **Deficiency:** Tay-Sachs: beta-hexosaminidase A only; Sandhoff: beta-hexosaminidose A and B
- **Accumulation:** Lysosomal GM2, especially in **CNS**
- **Predilection:** Ashkenazi Jews
- **Key features:** <u>Tay-Sachs</u>: infant with motor loss, hyperacusis (with **increased startle response**), macrocephaly (no hydrocephalus), **macular cherry-red spot**, seizures and **progressive neurodegeneration**; death before age 5 years. <u>Sandhoff</u>: similar to Tay-Sachs with prominent hepatosplenomegaly, cardiac involvement, and skeletal abnormalities

Gaucher disease
- **Deficiency:** Beta-glucosidase
- **Accumulation:** Glucosylceramide in **reticuloendothelial cells**
- **Pathology:** Gaucher cell in the reticuloendothelial system (especially bone marrow): intracytoplasmic inclusions that stain positively
- **Predilection:** The **most common of the lipidoses, and Gaucher**—*not* Tay-Sachs—**is the most prevalent genetic disorder in Ashkenazi Jews.**
- **Key features:** Most patients present by adolescence with a non-neuropathic form (infants with an acute, neuropathic form); **hepatosplenomegaly** (often with **huge spleen**), **bone marrow findings**, i.e., thrombocytopenia (bruising, mucocutaneous bleeding), anemia, and bone pain; and **skeletal abnormalities** with pathologic fractures.

Nieman-Pick disease
- **Deficiency:** Acid sphingomyelinase
- **Accumulation:** Sphingomyelin and other lipids in **monocytes and macrophages**
- **Key features:** Types A and C have **neurodegeneration**, and type B has systemic manifestations (pulmonary symptoms in adults; more variable); infants with **hepatosplenomegaly, lymphadenopathy, neurodevelopmental regression with severe psychomotor retardation**; death by age 3 years

Krabbe disease
- **Deficiency:** Galactocerebrosidase
- **Accumulation:** Galactosylceramide (myelin) in neural **white matter**
- **Key features:** Infant with irritability, **hypertonicity, opisthotonos**, seizures, **severe psychomotor retardation, and optic atrophy**; death by age 3 years

Metachromatic leukodystrophy

- **Deficiency:** Arylsulfatase A
- **Accumulation:** Sulfated glycosphingolipids in neural **white matter → demyelination and neurodegeneration**
- **Pathology:** Metachromatic neural inclusions that stain positively in white matter
- **Key features:** Most present in first to second year of life with **no walking**, little or no deep tendon reflexes, **hypotonia, and gradual muscle wasting**; then nystagmus, **loss of any speech, loss of hearing, myoclonic seizures, quadriparesis, and optic atrophy**; death in the first 10 years of life. Labs: increased CSF protein, urine sediment **metachromatic granules, MRI of brain:** diffuse symmetric attenuation of white matter

Lipoproteins

Examples of Hyperlipoproteinemias

Familial combined hyperlipidemia

- **Most common primary lipid disorder**; autosomal dominant
- Moderate increase in **LDL and cholesterol** and decreased HDL
- **Family history of premature atherosclerotic cardiovascular disease**
- Dx: two first-degree relative must have either LDL above the 90th percentile, triglycerides above the 90th percentile, or both
- **No xanthomas** (see below)
- Many with **metabolic syndrome** (see Chapter 16)
- Therapy: **diet + exercise**; consider pharmacotherapy if LDL remains significantly elevated

Familial hypercholesterolemia

- Autosomal co-dominant; mutations of LDL receptor (no receptor mutation more severe than defective receptor)
- Homozygous (2 gene copies): significant increase in **cholesterol**, with normal triglycerides and small decrease in HDL
  - History of **premature cardiovascular disease** in first-degree relatives
  - **Poor prognosis:** severe atherosclerosis by middle childhood
  - **Xanthomas** on tendons (Achilles tendon, hand extensors) or skin
  - Death during childhood, if untreated
  - Rx: **drugs** to decrease absorption and synthesis; selective removal of circulating LDL; liver transplant
- Heterozygous
  - Co-dominant with full penetrance → half of first-degree and 25% of second-degree relatives of the affected person will also be affected
  - **Cardiovascular disease symptoms** in the 40s for men and 50s for women
  - First- and second-degree relatives of any child with high cholesterol should be **screened**
  - Rx: diet modification, pharmacotherapy as above

Familial hypertriglyceridemia (Type IV)

- Autosomal dominant; unknown cause
- Very high **triglyceride** levels with or without mildly increased cholesterol and low HDL
- Mostly presents in adults; **less atherogenic**; **no xanthomas**; may present with **acute pancreatitis**
- Dx: requires at least one affected first-degree relative
- Primary Rx is dietary, unless with significant persistent elevations (no fibrates or niacin in children), mostly to prevent pancreatitis

FLUID, ELECTROLYTE, AND NUTRITIONAL MANAGEMENT

3

PART ONE: FLUID AND ELECTROLYTE MANAGEMENT

Total Body Water (TBW) and Fluid Compartment Distribution

- Term newborn has 75–80% TBW as a percentage of total body weight.
- TBW increases with decreasing gestational age.
- With the normal diuresis after birth, TBW decreases by about 5% (accounts for the weight loss after birth, which is typically regained by 10–14 days of life).
- TBW gradually decreases over the first year when it is at the adult level of about 60%.
  - Extracellular fluid space (ECF; 25% body weight)
    - Intravascular fluid (5%)
    - Interstitial fluid (15–20%)
  - Intracellular fluid space (ICF; 30–40%)

Composition

- **Intravascular fluid:** Most is Na^+, with its corresponding anions, Cl^- and $HCO3^-$; then small amounts of K, Ca, Mg (cations), and proteins and phosphorus (anions)
- **Interstitial fluid:** almost the same except for **decreased protein**
- **Intracellular:** The major cation is K^+, then small amounts of Na and Mg; the anions (in decreasing order) are phosphorus, proteins, HCO_3^- and Cl^-.

Maintenance of plasma volume

- Osmotic equilibrium between the extracellular fluid (ECF) and intracellular fluid (ICF) due to the permeability of the cell membrane to water.
- Size of each space depends on the **amount of water in each** (depends on the **osmolality** of each compartment).
- Plasma volume is maintained due to the presence of poorly permeable proteins (greatest influence per weight is **albumin**), establishes an **oncotic pressure to oppose the hydrostatic pressure** of the blood pumped from the heart; normal serum osmolality is maintained through **renal regulation of sodium and water**.

- ICF volume is greater than ECF volume and there are variations in electrolytes between them, **so the serum content of electrolytes (Na and K, primarily) does not reflect total body electrolyte content** (see below for further discussion).
- **Measured serum osmolality** (osm) is 285–295 mOsm/kg; osmolality can be calculated as:

$$\text{Serum osmolality (mOsm/L)} = 2 \text{ (Na in mEq/L)} + BUN/2 \text{ (mg/dL)} + glucose/18 \text{ (mg/dL)}$$

(Note: the 2 and 18 are conversion factors to obtain mOsm; Na is multiplied by 2 because of its two accompanying anions: Cl^- and HCO_3^-.)

- Urea contributes little to the osmolality since it can cross the cell membrane.
- With hyperglycemia, there is an effect on serum osmolality because it is not in equilibrium with the intracellular fluid.
- If the measured osmolality > than the calculated, there is an **osmolal gap (>10 mOsm/kg) unmeasured osmols** (e.g., ethanol, ethylene glycol).

Sodium Homeostasis Abnormalities

- Daily requirements for sodium and chloride are 3 and 2 mEq/kg, respectively.
- Water balance determines the serum [Na] through antidiuretic hormone (ADH) with a change in serum osmolality.
- The kidney excretes sodium based on effective plasma volume through the renin-angiotensin-aldosterone system and intrarenal mechanisms.

Hypernatremia

Definition: serum [Na] >145 mEq/L

Physiology: increased [Na] → ECF hypertonicity → movement of water out of cells → cellular dehydration; the **intravascular volume is preserved** so that **initially blood pressure and urine output are still normal** (when diagnosed, patient may already be **severely dehydrated**). There is a deficiency of water with respect to total body Na.

- Hypernatremia may occur from either a net loss of water, or a loss of both water and sodium (with the water deficit greater than the Na deficit), or a net sodium gain.

Signs and symptoms: with increasing [Na], the **central nervous system (CNS) symptoms** worsen (lethargy, irritability, weakness, hyperpnea, severe thirst)

- With **increasing osmolality**, more water moves out of brain cells → decreased brain volume and tearing of bridging and intracerebral veins → **brain hemorrhage**.
- **Central pontine myelinosis** and extrapontine myelinosis may occur (as well as with rapid correction of severe hyponatremia).

Etiology and Diagnosis of Hypernatremia

Na Gain

- Most causes:
  - Iatrogenic (hospital) hypertonic saline or sodium bicarbonate administration
  - Home: formula made incorrectly, salt poisoning, accidental ingestions
  - Hyperaldosteronism

- Diagnostic considerations:
  - **Do not show signs of dehydration**; will have some degree of volume overload (so must **ask about salt intake**)
  - With excess salt administration, the **fractional excretion of Na is elevated**.
  - Hyperaldosteronism: hypernatremia with hypokalemia and hypertension

Water loss

- Most causes:
  - **Imbalance** between Na intake and loss (e.g., high insensible losses in preterm infants) or **inadequate intake**
  - Central or nephrogenic diabetes insipidus (only if cannot control water intake)

- Diagnostic considerations:
  - With diabetes insipidus: high urine volume and inappropriately dilute urine
  - Imbalance or inadequate intake: **low urine volume with concentrated urine**

Water and Na loss:

- Most causes:
  - Renal causes:
    - Chronic renal disease
    - Diuretic phase of obstructive uropathy or acute tubular necrosis
    - Osmotic diuresis (e.g., with diabetes)

  - Extrarenal:
    - Losses through the skin (e.g., severe burns) or the gastrointestinal tract (with gastroenteritis if there is inadequate intake, i.e., persistent vomiting)

- Diagnostic considerations:
  - Extrarenal causes: there is Na retention by the kidneys (**urine Na <20 mEq/L**, i.e., a **low fractional excretion of Na**), and a **low, concentrated urine volume**
  - Renal causes: **higher urine Na (i.e., a high fractional excretion of Na) with increased and more dilute urine**

Hyponatremia

- **Definition: serum [Na] <135 mEq/L**
- **Physiology:** determined by total body water and total body Na; there is a decrease in [Na] with a low, normal, or high total body Na and water
  - Decreased serum osmolality → **water shifts into the brain ICF space**, which is responsible for most symptoms

- **Signs and symptoms:** depend on how fast the Na decreases and the degree of the resulting hypo-osmolality; CNS symptoms develop when serum **[Na] <125 mEq/L** (irritability, headache, lethargy, nausea and vomiting, hyporeflexia, seizures, and eventually coma)
- Two conditions to rule out:
  - **Factitious hyponatremia:** lab artifact due to increased proteins or lipids in the serum; water displaced by increased solids → decreases the serum sodium per liter, but the measured serum osmolality is not changed (can be avoided by using an ion-selective electrode to measure the sodium); an increase in triglycerides by 1 g/dL will decrease the Na by 2 mEq/L.
  - **Dilutional hyponatremia:** with increased osmols in the serum (e.g., hyperglycemia or mannitol), [Na] decreases due to water moving from the ICF → ECF; but there are no symptoms of hyponatremia because there is no decrease in the osmolality; an increase in blood glucose by 100 mg/dL will decrease the measured [Na] by 1.6 mEq/L.

Hypovolemic hyponatremia
- Na loss higher than water loss; compensatory water retention
- Most causes:
  - Extrarenal:
    - Gastrointestinal losses (**acute gastroenteritis** most common cause)
    - Skin losses (burns)
    - Third-space losses
  - Renal:
    - Kidney disease
    - Osmotic diuresis
    - **Diuretics (loop and thiazides)**
    - Cerebral salt-wasting
    - Hypoaldosteronism
- Diagnostic considerations:
  - Renal: **urine Na >20 mEq/L**
  - Extrarenal: **urine Na <20 mEq/L**

Hypervolemic hyponatremia
- Excess of total body water and Na, but increase in water is greater than that of Na; most with a decrease in effective blood volume (from decreased cardiac output or third-space fluids); compensation by:
  - Increased ADH secretion → water retention
  - Increased renin-angiotensin-aldosterone → sodium retention
- Most causes: **edematous states** (congestive heart failure, cirrhosis, nephrotic syndrome) and **acute or chronic renal failure**
- Diagnostic considerations: in the edematous states, **urine Na is <20 mEq/L** and in renal failure, it is **>20 mEq/L**

Euvolemic hyponatremia
- Decreased Na **without any clinical evidence of hypovolemia or fluid expansion; mostly with increase in body water** and slight decrease in total body Na

- Most causes:
  - Syndrome of inappropriate ADH secretion (**SIADH**)
  - Overtreatment with desmopressin for diabetes insipidus
  - Water intoxication (iatrogenic, accidental, purposeful); hyponatremia only if water intake is greater than renal elimination
  - Glucocorticoid deficiency and hypothyroidism: both cause renal water retention but the mechanism is unknown

---

SIADH

- No inhibition of ADH secretion → water retention and hyponatremia; increase in ECF → mild increased intravascular volume

- Kidney increases Na excretion (trying to decrease intravascular volume to normal) and therefore there is a mild decrease in total body Na.

Most causes: CNS (infection, tumor, postictal, psychiatric); lung disease, malignancy, **medications** (tricyclic antidepressants, salicylates, haloperidol, barbiturates, vinblastine, vincristine, cyclophosphamide, carbamazepine, and chlorpropamide)

Diagnosis: no evidence of dehydration; must have no diuretic use; no congestive heart failure, nephrotic syndrome or cirrhosis and no renal, adrenal, or thyroid deficiencies and:

- Serum [Na] <135 mEq/L
- Serum osmolality <280 mOsm/L
- Urine [Na] >25 m/L
- Urine osmolality >100 mOsm/L (often > plasma osm)

Disorders of acid-base metabolism

Normal physiology

- Lungs increase or decrease ventilation rapidly to keep the blood pCO_2 at 35–45 mm Hg (normal pH is 7.35–7.45).
- Kidney excretes acid (normal daily production of 2–3 mEq/kg depending on protein intake); neutralized by bicarbonate (HCO_3; normal blood level 20–28 mEq/L), regenerated by the kidney (through the secretion of H^+).
- The proximal tubule resorbs most of filtered HCO_3 (the rest is in the ascending loop of Henle); collecting duct is main location of H^+ secretion, coupled to the generation of bicarbonate (replaces the bicarbonate filtered)
- Proximal tubule generates ammonia (mostly from metabolism of glutamic acid), used as a urinary buffer; collecting duct H^+ pump cannot decrease the urine pH to <4.5, so buffers are needed (otherwise, huge volumes of water would need to be excreted daily).
  - H^+ excretion is adjusted as needed (the ECF pH is the most important regulator of acid excretion): if H^+ excretion is increased, then collecting duct H^+ secretion is increased and urinary pH becomes more acidic (but not to <4.5); if there are larger amounts of H^+ excretion, ammonia production is increased.
- With alkalosis, proximal tubule resorbs less bicarbonate in the collecting duct and there may be secretion of bicarbonate into the tubular lumen and H^+ into the blood.

Diagnosis of Acid–Base Disorders

Acidosis is a pathologic process causing an increase in hydrogen ions, and **alkalosis** is the opposite. **Acidemia** (pH <7.35) and **alkalemia** (pH >7.45) are the net results of these processes:

- An increase in pCO_2 or a decrease in $[HCO_3]$ → increased $[H^+]$ → decreased pH
- A decrease in pCO_2 or an increase in $[HCO_3]$ → decreased $[H^+]$ → increased pH

Compensation

Fast (12–24 hours; cannot completely normalize the pH):

- **Simple metabolic acidosis** → decreased pH → increased ventilation → decreased pCO_2 → increased pH
- **Simple metabolic alkalosis** → increased pH → decreased ventilation → increased pCO_2 → decreased pH

Slow (3–4 days, depending on acute or chronic):

- **Simple respiratory acidosis** → increased renal H^+ excretion → increased HCO_3 generation → increased serum $[HCO_3]$ → increased pH
- **Simple respiratory alkalosis** → increased renal HCO_3 excretion → decreased serum $[HCO_3]$ → decreased pH

If a patient does not have the appropriate compensation (see Table 3.1), then the disorder is **mixed**; e.g., a primary metabolic lactic acidosis + respiratory acidosis due to respiratory failure.

Table 3.1: Diagnosing Acid-Base Abnormalities

Acidemia → Metabolic Acidosis (decreased HCO_3)	Acidemia → Respiratory Acidosis (increased pCO_2)	Alkalemia → Metabolic Alkalosis (increased HCO_3)	Alkalemia → Respiratory Alkalosis (decreased pCO_2)
Low pCO_2: mixed metabolic acidosis and respiratory alkalosis	**Low HCO_3:** mixed respiratory + metabolic acidosis	**Low pCO_2:** mixed respiratory + metabolic alkalosis	**Low HCO_3:** mixed respiratory alkalosis and metabolic acidosis
Expected pCO_2 = $1.5 \times [HCO_3] + 8$: simple metabolic acidosis	**Expected HCO_3 =** increases by 1 mEq/L for each 10 mm increase in pCO_2 (acute) or increases by 3.5 mEq for each 10 mm increase in pCO_2 (chronic): simple respiratory acidosis	**Expected pCO_2 =** increased by 7 mm Hg for each 10 mEq/L increase in HCO_3: simple metabolic alkalosis	**Expected HCO_3 =** decreases by 2 mEq/L for each 10 mm decrease in pCO_2 (acute) or decreases by 4 for each 10 mm decrease in pCO_2 (chronic): simple respiratory alkalosis
High pCO_2: mixed metabolic + respiratory acidosis	**High HCO_3:** mixed respiratory acidosis + metabolic alkalosis	**High pCO_2:** mixed metabolic alkalosis + respiratory acidosis	**High HCO_3:** mixed respiratory + metabolic alkalosis

Metabolic acidosis

- Occurs as a result of **loss of HCO$_3$, decreased renal H$^+$ excretion or exogenous acid**
- **Anion gap** is normal or increased.
- With **normal anion gap** metabolic acidosis, the **HCO$_3$ is decreased** with no increase in **unmeasured anions**; it is a **hyperchloremic metabolic acidosis** (with changes in [HCO$_3$]), [Cl$^-$] must increase or decrease to preserve electroneutrality).

The Anion Gap

Anion gap = [Na$^+$] − {[Cl$^-$] + [HCO$_3^-$]}

- The normal is 4–11 (due to albumin)
- Increased with any unmeasured anions (e.g., lactate in lactic acidosis)

Table 3.2: Differential Diagnosis: Normal vs. Increased Anion Gap (unmeasured anions) Metabolic Acidosis

Increased Anion Gap	Normal Anion Gap
Ketoacidosis (ketoacids)	Diarrhea
Lactic acidosis (lactate)	Renal tubular acidosis
Renal failure (retention of phosphate, urate, sulfate)	Ammonium chloride intake
Drugs:	Urinary fistulae
Salicylates	Some inborn errors of metabolism (see Chapter 2)
Toluene	
Ethylene glycol	
Methanol	

- Symptoms proportional to the **degree of acidemia: tachypnea, hyperpnea**, lethargy to coma, impaired heart contractility, pulmonary vasoconstriction → pulmonary artery hypertension, weakness (increased protein degradation → decreased ATP), **hyperkalemia** and arrhythmias (K moves from the ICF → ECF); chronically: failure-to-thrive
- Treatment; correct the underlying disorder first, if possible; in certain conditions, bicarbonate may be indicated acutely and chronically; for acute correction, IV NaHCO$_3$ or Na-acetate administered as a bolus (1 mEq HCO$_3$/kg) or as part of IV infusion; examples of use: salicylate poisoning, renal tubular acidosis, acute and chronic renal failure, certain inborn errors.

Metabolic alkalosis

- **Increased serum [HCO$_3$]** with partial compensation (but can never have >55–60 mm pCO$_2$)
- Initially, separate causes based on **urinary chloride into low (chloride <15 mEq/L) and high (chloride >20 mEq/L)**

- Low urinary chloride = **chloride-responsive**
  - Maintained by **volume depletion** (decreased filtered HCO_3 → increased resorption of Na and HCO_3 in proximal tubule → decreased HCO_3 excretion
  - Increased aldosterone (due to volume depletion) → increased HCO_3 resorption and H^+ secretion in collecting duct; also leads to increased urinary potassium losses and movement of potassium from ECF → ICF during metabolic alkalosis (**hypokalemia**)

- High urinary chloride = **chloride-resistant**
  - Separated as to whether or not **hypertension** is present; hypertension due to any increase in **aldosterone** → increased [Na] → increased blood pressure; increased excretion of H^+ and K → **metabolic alkalosis and hypokalemia**; so there is **volume overload and therefore the urine chloride is low**

Table 3.3: Major Causes of Metabolic Alkalosis

Chloride-Responsive	Chloride-Resistant	
Gastric losses	High BP:	Adrenal hyperplasia (some forms)
Chloride-losing diarrhea		Adrenal adenomas
Thiazides and loop diuretics		Cushing syndrome
Cystic fibrosis		Renovascular
	Normal BP:	Bartter and Gitelman syndromes
		Administration of base
		Hypoparathyroidism (autosomal dominant)

Specific notes

- **Diuretics:** with volume depletion → increased angiotensin II → aldosterone → adrenergic renal stimulation; increased Na delivery to the distal tubule and collecting duct → increased H^+ secretion; also hypokalemia → increased H^+ excretion; causes a **contraction alkalosis,** i.e., the fluid loss is without bicarbonate, so the remaining bicarbonate is in a smaller fluid volume and therefore → increased $[HCO_3]$. Early with diuretic use there is increased chloride excretion, but then there is renal chloride retention due to volume depletion, so the **urine chloride may be high or low, depending on when it is measured with respect to the starting of the diuretic.**
- **Cystic fibrosis:** there are excessive losses of **sodium and chloride in sweat** → metabolic alkalosis with hypokalemia (increased urinary losses) and to some extent hyponatremia (sodium loss and renal water retention from ADH)
- Bartter syndrome (Gitelman is essentially milder, with different etiology): defect in sodium and chloride resorption in the loop of Henle → volume depletion → secondary hyperaldosteronism → hypokalemia metabolic alkalosis
- Most will present per the underlying disease; with volume depletion: thirst, lethargy, weakness, symptoms related to hypokalemia (arrhythmias), decreased ionized calcium (due to increased albumin binding) → tetany, decreased ventilation; hypertension if one of the diseases of chloride resistant alkalosis is underlying

- Treatment: primarily with the underlying problem with moderate to severe alkalosis; may need administration of NaCl and KCl; replacement of gastric losses, IV or oral potassium

Respiratory acidosis

- Pulmonary or non-pulmonary disease causing an increase in pCO_2; with acute acidosis, there is rapid titration of acid by non-bicarbonate buffers; chronically, there is more metabolic compensation by the kidneys with increased acid excretion over several days; increase in HCO_3 → decrease in body chloride, → **chloride-responsive partially compensated alkalosis** develops
- Signs and symptoms: proportional to the degree of acidosis (acute > chronic); **signs of hypoxia when there is respiratory acidosis**: headache, anxiety, dizziness, hallucinations, seizures, coma, decreased cardiac contractility; diagnosis based on presentation with appropriate use of tests for pulmonary or non-pulmonary causes; also treatment per underlying cause and support (e.g., oxygen, ventilation); pCO_2 should never be decreased rapidly with chronic hypercarbia.

Respiratory alkalosis

- Decrease in pCO_2; acute metabolic response in minutes is H^+ release from non-bicarbonate buffers and the chronic response is greater and takes longer—decrease in serum HCO_3. Chronic respiratory alkalosis is the only time when the compensation may be almost normal.
- Most causes from **hypoxemia** (need **arterial blood gas** for accurate determination) and/or stimulation of lung receptors: lung disease, congestive heart disease, cyanotic heart disease, hypotension, severe anemia, altitude, carbon monoxide poisoning; in the absence of lung disease, the **stimulation is centrally**: CNS disease, pain, anxiety, sepsis, pregnancy, liver failure (unknown mechanism), medications (salicylates, caffeine, progesterone)
- Signs and symptoms: chest tightness, palpitations, syncope (decreased cerebral blood flow with hypocarbia), seizures, muscle cramps and paresthesias (decreased ionized calcium); treat underlying cause

Potassium Homeostasis Abnormalities

- Daily requirements: **1–2 mEq/kg**
- The major intracellular cation, most in muscle; most extracellular K is in bone
- Major use for **electrical activity of nerve and muscle cells**
- **Plasma concentration does not always reflect total body K** because of changes in distribution between the ICF and the ECF; Na/K-ATPase: pumps Na out of cell and K in; insulin activates
  - **Acidosis** drives K out of the cell and alkalosis into the cell.
  - **Hyperosmolality** drives water to the ECF and K follows because of solvent drag (e.g., in diabetic ketoacidosis).
  - **Beta-adrenergic** stimulation drives K into the ICF.
  - **Alpha-adrenergic** stimulation drives K into the ECF.

- K is filtered in the kidneys and 90% resorbed before the distal nephron, where aldosterone acts to regulate secretion; increased [K] → increased secretion

Hyperkalemia

- Major causes:
  - **Factitious hyperkalemia**: from **hemolysis** with blood-drawing or prolonged tourniquet application; also with **thrombocytosis**, K is released from platelets during clot formation; and with **leukocytosis**
  - Increased intake, especially with **transfusions**
  - **Shifts from ICF → ECF** (as above, and during exercise, with hemolysis or rhabdomyolysis, and with certain drugs, e.g., beta-blockers, digoxin, succinylcholine)
  - **Decreased excretion**: renal failure, hypoaldosteronism, hyporeninemia (with lupus nephritis, renal transplant), tubular-interstitial disease, certain medications with underlying renal insufficiency (K-sparing diuretics, acetylcholinesterase inhibitors, nonsteroidal anti-inflammatories, heparin)
- Clinical findings: most significant problems are with **cardiac conduction** and **may begin abruptly** prior to other symptoms (ascending muscle weakness to paralysis, paresthesias)
  - **ECG findings in order**:
    - Peaked T waves
    - Lengthened P-R interval
    - Flattened P waves
    - Widened QRS complex
    - Ventricular fibrillation or asystole

- Diagnosis usually evident from underlying disorder; obtain CBC, platelets, other electrolytes, BUN, creatinine, blood gas, urine K (for high or low K excretion) and possibly aldosterone

---

Emergency Treatment of Hyperkalemia

1. Stop all sources of potassium

2. Continuous ECG monitoring

3. Reverse membrane effects with 10% **calcium gluconate**, 0.5. mL/kg (effects in 30–60 minutes)

4. Start removal of K (because effects will take time):

   a. Aerosolized **albuterol** (rapid intracellular movement of K; about 15–30 minutes) 0.5% solution: 0.01–0.05 mL/kg in saline

   b. Oral or rectal **sodium polystyrene sulfonate resin** with sorbitol (Kayexalate; excretion may take hours for effect) 1 g/kg

   c. 7.5% **sodium bicarbonate**, 2–3 mL/kg (30 minutes to several hours; movement of K into cell)

   d. 50% **glucose + regular insulin** infusion (1 unit per 5 g glucose; movement of K into cells)

Hypokalemia

- Most important causes:
  - **Factitious**: if plasma with very high WBC counts (leukemia) is left at room temperature, the WBCs take up K
  - **Shifts to the ICF** (see previous discussions)
  - Decreased intake—in **anorexia nervosa**
  - Non-renal losses: diarrhea, **laxatives**, excessive sweat
  - Renal losses:
    - ○ With metabolic acidosis: renal tubular acidosis, diabetic ketoacidosis
    - ○ Tubular-interstitial disease, diuretic phase of obstructive nephropathy
    - ○ Hypomagnesemia
    - ○ Penicillin sodium salts and derivatives
    - ○ With metabolic alkalosis (see previous discussions)

- **ECG findings** (especially with digitalis):
  - Flattened T waves
  - Depressed S-T wave
  - U-wave (between T and P waves)
  - Ventricular fibrillation or torsades de pointes

- Other signs and symptoms: **weakness, muscle cramps, paralysis**, decreased gastrointestinal motility, decreased bladder function, causes primary polydipsia and causes polyuria (impaired urinary concentrating ability)
- Diagnostic considerations: dietary intake, **IV fluids with K, gastrointestinal losses**, medications, presence of hypertension; same lab studies as with hyperkalemia
- Treatment: treat severe symptoms aggressively; particular **care with IV potassium** (0.5–1 mEq/kg over 1 hour); oral KCl (or K-acetate or citrate with acidosis); restoration of intravascular volume, stop K losses (e.g., use K-sparing diuretic).

Fluid Management in Dehydration and Shock

The process of fluid assessment and management is illustrated in the following diagram.

Rapid assessment of hydration status with history and physical;
draw and send blood and urine for pertinent studies

IMMEDIATE TREATMENT OF SHOCK FROM SEVERE DEHYDRATION

Calculation of maintenance and deficit water and electrolytes;
specific replacement dependent on type of dehydration present
(iso or hyponatremic or hypernatremic); careful monitoring of vital
signs, exam and lab values; make changes as needed

Monitoring and replacement of ongoing losses; continue monitoring
of vital signs, exam, and lab values; make changes as needed

Figure 3.1: Process of Evaluation and Treatment of Dehydration

Quantifying dehydration

The most exact method to determine the amount of dehydration present is performed if the **pre-illness weight** (i.e., the weight just before the onset of illness) is known; then:

Accurate Assessment of Percent Dehydration

% dehydration = (Pre-illness weight – Current weight)/Pre-illness weight × 100

This information is not commonly available, so the percentage of dehydration is typically estimated:

MILD DEHYDRATION

<u>INFANT (<5%)</u>

- Normal exam and vital signs (mild tachycardia) ± slight decrease in urine output

<u>OLDER CHILD (>1 year or >20 kg) TO ADULT (<3%)</u>

- Same findings

MODERATE DEHYDRATION

<u>INFANT (5–10%)</u>

- Lethargic
- Sunken eyes, fontanelle
- Decreased tears and dry mucous membranes
- Decreased skin turgor (pinch skin over abdomen → delayed elastic recoil)
- Cool, pale extremities with delayed capillary refill (≥2 sec.)
- Tachycardia
- Decreased or no urine output

<u>OLDER CHILD TO ADULT (3–6%)</u>

- Same findings (except for fontanelle)

SEVERE DEHYDRATION

<u>INFANT (>10%)</u>

- Obtunded, limp
- Very sunken eyes, fontanelle
- No tears and parched mucous membranes
- Cold and mottled extremities with capillary refill >3 seconds
- Tachycardia with weak pulses and hypotension (late finding)
- No urine output

<u>OLDER CHILD TO ADULT (>6%)</u>

- Same findings (except for fontanelle)

Figure 3.2: Assessing the Degree of Dehydration

Fluid Deficits

If the pre-illness weight is known, then:

Fluid deficit (L) = Pre-illness weight – Current weight

Example: if the pre-illness weight is 8 kg and the current weight is 7.8 kg, the fluid deficit is 8,000 – 7,800 = 200 g = 0.2 L deficit (200 mL)

If the findings in [Figure 3.2] are used, then every **1% dehydration = 10 mL/kg fluid deficit**.

Example: 5% dehydration = 50 mL/kg fluid deficit

Along with the water deficit, Na is lost (primarily from the ECF) and K is lost (primarily from the ICF).

Maintenance fluid

Easiest method of calculating maintenance fluid is the Holliday-Segar system, where **1 kcal of energy requires 1 cc of fluid for homeostasis**; fluid losses are primarily through the skin, airways, and urine; stool losses are negligible; all electrolyte losses are urinary; requirements are the same for all patients regardless of age because needs are based on basal metabolic rate and the ratio of electrolytes to water is fixed.

Daily Maintenance Calculations (Holliday-Segar System)

Weight	Total Maintenance Fluid/24 Hours
0–10 kg	100 mL/kg
10–20 kg	1,000 mL + 50 mL/kg for every kg >10
>20 kg	1,500 + 20 mL/kg for every kg >20

- Maintenance fluid must be adjusted **for increased water needs**: fever, burns, tachypnea, presence of a tracheotomy tube, gastrointestinal losses, third-space losses, increased urine output (insensible losses at 25–40% of maintenance + urine replacement volume for volume with solution based on urine electrolyte composition) and surgical drains, infants on radiant warmers or under phototherapy lights; maintenance fluids must be **decreased for**: decreased or absent urine output (insensible losses + urine output volume for volume with 0.45 normal saline, NS), ventilation with humidified oxygen, and an infant in an incubator
- Children typically can receive:
  - **<10 kg**: D5 0.2 NS + 20 mEq/L KCl (high water needs per kg and decreased renal concentrating ability)
  - **>10 kg**: D5 0.45 NS + 20 mEq/L
- These quantities, however, may need to be modified depending on the disease state, renal function, and therefore the alteration of normal homeostasis.

Table 3.4: Composition of Standard Electrolyte Solutions

Solution	Na	K	Cl	HCO$_3$	Ca	mOsm/L
D5W						252
D10W						505
NS (0.9%)	154		154			308
½ NS (0.45%)	77		77			154
D5 NS	154		154			560
D5 ½ NS	77		77			406
D5 ¼ NS (0.2%)	34		34			321
D5 RL	130	4	109	28	2.7	525
RL	130	4	109	28	2.7	273
3% NaCl	513		513			1027

Abbreviations: normal saline, NS; Ringer's lactate, RL

- Ongoing losses are replaced as they occur, and figures are available for electrolyte losses in diarrhea and for nasogastric losses; based on average diarrhea stool electrolyte, stool losses are replaced mL-for-mL with D5 0.2 NS + 20 mEq NaHCO$_3$/L + 20 mEq KCl/L every 1–6 hours; similarly, nasogastric losses are replaced with NS + 10 mEq/L KCl in the same manner.

Isonatremic (isotonic) and hyponatremic (hypotonic) dehydration

- **Isonatremic: [Na] 130–150 mEq/L**
- **Hyponatremic: [Na] <130 mEq/L**; may appear to be sicker as the hyponatremia produces significant fluid shifts from the ECF → ICF; may present with neurological signs

(1) Resuscitation phase (immediate treatment of shock from severe dehydration): **20 mL/ kg NS or RL over 20 minutes**

(2) **Reassess:** patient may need more boluses until intravascular volume is adequate, perfusion has improved, heart rate has decreased, and blood pressure has normalized.

(3) Give **additional 20 mL/kg isotonic saline over 2 hours** to assure restoration of intravascular volume.

(4) Calculate **maintenance and deficit** and add together.

(5) From this, **subtract the total of isotonic fluids** already given in restoration of the intravascular volume.

(6) Give the remaining fluid (maintenance) **over 24 hours**.

- *Do not* raise the [Na] **>12 mEq/L/24 hr (central pontine myelinosis)**
- With **hyponatremic seizures, must increase [Na] to at least 125 mEq/L and therefore use 3% NaCl**; for every 1 mL/kg of 3% NaCl, the [Na] increases by 1 mEq/L
- **No potassium until there is urine output**; adjust K in fluids based on initial [K] and renal function

(7) Replace **ongoing losses**.

Hypernatremic dehydration

- **Hypernatremic: [Na] >150 mEq/L**

(8) As above, **first restore the intravascular volume** with NS (*not* RL; too hypotonic) and monitor response.

- *Do not* decrease the [Na] by >12 mEq/L/24 hour (risk of cerebral edema; usually seen as seizures). Use 3% NaCl to rapidly increase [Na].
- The **rate of correction is dependent on the [Na]**, based on the amount of free water (water without Na): 24–48 hours for [Na] 145–196 mEq/L

- **Start with D5 ½ NS + 20 mEq/L** (after urine output) at 1.25–1.5 maintenance, and adjust as needed for follow-up [Na] (increase or decrease rate or IV fluid [Na]).

Oral Rehydration Therapy

- Used primarily for **mild to moderate dehydration** and not initially for shock or severe dehydration (IV intravascular volume repletion), intractable vomiting; not for gastric distention, ileus, coma; around the world → significant decrease in morbidity and mortality related to diarrhea illnesses and to malnutrition associated with diarrhea.
- Solutions based on **glucose/Na** transport coupling in the intestine. Number of available solutions, including the World Health Organization (WHO) oral rehydrating solution (ORS), Infalyte, Pedialyte, Rehydralyte, and others. Most solutions now have a **lower osmolality** (lower glucose and NaCl) compared to the original WHO RHS, and this appears to **reduce stool output and vomiting and decrease the need for IV fluids without any appreciable hyponatremia** (because of the lower [Na] compared to the original).
- ORS needs to be given **slowly**, e.g., 50–100 mL/kg over 4 hours for mild to moderate dehydration; and especially in the presence of **vomiting** (may start with only 5 mL and use a teaspoon or syringe; small volume may be needed to be given very frequently). Volume is increased slowly as tolerated, and additional volume must be given for **ongoing losses**.
- After hydration, **maintenance** volumes may be given along with any continued stool losses.
- **Early re-feeding** decreases the duration of diarrhea; after initial rehydration, breast-feeding or formula feeding should continue.

PART TWO: NUTRITIONAL MANAGEMENT
Nutritional needs of the preterm and low-birth-weight (LBW) infant
Breast Milk and Breastfeeding

✓ Breast milk is ideal in terms of quality of protein (whey > casein) but not in terms of quantity; in order to obtain the recommended 3.5 g/kg/day of protein, fortifier must be added to the breast milk or a preterm formula should be used.

✓ LBW infants **can absorb almost all of the lactose** from breast milk; preterm formulas, however, generally contain mixtures of lactose and glucose polymers (decreased osmolality).

✓ Preterm infant formulas are modified to be similar to breast milk in terms of fat content, but because the lipid system present in breast milk cannot be duplicated and because **long chain fatty acids are less readily absorbed** in preterm infants, there are added **medium chain triglycerides (MCT)**—easily hydrolyzed and **do not require bile acids for absorption**. They are **transported directly to the portal vein (and bypass the lymphatic system)**.

✓ Breast milk contains the **very long chain fatty acids linoleic and linolenic**, from which is made **arachidonic and docosahexaenoic acid (DHA)**; these are important components of phospholipids in the **brain and the RBCs** and are important for normal **growth and development**. Preterm formulas should contain 4.5–6 g/100 kcal of fats (40–54% of calories) and have **added linoleic and linolenic acid**; some have added arachidonic acid and DHA.

✓ Breast milk contains **too little Ca and P** to meet the needs in terms of intrauterine accretion rates, although they are more bioavailable in breast milk than preterm formulas; therefore, there is **added Ca and P in preterm formulas**; without this, bone resorption will be stimulated, which can result in **decreased bone density and rickets**; in addition, the ratio of Ca to P must be regulated carefully and **P intake must not be too great**, as this will cause hypocalcemia.

✓ **Breast-milk fortifiers** come in powder or liquid form, and certain quantities are added per specific volumes of breast milk to provide the necessary added nutrients.

✓ Recommendation from the American Academy of Pediatrics and WHO is that infants receive breast milk solely through the **first 6 months** and then continue to receive it along with other foods **through the first year**.

✓ Protective effects of breast milk:

- Passive immune protection from IgA and other antibodies
- Antimicrobial protection from lysozyme
- Decreased iron-dependent organisms because of lactoferrin
- Macrophages and lymphocytes
- *Lactobacillus bifidus* **promotes beneficial bacterial growth** and inhibits pathogens (also from ingested antibodies)

✓ Benefits from breast milk: lower incidence of **diarrhea, otitis media, respiratory infections**, and significant bacterial infections

✓ Drugs contraindicated while breastfeeding:

- Illicit drugs, nicotine, alcohol
- Radionuclides
- Lithium

- Methotrexate
- Bromocriptine
- Cyclosporine
- Cyclophosphamide
- Ergotamine
- Also possibly: antianxiety medications, antipsychotics, antidepressants (any with sedative properties may cause sedation in the infant), metronidazole, metoclopramide, chloramphenicol

✓ Breastfeeding contraindicated if following disease present in mother:

- PKU
- Galactosemia
- Untreated, active tuberculosis
- Hepatitis C
- HIV, **as long as there is safe formula available**

✓ Major differences between breast milk and cow's milk: both use **lactose** as the carbohydrate; both have the same energy density **(20 cal/oz)**; **human milk is whey-predominant; cow's milk is casein-predominant and contains more total protein** (increased **renal solute load**, and different amino-acid composition leading to potential toxicities with respect to early brain development; slightly less fat in cow's milk than in human). Both are **low in vitamin K** and every baby must receive parenteral vitamin K after birth to prevent hemorrhagic disease of the newborn; both are **low in Fe**, but **breast milk Fe is more bioavailable**; both **low in vitamin D**.

✓ **Vitamin D supplementation** is now recommended (AAP 2008 Updated Guidelines) at birth using 400 IU/day for breast-fed and partially breast-fed infant until infant is on 1 L (or quart)/day of vitamin D-fortified formula or whole milk.

✓ **Iron fortification** is recommended at **4–6 months of life**, preferably with the start of an iron-fortified cereal (age 4 months) and then addition of other solids at age 6 months.

✓ **No additional water** is needed.

✓ **No fluoride supplementation <6 months of age**; from age 6 months to 3 years, supplement only if the water source has less than 0.3 ppm; from 3–6 years, supplementation is for ≤0.6 ppm; and for 6–16 years, it is also for ≤0.6 ppm; therefore no fluoride supplementation is needed for water fluoride >0.6 ppm.

Formula Feeding

Important issues regarding infant formulas

✓ Term infants with normal gastrointestinal tracts should be fed an **iron-fortified cow's milk formula containing lactose** (examples: Similac, Enfamil, Carnation Good Start).

✓ Infants with diagnosed primary or secondary lactose intolerance should be fed a **lactose-free formula** (examples: ProSobee, Isomil, Enfamil LactoFree, Similac Lactose Free).

✓ With a concern of **milk protein allergy**, try a **soy formula** first (examples: Isomil, ProSobee); however, some patients with milk protein allergy are also **allergic to soy**.

✓ **Protein hydrolysate formulas** are recommended for infants who are **unable to digest and absorb protein, lactose, and/or fat**; for documented sensitivity to intact protein: use Nutramigen (hydrolyzed casein; also lactose- and sucrose-free); for those with fat and/or protein malabsorption: use Pregestimil (hydrolyzed casein; no lactose or sucrose; and fat from MCT, soy, corn, safflower oil; high in oleic acid) or Alimentum (hydrolyzed casein; no lactose or corn; fat from MCT, safflower, and soy).

✓ **Elemental formulas** (e.g., Neocate) are made from **predigested amino acids, or hydrolyzed protein, carbohydrate, and fat** (MCT or essential fatty acids); very little digestion needed with minimal stimulation of bile and pancreatic secretion; should be considered in **short-gut syndrome, severe malabsorption syndromes, and severe inflammatory bowel disease, and with fistulas**.

✓ **Follow-up formulas** are second stage for infants over age 6 months and who are receiving at least 12 Tbsp solid food per day; these formulas are also available in soy (examples: Carnation Follow-Up, Next Step Toddler).

✓ For **impaired fat malabsorption, a lymphatic disorder, or chylous effusion**, use a formula where almost all of the fat is from MCT (see previous discussion; example: Portagen).

✓ For **decreased renal function**, a formula with intact protein (decreased amount; whey protein concentrate and sodium caseinate) with low Fe, lower in Ca, and K (Similac PM 60/40).

✓ Formulas may be modified to increase calories by **concentrating the formula** (up to 24–26 cal/oz) or by **adding modular components** of proteins (e.g., ProMod; 3 g protein/Tbsp, 17 kcal), carbohydrates (Polycose; 23 kcal/Tbsp), or fats (MCT oil; 7.7 kcal/mL). Some reasons for increasing caloric density are heart disease, failure to thrive, chronic diarrhea, bronchopulmonary dysplasia.

✓ Infants who are fed **goat's milk** exclusively must be supplemented with **folic acid** (megaloblastic anemia).

Progression of Solid Food

✓ No solids <4 months of age; start with **single-ingredient food and add a new one every 3–4 days** to check for any possible reactions; at 4 months, the infant develops a true suck and increasing sequences of suck-swallow-breathe; foods are added with **increasing texture and sizes of pieces** based on development of appropriate tongue movements and tooth development for grinding, biting, and moving food to the back of the mouth. Too-early introduction of swallowing may lead to **choking and aspiration, later feeding difficulties, and later development of allergies**.

✓ **4 months**: begin Fe-fortified box cereals (rice, oatmeal); or can wait until 6 months; avoid wheat products through first year

✓ **6–8 months**: Add strained or mashed vegetables (dark-yellow or orange and dark-green; avoid corn through first year); mashed or strained fruits

✓ **8–10 months**: add hard breads (e.g., crackers or toast); increase cooked or mashed, fresh or frozen vegetables; increase fruit; if fruit juice, no more than 8 oz. per day (no citrus for the first year; too much fruit juice replaces calories with too much sugar and may lead to chronic nonspecific diarrhea of infancy); add lean meat (poultry; avoid fish for first year), egg yolk (no white for first year), cheese, yogurt, cooked dried beans

✓ **10–12 months**: add other starches (noodles, pasta, soft breads), fresh fruit (peeled and seeded), cooked vegetables (larger pieces), small pieces of meat or poultry; peanut butter after 12 months

✓ **By end of first year**, should be having three meals/day plus two or three snacks/day; self-feeding should be encouraged as soon as the infant is able.

Feeding after the first year

✓ Because the **growth rate decreases** at the end of the first year, **appetite** typically does so as well; this is important to realize to avoid feeding problems.

✓ **Self-selection and self-feeding** of food is important after the first year as long as the total daily nutritional needs are met.

✓ By **2 years of age**, the child should be on the same diet as the rest of the family.

✓ The **American Heart Association Step 1 Diet** is recommended (and the National Cholesterol Education Program; see later discussion); use the Food Guide Pyramid—offers wide selections; energy needs vary based on age and activity level.

✓ **Family and cultural determinants** can influence dietary intake, and this can affect growth.

✓ All children taking less than 1 L/day of vitamin D-fortified milk should receive 400 IU/day vitamin D (including adolescents).

Adolescent nutrition and sports participation

✓ Due to growth and activity level, adolescents need **more calories** (2,200–2,800 cal/day) and nutrients (**additional calcium and iron**); caloric needs and **protein requirement** increases with height (45–60 g/day).

✓ Lifestyle changes that have developed may lead to **many nutritional problems** from skipping meals, increased snacks, and/or eating fast foods high in saturated fat.

✓ Inadequate calcium (need 122 mg daily) intake → risk of **later osteoporosis**; highest incidence of **iron-deficiency anemia** (need 12–15 mg Fe per day); fast foods and increased low-quality snacks (should be low in fat and added sugar) → **obesity and obesity-related chronic disease.**

✓ Also at risk for **eating disorders** (fear of gaining weight, appearance-conscious, peer pressure)

✓ For adolescents participating in sports, the most important issue is to maintain a **balanced diet** with respect to all recommended daily allowances for age and the division of calories per the **Food Pyramid Guide**.

- Athletes need increased energy (mostly from **carbohydrates**); carbohydrate-based snacks should be eaten just before exercise or an athletic event and 2–3 hours prior as well.
- Protein **does not** need to be increased for sports activities; in fact, **increased protein intake can be dangerous**.
- Fat **does not** need to be increased (may be combined with carbohydrate snack).
- **Increased fluid** is needed prior to practice or an event and to replace ongoing losses (water); with increased sweat, there may be substantial **electrolyte losses**, and electrolyte-supplemented drinks may be used.
- There is no research that shows benefit from **supplements** (outside the jurisdiction of the FDA), and caution must be exercised with these.
- Female athletes (particularly ballet dancers, gymnasts, ice-skaters, and cheerleaders) have a higher incidence of amenorrhea, **decreased bone density, and anemia**; **female athlete triad:** overexercise, amenorrhea, eating disorders.

Vegetarian diets

✓ Definitions:

- **Semi-vegetarians** eat no beef or pork, but do eat: poultry and fish; dairy foods; all grains, nuts, seeds, vegetables, and fruits.
- **Lacto-ovo-vegetarians** eat no meat, but do eat all dairy and everything else listed above.
- **Lactovegetarians** eat no meat and no eggs, but do eat other dairy and everything else.
- **Ovo-vegetarians** eat no meat and no dairy except for eggs, and do eat everything else.
- **Vegans** eat no meat, dairy, or eggs, but do eat everything else.

✓ A balanced vegetarian diet can be appropriate for a child from infancy through adolescence.

- **Protein:** will not be deficient if a wide variety of non-meat foods are eaten to provide adequate calories

- **Calcium**: wide variety of non-dairy goods contain calcium (dried beans; green, leafy vegetables; juices)
- **Iron**: will not become deficient if Fe-rich and vitamin C-rich foods are eaten (dried beans; green, leafy vegetables; Fe-fortified cereals)
- All vegetarians need to receive a regular source of **vitamin B12** from fortified foods (some cereals, soy milk, and nutritional yeast) or from a supplement.

✓ A **vegan diet** is not appropriate for children **<2 years of age** (older children may be vegan with careful thought and planning).

Minerals and Deficiencies

Table 3.5: Essential Minerals and Deficiencies

Mineral	Function	Dietary Deficiency
Calcium	**Bone matrix**, muscle contraction, nerve conduction, blood-clotting	Decreased dietary Ca may lead to **rickets** in a child; especially if diet is **high in phosphorus** → further decreases dietary absorption of Ca; also seen in malabsorption diseases and in **rapidly growing premature infants with a low Ca or P intake**
Phosphorus	Intracellular anion used for many enzymatic reactions; needed for generation of **ATP**	P is present in **most foods**, so it is difficult to develop a dietary deficiency; may be seen in **malabsorption diseases**; if seen with rickets, the problem is usually a decreased Ca and/or vitamin D; presents with weakness, lethargy, anorexia, and decreased growth
Magnesium	**Extracellular-bone reservoir**; most intracellular in liver and muscle; cofactor for many enzymatic reactions; used for membrane stabilization, nerve conduction, **ATP** and GTP biochemistry	Decreased primarily from **gastrointestinal or renal disease**; causes **secondary hypocalcemia** by impairing release of parathyroid hormone and interfering with peripheral action; symptoms secondary to hypocalcemia; may also lead to hypokalemia
Zinc	Enzyme cofactor; aids in regulation of gene transcription	**Growth deficiency**, decreased immunity, poor wound-healing, **diarrhea**, **skin lesions** (all may be seen with genetic inability to absorb zinc = **acrodermatitis enteropathica**)
Copper	Enzyme cofactor	**Microcytic anemia** and neutropenia; **neurological dysfunction, osteoporosis, skin and hair depigmentation** (see Menkes disease, Chapter 2)
Chromium	Assists **insulin** action	**Glucose intolerance**, peripheral neuropathy, encephalopathy

Abbreviations: adenosine triphosphate, ATP; guanosine triphosphate, GTP

Vitamins, Deficiencies, and Hypervitaminosis

Table 3.6: Vitamin Deficiencies and Hypervitaminosis: Fat-Soluble Vitamins

Vitamin	Function	Deficiency	Hypervitaminosis
A	Must take in **carotenoids** from plants → converted to vitamin A in body; most important product is **retinoic acid**; regulates genes involved with cellular function → affects many processes: **vision**, immune function, bone development, maintenance of epithelial function	Most with **lipid malabsorption or severe protein malnutrition**; loss of epithelial function → airway obstruction, infections (urinary, GI, respiratory); decreased immune function, poor growth; **dry scaly skin patches; eye lesions (corneal: xerophthalmia), night blindness; increased intracranial pressure**	Skin lesions, alopecia, bony abnormalities, hepatosplenomegaly; dry mucous membranes, desquamation of palms and soles; **pseudotumor cerebri**: diplopia, headache, papilledema; vomiting, anorexia. Increased carotenoids = **carotinemia** → transient yellow skin
D	Produced in skin and dietary intake; needs to be hydroxylated in liver and kidney; needed for GI **absorption of Ca** and to a lesser extent P; direct effect on **bone resorption**	**Rickets**: unmineralized epiphyseal matrix prior to epiphyseal fusion; most are skeletal manifestations: **craniotabes, rachitic rosary** (costochondral junctions), **widening of epiphyses** (especially seen at wrists and ankles), soft ribs, difficulty walking, other **skeletal deformities, non-traumatic fractures; symptoms of hypocalcemia. Radiographic findings**: thick epiphyses, metaphyseal fraying (loss of a sharp border) with cupping (edge becomes concave), widening of distal metaphysis, decreased bone density	Always due to increased intake (never due to overexposure to sun); increased bone absorption with **hypercalcemia**: poor feeding, vomiting, abdominal pain, constipation, pancreatitis; **hypertension, shortened Q-T on ECG, arrhythmias**; many CNS findings from lethargy to coma; polyuria with dehydration and hypernatremia; **nephrocalcinosis** and renal failure
E	**Antioxidant** (main form is alpha-tocopherol); mostly in cell membranes and **prevents lipid oxidation and formation of free radicals**	**Hemolytic anemia**, wide variety of **neurological symptoms (especially cerebellar and posterior column)**, retinal problems; in **premature infants**: thrombocytosis, edema and hemolytic anemia (prevented with preterm formulas containing decreased polyunsaturated fatty acids, later introduction of Fe, and supplementation with vitamin E)	—

(continued on next page)

Table 3.6: Vitamin Deficiencies and Hypervitaminosis: Fat-Soluble Vitamins *(cont.)*

Vitamin	Function	Deficiency	Hypervitaminosis
K	Dietary sources and made by intestinal bacteria; needed for function of clotting **factors II, VII, IX, X**; limited stores	**Early bleeding** (maternal medications crossing the placenta and interfering with function), **classic hemorrhagic disease of the newborn** (see Chapter 1) and **late bleeding** (age 2 weeks–6 months): breast-fed infants, often with unrecognized malabsorption disease	—

Abbreviations: central nervous system, CNS; gastrointestinal, GI

Table 3.7: Water-Soluble Vitamins

Vitamin	Function	Deficiency
B6 (thiamine)	Coenzyme for thiamine pyrophosphate; NAD production, release of energy, acetylcholine production	Beriberi (mostly with severe GI or liver disease)
B2 (riboflavin)	Part of coenzyme system—FAD; electron transport; growth and tissue respiration	Rare by itself; if present, with other B-complex deficiencies
Niacin	Cofactors NAD and NADP; glycolysis and electron transfer	Pellagra (mostly where corn is the main staple; poor source of tryptophan)
B6 (pyridoxine)	Coenzyme for amino-acid metabolism and synthesis of neurotransmitters, histamine, heme	B6-dependent syndromes (e.g., homocystinuria)
Biotin	Coenzyme for enzymes of carboxylation reactions	Widely distributed so deficiency very unlikely unless on long-term TPN low in biotin
Folate	Coenzyme for DNA and protein synthesis	Risk increased **with rapid growth or increased cell metabolism; malabsorption syndromes, hemolytic anemias,** inborn errors of folate metabolism, certain medications (methotrexate); major finding is **megaloblastic anemia**
B12 (cobalamin)	Cofactor for enzymes in lipid and carbohydrate metabolism; also needed for folate metabolism, protein synthesis, and purine and pyrimidine synthesis	Almost exclusively from animal products; risk especially with strict vegan diets; may be seen in breast-fed baby of vegan mother or if mother has a malabsorption syndrome or pernicious anemia that has not been treated; also seen with bacterial intestinal overgrowth, decreased ileal absorption (Crohn, resected terminal ileum), and juvenile pernicious anemia; major problem is megaloblastic anemia and growth failure; treat with B12 injections until hemodynamically improved, then intranasal B12

(continued on next page)

Vitamin	Function	Deficiency
C	Dependent on **dietary sources**; formation of collagen, neurotransmitters, steroids, carnitine; **antioxidant** (electron donor) → functions to **maintain metalloenzymes reduced**; many hematopoietic functions (Fe absorption, transferrin → ferritin, tetrahydrofolate synthesis)	**Scurvy**: gum changes, skin and hair changes, anemia, swollen joints, edema, generalized tenderness, decreased wound-healing, muscle weakness, brittle bones, irritability and psychological changes

Abbreviations: flavin adenine dinucleotide, FAD; gastrointestinal, GI; nicotinamide adenine dinucleotide, NAD; NAD phosphate, NADP; total parenteral nutrition, TPN

Enteral Support and Total Parenteral Nutrition (TPN)

Total Parenteral Nutrition (TPN)

✓ **Indication**: with medical conditions where enteral feedings are contraindicated (e.g., surgical disorders requiring long periods before full restoration of enteral feedings, acute non-surgical gastrointestinal disease where there will be a time of no enteral feedings). **Decreased to absent enteral nutrition expected for at least 5 days**: peripheral TPN; if >7 days: central-line TPN.

✓ **Basic composition**: dextrose (5–30%) with electrolytes (Na, Cl, K, Ca, P, Mg), crystalline amino acids (1–3.5 g/kg/day), lipids (essential fatty acids and concentrated source of calories; start at 1 g/kg/day up to 3 g/kg/day and not more than 50% total calories), multivitamins (vitamin K, increased vitamin D and decreased B complex compared to adult), trace elements (Zn, Cu, Mn, Cr; others may be needed depending on the disease process)

✓ **Complications**: catheter-related, medication incompatibility, hypo- or hyperglycemia; electrolyte abnormalities, inadequate fluid, overhydration, displacement of bilirubin from albumin (fat emulsion), lipemia and hypertriglyceridemia, calcium-phosphorus complexes → phlebitis, thromboembolism; vitamin deficiencies, mineral deficiency

✓ **Monitoring**: plot weight, height, head circumference daily; daily fluid balance and vital signs (multiple checks); daily catheter function and insertion site checks (multiple checks); daily blood glucose, frequent urine glucose checks; weekly electrolytes as above + CO_2, BUN, Cr), weekly triglycerides, liver enzymes, pre-albumin, albumin, total protein, and bilirubin; periodic (as needed) Fe, Cu, Zn, and selenium

Enteral Support (Tube Feeding)

✓ The **basic indication** for tube feeding is the inability to take nutrition orally (prematurity, anatomical abnormalities, severe neurological impairment), inability to take full caloric needs by mouth (trauma, sepsis, burns, psychological disorders, anorexia), or alterations that require a modified diet (short bowel, pancreatitis, inborn errors, chronic diarrhea).

✓ Tube feedings may be given **intermittently (bolus) into the stomach or continuously into the small bowel**. Bolus feedings are used primarily to supplement oral intake, with swallowing disorders, and for anorexia (contraindicated with severe reflux or poor gastric motility). Continuous small-bowel feedings are used with delayed gastric emptying or anything that poses a risk of aspiration (contraindicated with intestinal nonfunction). Feeding pumps are used to deliver a slow, steady rate of feeding.

✓ There are many **advantages of enteral vs. parenteral feedings**: enteral is more closely related to normal nutrition, can help healing from mucosal damage, preserves/restores enzymes for digestion, **decreases** risk of metabolic abnormalities and infection, and is less expensive.

✓ There are also a number of **complications** (depending on gastric or intestinal): risk of aspiration, discomfort, tube-clogging, improper tube size/placement, perforation, residual volume prior to the next feed, obstruction, poor psychomotor development with long-term feedings.

✓ Use the best formula for age, diagnosis, and caloric/nutrient needs. **Types of formulas**: for **intact gut** (e.g., PediaSure, Boost, Ensure; intact nutrients; homogenized food); **lactose-free** (similar brands and composition without lactose; also used for diarrhea); formulas with **increased protein** (Ensure High Protein, Osmolyte HN); formulas where **volume needs to be restricted** (Boost Plus, Ensure Plus); added calories with increased protein and/or MCT oil so smaller volumes can be used; **specific formulas for various organ system dysfunction** and for **impaired digestion** (free amino acids, lactose-free, low fat with MCT oil, hydrolyzed protein; Pediatric Vivonex, Peptamen).

Obesity

Predictors of overweight/obesity

Increased birth weight (maternal obesity, infant of diabetic mother [IODM]), genetic weight regulation, overweight children more likely to be overweight adults (older the child is, the greater the risk); **strongest predictor is parental obesity**

Environmental contributors

High amount of convenience foods that are **high in calories, fats, simple sugars, and sodium**; increased snacks high in fat and simple sugars; increased sweetened beverages; increased sedentary lifestyle with lack of exercise; children and adults with schedules too busy for appropriate nutrition

Differential diagnosis

Some syndromes (e.g., Prader-Willi), conditions leading to inactivity (e.g., wheelchair-bound), hyperinsulinism, endocrine (Cushing, hypothyroidism)—*but* these account for an extremely small percentage of childhood obesity. **Normal linear growth precludes an endocrine cause** (children with moderate exogenous obesity tend to be tall for their age).

History and physical findings will help to determine an endogenous cause (short stature, hypogonadism, dysmorphic features, specific endocrine signs and symptoms).

Evaluation

The most reliable method of determining adiposity is the **body mass index** (BMI) + clinical assessment:

$$\textbf{BMI} = \textbf{wt (in kg)/Ht (in cm)}^2$$

BMI should routinely be plotted on BMI percentile curves. Children have changing adiposity; it increases over the first year, then reaches a low point at 5–6 years, then increases again (adiposity rebound); can identify children at risk.

BMI ≥85% but <95% defines overweight

BMI ≥95% defines obesity

Comorbidities

Metabolic syndrome: insulin resistance (with acanthosis nigricans), type 2 diabetes, central adiposity, hypercholesterolemia, and hypertension; also orthopedic and musculoskeletal abnormalities (slipped capital femoral epiphyses), sleep apnea, polycystic ovary syndrome, psychosocial problems

Management

No endocrine studies unless height velocity is low. **If there is evidence of genetic syndrome**, refer to geneticist.

Evaluate children who are overweight for **comorbidities** (follow blood pressure, blood fasting glucose, insulin level, lipid panel, liver enzymes).

First step: **intensive lifestyle changes** (dietary, physical exercise, behavioral modification)

Pharmacotherapy

Consider *only* with severe comorbidities in patients in whom intensive lifestyle modifications have been ineffective; only clinicians with expertise in antiobesity agents should prescribe (Sibutramine, Orlistat).

Bariatric surgery

Adolescents with BMI of [40–50] and comorbidities in whom lifestyle changes and pharmacotherapy have been unsuccessful; must have mastered healthy diet principles; cannot have an unresolved eating disorder or untreated psychiatric disorder; surgery must be performed by experienced surgeon and managed by a multidisciplinary team

Malnutrition

- **Height-for-age** (cumulative effects of undernutrition), **weight-for-age** (recent and longer-term undernutrition), and **weight-for-height** (recent undernutrition) less than 80–90% of expected are consistent with causes of undernutrition (but not specific for any particular cause).
- **Protein-energy malnutrition** (severe childhood undernutrition): may be primary (insufficient food) or secondary (increased needs, decreased absorption, increased losses)
- Severe childhood undernutrition (SCU):
  - **Marasmus:** non-edematous SCU with severe wasting: low plasma albumin; weight loss, irritability, lethargy, emaciation; loss of subcutaneous fat, abdominal distension, constipation, muscle atrophy and decreased tone; eventually hypothermia and brady-cardia
  - **Kwashiorkor:** edematous SCU: low plasma albumin; features similar to marasmus but early onset of edema, liver enlargement, dermatitis, depigmentation, loss of hair; eventually coma and death; unsure as to why some children develop edematous mal-nutrition vs. non-edematous
  - Marasmic-kwashiorkor: features of both

- Protein-losing enteropathy: excessive bowel protein loss → hypoalbuminemia; presents as edema; may be present with certain disorders causing bowel mucosal inflammation and in lymphangiectasia; screening test = stool for alpha-1-antitrypsin.

WELL-CHILD CARE: INFANCY THROUGH MIDDLE CHILDHOOD

NORMAL GROWTH: GROWTH ISSUES TO KNOW

- Average U.S. birth weight is **3.4 kg (7.5 lb)**; average length at birth is **50 cm**.
- Average head circumference at birth is **35–36 cm**, and circumference should increase as follows: about 2 cm/month over the first 3 months, then 1 cm/month until age 6 months, then 0.5 cm/month through age 1 year, then 0.25 cm/month through age 3 years, then 1 cm/year from age 4–6 years. Brain growth then slows, and head circumference increases another 2–3 cm during mid-childhood.
  - **Microcephaly:** head circumference <3 standard deviations (SD) below the mean for age and sex.
    - Etiologies: most are **familial and autosomal dominant** and chromosomal/genetic syndromes; also perinatal infection, drugs, oxygen deprivation, malnutrition, and inborn errors
    - Problem after age 2 years is less likely to cause severe microcephaly.
    - Need to make **serial head circumference** determinations and plot on graph; measure **head circumference of each parent**.
    - Note differences between **hydrocephaly (impaired cerebrospinal fluid [CSF] circulation/absorption with signs and symptoms) and macrocephaly (megalencephaly)** due to other reasons, including **familial** (no symptoms; family head circumferences are large and there are no neurological symptoms).
- Infants **lose up to 10% of birth weight over the first week of life** and **should regain it by the end of 2 weeks.**
  - Birth weight should then **increase by 20–30 g/day** over the first 3 months; and **double by age 6 months** and **triple by age 1 year.**
  - Birth length doubles by 3–4 years.
- Most track along a single percentile (except in first 2 years: birth size reflects the intrauterine environment; **size at age 2 years reflects the average of the parents' heights**); at age 6–18 months, may be a **shift up or down (genetic-driven), but should be on 2 large percentile bands.**

- During mid-childhood, there are irregular growth spurts (three to six per year; each about 8 weeks long).
- Head and trunk are large at birth with a subsequent increase in limb size; the **lower segment** is the distance from the pubic symphysis to the floor (heel), and the **upper segment** is the height minus the lower segment; the upper segment/lower segment ratio is about 1.7 at birth and goes to **1 by age 7 years**.
- Most preterm infants have **weight catch-up in the first 2 years** and **height catch-up by age 2.5 years**.

DEVELOPMENTAL SCREENING AND SURVEILLANCE

The American Academy of Pediatrics (AAP) states that **developmental surveillance** should be done at each visit to identify children with **possible developmental problems and delays**.

Standardized tool should be administered for **developmental screening at 9, 18, and 30 months**; it identifies children at risk but does not yield a specific diagnosis for the problem.

Developmental surveillance: done at each visit; in addition to information from the medical history (to identify risk factors), look for family functioning, observe child behavior and developmental skills, interview parents regarding concerns, and document and maintain a developmental history.

- Domains: gross motor, fine motor and adaptive, speech, language (expressive and receptive), social-emotional, cognition (language and visual-motor/problem solving)
- Used for determining referrals, providing education with respect to normal development, and monitoring effects of developmental therapy through **early intervention**
- Once a disability has been detected, refer for more comprehensive assessment and intervention.
- **Individuals with Disabilities Education Act (IDEA):** national system to identify children at risk for developmental problems or those who have been identified with delays; free-of-charge, IDEA-funded programs
- For continued special education enrollment, the school system is required to diagnose the disability by the time the patient is 8 years of age.

Examples of Recommended Developmental Screening Tests

✓ Parents' Evaluation of Developmental Status (PEDS): filled out by parents at home prior to visit, or done by interview; birth–9 years.

✓ Ages and Stages Questionnaire (ASQ): parents indicate skills on form; done at home or in interview; 4 months–5 years.

✓ Pediatric Symptom Checklist: behavioral and emotional screen; scoring system; 4–16 years

✓ Modified Checklist for Autism: second stage for problems identified on PEDS or ASQ; 18 months

✓ Bayley Infant Neurodevelopmental Screen: direct elicited items—neurological, developmental skills; cut-off scores; 3–24 months

✓ Comprehensive Inventory of Basic Skills: school performance screen; one to three subsets; computer or hand-scoring into percentiles

WELL-CHILD CARE VISITS: DEVELOPMENTAL MILESTONES, IMMUNIZATIONS, AND ANTICIPATORY GUIDANCE

Prenatal Visit

Recommended for high-risk parents, for first-time parents, and for any other parent who requests it; discuss medical history, family history, and social issues; give anticipatory guidance for neonate and discuss benefits of breastfeeding

Newborn Visit

- Full evaluation **within 24 hours** of birth; look at prenatal factors, peripartum and postpartum factors, maternal-infant attachment, parental interactions, and psychosocial issues; **support breastfeeding**
- Full **physical exam, developmental and behavioral assessment**; if hospitalized >48 hours, need a discharge exam; **assess for jaundice; document meconium passage**
- **Measurements**—Length, weight, head circumference, weight for length; plot on growth curves to determine appropriateness of growth for gestational age (i.e., appropriate for, small for, or large for gestational age [AGA, SGA, and LGA, respectively]).
- **Studies**—Newborn screen and hemoglobin/hematocrit (Hgb/Hct) as per state law; all screened for congenital sensorineural hearing loss.

Maturational Differences between Term and Preterm Infants

✓ Differences are related to decreasing gestational age and degree of illness plus degree of environmental stimuli in neonatal units → developmental influences occur out of sequence.

- Increased risk of disabilities; most may have delays without subsequent significant disabilities; more hearing and visual deficits

✓ Preterm infants with more extensor tone that may be decreased to various degrees

✓ Delays are dependent on whether or not one corrects for prematurity (i.e., uses postconceptional age for development); most correct for motor development through infancy (but pattern of improvement is more important).

✓ Many preterm infants with delays will have catch-up by age 2–3 years; most of the very and extremely premature infants will have catch-up by 4.5–5 years of age.

- **Anticipatory guidance**—Jaundice, breastfeeding and normal feeding, infant capabilities, sleep pattern; explain newborn screening tests, routine baby care, transition, siblings, family support and resources; safety (car seats, cigarettes, smoke alarms); return visit: if discharged <48 hours after birth, return to office within 48 hours (feeding, jaundice, meconium); otherwise return 48–72 hours after discharge
- **Development**—Flexion in prone, mostly flexed in supine, symmetric arm and leg movements (i.e., no side preference); can see 8–12 inches in front, should fix on bright object, especially face (prefers) with brief gaze back to mother; turns to voice or bell (but should habituate quickly); positive Moro, step, place and grasp reflexes
- **Immunizations**—Hepatitis B vaccine #1 before discharge

Post-Discharge Visit (48–72 hours)

- **How things have been since discharge**—Breastfeeding, passage of stool, and jaundice; answer any questions and address concerns; observe drying of umbilical cord and healing of circumcision.
- **Anticipatory guidance**—Parent roles, stress, health and depression, newborn transition, nutrition, review safety, newborn care (temperature-taking, skin care, handwashing)

Two-Week to One-Month Visit

- Interval history and full physical and developmental surveillance; behavioral and psychosocial assessment
- **Measurements**—As previously, and plot on growth curves
- **Studies**—Repeat newborn screen at 2 weeks

- **Development**—Over the first month: increase extension of legs in prone and chin up briefly; arms and legs flexed with head up briefly in ventral suspension; tonic neck (asymmetric) posture in supine; head lag with pull-to-sit; follows objects, watches person; starts to smile
- **Immunizations**—Hepatitis B vaccine #2 at 1 month (or can give at 2 months; use monovalent vaccine; or, if at 2 months, can use a combination product)
- **Anticipatory guidance**—Maternal health, child-care issues, breastfeeding plans (if return to work or school), sleep position, car safety, developmental changes, feeding routines

Two-Month Visit

- Interval history, full physical exam, developmental surveillance, behavioral and psycho-social assessment
- **Measurements**—As previously, and plot on growth curves
- **Development**—Head up in prone; head sustained with body plane during ventral suspension; continued tonic neck posture in supine; continued head lag (but less) in pull-to-sit; tracks an object or face 180 degrees; listens to voice; social smile; coos and vocalizes in response to another person. **No visual fixation by 2 months is abnormal!**
- **Immunizations**—Rotavirus #1 (first dose *only* between ages 6 weeks and 14 weeks, 6 days); DTaP #1 (minimum age 6 weeks; also for others); inactivated poliovirus #1 (IPV); *Haemophilus influenza* type b #1 (Hib; may use the combined vaccine with hepatitis B (HepB), and therefore give the second HepB here); pneumococcal conjugated vaccine #1 (PCV)
- **Anticipatory guidance**—Maternal well-being, infant behavior (sleep, developmental changes, calming, communication), parent-infant separation, nutritional adequacy, safety (drowning, water temperature)

Four-Month Visit

- Interval history, full physical exam, developmental surveillance, behavioral and psycho-social assessment
- **Measurements**—As previously, and plot on growth curves
- **Development**—Head and chest up in prone with weight on forearms; rolls front prone to supine; mostly symmetric posture now in prone with hands to midline; no head lag in pull-to-sit, and head steady in supported sit; in supported standing, will push with feet; reaches and grasps object with whole hand and brings to mouth; visually fixes on small object; laughs and squeals; initiates social contact; **continued head lag in pull-to-sit and unsteady head in sitting position is abnormal by 4 months!**
- **Immunizations**—Rotavirus #2; DTaP #2, Hib #2, IPV #2, and PCV #2
- **Anticipatory guidance**—Tummy time (time spent in prone position), infant self-regulation, social development, nutritional adequacy, teething/drooling, no bottle in bed, clean pacifier, safety (burns, choking, lead poisoning)

Six-Month Visit

- Interval history, full physical exam, developmental surveillance, behavioral and psychosocial assessment; oral health assessment; fluoride if needed
- **Measurements**—As previously, and plot on growth curves
- **Development**—Rolls both ways (7 months); sits with tripod support (hands in front between legs); bounces with supported stand; reaches and grasps large objects and transfers between hands; rakes in a small object; babbles (polysyllabic vowel sounds, then imitates consonants); turns directly to sound and voice; **failure to turn to sound of voice by 6 months is abnormal!**
- **Immunizations**—Rotavirus #3 (final dose no later than 8 months, 0 days); DTaP #3, Hib #3 (6-month dose not needed if combined dose with HepB was given; may be given anytime through 18 months); PCV #3; IPV #3 (between 6 and 18 months); yearly influenza vaccine (no earlier than 6 months; inactivated only <age 2 years) during flu season
- **Anticipatory guidance**—Infant development and parent expectations, feeding strategies and guidance, oral health (fluoride, no bottles in bed, soft toothbrush), review safety issues

Nine-Month Visit

- Interval history, full physical exam, developmental screening (note difference from surveillance; see previous discussion), behavioral and psychosocial assessment; oral health assessment
- **Measurements**—As previously, and plot on growth curves
- **Development**—Sits without support with back straight; pulls-to-stand and cruises (10–12 months); creeps/crawls; immature pincer grasp and pokes with forefinger; holds object in each hand and bangs together; feeds with fingers; object permanence (9–10 months); plays pat-a-cake and waves bye-bye; nonspecific Mama and Dada (i.e., repetitive consonant sounds); understands own name; recognizes common objects; **lack of consonant babbling by 9 months is abnormal!**
- **Immunizations**—None, unless this visit used for IPV #3 or influenza vaccine (if in season)
- **Anticipatory guidance**—Discipline, culture beliefs, changing sleep pattern, mobility, cognitive development, temperament, cup-drinking, self-feeding, safety (safety locks, window locks, guns, poisoning)

One-Year Visit

- Interval history, full physical exam, developmental surveillance, behavioral and psychosocial assessment; oral health assessment
- **Measurements**—As previously, and plot on growth curves
- **Studies**—Hgb or Hct, lead screen in high-risk, tuberculin test in high-risk (re-evaluate need every 6 months to age 2, then yearly)

- **Development**—Pulls-to-stand and cruises (10–12 months); walks holding one hand, with or without a few independent steps; plays simple ball game; full pincer grasp and release; Mama, Dada specifically, plus one other word; beginning of stranger anxiety
- **Immunizations**—Fourth dose of DTaP may be given at this time as long as 6 months have lapsed since the third dose; Hib #4 (12–15 months); PCV #4 (12–15 months); IPV #3, if not yet given; measles-mumps-rubella (MMR) and varicella (minimal age for each is 12 months; can be given at 12–15 months; both at same visit or separated by at least 28 days); may administer the first dose of hepatitis A (HepA) vaccine no earlier than 12 months; two doses 6 months apart, between 12–23 months of age); influenza vaccine, if in season
- **Anticipatory guidance**—Teeth-brushing, nap times, bedtime, nutritious foods, home safety

Fifteen-Month Visit

- Interval history, full physical exam, developmental surveillance, behavioral and psychosocial assessment
- **Measurements**—As previously, and plot on growth curves
- **Development**—Walks alone, stoops, crawls up stairs, plays ball; puts a small object into a bottle, builds a tower of two to three blocks; copies a line with crayon, drinks from cup; three to six specific words, uses jargon, follows simple commands, points to indicate; hugs
- **Immunizations**—If the fourth DTaP was not given at the 12-month visit, it may be given between 15–18 months; as above for the immunizations that were not given at 12 months: HepB, Hib, PCV, IPV, MMR, varicella
- **Anticipatory guidance**—Separation, communication of wants and needs, night waking, consistency and praise, fire safety

Eighteen-Month Visit

- Interval history, full physical exam, developmental screening (as done at the 9-month visit), autism screening (early identification of children with autism), behavioral and psychosocial assessment; oral health assessment
- **Measurements**—As previously, and plot on growth curves; after this visit, no further weight-for-length measurements need to be performed unless there is a concern for undernutrition.
- **Development**—Runs, walks up steps with one hand held, builds tower of three to four blocks; imitates scribble and a vertical stroke; seven to ten words, including words for need/want; imitates house task; knows one or more body parts, feeds self with spoon; kisses; may indicate when diaper wet; **inability to walk by age 18 months is abnormal!**
- **Immunizations**—Any immunizations from above lists that have a range of possible administration times and have not yet been given; yearly influenza in season
- **Anticipatory guidance**—Return to clinging, language use; encouragement of reading, singing, talking; toilet training readiness signs, falls

Two-Year Visit

- Interval history, full physical exam, developmental surveillance, behavioral and psychosocial assessment and autism screening; oral health assessment
- **Measurements**—As previously, and plot on growth curves; no further head circumference measurement necessary after this unless there is an abnormal pattern of head growth; begin yearly measurement of body mass index (BMI).
- **Studies**—Lead screening for high-risk (continue to re-evaluate based on risk factors); dyslipidemia screen for high-risk
- **Development**—Runs well, walks up and down steps one foot at a time; climbs on furniture, jumps with both feet off the floor; throws large ball overhand, kicks ball; builds tower of seven blocks; mimics horizontal stroke, scribbles in circles; 50-plus words, and puts three words together; points to named objects; uses "I, me, mine"; feeds self with fork and spoon; helps undress self; **failure to use single words by age 2 years is abnormal and needs further evalution!**
- **Immunization**—For children with high-risk underlying conditions, administer the pneumococcal polysaccharide vaccine (PPSV; unconjugated; Pneumovax®) beginning at age 2 years; meningococcal conjugated vaccine (MCV) for high-risk conditions only, beginning at age 2; give the HepA vaccine if it was not given per the recommended schedule after age 2.
- **Anticipatory guidance**—Communication skills, temperament and behavior, toilet training, television watching, safe play, bike helmets

Thirty-Month Visit

- The main purpose of this visit is to perform the third early developmental screen; this is done as described previously, with a full history, behavioral/psychosocial assessment, and physical exam.
- **Anticipatory guidance**—Interactive communication, limited reciprocal play with others, imitation of others. Readiness for early childhood programs, water safety, outdoor health and safety, pets.

Three-Year visit

- Interval history, full physical exam, developmental surveillance, behavioral and psychosocial assessment; refer for dental evaluation
- **Measurements**—As previously, and plot on growth curves
- **Studies**—Vision screen; begin yearly blood pressure check
- **Development**—Pedals a tricycle; stands briefly on one foot; broad jump; builds a tower of 10 blocks; imitates a cross and circle; has 75% intelligible speech; uses sentences of five to eight words; follows simple directions; knows age and gender; engages in parallel play (2–3 years; independent play side-by-side); helps dressing (unbuttons, puts on shoes); washes hands; repeats three numbers and counts three objects; **failure to speak in three-word sentences by age 3 is abnormal!**
- **Immunizations**—PPSV, MCV, HepA as needed (see above)
- **Anticipatory guidance**—Sibling rivalry, encouraging literacy activities, playing with peers, pedestrian safety

Four-Year Visit

- Interval history, full physical exam, developmental surveillance, behavioral and psychosocial assessment
- **Measurements**—As previously, and plot on growth curves
- **Studies**—Vision screen, hearing screen; blood-pressure check; dyslipidemia screen for high-risk
- **Developmental**—Stands on one foot for 3 seconds; hops on one foot; uses scissors to cut out pictures; copies cross and square; draws simple person (head plus two to four body parts); speech fully intelligible; counts four objects; tells a story, pretend play; asks "wh" questions; (e.g. where, when) plays with several children; uses toilet alone
- **Immunizations**—Preschool immunizations: final DTaP, final IPV, second MMR and varicella (these may be administered between 4 and 6 years of age); yearly influenza if in season; PPSV, MCV, HepA as needed
- **Anticipatory guidance**—School readiness, healthy daily routines, limits on-screen time, activities outside the home, belt positioning booster seats

Five-Year Visit

- Interval history, full physical exam, developmental surveillance, behavioral and psychosocial assessment
- **Measurements**—As previously, and plot on growth curves
- **Studies**—Hearing and vision screening; check blood pressure
- **Development**—Climbs steps alternating feet; copies triangle; draws a person with six body parts; dresses and undresses; ties shoes; knows four colors; counts 10 objects; asks about meaning of words; domestic role-play; plays board games and cards
- **Immunizations**—Preschool immunizations, as above; yearly influenza in season
- **Anticipatory guidance**—School readiness issues, temper problems, social interactions, routines, healthy eating, exercise, adequate calcium intake, dental visits, swimming safety, sexual abuse prevention, carbon monoxide detectors

Six-Year Visit

- Interval history, full physical exam, developmental surveillance, behavioral and psychosocial assessment
- **Measurements**—As previously, and plot on growth curves
- **Studies**—Vision and hearing screening (then every other year); blood-pressure check; dyslipidemia screen for high-risk
- **Development**—Rides bicycle without training wheels, writes name, knows left vs. right across the midline; names of colors, letters, and numbers; increased strength,

coordination, and stamina for complex movements. By 5 years, most have ability to learn in a school setting. A kindergarten-ready child:
- Must be able to separate from parents for hours
- Plays well
- Takes turns
- Follows directions
- Relates personal experiences
- Tells stories

- **Immunizations**—Preschool immunizations, as above
- **Anticipatory guidance**—After-school care and activities, friends, fears, pedestrian safety, helmets, swimming safety, fire-escape plan

Yearly Visits Through End of Adolescence

- Interval history
- Measure height, weight, BMI, and blood pressure
- Vision and hearing screening every other year, and as needed; dental referral as needed
- Developmental surveillance and behavioral/psychosocial assessment; alcohol and drug use assessment as needed beginning at age 11; sexually transmitted infection screening for any sexually active adolescents (and cervical dysplasia screening for sexually active girls)
- Complete physical exam
- Special studies as needed: Hgb/Hct, tuberculosis (TB) test, lead screen, dyslipidemia screen
- **Immunizations:** 11–12-year visit: Tdap, HPV (three doses for girls and boys), and routine MCV at this time; high-risk immunizations as indicated previously, plus any catch-up immunizations yearly; influenza through age 18, in season
- **Anticipatory guidance:** school, development and mental health issues, nutrition and physical activity, oral health, safety

WHAT TO KNOW ABOUT IMMUNIZATIONS
General Principles

- Vaccines produced by different companies are **interchangeable,** except where specifically stated. Most vaccines can be safely given **simultaneously** when indicated. *Exception:* Two or more live parenteral vaccines may be administered simultaneously, but if the decision is made to give them separately, they must be **separated by at least 28 days.**
- A lapse of immunizations requires catch-up only from the point where the schedule was interrupted. It does **not require beginning the whole series again.**

- Any patient with an **uncertain immunization status or without an official immunization record** (from the United States or another country) should be considered susceptible to those diseases for which the immunization is uncertain or undocumented and the **series must be given from the beginning**. Immunizations given outside of the United States must match the immunizations required.
- No reduced or split dose should be given **for low birth-weight or premature infants**. The schedule is followed as it is for term infants (except for HepB—see below).
- **Recent immunoglobulin administration** (immune serum globulin, specific hyperimmune globulins, certain blood products, IV immunoglobulin [IVIG]) has been shown to inhibit the response of live vaccines (but not the response of inactivated vaccines or toxoids). There is, therefore, a recommended **interval** to wait (3–11 months, depending on product and specific use; tables available) between immunoglobulin administration and live vaccines (MMR and varicella).
- All U.S. licensed vaccines are **safe and effective**. Minor adverse reactions are common (fever, swelling, erythema, tenderness).
  - There is **no credible evidence that there is a causal link between the MMR vaccine and autism** (and this has now been refuted).
  - Thimerosal (Hg-containing preservative) has now been removed from all vaccines in the childhood and adolescent immunization schedule; however, the evidence **does not support a causal relationship between thimerosal and neurodevelopmental disorders**.

Precautions and Contraindications

- A **minor illness, regardless of fever,** is not a contraindication to vaccine administration.
- For **moderate to serious illness, regardless of fever,** the child should be immunized when recovered.
- The current DTaP vaccine has a significantly **decreased rate of adverse events compared to the older DTP** (see discussion under DTaP). Previous reactions that involved only minor, local adverse effects or temperatures <105°F (40.5°C) are not contraindications.
- The MMR is derived from chick embryo fibroblast tissue culture and contains **no significant egg protein**; therefore, documented **egg allergy is not a contraindication** for administration. **Influenza and yellow fever vaccine do contain egg proteins** and, in general, egg-allergic children with previous systemic reactions should not receive these vaccines (may skin-test first). Antibiotic reactions (certain vaccines contain trace amounts) are seen, e.g., with IPV (**polymyxin B, streptomycin, neomycin**); reactions have also been documented to other vaccine components, including the infectious agent itself.

- **Vaccine viruses in the MMR and varicella are not transmitted by vaccine recipients** (rare with varicella and asymptomatic or mild reaction), and therefore the **vaccines may be given safely to a child of a mother who is pregnant (or with any other pregnant household person)**.
- The only absolute contraindication is **previous anaphylactic reaction** to a vaccine.

Immunocompromised Children

In general, no live vaccines except for specific circumstances:

- **For primary B-cell deficiencies:** no live vaccines, except consider measles and varicella (but effectiveness is doubtful)
- **For T-cell deficiencies** (severe combined immunodeficiency disease [SCID]): no live vaccines (MMR, OPV, varicella, rotavirus, smallpox, bacilli Calmette-Guérin [BCG], and *Salmonella typhi* Ty21a)
- **Complement deficiency:** no contraindications
- **Defective phagocytic function:** no live bacterial vaccines (BCG and Ty21a)
- **HIV/AIDS:** no OPV, smallpox, BCG; **may administer MMR and varicella if child has no AIDS-related illness and CD4 count is at least 15%** (absolute counts vary per age, based on percentages of total)
- **Malignancy, transplantation, immunosuppressive or radiation therapy:** no live or bacterial vaccines, depending on immune status
- Household contacts of a person with an immunodeficiency should not receive **OPV (no longer available in the United States)** because the virus may be transmitted; **however, administration of the MMR and varicella to household contacts is not contraindicated** (see above). Household contacts at least 6 months of age should receive inactivated influenza during the season.

Postexposure Prophylaxis to Susceptible Contacts

Susceptible contact = unimmunized, has not had the disease

- **Measles:** live virus vaccine within 72 hours of exposure to immunocompetent contacts (problem is determining the time of exposure); for immunocompromised, pregnant, or infants <1 year: give IM immune globulin within 6 days of exposure
- **Varicella:** for immunocompetent contacts, give the vaccine within 3 days of appearance of the rash in the index case. For immunocompromised, give varicella zoster immune globulin (VZIG) as soon as possible after exposure. See further discussion below.
- Immunization with the vaccine and **HepB immune globulin (HBIG)** is very effective for postexposure prophylaxis; in this case, the HBIG does not inhibit the response of the vaccine (see further discussion below).
- **Mumps and rubella:** postexposure prophylaxis does not necessarily work; however, the live-virus vaccine is indicated for exposed adults born in the United States during or after 1957 who have not been previously immunized.

- HepA: give the vaccine within 2 weeks of exposure; follow with second dose 6 months later.
- Tetanus: see specific vaccine below

International Travel

Vaccination may be required or recommended, depending on destination (HepA, yellow fever, meningococcal disease, typhoid, rabies, Japanese encephalitis). Information may be obtained and vaccines administered through local health departments; all children should be up-to-date on routine immunizations according to their age.

Specific Vaccines

HepB (recombinant DNA-produced HBsAg)

- If **mother is HBsAg-positive** at time of giving birth, the baby should receive the **first dose of the vaccine and a dose of HBIG simultaneously at two different sites within the first 12 hours of life**. Test the infant for HBsAg and the antibody after the three vaccine doses (age 9–18 months).
- Medically stable, preterm infants with **birth weights <2,000 g** show good antibody responses to the vaccine starting at 30 days of age; therefore, the series may be **started at 1 month of age**. But all preterm and low birth-weight (LBW) infants born to mothers who are **HBsAg-positive are treated as described above for term infants**, except that the birth dose is not counted **and three more vaccine doses** are given, starting at 1 month of age (so a total of four doses are given).
- **Catch-up:** administer the three-dose series for anyone who is behind; the adult two-dose series may be used for children >11 years of age; refer to catch-up immunization schedule for minimum dosing interval between each dose.

DTaP (toxoids—single antigen that is a highly defined constituent—and inactivated bacterial components

- Rarely, **more serious events** that once were associated with the DTP (whole-cell pertussis; encephalopathy) **occur less frequently**.
- **Catch-up:** if the fourth dose is given after age 4 (because of delay for whatever reason), the fifth dose is not needed; otherwise, catch-up all children who are behind, per the recommendations, with the minimal dosing interval between each dose.
- If there is a contraindication to pertussis vaccine, then further doses are contraindicated (encephalopathy within 7 days, immediate anaphylaxis, unstable/active central nervous system [CNS] disease; *but* is *not* contraindicated with stable CNS disease, family history of seizures, a sibling who died of sudden infant death syndrome [SIDS]; a subsequent decreased volume of the vaccine is inappropriate). If the pertussis is contraindicated, use **DT** (full doses each of diphtheria and tetanus). Also, other than indicated below, if there is any catch-up after the **7th birthday, no further full-dose pertussis is given**.

- Once the primary series is completed, administer **Tdap** (tetanus and diphtheria toxoids and acellular pertussis vaccine) at the **11–12-year visit**; persons age 13–18 who have not received the Tdap should receive a dose. If the child received a previous Td (adult formulation tetanus and diphtheria toxoids), then wait 5 years to give the Tdap. This recommendation began in 2008 as a result of **increasing pertussis infections** (it is now known that with immunization or disease, pertussis immunity wanes).
- **Postexposure wound prophylaxis:** tetanus-prone wounds are those contaminated with dirt, rust, saliva, feces, soil, and puncture wounds; avulsion wounds; crush, burn, frostbite, and missile wounds. All others are designated clean, minor wounds.
  - If there have only been **one or two previous absorbed tetanus toxoid immunizations**, then for a **clean, minor wound**, only **Td is** administered; in the same category, if the **wound is at-risk**, then **both Td and a dose of tetanus immune globulin (TIG; no permanent immunity)** are administered.
  - If there is a history of **at least three previous absorbed tetanus toxoid immunizations** and the wound is **clean** and minor, then no tetanus immunization is needed (and no TIG) **unless it has been more than 10 years** since the last dose; for **at-risk wounds**, no Td is needed unless it has been **more than 5 years** since the last vaccine; no TIG is needed.
  - Administering **too many doses or increased volume** is related to **increased risk** of severity of adverse events, including arthus reaction, Guillain-Barré, and brachial neuritis.

Rotavirus (oral, live, pentavalent)

- The first of three doses (2 months apart) can be administered between 6 weeks and 14 weeks, 6 days; and the final dose by 8 months, 0 days.
- An older rotavirus vaccine was withdrawn due to a high incidence of **intussusception**.
- Live virus contraindications

Inactivated poliovirus vaccine (IPV)

- Poliovirus occurs only in humans and is spread by the fecal-oral and respiratory routes; the last reported case in the United States attributed to indigenously acquired wild-type virus was in 1979. All other cases have been **vaccine-associated paralytic poliomyelitis (VAPP)** from the **previous oral polio vaccine**. The IPV (since 2000) has ended the occurrence of VAPP.
- **IPV is the only polio vaccine now in the United States** (but the oral polio virus [OPV] is the only one recommended for global eradication). There are no serious adverse events reported.
- A fourth dose is not needed if the third dose was given on or after age 4 years (unless a combination of OPV + IPV was used).
- **Catch-up** all children through age 18 who are behind in any doses. For adults, catch-up is recommended only for certain people who are at high risk of exposure to wild-type polio.

Haemophilus influenza type b conjugate vaccine (Hib, inactivated; type b only)

- Hib capsular polysaccharide covalently linked to a carrier protein
- There are few adverse reactions.
- **Catch-up:** for initiation of series at 7–11 months, only three doses are used; and for initiation at 12–14 months, only two doses are given. However, if initiated at 15–59 months a **single dose** is given; **no further dosing is given after the 5th birthday** (except for unimmunized children with an underlying disease predisposing to infection with Hib).
- Because there has been widespread use of the conjugate vaccine for about 30 years, the **incidence of Hib infection in the United States has decreased by 99%.**

Pneumococcal conjugated vaccine, (13-valent, PCV13 as of March, 2010)

- **PCV13:** purified polysaccharides of 13 serotypes conjugated to a diphtheria protein; benefits include protection against pneumococcal pneumonia and meningitis **but less so with respect to otitis media**
- Also available is the **23-valent pneumococcal polysaccharide vaccine (PPSV):** 23 capsular polysaccharides; because it is not conjugated (and is a polysaccharide vaccine), it does **not induce protective antibody responses in children <2 years of age** (also, no reliable booster response or long-term immunity), whereas the PCV13 does. In addition to routine immunization with PCV13, children at **high risk for pneumococcal disease** (functional or anatomic asplenia, cochlear implants, chronic lung disease, HIV, congenital immune deficiencies, chronic cardiac disease, cerebrospinal fluid [CSF] leaks, chronic renal insufficiency, immunosuppressive therapy, diabetes mellitus) **should also be vaccinated after age 2 with the PPSV.**
- **Catch-up** (AAP 2007 revised guidelines):
  - All healthy children between 24–59 months of age who have not completed the PCV13 schedule should receive one dose.
  - All at-risk children between 24–59 months of age who have received three doses should receive one more.
  - All at-risk children between 24–59 months of age who have received fewer than three doses should receive two additional doses, given at least 8 weeks apart.

Measles-mumps-rubella (MMR; live attenuated vaccine)

- The second dose may be administered prior to age 4–6 years as long as at least 28 days have elapsed from the first MMR (no earlier than 12 months of age).
- All children should be **caught up with two doses** if behind (consider susceptible unless both doses have been administered).
- Any infant **immunized at <12 months of age should be considered unimmunized,** and the two-dose schedule still should be administered.
- During a **measles outbreak, monovalent measles** (also available as measles-rubella; the MMR is the preferred vaccine) vaccine may be given to infants **as young as 6 months;** re-immunization with MMR is needed as described above. For others, immune serum globulin within days of exposure may prevent or modify the disease.

Varicella (live, attenuated vaccine)

- The second dose may be given prior to age 4–6 years as long as at least 3 months have elapsed since the first dose.
- MMR and varicella may be given as a single MMRV vaccine; AAP states no preference but MMRV appears to be associated with increased incidence of febrile seizure compared to each individually.
- All children **need to have both doses for appropriate immunity**, and therefore catch-up should occur when a deficiency is found (minimal dosing interval: 3 months for those <13 years, and 28 days for those 13 years and older).
- In a small number of immunized people, a **varicella-like rash occurs** (several lesions); also is associated with the **development of zoster** in both immunocompetent and compromised persons from as little as 3 weeks up to 2 years after administration of the vaccine.
- Also for **prophylaxis:**
  - **Administer VZIG** to a newborn whose mother was diagnosed with chickenpox from **5 days prior to delivery to 48 hours after delivery** (inadequate transplacental IgG and newborn IgM); onset of the rash prior to 5 days before delivery or more than 48 hours after delivery does not require prophylaxis (no added benefit).
  - With any significant exposure: any hospitalized premature infant born at least at 28 weeks' gestation where there is no reliable history of chickenpox in the mother or serological evidence of protection against varicella
  - With any significant exposure: hospitalized premature infants under 28 weeks' gestation or ≤1,000 g birth weight regardless of maternal history or serology

Meningococcal conjugated vaccine (MCV; inactivated, conjugated polysaccharide vaccine)

- **Tetravalent vaccine: covers serogroups A, C, Y, and W-135; does not cover B** (one-third of all cases and the most common in infants)
- The vaccine should be given routinely at the **11–12-year visit** and a second dose at age 16 years.
- If not previously vaccinated, administer at **age 13–18** (as early as it is noticed that the patient is not vaccinated); also give to any **college freshmen living in dormitories** who have not been previously vaccinated.
- Recommended for children **2–10 years** with terminal complement component deficiency or anatomic or functional asplenia, and for others at high risk for meningococcal disease
- Children who received the older polysaccharide vaccine (MPSV, meningococcal polysaccharide vaccine) at least 3–5 years earlier and who remain at increased risk for meningococcal disease should be revaccinated with the MCV.

Human papillomavirus vaccine (HPV)

- Inactivated **quadrivalent vaccine covering HPV types 6, 11, 16, and 18** (covering the majority of types causing genital warts and cervical cancer)
- Currently recommended for **females between 11–12 years of age** and now boys beginning at age 9 (prevention of genital warts) (March, 2010). Three doses are given (the second dose 2 months after the first; and the third, 6 months after the first).
- Give at 13–18 who have not been previously vaccinated.

Influenza vaccine: trivalent inactivated vaccine (TIV) or live attenuated influenza vaccine (LAIV)

- Contains antigens for **influenza A and B and H1N1 (strains change annually)**.
- Recommended: yearly administration for every child from **6 months through 18 years during the influenza season**
- For children who are **healthy** (without underlying conditions that predispose to influenza complications), are not pregnant, and do not live with anyone who has a primary or secondary immune deficiency, the **live attenuated intranasal** (both nares) **mist may be given, but only between the ages of 2 and 49 years**.
- Children **under 3 years** receive 0.25 mL of TIV; age ≥3 years receive 0.5 mL
- If a child is **less than 9 years and receiving the influenza vaccine for the first time, two doses are given, 4 weeks apart**; children should also receive two doses if they were vaccinated for the first time the previous season but received only one dose (in error). Thereafter (or for any child ≥9 years), they receive only a single dose per season.
- If there is a vaccine shortage during any season, all high-risk people (children; any person with chronic illness or immune deficiency, or who is elderly or pregnant) receive the vaccine first; if there is vaccine remaining, it may be administered to people without these high-risk conditions.
- Vaccinate household members and out-of-home care providers of all children who are at high risk.
- **Contraindications** to both vaccines include moderate to severe febrile illnesses, egg hypersensitivity, and/or a history of Guillain-Barré syndrome within 6 weeks of administration of a previous influenza vaccine.

WELL-CHILD CARE: ANTICIPATORY GUIDANCE, SAFETY, AND PREVENTION

Blood-Pressure Screening

- Blood pressure (BP) of a premature infant ranges from 55–75/35–45 mm Hg, depending on the gestational age; in the first 3 months of life, BP of a term infant is 65–85/45–55 mm Hg; thereafter, it rises steadily so that pressures of 100–120/60–75 mm Hg are reached between **6 and 12 years of age**, and 110–135/65–85 mm Hg after age 12 years.

- The appropriate cuff size should be one-third of the upper arm and should completely encircle it; if an elevated BP is found, measurement should be repeated twice more over a 6-week period; a persistently elevated BP (>95% for age) needs to be evaluated. The first step is to perform four extremity blood pressures.
- Start checking BP at **age 3 years**, or earlier if there is any reason to suspect the child may have elevated BP. BP may be taken seated or supine, but subsequent BPs should be taken in the same position.

Hemoglobin (Hgb) and Hematocrit (Hct)

- Check routinely at the **12-month visit**; note elevation (hemoconcentration) if a peripheral (heelstick) blood draw is performed.
- The average Hgb at 6 months–6 years of age is 12 g/dL (10.5–14 g/dL); average Hct is 37 (33–42); the MVC typically ranges between 70–74 FL.

Lead Screening

- Screen for lead at the **12- and 24-month visits** (and before and after, when needed) for any high-risk child: all Medicaid recipients, children who live in or regularly visit a house that was built before 1978 (when lead was taken out of paint) and has recent (within 6 months) or ongoing renovations; children who live near lead smelting plants; children who have a sibling or playmate with lead poisoning.
- Upper limit of normal is **5 µg/dL** (as of 2012); any abnormal value needs to be followed up with a good venous sample for blood lead level.

Vision Screening

- Infants are hyperopic, which increases until age 7 years and then decreases toward myopia until age 14 years; if this continues, the child develops myopic vision and needs corrective lenses.
- Visual acuity in a newborn is about 20/400; by age 2–3 years it is 20/40; at age 4, 20/30; and **by 5–6 years, 20/20.**
- Visual screening should begin at the 3-year visit.
  - Tests at 2.5–3 years involve **illiterate eye tests** using schematic pictures. Test each eye separately.
  - Preschoolers may be tested with the **E test** in which child points in direction of letters (most can do this at age 3–4 years).
  - The **Snellen chart** can be used at age 5–6 years if letters are known.
- Ocular alignment: test with the **unilateral cover test** at 10 feet; any eye movement of the uncovered eye is abnormal; for young infants, the **corneal light reflex** can be used.
- Conditions which may be found through periodic eye evaluations (simple ophthalmoscopy): cataracts, retinoblastoma, retinopathy

Screening for Lipid Disorders (U.S. Preventive Services Task Force, 2007)

- Abnormal lipid levels are strongly correlated with the **risk of coronary heart disease** in adults; children with lipid disorders are at risk for becoming adults with lipid disorders.
  - Negative influences on risk of coronary heart disease: poor diet, lack of exercise, smoking, alcohol, diabetes
  - Positive influences: vitamin D and calcium intake, weight-bearing exercises
- Simply screening via family history has been found to have high rates of false-negative results.
- Treatment in childhood has been shown to be effective in lowering lipid levels in select populations.
- Current AAP recommendations are: selective screening, beginning at the 2-year visit, of children and adolescents with a family history of premature coronary heart disease or at least one parent with a total cholesterol >240 mg/dL. Other children may be tested who are deemed to be at high risk regardless of family history (e.g., **obesity**).

Screen Time

- There have been increasing rates of children performing sedentary activities such as television-watching, computer and video play (4–6 hours per day).
- This is correlated with the **childhood obesity epidemic**.
- Recommendations are: limit screen time to **2 hours per day** (aside from what is necessary for schoolwork on computer), remove the television from the child's bedroom, and monitor children closely.

Sleep Hygiene

- **Set bedtime and routine**; no difference greater than 1 hour in bedtime or wakening time between school nights and non-school nights
- **Quiet time** prior to bed at night
- **Do not allow a child to go to bed hungry** (light snack); **no caffeine** for several hours prior to bedtime.
- Bedroom should be quiet and dark, with a temperature no greater than 75°F (23.8°C).
- **No television in bedroom**; no time-outs in bedroom
- The child should spend some time outdoors every day.
- **AAP Back to Sleep** recommendations for infants birth to 6 months (see also Chapter 7)

Safety Issues

Important safety issues by age

- **Newborn:** car seats, tap-water temperature, smoke detectors
- **Infants:** car seats, tap-water temperature, bath safety, stairs, and infant walkers
- **Toddlers/preschool:** car seats, pedestrian skills, water safety, childproof caps

- **Primary school:** pedestrian skills, water skills, seat belts, bicycle helmets, removal of firearms from home
- **Middle school:** seat belts, firearms, pedestrian skills
- **High school/adolescent:** seat belts, safe driving, alcohol/drug use, firearms, occupational injuries

Most common injuries

- **Infants/toddlers:** burns, drowning, falls, poisoning
- **School age:** pedestrian injuries, bicycle accidents, motor vehicle occupant injuries, drowning, burns, intentional trauma
- **Middle adolescence:** motor vehicle accidents (especially with alcohol/drug use by self or friends), work-related injuries

Car seats

- **Premature infants:**
  - AAP recommends pre-discharge monitoring (heart rate, pulse oximetry) of all infants born at <37 weeks; may need oxygen or alternative method for car-riding (car bed, reclined seats)

- **Infants 0–1 year (up to 20–22 lb)**
  - Infant seat or **rear-facing** convertible seat only
  - **Rear seat** only
  - Harness straps at or below the shoulder level

- **Toddlers (>1 year and 20–40 lb)**
  - Convertible or **forward-facing seat**
  - Rear seat only; back middle seat is safest
  - Harness straps at or above shoulder level

- **Young children (>40 lb and <4 ft 9 in tall; generally, 4–8 years old at 40–80 lb)**
  - Belt-positioning **booster seat**
  - **Forward-facing**
  - **Back seat until >13 years old**
  - **Both lap and shoulder belts**; lap: low and tight across lap/upper thigh; shoulder: fits well across chest and shoulders (young children have incomplete pelvic development and seat belt rides up into abdomen, which can result in severe injury—i.e., abdominal, fracture of lumbar spine); therefore, booster seat is required with proper placement of the lap belt.

Bicycles

- Most injuries secondary to head trauma
- **Helmets:** provide significant decrease in injuries to head and mid-to-upper face; needs a **firm, polystyrene liner** to allow good fit to the head; never buy a larger size, expecting a child to grow into it.
- Best riding areas are designated bicycle paths.

Poisoning

- Begin discussions at **6-month visit**.
- **Child-resistant packaging/caps** and decreased doses per container
- **Store out of reach**; use **childproof drawer and cabinet locks**.
- "Mr. Yuk" stickers are not effective; more effective is the **poison control emergency telephone numb**er on the stickers.
- **No more home use of ipecac**

Firearms

- Increased risk of **adolescent suicide and homicide**
- Greater chance of risk to household occupants than using the firearm on an intruder (handgun = greatest risk)
- **Lock and unload** all firearms; **store ammunition in a locked box in a different location**.
- Best option: remove all firearms from home

Drowning

- With swimming pools: best way to prevent drowning is to **fence in the pool completely; fence at least 5 ft high with locked door plus constant adult supervision**
- **No alcohol/drug** use in/around pools or bodies of water
- No alcohol/drug use while **boating**; everyone wears **personal flotation devices**
- In bathtubs: careful**, constant attention** to toddlers and young children, and to any child with a seizure disorder

Fires/burns

- Highest injuries in first decade; more male, and higher with decreasing socioeconomic status
- Federal Flammable Fabric Act (1967) mandated child **sleepwear to be flame-retardant** (but these types of burns represented a small fraction of total).
- **Scald burns** are more common in <5 years.
  - Decrease water temperature to **125ºF (51.6ºC)**.
  - Keep children away from the stove when boiling liquids/heating foods.
  - Do not use long cords that may trip children (and/or pull a hot substance over on them).

- No infant walkers in the kitchen
- Do not drink hot liquids while holding an infant.
- Install **smoke detectors**.
- Use fire-safe, **self-extinguishing cigarettes** (better yet, don't smoke).
- Avoid bright sunlight (10 A.M.–3 P.M.), wear protective clothing and hat, use sunscreen

Sunburns

- **Highest risk**: red hair, freckles, Celtic background (type I); fair hair and skin, blue-eyed, white (type II); dark skin, white (type III); least risk is black skin. All of these groups need a skin protective factor **(SPF) of at least 15**.
- Best sunscreens are chemicals (PABA, salicylates, dibenzoylmethanes): absorb damaging radiation; block UVA and UVB range; if vitamins C and E are added, there is a decrease in reactive oxygen species.

DEVELOPMENTAL, BEHAVIORAL, AND MENTAL HEALTH DISORDERS

5

PART ONE: DEVELOPMENTAL ABNORMALITIES

Disorders of Intellect

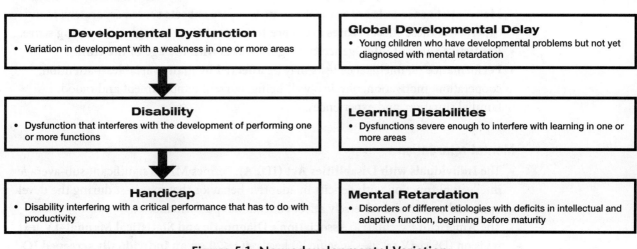

Figure 5.1: Neurodevelopmental Variation: Atypical Pattern of Neurodevelopmental Function

Intellectual ability

- Factors involved in **neurodevelopmental dysfunction**: physical health, family circumstances and events, individual temperament, culture, environment.
- **Language development** in infancy and early childhood is a **better predictor of cognitive function** than is motor development.
- **Age of presentation of a child with an intellectual disability varies with the severity.**
- **Majority of children with intellectual disabilities are in the middle range of impairment.**
- Mild intellectual disabilities and borderline intelligence may be **difficult to diagnose prior to school entry**; younger children **may show cognitive problems without deficits in adaptive behaviors.**
- **Mild mental retardation** diagnosed early in life may not be a lifelong condition— but **most have stabilized by adolescence**. Most mildly retarded people can live

independently or in a supervised setting, can develop social independence, and are literate.

Intelligence Quotient (IQ)

- The ratio of mental age to chronological remains essentially **constant with age**:

    IQ = Mental age (MA)/Chronological age (CA) × 100

- MA stops increasing at about age **16 years**.
- The average IQ of a population as a whole is **100**, by definition (50% fall between 90–110; 70% fall between 85–115; 95% fall between 70–130 and 99.5% fall between 60–140).
- IQs near the center (75–125) are represented by a bell curve; IQs <75 do not fit into this distribution, as there are people who increase the number with significant retardation due to brain damage; same is true for IQs >125, felt to be due to uneven rates of mental growth.
- Many intelligence tests are available; some measure **subsets** scored separately; many experts feel these **subset scores are more important than a single underlying score**.
- **Predictive value of intelligence testing increases with the age of the child.**
- **Performance** on intelligence tests may be **affected by many variables**—attention, cooperation, motivation, physical well-being, current temperament and mood, familial situation, and experiences.

Mental retardation

- The **Individuals with Disabilities Act (IDEA)**: defines MR as significant sub-average intellectual function with deficits in adaptive behavior that manifest during the developmental period and adversely affect educational performance.
- The **American Psychiatric Association's Diagnostic and Statistical Manual–IV** text revision (DSM-IV-tr) uses specific IQ levels: **IQ ≤70 on an individually screened IQ test** or by observational testing in an infant with **adaptive impairments in at least two areas** (e.g., home living, safety, self-care, use of community resources).
- The **American Association of Mental Retardation** uses **levels of support needed** (intermittent, limited, extensive or pervasive) in areas of adaptive function.
- Definitions of severity of MR based on IQ:

  - **Mild:** 50–55 to 70 — Educability 3rd-to-6th-grade at lower end, 6th-to-8th-grade at upper; can perform very simple tasks; needs supervision; may have basic job skills and live independently; may use public transportation.
  - **Moderate:** 35–40 to 50–55 — 1st-to-2nd-grade educability; can perform simple, non-critical household chores; some self-care skills and perhaps some simple job skills.
  - **Severe:** 20–25 to 35–40 — Illiterate, unemployable, and institutionalized in the lower end.
  - **Profound:** <20–25 — Limitation of self-care and continence, mobility.

- **Clinical presentation: may present differently and at different times** depending on the underlying etiology.
  - **Frequently associated defects:** speech and language delays/deficits, hearing impairment, gross motor deficits/delays (e.g., with cerebral palsy), visual abnormalities, seizures, orthopedic problems, and behavioral/emotional disorders (**the greater the MR, the greater the severity of other impairments**).

Table 5.1: Major Etiologies of Mental Retardation and Studies to Consider for Diagnosis

Presentation	Possible Diagnoses	Most Important Studies/ Evaluations	Examples
IUGR, low Apgar scores, problems with intrapartum monitoring, hypotonia; seizure; prematurity with severe medical problems (e.g., intraventricular hemorrhage)	Perinatal insults, fetal nutritional/ oxygen deprivation; intracranial hemorrhage/ periventricular leukomalacia/cystic leukomalacia	Evaluate prenatal, intrapartum, and postpartum factors; **CT scan** for intracranial hemorrhage, infarct; **ultrasonography** for premature infant with intraventricular hemorrhage; **EEG**	Hypoxic-ischemic encephalopathy, cerebral infarction, premature with periventricular leukomalacia
Severe head trauma, anoxia, CNS infection, shock states; seizures	Acquired (postnatal)	History of event and physiologic response; **CT of brain** (MRI if needed for better anatomical/ pathological delineation); **EEG**	Head trauma, meningoencephalitis, septic shock, near-drowning
Small head, poor growth, dysmorphic features; specific pattern of malformations; family history of multiple anomalies or specific family diagnosis; history of mental retardation	Chromosomal abnormality/ genetic syndrome; teratogenic syndrome (prenatal exposure to drugs/ medications taken by the mother); specific brain abnormality; congenital infection	Prenatal history including medications/drug use; careful exam for characteristic dysmorphic features which may suggest a particular syndrome; **karyotype**, molecular genetic analysis; dysmorphology/ genetics consultation; MRI	Trisomies, Klinefelter syndrome, fragile X syndrome, Prader-Willi syndrome, Williams syndrome; familial retardation; prenatal drug abuse, fetal alcohol syndrome, holoprosencephaly, lissencephaly, TORCH infection
Progressive neurological disorder and/or acute neurobehavioral changes; neonate or infant with presentation for inborn errors (see Chapter 2); seizures	Inborn errors of metabolism, neurodegenerative diseases	**MRI**, ophthalmoscopic exam, review neonatal screen, serum amino acids, serum and urine organic acids, lactate, ammonia, tissue culture/biochemistry for diagnosis of specific disease; genetics evaluation; **EEG with neurological consultation**	Aminoacidemias, organic acidemias, other metabolic problems including rarer neurodegenerative diseases (see Chapter 2)

Abbreviations: central nervous system, CNS; intrauterine growth retardation, IUGR

Note: All children also need to be evaluated for hearing, vision, speech, and language.

- **Mild MR (IQ >50) is more often associated with environmental and genetic factors,** e.g., low parental educational level, low socioeconomic status (SES), mild MR in first-degree relatives; the specific cause is identified in <50% of patients. **More severe MR (IQ <50) is often due to biological causes** (see below).
- **Etiology and evaluation:** Evaluation should be based on an initial thorough history (prenatal, intrapartum, postnatal, and subsequent medical course), complete family history, and physical exam including a thorough neurological and developmental exam.

Formal testing—Administer individual tests of intellect and adaptive function.
- **Bayley Scale of Infant Development-II (BSID):** from 1 month to 3 years; most commonly used; measures gross and fine motor skills, language, behavior, and visual problem-solving; yields a mental developmental index (MDI) and psychomotor developmental index (PDI)
- **Wechsler Scales** (Wechsler Preschool and Primary Scale of Intelligence and Wechsler Intelligence Scale for Children): for children with mental age between 2.5–7.3 years and >6 years, respectively; verbal and performance area subtests
- **Vineland Adaptive Behavior Scale:** interviews with parents, caregivers, and teachers; measures adaptive behavior in motor skills, socialization, communication, and daily living

General therapeutic principles
- Intervention/management of associated impairments
- Treat behavioral problems and mental illness
- **Interdisciplinary management** (psychologist/psychiatrist, physical therapist, occupational therapist, speech pathologist, audiologist, nutritionist, geneticist, neurologist, social worker)
- Create an **Individual Family Service Plan (IFSP)** specifically designed to the needs of the child and family
- Periodic reevaluation (every 6–12 months) and particularly with transitions, e.g., to adult care (IDEA of 2004 recommends doing this at age 14; transfer to adult care by age 21).
- Education is the most important part of therapy; must create (per IDEA) an Individualized Education Program (IEP) for school-aged children
  - Include **social, leisure, and recreational activities**—important for physical activity, socialization, play, and **self-esteem**

Long-term goals/outcomes—Outcome depends on underlying cause of the MR and associated morbidities, along with severity of developmental impairments and support from family, school, and community. Major goals are to enhance adaptive abilities, teach appropriate living skills, and train for employment skills.

Autism spectrum disorder (pervasive developmental disorders; PDD)

Etiology—Unknown; **strong genetic influence:** 100 genes in all chromosomes except numbers 14 and 20 which interact with a number of (and variable) environmental factors (multifactorial); is linked to other neurodevelopmental disorders

Diagnosis—Clinical presentation varies with severity; better outcome with higher intelligence, functional speech, and less severe behaviors; must have:

- **Qualitative impairment in social interaction:** decreased or absent nonverbal behaviors, no social or emotional reciprocity, no peer relationships
- **Qualitative impairment in communication:** delay in language or no speech; stereotypic, repetitive language (e.g., echolalia); does not initiate or sustain conversation
- **Restricted, repetitive, stereotyped patterns of behavior and interests:** inflexible adherence to rituals (preservation of sameness), repetitive motor mannerisms, preoccupation with at least one restricted interest
- Abnormality of at least one of the following: **social interaction, language for communication, or imaginative play prior to age 3 years**
- Children with **isolated speech and language delay, intellectual disabilities, or profound hearing loss** will have presentations diagnostic of those particular problems but will not show the other findings needed for diagnosis of autism.

Most common clinical findings—No eye contact, pointing, pretend play; completely withdrawn to intermittent engagement; nonverbal to advanced speech (echolalia and other verbal mannerisms); from mental retardation to high intellect in certain skill areas (but with testing, usually found in the retarded age because of language and social deficits); stereotypical/repetitive body movements; preservation of sameness; abnormal social/emotional development evident usually by 1 year of age (before onset of other behaviors)

Diagnostic tools (screen routinely at ages 18, 24, and 30 months)—**Modified Checklist for Autism in Toddlers (M-CHAT):** 18-month well-child care visit screening; parental response to brief interview; also Pervasive Developmental Disorders Screening Test: 0–3 years; further evaluation: thorough history and physical exam, including neurological and developmental; hearing, speech, and language evaluations; MRI only with abnormal head size/shape; genetic referral for any dysmorphic features or anything suggesting a syndrome

Major therapeutic issues—**Intensive behavioral therapy**, especially with speech and language (increases language abilities and later social functioning); work with families with respect to behavioral training, management, coping; **alternative education** (start early, by age 2–4 years); **social skills training; psychotherapy, medications for psychiatric symptoms** (e.g., hyperactivity, aggression, anxiety, obsessive-compulsive disorder) may improve certain behaviors

Asperger syndrome

- Similar to autism but **without severe language impairments** (normal history of speech milestones); **appear peculiar and awkward** to others; **clumsy, unusual gait**
- **Impairment in social interactions and restrictive/repetitive behavioral patterns** and interests as seen in autism
- High risk for comorbidities: **mood and oppositional-defiant disorders**
- Most effective therapy: **group social skills training**

Childhood disintegrative disorder

Normal development until age 2–4 years, then **severe deterioration** over next several years (before age 10): regression of mental and social functioning and loss of bowel and bladder control; often with seizures; **very poor prognosis**

Rett disorder

- Genetic mutation of the MECP2 gene; X-linked dominant, but mostly seen in girls
- Development is normal for first 6 months, then **rapid regression through age 3–4 years**.
- **Acquired microcephaly**, regression of hand skills (with **midline hand-wringing**); loss of socialization; **ataxia**; severe **psychomotor retardation** (**wheelchair**; profound mental retardation); **bruxism,** scoliosis

Speech and language disorders

- There is **normal variation** among children for rate of development of infant speech and word understanding, usage, and combination in the first 2–3 years.
- Normal disfluency of language during the second to third year, and articulation of all consonant sounds is not complete until age 5–6 years.
- Influences of language development: complexity of grammar structure, **use of more than one language at home**, **early communication with the infant**, language usage by parents and other caregivers; generally, **language development parallels cognitive development**.
- The majority of children with language impairment do not have risk factors for neurologic injury. **Genetic factors play the major role** (language disorders tend to occur in families); therefore, **family history** is very important in the evaluation of a child with a language impairment.
- Whatever the underlying cause of a communication disorder, it **interferes with academic or occupational achievement or with social communication**.
- **Hearing loss** may also be a contributing factor, so any child with language impairment needs to have an **audiology assessment**.
- The majority of preschool children with a language delay (and normal nonverbal skills) continue to have problems **into early adulthood**; half have a **reading disorder**; many have **later emotional dysfunction**.

Other major clinical etiologies

- **Specific language impairment** (developmental language disorder): functional language level is significantly decreased compared to overall cognitive level and nonverbal skills; may display any of a number of specific problems related to spoken language, but do learn visually; tend to improve with treatment
- **Pragmatic language disorder:** difficulty interpreting higher-order, more abstract aspects of communication (e.g. inability to draw proper inferences); can be a symptom of many disorders (e.g., Asperger) or as part of a specific language impairment
- **Isolated expressive language disorder (late-talker):** variant of normal; greater in boys, often with a family history; have age-appropriate skills; once they talk, there are no speech problems and no increased risks.
- **Selective mutism:** failure to speak only in particular situations; most seen with underlying chronic anxiety disorder and as part of a familial trait.
- **Motor speech disorders (dysarthria): neuromotor disorders** which may affect speech and other oral functions; anywhere from slow, labored speech to slurred/distorted speech to unintelligible speech
- **Stuttering (disfluency):** involuntary, frequent repetitions of syllables or sounds; or lengthenings or arrests in the production of sounds; gets worse with increasing sentence complexity; represents a clinical disorder seen after age 3–5 years; common in families

    - **Preschool disfluency** is normal (age 2–3 years); resolves by school age and involves much fewer words, without silent pauses after the disfluency, with no interruption of airflow and no vocal tension; observe the child and **reassure the parents**

Screening

Should be **part of developmental surveillance for the well-child care visits**; developmental screening tests; **specific language screening tools** may be used if there is an indication of impairment (e.g., Clinical Linguistic and Auditory Milestone Scale).

Therapy

- Complete thorough history, family history, physical exam, developmental evaluation, and neurological exam
- If possibility of delay/impairments, **refer to a speech and language pathologist in conjunction with audiologic testing**.
- Psychological/psychiatric assessment may be warranted (look at nonverbal abilities, social behaviors, learning disorders, emotional disorder).
- With **true stuttering:** behavioral and speech therapy; most effective if started preschool.

Learning Disorders

Definition: disorders of reading, math, or written expression

- **Observed difference between intelligence test scores and tests of achievement**; this is used to determine **eligibility for special-education services**
- Neurodevelopmental function in broad areas (memory, gross and fine motor function, verbal-spatial relationships, language, critical thinking and problem-solving) are needed for academic achievement, and a **problem in one or more of these areas may lead to a specific disorder.**
- **Certain errors are normal through specific ages** (e.g., letter reversals, such as a B for a D, are common through age 7 years).
- Learning disorders have a **genetic component**, so (as usual) **family history** is very important; in any child there is **usually a combination of factors: genetic, environmental, medical, and social.**
- Cognitive abilities and academic skills develop at different rates among children.
  - A learning disorder may **present at any time** throughout school.
  - The child may initially present with **attention-deficit.**
  - **Factors other than intellect and learning disabilities may lead to academic underachievemen** e.g., physical impairments; chronic illnesses; medications; emotional problems; socioeconomic problems; parental education, culture.
- Children with **central nervous system (CNS) chronic conditions** have a higher incidence of learning disorders; acute CNS injury may also lead to temporary learning problems.
- With appropriate interventions, a child may show improvement in various areas; however, **learning disabilities are not completely outgrown.**
- Learning disorders have **many potential effects:** avoidance of reading, excessive anxiety about performing, clinical depression, decreased self-esteem, difficulty with peer relationships, drug use, delinquency, school dropout, and long-term occupational consequences.

Most common problems

Reading disabilities (dyslexia)—Most common learning disorder; problems decoding individual words (but vocabulary and syntax are appropriate and listening comprehension is good) with slow, labored reading and many pauses and mispronunciations; **familial** (one of the most important risk factors); **may occur with ADHD**

- Examples: spelling problems, dysgraphia (writing problems), dyscalcula (math), and content area subjects (science, social studies).

Screening and diagnosis

- **Rule out medical causes**—thorough history, physical, and neurosensory exams; and developmental assessment of memory, attention, and language
- Use standardized screening questionnaires (**Child Behavior Checklist, Behavior Assessment System for Children**) and direct questions to the parents.

Individuals with Disabilities Act

✓ Covers children with disabilities from **birth to age 21 years**

✓ **Early Intervention (age 0–3 years)**

- Identification at the time of diagnosis

  - Eligibility: developmental delays, medical conditions (cerebral palsy, Down syndrome), those at risk for significant delays if services are not provided

  - Referral to appropriate state agency (**each state must have an Interagency Coordinating Council** that assures multidisciplinary services are available)

  - **Each state may determine its own criteria.**

- Assessments to determine extent of need, then all parties (professionals and family) prepare an **Individualized Family Service Plan (IFSP)**

- Direct services for the condition, at home and in the community: family training, counseling, home visits, speech therapy and audiology, physical and occupational therapy, diagnostic medical services and other health services, case management, psychological services, social work, vision services, assistive technology and transportation (again, **states may determine which services are discretionary or mandated**)

- Preventive services to avoid secondary disability

✓ **Special Education (age 3–21 years)**

- States must provide a full appropriate public education for all children with disabilities (mentally retarded, hearing impaired, speech impaired, visually limited, serious emotional impairment, health impairments or multiple disabilities, and children with learning disabilities).

- State is required to identify, locate, and evaluate all children with disabilities, and to prepare and implement **individualized education plans (IEPs)** for these children. Individualized plans are created for the child by: parents, teacher, child, special education representative, and others identified by the parents or the agency (the physician).

  - Ensure placement in the **least restrictive environment** possible that will also maintain safeguards for children in public schools.

  - Major service is **special education**.

  - Need to provide **related services** (transportation, counseling, developmental therapy, sensory therapy, school health services)

- Obtain **assessments from school; interview teachers.**
- **Listen to the child read aloud**, and administer diagnostic writing exercises (spelling assessment and writing problems).
- Requires a **multidisciplinary assessment**: psychologist or psychiatrist, psychoeducational specialist (detailed analysis of skills; intelligence testing with subtests); other specialists as needed based on the individual (e.g., speech pathology, neurology)
  - As the discrepancy between verbal and performance IQ scores increases, so does the likelihood of learning dysfunction in the child.
  - **Achievement tests** measure what the child already knows in specific areas; both achievement and IQ tests are valuable in the evaluation of a child for learning disability—**subnormal scores on achievement tests with normal overall intelligence may indicate a specific learning disability.**
    - Neuroimaging studies only if history and examination strongly suggest a particular diagnosis where it is likely to demonstrate a CNS abnormality.
- Intervention and therapy: **multidisciplinary approach**
  - Use strategies to **accommodate to the child's needs** (calculator for math problems, texts on tape, use of word processors and spellcheck features, oral presentations and exams instead of written).
  - **Skills remediation at school and at home**: private/public tutoring; use of special services at school (**self-contained classrooms, resource rooms**) requires that children be **classified as learning disabled.**
  - Alteration in school curriculum
  - **Developmental therapy**: speech, physical, occupational therapy
  - **Exploit strengths**, e.g., artistic, musical, athletic skills
  - **Behavioral modification**: selected interventions can be used to address specific needs
  - **Counseling**: individual and parents (e.g., adolescent problems, transitions and losses, expectations for quick solutions)
  - Use of **community resources**: academic, recreational, and leisure programs for people with learning disabilities; special camps
  - **Medications** for ADHD, specific psychiatric problems
  - **Therapies with no scientific proof**: dietary (including Feingold diet, sugar restriction, food allergies), neurophysiologic therapies (patterning, sensory integration, vestibular medications and therapies, auditory processing training, visual therapies), cranial manipulation and facilitated communication

Sensory Disorders

Hearing impairment

Hearing impairment is generally to be considered with a **>25-dB hearing loss**, and is graded from mild to profound, depending on the range of hearing loss measured in decibels, from 26–40 dB at the mild end to >90 dB at the profound. **Profound hearing loss is rare; milder forms are common.**

- **Conductive hearing loss:** due to any interruption in the structures of the ear from the pinna and external canal through to the middle-ear cavity; child has losses across the entire range of frequencies, but can generally hear speech if it is loud enough
- **Sensorineural hearing loss:** loss from problems at the cochlea through to the nerve pathways; includes higher frequencies
- **Developmental effects of hearing loss are greater with:** more profound loss, certain etiologies (children with inherited deafness with hearing loss in parents seem to do better than those with acquired hearing loss), age at onset (children with onset of deafness at <2 years do significantly worse than those with onset >5 years of age in terms of language development and other developmental problems); better adaptability and increased communication when born to families with hearing impairment; with early diagnosis and interventions, there is a better outcome.

Clinical presentation/common causes—**Hereditary:** positive **family history of hereditary hearing loss**, abnormal newborn screen, with or without dysmorphic features (e.g., craniofacial anomalies and others)

- **Sensorineural:** half have a genetic basis; 80% are autosomal recessive; of the cases with a genetic basis, half are nonsyndromic (many may be in the class of undetermined etiology); others may have specific features suggestive of a syndrome specifically associated with hereditary hearing loss (**Waardenburg, Alport**); X-linked (**Hunter**) and non-Mendelian syndromes.
- **Conductive:** autosomal recessive causes (very rare), autosomal dominant (**Treacher Collins syndrome**), X-linked, and non-Mendelian syndromes

Acquired:

- **Sensorineural:**
  - prenatal problems: **TORCH** (presentation with clinical findings in the newborn)
  - perinatal: **prematurity, hypoxic-ischemic encephalopathy, hyperbilirubinemia**
  - postnatal: **meningoencephalitis**, severe injury, tumor, **ototoxins**, neurofibromatosis-II

- **Conductive:** otitis media with effusion, tympanic membrane disruption

Screening and diagnostic evaluation
- Thorough history and physical exam including neurological; careful attention to any dysmorphic features, **craniofacial anomalies; thorough family history;** depending on the findings, an otolaryngology, genetics, or neurology referral may be appropriate.
- **If there is any question as to hearing impairment, an audiology referral needs to be made promptly.**
- **All children with hearing impairment should have a formal assessment of language, cognitive, and social abilities by experts in evaluating hearing-impaired.**

Therapy

- Primary care for well-child care and management of medical problems; specialty care as needed for other problems
- Hearing aids, cochlear implants (in select children with profound hearing loss), tele-communication devices for the deaf, environmental modifications (visual signals to sound producers)
- Education: **early intervention, focus on language-communication skills; factors for optimal development:** language interaction with parents and others from an early age, active exploration of the environment, and social interactions

Visual impairment

- The U.S. Public Health Service definition: **the best corrected acuity in both eyes of 6/60 meters or visual fields <20 degrees bilaterally.** The World Health Organization divides the impairment into subsets with worsening vision including visual impairment, social blindness, virtual blindness, and total blindness (no light perception).
- Children who are blind at 1–2 years of age tend to do better developmentally than those with congenital blindness (e.g., better performance on spatial-perception tasks).

Most causes—Leading causes are **retinopathy of prematurity and cataracts**; others include accidents, brain trauma, **neoplasms affecting the visual system**; macular degeneration, optic nerve atrophy, **congenital glaucoma, chorioretinitis (congenital infections)**; wide range of visual disturbances due to **amblyopia** (from many causes, such as strabismus), nystagmus, and problems with the cornea, sclera, and vitreous

Screening and diagnostic evaluation—Routine developmental surveillance and **formal visual screening** (with the age-appropriate tools) as discussed in Chapter 4; examinations in infancy to detect strabismus, or any problem which may interfere with appropriate retinal images (**retinoblastoma, cataract**)

Therapy

- Early recognition of any eye pathology that may have resulted in or could result in visual impairment needs to be referred **promptly to an ophthalmologist**
- Any congenital condition that may involve visual impairment requires consultation from an ophthalmologist (**prematurity <34 weeks, TORCH infections**)
- **Older children who fail vision screens** should be referred for a full ophthalmological evaluation
- Complete developmental evaluation should be performed to look for other developmental dysfunctions so that interventions may be initiated.

Educational issues

- Read large-print material.
- Alternatives (e.g., teaching and use of **braille**, "talking book" program).
- Issues with **orientation and mobility**: long cane, guide dog, sensory aids.

- **Local districts for schooling** (residential schools usually contain severely visually impaired children with other disabilities): self-contained classrooms.
- Provisions through **local Committee on Special Education and Commission for the Blind**.

PART TWO: BEHAVIORAL AND MENTAL HEALTH DISORDERS

Behavioral Issues from Infancy Through Middle Childhood

Table 5.2: Behavioral Issues: Infancy–Middle Childhood

Behavioral Issue	Major Concepts
Feeding	Infants self-regulate to breastfeeding 8–12 times per day (about every 2–3 hours); with bottle-feeding, start with 2 oz formula every 2–3 hours and increase based on feeding cues of continued hunger; stop when infant indicates satiety (usually consumes 16–24 oz. per day in first weeks); by age 2 months, will want 6–8 feeds per day (even though sleep is 4–5 hours at night); with further increase in age and introduction of solids, volume per feed increases and frequency decreases (24–32 oz at 6 months, and then less with further solids).
Temperament	Ways that behaviors are influenced by the environment; range from regularity (predictability of sleep–wake cycles, feeding), and adaptability (mostly positive mood and mild to moderate intensity with environmental changes) to irregularity of functions and non-adaptability (slow or none: negative responses to new stimuli and usually negative intense mood changes).
Rocking movements	Rhythmic behavior for self-consolation; average age at onset is 6 months; majority of infants have some degree in first year, then decreases over next year with very few at 2–6 years of age. Usually when left alone, and episodes are short (<15 minutes); persistent long periods of rocking may indicate lack of environmental stimuli: may be seen in developmental disorders and visual impairment.
Head-banging	Banging of head against a solid surface, usually when quiet and relaxed (tired, alone) or when upset. Each episode is short (<15 minutes). Rapid decrease in episodes after age 18 months (very small number at age 3 years, some of which will persist by age 7 years). Does not result in physical injury and is usually not associated with developmental or emotional problems; best management: pad surfaces with soft material; ignore episodes (especially if related to tantrums).
Thumb-sucking	Onset in utero as early as 29 weeks, and present in almost every newborn within hours of delivery (100% through age 1 year, peaking at 18–21 months; continues in 50% by age 2 years, and in up to 20% by age 5 years; self-regulatory behavior at first, but with persistence becomes a coping response to stressors; mostly extinguished by 4–5 years, if ignored (child substitutes other mechanisms to cope). Problem only with persistent, extensive sucking after eruption of permanent teeth—dental abnormalities, thumb/finger deformations, paronychia, psychosocial problems. Management: no negative comments, manage stressors and anxiety, positive reinforcement and negative physical barriers to sucking (benign aversive taste substance on thumb, oral appliance to prevent seal), dental evaluation.

(continued)

Table 5.2: Behavioral Issues: Infancy–Middle Childhood *(cont.)*

Behavioral Issue	Major Concepts
Tantrums/ Discipline	Infants want autonomy → varying degrees of negative situations; common at end of second year; response to parents setting limits; if limits are not set, overly indulged children can exert control over the parents, and constant tantrums may result. Best management is ignoring, with a "time-out" in a safe place out of sight of caregivers (but not in the child's bedroom) until calm (younger children may not be able to regain control with this and may need to be held); parents must always exercise firmness, consistency, with appropriate use of positive and negative reinforcement.
Fears/Phobias	Preschool children have many common fears (e.g., darkness, monsters), may persist to some degree through early school years. Difference in fear vs. phobia is the degree of anxiety, how much the child is willing to do to avoid the fearful situation, and whether or not this results in functional impairment. Appears to be related to parental anxiety and traumatic occurrences. Must deal with fears with child (naming and confronting them; education) in order to decease or eliminate them.
Lying/Stealing	Preschool children tell stories consistent with understanding of a situation (they do not lie with the intent of making things up); they do not start to understand abstract principles (truth) until the beginning of school age. Also, young children may take things that are not theirs without realizing that this is inappropriate behavior (unless it is met consistently with negative reinforcement).
Masturbation	Spontaneous erections are seen in male infants as early as 2 days of life (occur in infancy during periods of sleep); self-exploration and interest increases in mid-childhood to adolescence, which is normal behavior, and various forms of masturbation are felt to be developmental learning experiences; stimulation in both sexes has been shown to lead to arousal. Problem only if adults overreact, or if masturbation is extreme and excessive.
Sex education	When child is in mid-childhood, parents need to provide accurate information (sex differences, pubertal changes, and allow for questioning). Pediatricians should perform a sexual maturity rating when child is age 7–10 years. Children should be told that it is all right to touch themselves, but not at certain times or in certain places. Children also need to understand that it is inappropriate for others to touch them in certain ways and that if this occurs, they should tell the parents about it immediately.

Unexplained Early Infant Crying (colic)

✓ Should no longer be referred to as colic; this denotes a gastrointestinal pathology, and this has not been found.

✓ Prolonged and excessive crying in young, healthy, and growing infants (from shortly after birth to 3–4 months, when it typically ceases), which is intense and may last for hours; infant may draw legs up to abdomen (nonspecific) and pass large amounts of flatus (probably secondary to forceful crying); is not quieted by further feedings or caregiver attempts at soothing.

✓ **Normal crying**: average 2 hours/day at age 2 weeks, 3 hours/day at age 6 weeks (peak), and 1 hour/day at age 3 months (increasing longest sleep time and total sleep)

✓ Based on temperament, infant may **not be able to organize and self-regulate in response to environmental factors (i.e., has a low sensory threshold)**

✓ Caregivers trying to soothe may end up **overstimulating the infant**, and the problem gets worse; this leads to increasing parental anxiety and a further worsening of the situation.

✓ **With first visit, evaluate**: feeding methods and appropriateness, observe infant's temperament and parent interactions with infant, explore psychosocial stressors; physical exam should concentrate on ruling out **certain medical/surgical problems which may result in excessive crying**, e.g., inguinal hernia, circumferential digital hair, hydrocephalus (bulging fontanelle), otitis media, corneal abrasion. No lab studies unless specifically indicated by features of the history and physical.

✓ **Most effective course of management is counseling**: education as to the fact that the infant is healthy; explanation of cause of crying, and ways to appropriately soothe: not picking him up every time he cries, swaddling, quiet environment with decreased sensory stimuli, the use of white noise, a hot-water bottle (warm temperature, and wrapped in cloth), pacifier use. *Do not* change the composition of feeds; there is no evidence that milk allergy (or anything else in the formula) is a related cause.

✓ In **extreme cases** (severe loss of sleep, inability to cope, increasing crying), may use 1–2-week course of phenobarbital or diphenhydramine elixir; in worse cases, short-term separation of infant from parents (care by another person, unless breastfeeding).

✓ If above is followed, results usually appear **within 2–3 days.**

Breath-Holding Spells

✓ Infant is typically provoked by a minor injury, fear, or anger; and then cries intensely, stops at expiration, and becomes apneic with paleness or cyanosis.

✓ A **simple breath-holding spell** resolves and the child takes a breath. If the spell continues, however, it may result in **loss of consciousness and a short seizure** with a postictal drowsy period.

✓ **Cyanotic spells** are more common and result in an abnormality in respiratory regulation, resulting in an expiratory apnea. **Pallid spells** are due to an overactive vagal response with bradycardia or even asystole.

✓ Management is **reassurance**: the spells do not result in brain injury. If there is loss of consciousness, the infant will then breathe; however, with severe and recurrent pallid spells, **atropine** may be useful (decreases frequency of seizures).

✓ Other diagnoses to consider, depending on the history and physical and the nature and timing of spells: arrhythmia (e.g., long Q-T), anemia (especially with pallid spells), seizure disorder, brain-stem dysfunction. These are rare causes and **usually no lab studies need to be performed**.

Toilet Training

✓ **Start discussion at age 18 months but in-depth discussion at 2-year-old visit.**

✓ Range of bladder control is **18–60 months** and bowel control is **16–48 months; daytime control** (average 30 months) usually precedes nighttime.

✓ Start when child:

- Is dry for 2-hour periods
- Knows the difference between wet and dry
- Can pull own pants up and down
- Wants to learn
- Can say when he is about to have a bowel movement

✓ Management:

- **No negative reinforcement**
- Read books about "going to the potty"
- Use much **positive reinforcement**
- Establish **daily routine**; place on potty every 1–2 hours
- Provide a relaxed atmosphere
- Use easy-to-remove pants

Externalizing Behaviors and Conditions

Aggressive behaviors

- **Mild and intermittent aggressive behavior is common in young children** (mild biting, kicking, verbal abuse) and may not be a concern, but it **needs to be discussed and behavioral modification employed to avoid escalation.**
- Many possible causes: attention-seeking, retaliation, family problems, poor parenting, low SES, parental abuse; **increased spanking worsens aggressive/antisocial behaviors later.**
- Treatment is needed **depending on the behavior's frequency, duration, and intensity, and the presence of emotional problems**: initially avoiding corporal punishment, learning **appropriate methods of discipline**, the use of "time-outs"; parents and child need to be taught skills related to **anger management and impulse control.**

Aggressive-oppositional problems and disruptive and antisocial behaviors—
Pattern of behavior that is verbally or physically harmful to property, animals, or other people, and the behavior is contrary to social expectations

*Contributors and associations—***Genetics (biological markers) + environment**

- Problem levels of aggressive behaviors may **run in families; e.g., parents with criminal records.**
- Increasing corporal punishment (especially with no positive reinforcements) tends to increase later antisocial behaviors.
- Physical (parental rejection, neglect, abuse) or sexual abuse is correlated with subsequent aggressive/antisocial behaviors.
- Inconsistent supervision, frequent changes in caregivers, early institutional living, association with delinquent peer groups.
- **Violence in the media is a suggested causal link.**
- Increased with **learning disorders**
- Low self-esteem, **increased suicidal ideation**, and attempted/completed suicide
- Antisocial behaviors at an early age; cruelty to animals and fire-starting are never normal behaviors and may indicate an underlying psychiatric disorder.

Table 5.3: Aggressive-Oppositional and Conduct Disorders

Aggressive/Oppositional Problem	Oppositional Defiant Disorder	Conduct Disorder—Childhood or Adolescent Onset
Problem when levels of aggression interere with family routines, when there are negative responses from others and/or cause school disruption	Hostile, defiant behavior towards others of at least six months' duration that is developmentally inappropriate	Repetitive and persistent pattern of behavior where rights of others and societal norms are violated; onset usually in late childhood and adolescence
Infants: frequent crying, kicking, biting, hair-pulling **Early childhood:** grabs others toys, shouts, verbally abusive, hits/punches **Middle childhood:** intermittent fights, uses bad language, may hit or hurt self (frustration, anger) **Adolescence:** hits others, uses bad language, verbally abusive, inappropriate suggestive sexual behavior	**Infants:** not possible to diagnose **Early childhood:** extremely defiant—will not follow rules/instructions, sasses parents and others, throws tantrums **Middle childhood:** refuses to comply with requests, often argues and purposely annoys others **Adolescence:** has frequent severe arguments, is extremely defiant, has negative attitudes, is unwilling to compromise, and may use alcohol, tobacco or drugs.	**Infants:** not possible to diagnose **Early childhood:** rare to diagnose due to symptoms that are not intense **Middle childhood:** may lie, steal, fight with peers, is cruel to people/animals, displays inappropriate sexual behavior, bullies, engages in destructive acts, violates rules, has academic problems and school truancy **Adolescence: delinquent,** aggressive behavior, harms people and property, has deviant sexual behavior, uses illegal drugs, is suspended or expelled from school, has difficulties with the law, runs away from home, has academic problems and has problems with work.

Delinquency—More of **a legal term**—a youth commits an illegal act, then comes before the police and courts.

- High rates of significant family stress, low SES, parents with psychopathological behaviors and higher rates of alcohol and drug use.
- Manifest with learning disabilities, poor school performance, ADHD, truancy, and lack of school completion.
- Anticipatory guidance: discussions and **screening questions on violence** should be part of each well-child care visit; discussions with parents about **discipline, appropriate parenting skills, the use of corporal punishment, and supervision;** gather family information and information from teachers; interview the child
- Rating scales and questionnaires
  - **School Social Behavior Scales (SSBS),** rating scale designed for teachers to assess social competence and antisocial behavior from kindergarten through 12th grade
  - **Pediatric Symptom Checklist,** 35-item parent-child questionnaire with respect to psychosocial functioning

- **Behavior Assessment System for Children–2 (BASC-2)**, rating scales for use by parent and teacher
- **Consider an ADHD tool**: e.g., Connors Rating Scales–Revised (CRS-R)—uses observer ratings and self-report ratings to help assess ADHD and evaluate problem behavior in children and adolescents; or the Vanderbilt ADHD Diagnostic Teacher Rating Scale.
- **Alter child functioning in everyday life**
  - **Parent management training** (alter parent-child interaction at home)
  - **Problem-solving skills** training to child (responses to situations, anger control training—individual and group)
  - **Family therapy** (interaction, communication, and problem-solving among all family members)
- Severe cases (e.g., rage): medication, but not as a substitute for therapy
- **Interdisciplinary team** of teachers, guidance counselors, and social workers to work with families to provide services to help in all aspects of child's life
- **Conduct disorders may be resistant to treatment**
- **Prognosis:** The longer the antisocial behaviors persist, the less likely they will be amenable to treatment; if by age 8 a child has not learned appropriate goal-seeking behaviors, he has a high chance of lifelong antisocial behavior.

Internalizing Disorders and Conditions

Anxiety disorders—Mood characterized by excessive worriedness or fearfulness, accompanied by autonomic nervous symptoms such as tachycardia and sweating. When it is to the degree that **interferes with functioning**, it is problematic.

- **Normal developmental anxiety** (worries): beginning at 7–9 months of age with unfamiliar people and circumstances; preschool children have fears of the unknown and the imaginary that are often replaced by other more concrete fears during childhood; adolescence: general worrying about the various aspects of their lives
- **Genetic and environmental influences:** family history of anxiety disorders, maternal overinvolvement, history of trauma and traumatic events; infants and young children who are very clingy with extreme fear of separation have a higher rate of anxiety disorder.
- **Coexisting conditions: mostly depression**, conduct disorders, and some personality disorders
- **Screening tools:** Anxiety Disorders Schedule for Children (ADIS-C), Children's Yale-Brown Obsessive-Compulsive Scale (C-YBOCS); Screen for Child Anxiety-Related Emotional Disorders (SCARED), and the Multidimensional Anxiety Scale for Children (MASC).

Table 5.4: Types of Anxiety Disorders in Children

Disorder	Description	Preferred Therapies
Separation anxiety disorder (SAD)	Unrealistic fears/worries about separation from parents/caregivers and being left alone; may have somatic complaints and develop into a panic attack	Preferred use of selective serotonin reuptake inhibitors (SSRIs) with recurrent, severe anxiety, plus cognitive behavioral therapy involving the parents also
Childhood-onset social phobia	Marked and persistent fear of being exposed to unfamiliar people: avoidance, anticipation, and distress from a possible situation lead to impairment of functioning; may develop into a panic attack	SSRIs are the treatment of choice; antianxiety agents are not effective.
Generalized anxiety disorder (GAD)	Excessive anxiety/worry on most days about many **general activities or events; associated with sleep problems, irritability, muscle tension, fatigue; leads to impairment in function;** may not manifest until puberty; more common in middle-to-upper-class white children	Cognitive behavioral therapy; with severe symptoms, try an SSRI or buspirone
Specific phobias	Excessive, persistent unreasonable fear about a **specific object or situation;** exposure leads to **immediate anxiety and possibly a panic attack;** avoidance and distress may lead to functional disturbances	Systematic desensitization
Panic disorder	Recurrent unexpected panic attacks (an intense period of fear or discomfort with severe physiological somatic and autonomic complaints) with a significant change in behavior and persistent worry over additional attacks and their consequences	SSRIs are effective in adolescents.

(continued)

Disorder	Description	Preferred Therapies
Post-traumatic stress disorder (PTSD)	Person exposed to a **traumatic event** where **life has been threatened** with severe injury or death (or actual death of another person); response was **intense fear, helplessness, and horror;** traumatic event is **persistently re-experienced** in number of ways (e.g., recurrent, distressing dream) with **persistent avoidance** of any stimuli related to the event and **persistent symptoms of increased arousal** (e.g., difficulty falling asleep).	**Active outreach and screening in children and adolescents after a traumatic event;** aggressive treatment of acute pain and return to comforting routines; individual, group, family, and school therapy, plus selective use of pharmacologic agents for sleep and hyperarousal (e.g., clonidine), depression (SSRIs)
Obsessive-compulsive disorder (OCD)	Either **obsessions**—recurrent or persistent thoughts, images, impulses that are intrusive and inappropriate and cause marked anxiety or distress (not worries about real-life problems); person tries to suppress, ignore, or neutralize these thoughts OR **compulsions**—repetitive behaviors or mental acts that the person feels are necessary to perform; they cause marked distress, are time-consuming, and interfere with normal daily functioning; most common are touching things, checking locks, and hand-washing. **May present in preschool or later.**	Cognitive behavioral therapy plus SSRIs; referral to a mental health expert is always indicated

Disorders of mood and affect

Major depressive disorder (MDD)

- **Depressed mood and/or loss of interest or pleasure** nearly every day and most of the day with **somatic symptoms:** weight changes, loss of appetite, insomnia or hypersomnia, psychomotor agitation, loss of energy; also feelings of worthlessness/guilt, decreased concentration, recurrent thoughts of death/suicidal ideation; symptoms cause **significant functional impairment**

- May present as acting-out, oppositional problems, or school problems rather than with the vegetative symptoms; mood swings more common in adolescence
  - **Earliest findings in infants**: withdrawal, lethargy, crying silently, apathy, hard to console
- **Recurrent disorder with an increased likelihood of adult depression.** In prepubertal children, it occurs equally in boys and girls; **in adolescence—marked female preponderance**; prevalence increased with age—highest in adolescents.
- **Causes and associations: genetic, familial, and environmental factors**; MDD in a parent (or first-degree relative), family instability, stressful events/trauma, chronic illness, abuse/neglect, decreased positive peer relationships
- **Major associations:** decreased school performance, decreased social functioning, increased risk of substance abuse, correlation with suicidal behaviors; increased in children with complex, chronic illnesses; higher rates of anger/hostility and anxiety disorders; more common in adolescents with sexual orientation issues
- **Assessment and screening:** primary-care provider and school professionals observe/ask about mood, somatic symptoms, changes in baseline behavior, negative self-concepts. There are a number of standardized rating scales (**e.g., Children's Depression Rating Scale (CDRS; age 6–12 years), Beck Depression Inventory (for age ≥13 years).**
- Distinguish MDD from **dysthymic disorder** (dysthymic has less severe but more insidious and longer-lasting episodes for at least 1 year; other symptoms of MDD may be present), **adjustment disorder** (emotional or behavioral reaction to an identifiable stressful event or change in a person's life that is maladaptive), and **bipolar disorder** (alternating depression and mania).
- **Therapy:** best response is with **cognitive behavioral therapy** (identification and influencing of dysfunctional emotions, behaviors, and thoughts through a goal-oriented systematic procedure) **plus an SSRI** (e.g., fluoxetine).

Bipolar disorder

- **Alternating depression and mania** (distinct period of elevated mood for at least 1 week with grandiosity, decreased need for sleep, increased talking, flight of ideas, distractibility, psychomotor agitation, and excessive involvement in pleasurable activities that have a potential for negative consequences) or rapid cycling of mood (more common in children and younger adolescents; may also present with delusions and hallucinations).
- Also has a genetic basis.
- Comorbidities: obesity, metabolic syndrome, anxiety disorders, substance abuse; increased suicidal ideation.
- Need to refer to psychiatrist—combination of psychotherapy and mood stabilizer (e.g., lithium carbonate, divalproic acid).

Suicidal Behavior

- In the United States, suicide is the third leading cause of death in ages 10–24 years (injuries and homicides are first and second); highest rate for age 15–24 years; rates for ages 5–14 years have increased over the past 30 years.

- 90% of suicides have some form of mental illness (most have MDD).
- Females make more attempts but males are more successful (more lethal methods).
- Self-poisoning after age 6 years is *not* likely to be accidental.
- Self-inflicted harm in any child may be a sign of a suicidal attempt.
- Publicity regarding suicide may prompt other adolescents to attempt suicide.
- Psychological intent does not always correlate with the seriousness of the attempt—all attempts must be taken seriously.

Risk factors for suicide completion

- Mood disorders (but among prepubertal children with completed suicide, this is usually not a contributor; **in female adolescents, the presence of major depression is the most significant risk factor**)
- **Family psychological diagnoses/dysfunction**
- History of **abuse**
- Past attempts (**in males, this is the most important predictor**)
- **Substance abuse** is a significant factor.
- **In-home presence of lethal means (especially firearms)**
- Gay and lesbian youth
- Feelings of hopelessness, hostility, negative self-concept
- Combination of mood disorder and disruptive behavior
- Surviving family members are at risk for depressive disorders and suicide.

Assessment and management—All of the above issues for depression and specific screening/rating questionnaires (suicide is preventable). Most potential suicides give definite warnings of intentions, but often friends/family are unaware of the significance of the warnings or do not know how to respond to them; **asking a person about suicide does not cause that person to become suicidal**.

- The initial evaluation after an attempt needs to **focus on clearly defining the intent**.
- **Outpatient management, as long as *all* of the following conditions are met (otherwise, hospitalize):**
  - No inpatient medical treatment is needed for psychiatric conditions.
  - No previous suicide attempts or psychiatric disorders
  - Is not actively suicidal
  - There is an adult in the home who has a good relationship with the child/adolescent *and* agrees to closely monitor the patient *and* agrees to remove all lethal modalities from the home.
  - Both adult and child have clear understanding of emergency contacts and follow-up.
  - Further outpatient care has been arranged.
  - Both patient and adult agree with the plan and state they will comply with all recommendations (a treatment contract serves to decrease short-term risks).

- Ongoing management to deal with underlying problems (medical and psychological); limit availability and access to lethal means of suicide; integrated prevention strategies; skill-based school programs; medication for comorbid conditions

Childhood Schizophrenia

Characteristic symptoms present for at least 1 month (**active-phase symptoms**: delusions, hallucinations, disorganized speech, grossly disorganized or catatonic behavior) and negative symptoms (e.g., flattened affect) period and continuous signs for at least 6 months (**prodromal or residual symptoms**: attention deficits, impairment in memory and language, poor gross and fine motor skills); at least one major area of social/occupational dysfunction

- Must exclude schizoaffective and mood disorders (with psychotic features): no major depressive, manic, or mixed episodes with the active-phase symptoms; and is not due to a drug, medication, or effects of a medical condition.
- **Early onset before puberty is rare** (show **progressive ventricular enlargement** with decreasing brain volume and decreasing intellectual function); **typical age of onset is late adolescence to early adulthood**.
- Prior to diagnosis, most show: developmental delays (greater global impairment), speech and language problems, social withdrawal and disruptive behaviors (violent aggression), fewer friends
- **Multimodal therapeutic approach:** parent training to teach ways to modify child's behavior in order to improve social functioning; individual therapy, school and community liaison work, **newer antipsychotics** (risperidone, olanzapine)

Disorders of Attention and Impulse Control

Attention-deficit hyperactivity disorder (ADHD)

- Prevalence is **higher in boys than girls**.
- Anxiety and depression can present as hyperactivity or inattention.
- In very young children, the diagnosis is more difficult.
  - The diagnosis of combined type (see below) peaks in early elementary school (most with hyperactivity and impulse control), but the inattentive type may not be identified until later in school.
  - Often **undiagnosed** in children and adolescents, and undertreated

Risk factors and associations

- **Strong genetic component:** dopamine transporter gene (DAT1) and dopamine 4 receptor gene (DRD4) plus other possible contributing genes
- **Prenatal and perinatal factors:** prenatal drug or alcohol use, long labor, toxemia, complicated delivery

At least **6 symptoms** of **inattention** for at least **6 months** that are **maladaptive and inconsistent with developmental level:**
- Distracted, forgetful with respect to daily activities, makes careless mistakes, does not follow through with instructions
- Does not listen when spoken to
- Does not pay attention to details, has problems organizing tasks and activities, often loses things needed for daily activities
- Avoids and dislikes tasks requiring sustained mental effort

AND/OR at least **6 symptoms** of **hyperactivity/impulsivity** for at least **6 months** that are **maladaptive and inconsistent with** developmental level
- Fidgets and squirms, leaves seat when inappropriate, runs and climbs excessively when inappropriate
- Difficulty in engaging in leisure activities quietly, always active, talks excessively
- Blurts out answer before question is completed, interrupts or intrudes on others, cannot wait for turn

PLUS:
- Some amount of consistent symptoms causing impairment prior to age 7 years
- Impairment from symptoms in 2 or more settings (school, home, social)
- Clear evidence of clinically significant impairment in academic, social, or occupational functioning
- Symptoms are not accounted for by another disorder

Figure 5.2: ADHD Diagnostic Criteria

- **Postnatal factors:** abnormal brain structures (with or without identifiable brain injury), psychosocial family stressors (inappropriate parenting, parental psychopathology, abuse), response to inappropriate classroom setting; **medical conditions:** hearing/visual deficits, thyroid disorders, heavy metal exposure (lead), medication effects, effects of substance abuse, seizure disorder, post meningoencephalitis, neurodegenerative disorder
- **Comorbid psychiatric conditions:** anxiety disorders, oppositional defiant disorders, conduct disorders, depression, and learning disabilities
- **Diagnoses that have ADHD behaviors:** fetal alcohol syndrome, PDD, OCD, fragile X syndrome, Tourette syndrome, schizophrenia

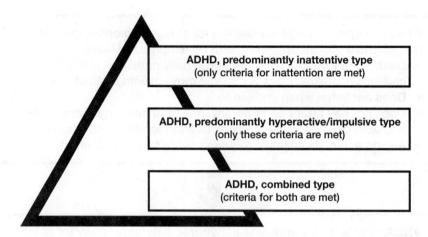

Figure 5.3: Types of ADHD

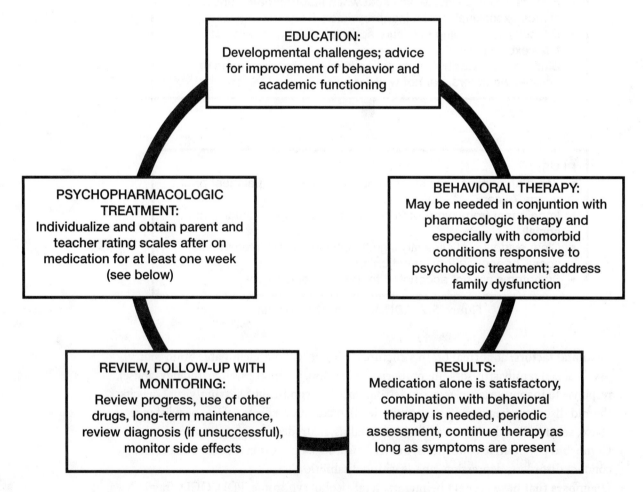

Figure 5.4: Management of ADHD

Evaluation and diagnosis
- **Screening:** As part of developmental surveillance, ask about symptoms of inattention, hyperactivity, and impulsivity; **if positive responses, evaluate for ADHD.**
- Perform detailed interview with parents/caregiver and child with respect to **each of the diagnostic symptoms** (see below); **review other possible psychiatric problems**, assess family and social issues; review complete past medical history and family history; review developmental milestones (**no lab or neurological studies if medical history is not suggestive**).
- Parents/caregiver and teacher should complete standardized rating scale; look at homework samples and report card.
  - Conners Parent Rating Scale-Revised (CPRS-R), Conners Teachers Rating Scale—Revised (CTRS-R), and others
  - Perform, or refer for, **psychological testing** if low achievement in language or mathematics relative to intellect.
  - Determine if **comorbid conditions** exist and whether they are primary disorders or secondary to ADHD; selection of treatment program is often influenced by comorbid conditions.

Management—Identify target behaviors and develop treatment plan with **alliance** of patient, clinician, family, teachers, and **community support**; provide systematic reviews and follow-up.
- Selection of initial agent is **choice of family and clinician** but may be influenced by comorbid behaviors.

Amphetamines

- **Short-acting:** Adderall, Dexedrine; need BID-TID dosing
- **Long-acting:** Adderall XR, Dexedrine Spansule; single daily dosing; more effects on evening decreased appetite and insomnia

---

Methylphenidates

- **Short-acting:** Focalin, Ritalin; BID-TID dosing
- **Intermediate-acting:** Ritalin LA, Metadate CD; usually QD dosing
- **Long-acting:** Concerta, Focalin XR; QD dosing; increased side effects as with amphetamines

---

Atomoxetine

- Selective norepinephrine reuptake inhibitor
- QAM or divided BID dosing
- Use as initial therapy or with side effects/abuse of a stimulant drug
- Effects on late evening behavior with divided dosing; monitor for suicidal thinking or unusual changes in behavior

Figure 5.5: Pharmacology of ADHD

- Start with low dose and titrate up every 1–3 weeks until maximum dose is reached, symptoms abate, or there are unacceptable side effects.
- **Common side effects** of stimulants: decreased appetite, weight loss, insomnia, headache, tics, emotional lability, irritability; may need to reduce dose, change medication, try a nonstimulant, or add a medication for side effects
- May need adjunctive medication for comorbid conditions (with referral to mental-health specialist)
- Medications are useful through adolescence and adulthood (and improve attention in normal individuals).
- Patient may not need medications in after-school hours/times, depending on level of daily functioning.

PSYCHOSOCIAL ISSUES/ PROBLEMS AND ETHICAL ISSUES IN PEDIATRICS

6

PART ONE: PSYCHOSOCIAL ISSUES AND PROBLEMS

Family and Environmental Issues

Divorce

Custodial issues: With joint custody, the goal is to have both parents in the child's life.

- **Joint legal custody:** both parents share in the legal responsibilities of raising and caring for the child; both parents must give consent and must agree on issues where consent is needed (e.g., medical procedures)
- **Joint physical custody:** one parent has primary legal custody but both share in responsibilities of caring for the child, accompanying the child to events, and providing transportation
- **Sole custody** may be granted if there is ongoing parental fighting that results in escalating tension and psychosocial problems for the child. Prior to granting sole custody, the courts may first rule for counseling, mental health evaluations, or mediation.

Developmental stage and effect on child
- **<3 years old:** may present with crying and irritability, separation anxiety, sleep problems, regression
- **4–5 years old:** crying, sleep problems, sadness, withdrawal, self-blame; somatic symptoms may occur
- **School age:** moodiness, anger, aloof or overtly aggressive behaviors; decreased school performance; somatic complaints
- **Adolescent:** increased generalized worries; aggressive or antisocial behaviors; may spend more time with peers and out of house; somatic complaints; engagement in sexual activities; higher number leave home at an earlier age

Blended families
- Children living with a **new stepparent** adapt more easily when the new situation occurs **at <8 years of age**; older children have **more conflicts**; girls tend to do worse

135

with a new stepfather. Older children and adolescents: more **resentment and problems with attachment** to the new stepparent.

- Higher amount of **anxiety**, perceptions that the stepparent (especially a young step-mother) is **responsible for the parents' break-up; fears of being excluded**

Long-term outcome
- Divorce when child is in late childhood or early adolescence: associated with **intimacy issues as an adult and decreased readiness for marriage**
- **Improved outcome** with parents who can get along and work together for the sake of the child, and if the child has a good relationship with the primary custodial parent
- Older children and adolescents in a blended family who have resentment toward the new stepparent are more likely to **leave home at an earlier age**.

Death

Grief
- Grief is normal but should never be ignored or neglected; may manifest as **shock, anger, denial, disbelief, or sadness**, and the expression of grief may change over time and may be nonlinear.
- Grief is problematic if: associated with unusual (acute or violent) circumstances of death; if there are significant changes in family functioning; if there are psychiatric symptoms; if there are school or work problems; or if there are persistent somatic symptoms.

Developmental stage and response to death of a parent —**Very young children** acutely affected by the **overwhelming sadness of a surviving parent or caretakers**; preschool children tend to work through their experiences with **play**; the child may not understand the feelings of the surviving parent, and may feel that it has something to do with his own behavior; children may also feel that the death of a parent is punishment to them because they were bad. **School-age children** may present with **nonspecific pains, nausea, stomachache, and headache**; may show **regression** and become more dependent on the surviving parent. **Adolescents** tend to have feelings of **guilt and resentment**; may turn to other adults outside the family for support and guidance.

Family responses to the terminal illness of a child
- **Parents** may blame themselves for a child's terminal illness; often feel a **total loss of control** with overwhelming situations (care, appointments, finances, taking care of other family members); may spend a lot of energy looking for **miracle cures; intense stress** (marital problems, managing everyday life while caring for a dying child), shock, **mood swings**
- **Healthy siblings** may feel that they are being **ignored or neglected**, which may lead to feelings of **resentment and anger**; younger children may have **magical wishing** that the sibling either is cured or dies; **high amount of somatic complaints**; peer relationships (friends may not understand how they are feeling) and school performance tend to decline.

Counseling

- **Re-engage** in appropriate activities as soon as possible.
- Watch carefully when grief has become **depression** and refer to **mental health professional**.
- Use a **multidisciplinary approach**: e.g. support from extended family, religious groups, **community bereavement groups**.
- Need **ongoing assistance in remembering and knowing** the person who has died; encourage talking about the person and sharing positive memories and experiences.

Sibling rivalry

- Sibling rivalry is **common and normal** but may be frequent and may develop into more severe problems: hurtful teasing, humiliating and insulting behaviors; at times physical harm (hitting, shoving); leads to **potential of longer-lasting emotional injuries**.
- Physicians should offer **advice and education** to parents on decreasing these types of behaviors and **anticipatory guidance with respect to the birth of another child**: discuss the new baby with the sibling by the second trimester; **offer special roles** in helping to care for the new baby; **protect the less dominant child** but not by consistently blaming the more dominant (older, perhaps) child.
  - If **psychological/behavioral problems** are identified, they need to be addressed through appropriate counseling and interventions.

Gifted child

A child with **superior abilities and the capability for high performance in one or several areas; require educational programs beyond what is offered** in order to realize their potential.

Parents may develop difficulties relating to the gifted child (child is brighter, parent is inadequate), and may lead parents to **treat the child differently** in terms of exercising **limits/discipline** and differently from other siblings; parents must be taught to treat child consistently with respect to same rules set forth for siblings.

- Parents may **push the child too fast** and not leave any time for play; need to advise parents to allow time for child's other, nonacademic interests.
- Too many, or all, areas may be encouraged; child may become **overwhelmed or even disinterested; child needs to make the decision** about which areas are of interest and the proportion of time spent in each.
- If parents consistently label child as "gifted" in front of her or his siblings, child **may feel special/superior**; especially problematic with **perceived differences to other siblings**.
- Child may have **increased pressure to always perform** well, and this may lead to **somatic complaints**; parents need to stress that the child should do as well as he is able.
- Gifted children **often play with older children** (more developmentally appropriate) and they may be friends of an older sibling, which can cause anger and resentment

and strain the peer relationships of the older child; siblings may also have **adjustment problems, anxiety, and decreased self-esteem**.

Pain

- Child's response is dependent on the **developmental status**; neonates and young infants show changes in **facial expression** (close eyes, furrow brows), cry, increase body movements, and have physiologic responses (increased heart rate, respiratory rate, blood pressure, change in skin color, dilated pupils); preschool children will scream and grimace, and will usually indicate where the pain is; between age 3–7 years, a child can generally state the location, quality, and intensity of the pain; at age 8 and older, they can use verbal or visual pain scales to relate the intensity of the pain.
- Managing pain depends on its nature (procedural, traumatic, chronic, recurrent, localized, or generalized), the severity, and the developmental response. For less severe and more acute pain, various **nonpharmacological methods** may be used (cognitive behavioral therapy, relaxation, distraction); for chronic recurrent pain, some children and families may be taught biofeedback, hypnosis, massage techniques, or yoga, or special techniques may be used (acupuncture, physical therapy); however, **any significant pain**, whether brief or chronic, must be controlled adequately with pharmacological agents.

Foster care and adoption

Physician's role in foster care and adoption

- Children placed into foster care need a screening evaluation by a physician within 72 hours and a comprehensive evaluation within 30 days of placement, including mental health and developmental/educational assessments.
- Children in foster care should consistently be seen by one primary-care physician, who provides **care coordination and case management** and has regular communication with the team.
- Children in foster care have special health-care needs: high rates of familial dysfunction, psychosocial problems, developmental problems, learning disabilities and academic underachievement, medical and dental problems.
- Physician needs to work effectively with adoptive families and agency: pre-adoption visits, review child's history and potential problems; advise parents, work with community social services, refer to specialists for any identified needs.
- **For international adoptions:** evaluate the health and developmental history from the available records, plot available growth points on U.S. growth charts, advise agency and parents about any special problems or needs. After adoption, provide a **comprehensive evaluation** (including evaluation for anemia, hepatitis B and C, fetal alcohol syndrome, lead, tuberculosis, birth defects, strabismus, feeding issues, developmental delay, psychosocial problems, and need for catch-up immunizations).

Foster care system

- Per the **Adoption and Safe Families Act**, a permanent plan must be made no later than **12 months** from child's entry into foster care.

- A **petition to terminate parental rights** must be filed to free a child for adoption if the child has spent **15 of the last 22 months in foster care**.
- The majority of children in foster homes have a history of **abuse or neglect**; majority have **behavioral and/or adjustment problems**, instability in the home.
- For youths aging out of the foster system (age 18 years or completion of high school), there is a high risk for **homelessness, incarceration, teen pregnancy, and drug/alcohol abuse**; prior to the youth's leaving the system, much attention needs to be given to independent living skills, job-procurement/training, and social support.

Cultural issues

- Physicians must be aware of cultural issues for **effectiveness in diagnosis and treatment.** Variability among different people and communities with respect to the seeking of health care.
- Differing and the perceptions of what constitutes bad health and the type of treatment that is needed.
- Physicians must develop diagnostic and treatment plans that **respect these beliefs but must still exercise good/safe medical judgment**.

Impact of mass media

- In the United States the average 2–5-year-old watches **20–30 hours of TV per week**.
- The recommendation of the American Academy of Pediatrics (AAP) is **to limit TV and other similar media to no more than 2 hours per day for children >2 years of age (no TV time for those under age 2 years)**.
- **Negative effects of TV and other media:** increased sedentary behaviors leading to decreased exercise and obesity; leads to aggressive and antisocial behaviors, fears; desensitizes to meaning and impact of violence; obscures fantasy vs. reality; trivializes sex and sexuality; **greater number of hours watched = greater stress**.

Violence

First childhood exposure to violence in the United States is usually **domestic violence**.

- **Highest during pregnancy**
- If wives are assaulted, higher likelihood that child will also be (including corporal punishment)
- Findings that may indicate violence in the home: child's depression, physical injuries, substance use; efforts by women to leave the home; initiation of separation or divorce
- Children living in high-crime-rate communities observe death more often and at younger ages.
- **Highest risk in these children with increased exposure to violence in media (TV)**
- **Risks with increasing violence exposure:** more injuries, psychosocial (especially anxiety and depression) and behavior abnormalities, **fear** of the world; decreased school performance; **increased violence in personal relationships**; decreased peer relationships, decreased self-esteem; **increased impulsive, risk-taking behaviors**

Specific Problems and Conditions

Enuresis—Child continues to wet himself **past the developmental age** when continence should have occurred, i.e. mental age of 5 years; it is a symptom with **many possible causes**; is **common in school-age children** (7% of 8-year-olds); **boys are more commonly affected** than girls.

Classification

- **Primary:** the child has never been consistently dry
- **Secondary:** the child was toilet trained (6 months of consecutive dryness) and has begun wetting again; more likely to have **psychological causes** (most) or organic causes (less common)
- **Nocturnal:** bedwetting at night and during naps; **more common** than diurnal
- **Diurnal:** daytime wetting

Etiological factors

- **Genetics:** strong familial tendency for **nocturnal enuresis**; always ask about family history
- **Psychosocial factors:** most children with enuresis do not have psychological problems; increased incidence of enuresis with lower socioeconomic status (SES), **family dysfunction/stress** (death, divorce, birth of a sibling)
- **Sleep and arousal:** studies have shown decreased arousal in some children with nocturnal enuresis
- **Urine volume:** some children with large, dilute urine volumes (decreased diurnal variation of antidiuretic hormone [ADH])
- **Bladder capacity:** decreased capacity
- **Constipation:** stool may impinge on bladder

Table 6.1: Differences between Diurnal and Nocturnal Enuresis

Diurnal	Nocturnal	Nocturnal + Diurnal
More common in girls; rare after age 9	Genetic: **decreased arousal and maturational bladder delay**	More likely to have **urinary tract abnormalities** (uncommon with either alone)
Most common cause is **waiting too long** to void	Secondary may be related to **psychosocial stressors or recent environmental changes**	
Secondary diurnal needs to be evaluated: **UTI, constipation, diabetes, chemical urethritis, stress incontinence**		

Abbreviations: urinary tract infection, UTI

Evaluation

- The most important part of the evaluation is a **careful history and physical**: pattern of enuresis (calendar is helpful) and stooling (constipation), developmental history and exam, psychosocial history and behavioral observations, sleep pattern and arousal, **family history**; how the parents have responded, and interventions tried so far
- **Lab findings in the absence of specific features of the history and physical are unlikely to be positive**; the only test to consider initially is a **urine analysis and culture**. If these are negative and the history and exam suggest no specific diagnosis, then no further lab tests are warranted.
- With **secondary enuresis, severe dysfunction, or a previous urinary tract infection (UTI), or when combined with encopresis, further workup should be performed:**
  - **Ultrasound** of the urinary tract, **voiding cystourethrogram** and **lower spine plain x-rays**
  - If these are negative, no further evaluation is needed.
  - If positive: **urological evaluation, neurological evaluation (depending on findings)**

Treatment

- First: **support and education (no punishment for accidents)**
- **Behavioral management is the mainstay:** voiding prior to bed, regular daytime trips to the bathroom, no fluids for several hours prior to bedtime, decrease carbonated beverages high in sugar, chart dry nights/days, **positive reinforcement**
- **Nocturnal enuresis:**
  - **Best method is conditioning with an alarm** (many available; probe placed on clothing in front of urethra senses initial drops of urine and sends signal to alarm); works as an **aversive stimulus**; when alarm sounds, child learns to respond, generally in 3–5 months; holds greater volumes of urine and eventually sleeps through the night.
  - Pharmacotherapy:
    - **Imipramine** (tricyclic antidepressant): **lightens sleep** enough that child can detect distended bladder; decreases frequency of nighttime wetting but gives **symptomatic relief**, is not a cure; side effects: insomnia, behavioral changes, arrhythmia with overdose
    - **1-Desamino-8-D-arginine vasopressin (DDAVP): decreases urine volume**; side effects—headache, nasal stuffiness, abdominal pain; potential for water intoxication; expensive; can be used safely for a year (**symptomatic relief,** not curative)

- **Diurnal enuresis:**
  - **Treat constipation first.**
  - **Small bladder**: responsive to **stretching exercises** (express a measured volume of urine; then stop the urine stream, hold as long as possible, and start again; measure increase in urine volume per void over time; offer positive reinforcement)
  - A **lazy bladder** (urgency but infrequent voids) is more responsive to **timed voiding** every 90–120 minutes.

Encopresis—Passage of feces into an inappropriate place after **age 4 years or the developmentally equivalent age**

Classification
- **Primary:** from infancy onward
- **Secondary:** after toilet training has been achieved
- **Retentive with constipation:** hard stool with overflow incontinence; **most cases**
- **Nonretentive:** without constipation

Etiological factors
- Under age 4 years, equal in boys and girls; school age: more common in boys
- **Associated with enuresis, UTI**
- **Possible organic causes:** Hirschsprung disease, spinal dysraphism, diarrhea, drugs, endocrine
- Behavioral/environmental causes and psychosocial problems: primary encopresis in males, usually with global delays; secondary in all children: higher amount of psycho-social problems and conduct disorder

Physiological effect of stool retention
—Hard stool impacted in rectum → overdistention of rectum → chronic stretching of rectal walls → distortion of tissues → loss of sensation (megacolon); after a maximal rectal capacity, there may be an explosive stool, or newly formed stool proximal to the impaction that is liquid, seeps around, and leaks out.

Evaluation and treatment
- **Assess fecal retention**; finding of impacted stool on rectal exam is sufficient; however, without that finding, a **plain x-ray** is needed.
- Constipation management:
  - **Clear fecal impaction:** short-term use of **enema and laxative** *plus* behavioral **management**
    - **Regular toilet use** after eating
    - **Positive reinforcement (no punishment)**
    - Ongoing behavioral management and **high-fiber diet**
    - If psychological problems: refer to mental health professional for evaluation and possible therapy
    - Biofeedback may be helpful in some cases of abnormal anal sphincter tone.
    - **No long-term laxatives!**

Rumination
- Definition: **weight loss or failure to gain weight due to repeated regurgitation** of food without nausea or any gastrointestinal pathology
- Rare; more in males; most present at age 3–14 years; can be fatal
  - **Psychogenic:** infants often with failure to thrive, disturbed parent–child relationship; otherwise normal development
  - **Self-stimulation:** seen mostly with mental retardation (even without any parent–child problems)

- Must **rule out repeated vomiting due to organic causes:** congenital gastrointestinal anomalies, pyloric stenosis, central nervous system (CNS) causes, inborn errors of metabolism
- Rx: behavioral therapy, parent counseling, family therapy

Pica

- Repeated chronic ingestion of nonnutritive materials; needs to be investigated if occurs after age 2 years
- Factors: lower SES, poor supervision, neglect, family disorganization, poor parenting skills, mental retardation; high in autism and other behavioral disorders
- Increased risk of **lead poisoning, iron deficiency anemia, and parasitic disease**

Failure to thrive

- Child who has **not grown at the expected rate for age and gender**
- Infant or toddler with weight >2 standard deviations (SD) below the mean for gestational-corrected age and gender (<5th percentile)
- Abnormal weight velocity: weight has decreased at least 2 major percentiles
- With ongoing problems: further decrease in height, head circumference, and development
- Abnormal weight velocity is disproportionate to that of the height velocity decrease

Etiology—The basic cause is **nutrition that is inadequate** to meet the needs of continuing weight attainment and growth.

- **Nonorganic causes:** majority of cases; multifactorial; problem with **parent–infant interaction/relationship**; overt neglect is not common. Many contributors: parental emotional, social, or physical problems; problems in the home environment and lack of support; infants that may be more difficult to care for (premature, multiple medical problems, small-for-gestational age [SGA]).
- **Organic causes:** any medical condition that is severe enough to interfere with weight attainment and to cause decreased growth; due to inability to take in enough calories (e.g., CNS disease), inability to absorb sufficient calories (e.g., malabsorption syndrome), or increased caloric needs due to disease causing increased caloric expenditure (e.g., severe persistent asthma)
- Mixed: combination of organic and nonorganic causes.

Observational clues to diagnosis—Early in the **first year:** more likely to present with **vomiting and diarrhea** (or a specific organic cause) **and developmental delays** (if it goes on over the course of the first year of life, it is likely to have long-term developmental effects); presenting **after 8 months, more likely with issues of control over feeding;** often with introduction of solid foods; mealtime behavioral problems, extreme dislikes of many foods, atypical eating behaviors; for the child >2 years, there may be complaints of **no appetite or child does not want to eat;** development is mostly normal, but may have **behavioral problems.**

Evaluation

- Document weight, height, head circumference, and weight-for-height on the appropriate growth curves.
- **Thorough medical history and physical exam:** identify any signs or evaluate for symptoms that might point to a specific condition; signs of child abuse
- **Development and behavioral assessment** (including oral motor assessment), family history (for any potential inherited problems); note parental sizes
- The results of the **history and physical (H&P) determines the use of laboratory studies** (H&P detects most causes of failure to thrive); only labs that may initially be helpful would be those to help document nutritional status (total protein and albumin); **no routine endocrine studies**
- **Nutrition and feeding evaluation:** amount and type, methods, preparation of infant formula; observe feeding and note interaction between parent and child; 3-day diet history
- **Social history:** mother's relationship with father; history of parents' childhood problems, support system; alcohol/drugs, major stresses, cultural practices
- Parent–child interaction: best way to observe is a **home visit**
- Possible psychiatric referral

Management

- Most can be accomplished with a **multidisciplinary team** (physician, nutritionist, speech/feeding therapist, social worker) in an **outpatient setting** (office visits and home visits)
- **Basis of management is nutritional:** start with up to 2 times the necessary calories for age to allow for catch-up and continued growth; eliminate poor nutritive intake and provide vitamin and mineral supplementation; may need to start with nasogastric feedings due to the larger caloric intake; monitor weekly weight gain. Also work on **improving parent–child interactions; provide support for social/family problems;** refer for mental health support as needed; provide developmental therapy for delays.
- **Need to hospitalize if:** concern about abuse, severe malnutrition, or extremely problematic relationships; or after failure of outpatient management

School refusal

- **Separation anxiety** is developmentally appropriate in the preschool child and for the first few months of kindergarten and first grade.
- The younger, **more anxious child** is more likely to have separation anxiety disorder; older children usually refuse because of school phobia (this is not the same as truancy, seen in adolescents); may also be associated with **depression and oppositional-defiant disorder;** typically interferes with daily functioning
- Somatic symptoms and family stress and disorganization are common.
- Management: parenting skills management, family therapy; child needs special attention—send to school daily and reward for each day spent there; if problem continues, need mental health referral

Vulnerable child syndrome—Caused by an early childhood event that a parent considered to be life-threatening; plus a continued unrealistic belief that the child is particularly susceptible to illness or death (based on parent's understanding and beliefs); and this has created a behavioral or learning problem in the child (all three are needed for diagnosis)

- In general, the earlier the event occurs, the more likely the syndrome.
- Higher prevalence with unmarried women, younger and less educated mothers, lower SES, decreased social support system, postpartum depression, and lack of emotional warmth

Etiologic factors—Pregnancy and delivery complications, preterm birth, neonatal illness/congenital anomalies, any serious illness, hospital admission, death of a previous child or relative early in life, prior miscarriage or stillbirth

Management—Primary prevention at time of health crisis (recognize anxiousness and deal with fears); clear statements of physical health after evaluations; do not use terms that are not supported by the diagnosis; help parents understand the relationship between the present problem and any past anxieties; advise interacting with the child in an appropriate manner; mental health referral, if necessary

Sleep problems

Normal developmental progression of sleep patterns:

- Newborn sleeps **16–18 hours per day**; majority is **REM sleep**.
- Through infancy, there are increasing periods of wakefulness with frequent naps.
- Consolidation into longer sleep (with sleeping through the night) may not occur **until age 1 year or later**.
- No further naps by mid-childhood; a **7-year-old sleeps about 10 hours at night**.
- **Adolescents sleep about 7–9 hours** (like adults), but may have problems with **delay in sleep phase** (due to erratic schedule or staying up late, especially on weekends).
- **REM sleep is more prominent in the last hours of sleep**, prior to awakening, and gradually decreases with age; **slow wave sleep (SWS; stage III and IV) is more prominent in the first third of the night**, peaks in early childhood and then drops off gradually.

Sleep refusal, sleep onset, and maintenance problems
- Common in young children; even with frequent awakenings, it is **rare for a child to become sleep-deprived**; the major problem is **sleep deprivation in the parents**.
  - **Sleep fragmentation and frequent night awakenings are normal in infants and toddlers**; contributors: nighttime feeding, excessive infant crying, certain medical conditions (gastroesophageal reflux, neurological disease, chronic illness) and medications; continued awakenings may be a sign of separation anxiety disorder
  - Older children (preschool and older) have **bedtime resistance and trouble falling asleep (limit-setting sleep disorder)**: inadequate sleep duration

- Major factors in the continuation of the behavior (leading to significant stress, fatigue, and psychological problems) are the **parents' reaction to the sleep problem and how they respond to it**.
- **For sleep fragmentation and awakenings, best treatment:** gradual or rapid withdrawal (**extinction**) of parental assistance at sleep onset and with any awakenings (increasing the interval of frequent checks, taking longer to respond to awakenings; insistence on child remaining in bed; slowly eliminating nighttime feedings); also, **positive reinforcement** to older children who do remain in bed; can also set bedtime closer to actual sleep time and then gradually advance the time (particularly useful with delayed sleep phase)
- For **limit-setting sleep disorder:** parent education regarding **appropriate limit-setting**, consistent bedtime routines, and positive reinforcement

Parasomnias

- Intermittent sleep behaviors involving **cognitive disorientation and autonomic and skeletal muscle disturbances**
- **First third of the night** (during SWS) **partial arousal parasomnias** (more common in preschool and young school-age children):
  - **Sleep terrors:** highly frightening event with extreme agitation and autonomic arousal; may be out of bed and may have repetitive/stereotypical behaviors; high threshold to arousal, but agitated if awakened; little or no recall and no daytime sleepiness; incidence is rare, but often with a family history
  - **Sleepwalking:** usually displaced from bed during the event, often with complex stereotypical/repetitive behaviors; low agitation and autonomic arousal; high arousal threshold and agitated if awakened; no or little recall and no daytime sleepiness; incidence is common with a positive family history

- **Last third of the night**, during REM sleep:
  - **Nightmares:** mild to high agitation and autonomic arousal with little motor behavior; low arousal threshold, awake and agitated after event; if prolonged, may have daytime sleepiness with vivid recall; very common with no family history

- Management: **Parental education and reassurance; avoid any exacerbating factors** (use good sleep hygiene principles); institute **safety precautions** for possible displacement from bed; rarely require any other form of therapy **unless frequent and persistent; evaluate for anxiety disorder, possible abuse**

Psychosomatic disorders

Conversion disorder—Symptoms or deficits that affect **voluntary or sensory function**; suggests a neurologic or medical problem, but after a thorough evaluation, the findings are not compatible with a neurological disorder, organic medical disorder, or direct effects of a substance. Examples: paralysis, blindness, amnesia, difficulty walking, unresponsiveness.

- Initiation of the symptom is not produced intentionally or pretended, and is preceded by conflicts or other stressors (and psychological factors)
- Causes **clinically** significant distress or impairment in functioning.
- Patients are said to have a relative lack of concern about the symptoms (*la belle indifference*)
- Theorized that the patient derives primary and secondary gains; **primary gain:** the symptoms allow the patient to express the conflict (leading to the conversion, and has been repressed subconsciously); **secondary gain:** symptoms allow the patient to avoid unpleasant situations or obtain support from others that would otherwise not be possible.
- Increased **anxiety, family disturbances, highly suggestible; history of physical or sexual abuse**; may have observed symptoms in a person close to the patient who had an actual medical condition.

Psychophysiologic disorder—Patient has a physical symptom which is known to be caused by a physiologic mechanism; the symptom is **stress-induced** and the **patient may recognize this** relationship. The symptom **responds to medication or stress reduction.**

Hypochondriasis—Preoccupation with **fears of having a serious disease** based on **misinterpretation of symptoms,** i.e., the physical signs and symptoms are normal; **fears persist** despite a **medical evaluation and reassurance;** causes distress or impairment in function; may be related to **anxiety or depression.**

Somatization disorder—Presents with **multiple somatic symptoms** in association with **general anxiety**; symptoms are not caused by known mechanisms; symptoms **persist despite therapy.**

Somatoform pain disorder—**Recurrent, ongoing pain** is the primary problem (e.g., headaches, abdominal pain); causes **distress and impairment in function; there are no positive physical findings.**

Factitious disorder—Deliberately fabricated; intentional production of or pretending of physical or psychological signs and symptoms; the motivation is to **maintain the sick role without any external incentives; if there is a clear potential for gain, the condition is called malingering.**

Chronic/recurrent pain—In **majority of children, a specific cause is never identified;** physician must tell the parents from the start that the child's care will occur without an identified etiology.

- **Recurrent abdominal pain:** highest in **school-age girls**; ill-defined, poorly localized, or **periumbilical**, with no systemic signs; may have **constipation** and left lower quadrant pain; occurs at least once per month for at least 3 months; exam (including rectal and neurological), growth and development, and lab screens are all negative; most resolve over time.

- **Recurrent chest pain:** average age of 12 years with equal prevalence in boys and girls; adolescents most often **psychogenic;** younger children with **musculoskeletal or pleuritic pain;** increases with inspiration or direct pressure.
- **Recurrent limb pain:** most are **"growing pains";** occurs late in the day or awakens from sleep; not joint-related; severe enough to interfere with activity; at least one time per month for at least 3 months; intermittent, with symptom-free periods; normal physical exam.
- **Recurrent headaches:** majority of headaches in children are either **migraine or tension;** the most concerning is acute-onset and progressive, frequently localized and associated with systemic and neurological findings. Recurrent, nonprogressive headaches are less likely to be associated with pathology.

Evaluation and management

History

- Thorough psychosocial evaluation (temperament, emotional state, school history, and peer relationships), recent stressors, and problems (observe behaviors and interactions), others who are ill with specific disease.
- Assess parental anxiety and parental pressure for a child to perform, as the psychosomatic disorder may be a manifestation of this.
- **School attendance/absenteeism** must be assessed.
- Look for possible gains from being sick.

Laboratory studies—Should be **based on documenting physical findings** to substantiate complaints of signs and symptoms; need to be cost-effective, otherwise there is a potential for a very costly and invasive investigation.

Management—**Avoid treatments that may have adverse effects** (placebo therapy is not reliable); **establish appropriate expectations at the first visit;** best is education and addressing psychological factors (possible therapy); return to normal activities; careful follow-up and reassurance.

Chronic illness and handicapped children—Emotions are similar to those seen in separation and loss: shock, disbelief, grieving and anger, stabilizing period, and acceptance. (Sequence is not necessarily linear, and some stages may be repeated.)

- **Effects on siblings:** some may enhance their own maturity and development by having the experience of helping; in others, **their own neglect is a major problem** and may lead to depression, aggression, acting-out, decreased school performance, and psychological problems.
- Extra burdens of care may affect **family cohesion** and may lead to **overt dysfunction and breakdown;** increased marital problems; overt psychological disturbances.
- **Psychosocial effects of home technology** (e.g., ventilator assistance, intravenous nutrition and medications); may require frequent/daily in-home nursing care; parents generally feel good about having the child at home instead of a hospital, but they also have negative feelings about loss of privacy, loss of control of parenting and care, and independence issues.

- There is an **increased rate of child abuse with chronic illness**.
- Physicians need to be supportive: provide all aspects of well-child care; recognize and help with psychosocial problems, family stresses, and coping skills; provide appropriate referrals to other professionals, community support groups, nursing services, social services, education, and placement.

Child Abuse and Neglect

Epidemiology

- Greatest number **between age 0–3 years**, with the **most deaths <1 year of age** (majority caused by a **parent or stepparent**); child abuse is significantly **underreported**.
- Most common form is **neglect**; common presentation is failure to thrive; adolescents are more likely to have physical abuse.
- **Siblings of an abused child are at increased risk of abuse**; the **mentally retarded** are at greater risk.
- **Other forms of domestic violence** frequently accompany child abuse.

Etiology and risks

- Child abuse is related to **child stressors** (chronic illness or handicap, attention-deficit hyperactivity disorder [ADHD], other child psychological problems or developmental disability), **social/situational stressors** (family problems, parent–child conflicts, low SES, multiple births, isolation), and **parent stressors** (depression, a **parent who was abused as a child, substance abuse**).
- Parents of abused children often have severely unrealistic expectations for their children's behavior.
- Abused/neglected children have increased risk of criminal behaviors, increased drug and alcohol use, and behavioral and functional disabilities, including social maladjustment and relationship problems.
- Abuse/neglect may be **physical abuse** (intentional injuries), **physical neglect** (lack of providing basic necessities such as food and clothing), **psychological neglect** (not providing love and support), **psychological abuse** (terrorizing, insulting), or **sexual abuse** (any act that is performed by an adult on a child with the intention of sexual gratification for the adult).

Physical abuse

- Suspect abuse when injury/injuries do not seem plausible with the explanation of how they were received, or injury/injuries are incompatible with the history or the child's level of development, or there is a delay in seeking care for significant injuries.
- Ultimately, the legal system determines whether or not there has been abuse or neglect.

Evaluation

- Record everything thoroughly, including environmental and developmental variables.
- Draw diagrams and label; **photograph everything**.

Table 6.2: Types of Physical Abuse and Important Issues

Type of Abuse	Important Features
Bruises	Most common; accidental bruises/skin injuries occur on surfaces of bone edges; **less likely areas are abdominal, back, genital, buttocks, neck**; if an object has been used, a **recognizable pattern** may be discerned on the skin. **Multiple bruises at different sites and at different stages of healing are significant.**
Fractures	Highly suggestive of abuse are multiple fractures at different stages of healing; bilateral fractures; complex skull fracture; fractures of the ribs, scapulae, sternum, and vertebrae; metaphyseal or femoral fractures in a child prior to the onset of walking; more likely to have a metaphyseal corner chip fracture from wrenching/pulling and a spiral fracture from twisting of an extremity. Suspect osteogenesis imperfecta if multiple fractures with blue sclera, short stature, bowing of long bones, osteopenia, and a positive family history.
Burns	Shape or pattern of burn may be diagnostic (cigarette with round, punched-out center); **immersion burns** into very hot water (bathtub) have **lines of demarcation with no splash marks**; there may be a glove/stocking pattern and failure of flexion creases; this is not compatible with falling into a tub of hot water.
Ingestions	Always think of the possibility that an ingestion of a toxic substance may be forced.
Intentional head trauma	**Most common cause of death from abuse**, and accounts for most serious head trauma in the first year of life; there may be no cutaneous findings; **retinal hemorrhages** are present in most young infants who are **shaken** (and are rarely seen with other forms of intracranial hemorrhage); this may be the cause of coma in a young infant without any cutaneous findings. Most common is **subdural hematoma**.
Abdominal injuries	Second most common cause of death from abuse; may present with any gastrointestinal findings; the **overlying skin may be free of bruises, or fist marks may be seen**; may cause **rupture** of the liver or spleen, **perforation or laceration** of the intestines, or **obstruction** from an intramural hematoma.

Table 6.3: Studies to Perform in the Evaluation of Physical Abuse

Type of Abuse	Diagnostic Studies
Bruises/ bleeding	Complete blood count, PT, PTT, platelets, bleeding time, INR
Fractures	Obtain a **bone survey** (not a single whole-body x-ray, but individual x-rays of all skeletal regions) in a **child <2 years** when there is any possibility of physical abuse, and only with bone tenderness or limited range of motion in older children; repeat in 7–10 days for callus formation; also for any child with an obvious fracture and the possibility of abuse; may also use **bone scan** to look for new fractures of the hands, feet, ribs, or vertebrae, or for subtle nondisplaced fractures of long bones.
Intentional head trauma	**CT initially (and skull films)** may need an MRI, depending on diagnostic features of the CT; **ophthalmological exam** for retinal hemorrhages
Abdominal trauma	Liver enzymes, amylase/lipase, stool for blood, urinalysis (for possible renal injuries), **abdominal CT with contrast**

Abbreviations: international ratio, INR; prothrombin time, PT; partial thromboplastin time, PTT

Management
- First, take care of any **medical, surgical, or psychiatric emergencies**.
- **Separate the child from the caregivers** (in the absence of the parents, a child older than 3 years may talk freely to an adult).
- Report to **Child Protective Services** (in most states, they must investigate within 24 hours; a detailed written report is required within 48 hours with a plan to eventually return the child to a safe home, preferably with the parents) and, depending on state laws, to the **police**.
- Physicians are **legally obligated** to report suspected abuse/neglect based on best medical judgment, but are protected if the court does not agree that there has been abuse or neglect.
- The **standard of proof in a civil court is the preponderance of evidence** (i.e., a lesser standard than in criminal proceedings with respect to child abuse).
- The child should be **hospitalized** for any medical or surgical treatment requiring inpatient management, if the diagnosis is unclear or if **no alternate safe place is available**; in most cases, the child will be placed into a safe home (relative or licensed foster placement); the child is appointed a guardian ad litem (child advocate); if the parents refuse, must obtain an **emergency court order**.
- Siblings and other children who have been watched by the suspected abusers should have full physical examinations within 24 hours to rule out abuse.
- Parents are provided with social services, interventions, and supervised parent visits (encouraged to do so).

Sexual abuse

Epidemiology
- Most common is sexual mistreatment by a **family member or nonrelative known to the child;** least common is abuse by a stranger; majority of offenders are male; girls are more commonly abused in child-care settings
- Significantly greater risk with stepfather than biological father
- Abuse of a daughter by a father or stepfather is the most common form of **reported** incest (but brother–sister incest is the most common overall).
- Approximate age distribution: one-third are <6 years of age, one-third are age 6–12 years, and one-third are >12 years.
- **Violence is not common**, but increases with the age and size of the victim and is more common with a single-stranger incident.
- Absence of a protective parent from the home increases the risk.
- Sexually abused children may also be physically abused and vice versa.

Presentation
- Historical: complaints of vaginal, penile, or rectal pain; genital discharge, bruising, bleeding, erythema; also consider with chronic dysuria, enuresis, or encopresis
- Explicit description or imitation of sexual behavior may indicate victimization or observation of sexual acts; also, drawing of genitalia by a child may indicate abuse.

- Physical exam:
  - Bite marks (measure, take wax impressions, wipe for saliva)
  - Abdominal exam: look for possibility of **pregnancy**; careful **rectal exam** for trauma
  - Separate labia and buttocks: a resistant young girl may be examined on her mother's lap, but the **best is a supine frog-leg exam to expose the hymen** (under good light with magnifying equipment).
  - Any postpubertal girl or any-age girl with major trauma or nonmenstrual bleeding (hymen with new or healed lacerations or transections, hymenal absence or remnants, posterior fourchette lacerations, vaginal wall tears, perianal lacerations) should have a **speculum exam and collection of specimens**; also any obvious sperm, semen, or pregnancy.
  - **Straddle injuries** to the labia and clitoris; scarring tears of labia minora
  - Labial adhesions, vulvar erythema, and anal tags are not signs of abuse.
  - Anal diameter >20 mm without the presence of stool
  - Genital trauma in boys is usually accidental or due to physical abuse: transient, non-specific erythema of penis.

Evaluation and management

Diagnostically critical is the first recorded forensic interview (notify the police); should be conducted with the **child alone on one occasion by experienced interviewers with law enforcement and social work (watching by closed-circuit TV).**

- **Avoid repetitive interviewing** as it increases the likelihood of leading questions, increases the chance of learned responses, is stressful, and increases the chance of inconsistency.
- Verbatim statements of the child may qualify as evidence in a criminal court.
- Questioning should start generally, and gradually become more specific; **anatomically correct dolls** may be used for a child who is nonverbal (the child can point).
- With DNA amplification, **forensic exam** may be useful for at least 4 days after the assault. There must be an **unbroken chain of evidence**.
- The presence of a **sexually transmitted disease** may indicate sexual abuse—semen, non–pregnancy related syphilis, gonorrhea, chlamydia, herpes II, or HIV; condyloma acuminata or *Trichomonas vaginalis* after age 3 years are probably diagnostic, but **herpes I and nonvenereal warts may be innocently inoculated with routine care in young child**.
- Specific recommendations for prophylactic treatment of sexual assault:
  - Treat once with intramuscular ceftriaxone for **gonorrhea**.
  - Treat once with oral metronidazole for ***T. vaginalis***.
  - Treat once with oral azithromycin for **chlamydia**.
  - Make sure **hepatitis B** immunization is completed.
  - For **pregnancy prevention** (within 120 hours of the assault): oral levonorgestrel; document pregnancy status
  - **Consider HIV prophylaxis** when there is oral, vaginal, or anal mucosal exposure. Test for HIV; if negative, prophylaxis may be stopped.

- **Do not assign blame to the victim** in helping families cope with sexual abuse; referrals should be made to rape crisis care centers, to mental health professionals for counseling, and to appropriate community support services.

Factitious disorder (Munchausen syndrome by proxy)

- Most commonly, a **mother simulates or produces disease in a child:** exposure of a child to toxic substances or medication, partial asphyxiation by smothering, producing recurrent fever with a hot-water bottle or heating pad, producing trauma to the skin to simulate rashes, or altering lab samples (urine or blood); **may continue while the child is hospitalized.**
- Victimized child is unable/unwilling to prevent this from happening and to identify the person who is causing the problems; **more common in very young children** but can occur in any-age child.
- With ongoing abuse, children may have **significant emotional and long-term psychological problems**, chronic medical disability, and even death.
- **Mother may have a history of Munchausen syndrome** and appears as an ideal parent.
- Physician must have a high index of suspicion so that unnecessary tests are not performed; must maintain **chain of evidence** for collection of all specimens, and they should be **evaluated for foreign substances**; search for **records from other medical facilities** (and for siblings); **careful observation** (concealed video) of hospitalized children
- After the diagnosis of Munchausen by proxy is made, physician and staff must confront the offending parent in a non-accusatory manner and offer help. Report to **Child Protective Services** immediately. The parent needs ongoing evaluation, therapy, counseling, education, and support.

PART TWO: MAJOR ETHICAL ISSUES IN PEDIATRICS

Withholding or Withdrawing Life-Sustaining Medical Treatment (LSMT)

- **Futility**—unilateral withdrawal or withholding of life-sustaining medical treatment (LSMT) by health-care professionals against the objections of the family
- **For conditions in which therapies have not been shown to deliver a positive response.**
- Medical therapies not medically indicated should be **withheld or withdrawn**
- Decisions are generally made in cooperation with the family.
- Most physicians consider it better to withdraw (as opposed to withhold) a therapy after the patient has failed to respond to it.
- Initial discussion should be on **"do not resuscitate"** (DNR) orders.
- **Address separately** the use of mechanical ventilation, intubation, cardiac medications, chest compression, and cardioversion. The orders need to be tailored to the **child's clinical condition; reviewed periodically.**

- Some states require clear evidence of a patient's **prior wishes in order to withdraw hydration and nutrition;** however, legal rulings have been for adults.
- Decisions by the child's parents after discussion with health-care professionals, the hospital ethics committee, and the parents' support system (other family members, clergy); and thorough consideration of moral and legal issues.

Palliative Care

- Involves the relief of symptoms/conditions interfering with any reasonable quality of life (relief of pain).
- Double effect—withholding or withdrawing palliative medications may hasten the patient's death while the **intent is to relieve pain**, increasing the dose of a narcotic analgesic to control pain may hasten death
- Does not mean the physician increased the dose to cause the patient's death in a shorter period of time (It was the ethical thing to do, regardless of the unintended outcome).
- **The AAP does not support physician-assisted suicide/euthanasia.**

Futile Care and Disabled Infants

- Federal child-abuse laws (1984) **prohibit withholding beneficial medical treatment from disabled infants except under certain conditions:** permanent unconsciousness, or the treatment would prolong dying or would be futile.
- "Baby Doe" rules—dismissed by the Supreme Court in 1986.
- Civil rights laws of 1989 mandate medical care for every child but state that it is inhumane to provide continuing therapy if **virtually futile** (some variation from state to state).

Delivery Room Decisions

- The ideal decision for CPR in the delivery room is to have sufficient antenatal information to discuss a decision with the parents upon delivery of the infant.
- In emergencies, need to **avoid unilateral decisions, respect parental authority**, and **not change course.**
- Decision to resuscitate **must not be delayed or partial.**
- Situations when resuscitation may be withheld: confirmed gestational age <23 weeks or birth weight <400 g; gestational age 23–24 weeks determined by assessment and with parental choice; when the outcome is known to be lethal or result in severe disability and parents have had the chance to participate in the decision.

Pregnancy Decisions

If a **pregnant woman** refuses therapy that may benefit a fetus at risk for death or severe disability, the courts may need to intervene.

- Physician should not oppose the woman's decision unless the risk to the woman is negligible, and the intervention is a proven therapy, without which there will be irreversible harm or death to the fetus or infant.
- **Last resort** should be to go to the court after seeking to persuade the woman and try other methods of conflict resolution (e.g., hospital **ethics committee**).

Organ Donation

Requests for **organ donation** should be separate from discussions of brain death or LSMT.

- Two rules governing the timing of organ donation: (1) Issue of **irreversibility**, (**no spontaneous return of circulation after CPR is performed, rather than failure to restore neurological function in spite of any intervention**). (2) **Absence of a conflict of interest** on the part of any person involved with organ procurement.
- For a **non–heart-beating donor (NHBD)**, the timing of organ procurement depends on the **time for asystole to occur after the withdrawal of LSMT** (usually 1–2 hours).
- Institutions and states have policies for **brain-death criteria.**

Ethics Committees

- **Institutional ethics committees** (IECs) are for voluntary consultation.
- Write and review hospital ethics policies.
- Educate professionals, patients, and families.
- Serve in individual case consultation and conflict resolution.

Patient–Parent–Pediatrician Relationship and Professionalism
Assent and Consent

- Legal age for informed consent varies among states. **Parents' right to direct a child's medical care is more limited than that of their own medical care**.
- Physicians have an **independent obligation** to act in the child's best interest (not just the parents' decision).
- Consent required for each procedure, must include all information and adverse effects, and must be obtained by the person performing the procedure.
- Informed consent requires the physician to involve the child at any given developmental level into decision-making despite immaturity; the child should express her **assent or dissent**, but parents supply the consent. (The **right of a minor to consent varies per state**.)
- Right for self-consent does occur in some situations: exam (including pelvic exam) in a sexually active adolescent, care for drug and mental health problems (in many states), contraception (most states), and abortion without parental consent (varies from state to state).
- Minors do not need parental consent for: emergencies; in cases involving emancipated minors (no longer subject to parental control and support); or with the mature minor rule (sufficiently mature and responsible to understand their illness and potential risks; mostly with low-risk care).

Code of Ethics

In the **AAP Code of Ethics**, physician has the duty:

- to be **intellectually honest and straightforward** in interactions with patients and in all professional communications
- to represent **reliability and accountability** to children and their families
- to treat all patients with **respect and sensitivity**
- to understand children's and families' reactions from their point of view (**compassion and empathy**)
- to make a lifelong commitment to **self-improvement**
- to maintain **self-awareness and knowledge of limits**
- to offer effective **communication and cooperation** in working as a team
- to have **unselfish regard** for the welfare of others
- to hold all information in strictest **confidence** (No medical information can be passed on to anyone without the direct consent of the patient.)
- to avoid behaviors that patients and parents might misunderstand as having sexual or inappropriate social meaning
- to accept only modest gifts from patients and families (Value of the gifts must never appear to influence the physician's professional judgment.)

Research with Children

- Should not be included in research **unless it is scientifically necessary**.
- Approval obtained from **Institutional Review Boards (IRBs)** prior to implementing studies.
- Must be protected by carefully **determining that the potential benefits outweigh the risks**.
- Involve children in the decision to enroll them, and ensure all procedures are done as safely as possible with no untoward psychological effects.
- For nontherapeutic research, no expected direct benefit for the subject and therefore any risk may present an unfavorable risk-to-benefit ratio.
- Federal regulations allow children to participate in **minimal-risk research** (i.e., slightly more than the risk of experiences of everyday life or from routine physical and psychological exams and tests).
- For **therapeutic research** the risks can be **more than minimal**, but must be **justified by the expected benefit**.
- **Innovative therapies** are new or unproven therapies which may provide no benefit to the patient, and there are no federal regulations with respect to these (generally sought out as a last resort).

RESPIRATORY DISORDERS

Select Signs and Symptoms

Stridor

Coarse, vibratory sound, **loudest on inspiration; extrathoracic airway obstruction**; anywhere from low/medium to high-pitched. **Critical obstruction occurs if present in both phases of respiration.**

Most common causes of congenital stridor—Nasopharyngeal malformation/stenosis/mass (cyst, hemangioma); neck masses (**bronchial cleft cyst, cystic hygroma**); **laryngotracheomalacia**, vocal cord dysfunction/paralysis, **subglottic stenosis**; extrathoracic vascular ring/sling

Most common causes of acquired stridor—Infectious (**croup [or spasmodic croup], epiglottitis, bacterial tracheitis, retropharyngeal/peritonsillar abscess**); foreign-body aspiration (lodged in extrathoracic structure); trauma (subglottic stenosis secondary to **intubation, vocal cord paralysis after neck or thoracic surgery**, burns or scalds of the larynx; metabolic (hypocalcemia or hypomagnesemia); allergic reaction

Diagnostic studies—Most acute infectious causes may be diagnosed on the basis of history and physical, and in many cases **radiographic studies may be contraindicated** (e.g., croup). Without evidence of severe airway obstruction, **first tests for chronic or recurrent stridor are AP and lateral neck x-ray/fluoroscopy, chest x-ray and barium swallow.** In most cases (**most accurate test**) laryngoscopy is necessary for diagnosis. A CT or MRI with contrast is best for vascular abnormalities.

Wheezing

Represents an **intrathoracic obstruction; worse on expiration; significant disease can lead to obstruction in both phases of respiration.** Obstruction of a larger airway produces a low to medium-pitched, focal (**monophonic**) wheeze, while peripheral airway obstruction is characterized by diffuse, medium to high-pitched (**polyphonic**) wheezes.

Congenital/recurrent wheezing—Primary intrathoracic tracheobronchomalacia, tracheal stenosis, webs or clefts; **tracheoesophageal fistula (TEF)**; extrinsic airway compression **(vascular rings/slings, double aortic arch); cystic fibrosis (CF); dyskinetic cilia syndrome**

Causes of acquired recurrent wheezing—**Asthma** and allergy (allergic bronchopulmonary aspergillosis)*;* **vocal cord dysfunction**; infection (**bronchiolitis**, bronchiectasis, pneumonia); **gastroesophageal reflux** (GER; from aspiration or reflex bronchoconstriction); **foreign-body aspiration (asymmetric wheezing and breath sounds)**; extrinsic airway compression (lymph node, lung abscess); **pulmonary edema** (congestive heart failure); mass (hamartoma, mediastinal mass, sarcoma)

Exercise intolerance
Most commonly seen for evaluation of inability to tolerate an exercise program at school or at play, **most commonly related to deconditioning in a child who is obese and sedentary** or is secondary to a primary illness.

Secondary causes—**Exercise-induced asthma (leading cause);** chronic lung disease; anemia; congenital or acquired heart disease; neuromuscular disease, primary myopathy; endocrine (hypothyroidism, diabetes)

Tachypnea
Sensitive but **nonspecific indicator of respiratory disease. Respiratory rates vary with age and varies with sleep, eating, and activity**; may also occur with fever, metabolic acidosis, or a primary respiratory center abnormality.

Hemoptysis
Approach to diagnosis—(1) **history of trauma or a recent procedure**; (2) **preexisting illness** may be responsible for the bleeding; (3) determine if the blood is from the lower respiratory tract, upper respiratory tract, or gastrointestinal (GI) tract (bright-red blood is from the respiratory tract vs. darker blood from GI tract).

Major causes of hemoptysis—Trauma or procedural (external or penetrating chest-wall injury/lung contusion; diagnostic procedure, therapeutic procedure, post-op complication); **severe coughing** from any cause; epistaxis, severe sinusitis, severe pharyngitis; infection (pneumonia); CF (**most common chronic condition with hemoptysis in children); foreign body**; toxic inhalations; congenital/acquired heart disease (chronically elevated pulmonary venous pressures); arteriovenous malformations; pulmonary hemosiderosis; vasculitis secondary to immune or connective tissue disorder

Initial management—Most important first step is **volume resuscitation and transfusion of blood with maintenance of an adequate airway. Bronchoscopy** is used with active bleeding to provide suctioning, for removal of debris, or removal of a foreign body and bronchial artery embolization. For more diffuse bleeding, corticosteroids and other immunosuppressive agents.

Clubbing—Thickening/broadening of ends of fingers and toes due to connective-tissue hypertrophy and hyperplasia with increased vascularity.

Causes—**Intrapulmonary shunting and inflammation:** severe infection, bronchiectasis, interstitial lung disease, malignancy; cyanotic heart disease and bacterial endocarditis

Cyanosis

Need at least **5 g of desaturated** (reduced) hemoglobin; occurs first in tissues with low blood flow or high oxygen extraction (peripheral cyanosis). Cyanosis is **not a sensitive indicator of oxyhemoglobin desaturation** because **oxygen content** is dependent on the total hemoglobin concentration (oxygen content in a patient with cyanosis who is polycythemic may be normal, and a patient with anemia may have a low oxygen content and not be cyanotic). **Best way** to verify a clinical observation of cyanosis is with arterial blood gas and oxyhemoglobin saturation.

Most common causes of central cyanosis—**Arterial hypoxemia** (primary pulmonary disease, pulmonary vascular disease, atrioventricular [AV] malformations); **cyanotic congenital heart disease** (right-to-left shunt); **hypoventilation** and apnea/respiratory depression; **methemoglobinemia** and other hemoglobinopathies

Chronic cough

Etiologies of chronic/persistent cough—**Postinfectious** (weeks of coughing after adenoviral, influenza infections); **sinusitis; asthma** (cough may be the only manifestation); **allergic rhinitis** (postnasal drip); **CF; tuberculosis (TB)**, fungal infection; **severe GER with or without aspiration**; hypersensitivity pneumonitis (physical/chemical irritation from environmental exposures); **foreign-body** or liquid aspiration; **trauma** (pulmonary contusion); congenital anomalies; mediastinal masses; immunodeficiency, ciliary dyskinesia, HIV; **psychogenic cough tic** (**habit cough**: a harsh, barking cough in a school-age child; refractory to treatment; does not occur during sleep; child appears well and is not bothered by the cough; often with family or school dysfunction/stresses)

Diagnostic tests—Initial screening tests should be a **chest x-ray, TB skin test, spirometry, and sweat test** before resorting to other tests.

Respiratory failure

Impaired ability to maintain adequate oxygen and carbon dioxide exchange. **Hypoxemic respiratory failure**: PaO_2 <60 mm Hg with an FIO_2 >0.6 without evidence of cyanotic heart disease. **Acute hypercarbic respiratory failure**: $PaCO_2$ >50 mm Hg. Acute respiratory failure (minutes/hours) is immediately life-threatening; chronic respiratory failure (months to years) may be life-threatening.

Signs and symptoms—**Acute hypercarbia**: tachycardia, headache (dilatation of cerebral vessels), agitation, confusion, flushing (peripheral vasodilatation with moderate to severe hypercarbia); **acute hypoxemia**: lethargy, confusion alternating with agitation, restlessness, dizziness, cold extremities (peripheral vasoconstriction), impaired cognition; **chronic hypoxemia**: polycythemia, pulmonary hypertension, cor pulmonale; **chronic hypercarbia** is compensated by renal mechanisms.

Physiologic mechanisms—**Hypoventilation** (respiratory depression from central nervous system [CNS] disease, neuromuscular disease); **right-to-left shunt** (venous blood enters the aorta from intracardiac shunts); **ventilation/perfusion inequalities** (most important cause; alveoli that are perfused but not ventilated results in intrapulmonary shunting; e.g., atelectasis, pneumonia, acute/adult respiratory distress syndrome [ARDS]); **diffusion block** (any reduction in the alveolar-capillary gradient, thickened alveolar-capillary membranes, or decreased rate of gas transport; e.g., pulmonary edema)

Etiologies—**Pulmonary disease, CNS disease** (hypoventilation), **neuromuscular disease** (weakness), **chest-wall abnormalities** (flail chest, severe kyphoscoliosis)

Management—**Oxygen to all with acute respiratory failure, and eliminate initiating factors as quickly as possible.** Provide oxygen **carefully with exacerbation of chronic respiratory insufficiency** (potential to decrease the compensatory respiratory drive). Ventilatory support is needed for worsening/persistent gas exchange abnormalities. **Goal is not to normalize the blood gases** but to maintain adequate oxygenation and ventilation with permissive hypoxemia and hypercarbia. Immediate ventilation is not necessary if a diagnosis of respiratory depression is secondary to a cause that may be quickly reversed (narcotic ingestion).

Diagnostic Testing for Pulmonary Disease

Table 7.1: Select Diagnostic Modalities

Diagnostic Study	Value
Spirometry (pulmonary function testing)	Measures vital capacity and expiratory flow rates; FEV_1 correlates well with severity of obstruction. Maximal midexpiratory flow rate (average flow during the middle 50% of FVC) is a more reliable indicator of mild airway obstruction.
Pulse oximetry	Measures oxygen saturation, not reliable <70%; accuracy depends on adequate tissue perfusion; may be erroneous values with very dark skin; not significantly altered with hyperbilirubinemia.
Capillary blood gases	If performed well, gives results similar to an arterial blood gas (pH best, PO_2 worst); best to correlate PaO_2 values with pulse oximetry.
Imaging:	
PA and lateral upright chest x-ray in full inspiration	Ideal method for chest x-ray
Lateral decubitus film	If pleural fluid suspected
Inspiratory and forced expiratory film	If a foreign body suspected
Lateral and AP neck	For upper airway obstruction, supra or subglottic spaces
Fluoroscopy	For stridor, diaphragm movement, to direct procedures
Barium swallow	TEF, vascular rings/slings, recurrent pneumonia, persistent cough, persistent stridor or wheezing
Chest CT (with contrast to enhance vascular structures)	Best for mediastinal or pleural lesions, solid or cystic parenchymal lesions, bronchiectasis, pulmonary embolism
MRI	Better for hilar and vascular anatomy associated with vascular rings/slings
Radionuclide lung scan (Tc-99m)	Pulmonary embolism

Abbreviations: forced expiratory volume in 1 second, FEV_1; forced vital capacity, FVC; tracheoesophageal fistula, TEF

Upper Airway Disorders

Infectious croup

Acute laryngotracheobronchitis, mainly causing **subglottic narrowing** from inflammation and edema; most commonly due to **parainfluenza**, influenza, respiratory syncytial virus (RSV) or adenovirus; ages **6 months–5 years** and occurring in the **autumn**; may last 7–14 days.

Key diagnostic words—Young child with **upper respiratory infection (URI) symptoms** with or without low-grade fever, then **barking cough** and **stridor** (primarily inspiratory); **moderate to severe croup if**: increased respiratory rate, retractions, stridor in both phases of respiration, stridor at rest, hypoxia

Diagnostic steps—**None are necessary** (except for pulse oximetry during assessment). If an airway x-ray is to be performed (because of uncertainly of the diagnosis), a person expert in airway management needs to accompany the child to radiology; the classic finding is **steeple sign** (subglottic air column coming to a point).

Management of mild croup—**No treatment is necessary**; supportive care; no benefit has ever been demonstrated with the use of cool or warm mist. Most important is observation for any signs of worsening and to ensure adequate hydration.

Management of moderate to severe croup (as defined above)—**First give oxygen** (if room air saturation <93%), then:

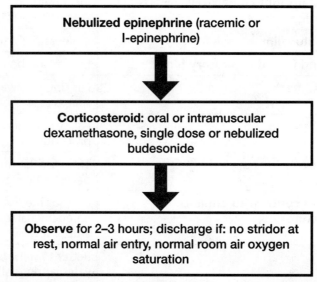

Figure 7.1: Management of Moderate to Severe Croup

Hospitalize if: Progressive stridor, severe stridor at rest, any respiratory distress (increased work of breathing), hypoxia, poor oral intake, or evidence of dehydration

Epiglottitis

Acute bacterial infection of **epiglottis and supraglottic** area causing **severe airway obstruction**; now **uncommon** in the United States due to long-term use of *Haemophilus influenzae* type b immunization; most causes now in vaccinated children are *S. pyogenes, S. pneumoniae, and S. aureus*.

Key diagnostic words—Young child with **acute onset of high fever and extremely sore throat with dysphagia**; quickly appears **toxic** and has **trouble breathing**; is in the "sniffing position" (tripod sitting, leaning forward with **neck hyperextended**, nose raised, **mouth open**) and **drooling. Stridor is a late finding** (near-complete airway obstruction).

Diagnostic steps—The history and appearance are classic. **No examinations or tests are needed, nor should they be done** (may provoke the child and lead to complete airway obstruction). In cases where the diagnosis is uncertain and neck x-rays are obtained, a person skilled in intubation must accompany the child to radiology. The finding may be the **"thumb sign"**, i.e., the swollen epiglottis. The most accurate diagnostic test is **direct laryngoscopy** (visualizing the "cherry-red" epiglottis) and performing **tracheal cultures** for microbiological diagnosis and antibiotic sensitivities.

Management—Allow the child to **stay comfortably in the mother's lap** (without doing any unnecessary exams), **arrange immediately for airway management**; if in a setting away from a hospital, arrange for **emergency medical transport** to a hospital with professionals expert in airway management.

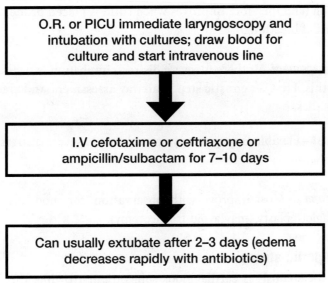

Figure 7.2: Management of Epiglottitis

Bacterial tracheitis

Bacterial complication to a viral upper respiratory infection (mostly laryngotracheitis); most causes are from ***S. aureus*** (then *Moraxella catarrhalis*, non-typable *H. influenzae*, and anaerobes). Most pathology from **swelling at cricoid cartilage** with thick secretions and possibly a pseudomembrane (like diphtheria).

Key diagnostic words—Child of 5–7 years (average age) with viral **URI symptoms, then getting worse: brassy cough and high fever, appears toxic but no drooling; can lie supine, and no dysphagia** (differences from epiglottitis)

First step in diagnosis—Usually none is needed, but an airway x-ray is reasonable; shows a narrowed, ragged-appearing trachea.

Next step in management—First, an airway may be needed for moderate to severe distress; otherwise, all patients need to be hospitalized for **IV broad-spectrum antibiotics** with staphylococcal coverage.

Laryngomalacia

Most common cause of congenital stridor; decreased cartilaginous support leads to **collapse of supraglottic structures during inspiration**, from little or no to severe respiratory distress

Key diagnostic words—**Inspiratory low-pitched stridor in a newborn beginning in the first 2 weeks of life**; stridor is made worse with any stress (e.g., crying) and is worse in the supine position (and therefore **improves when child is placed prone**); may or may not be increased work of breathing.

First step in management—If there is severe distress, intubation is necessary; most cases will not require this. **First diagnostic step is airway assessment and chest x-ray for any associated anomalies.**

Most accurate test—**Flexible laryngoscopy**; if moderate to severe distress, need **complete bronchoscopy**.

Further management—Most improve with **observation**; for moderate to severe cases, endoscopic supraglottoplasty (may avoid tracheotomy).

Congenital subglottic stenosis

Primary subglottic stenosis is cartilaginous subglottic narrowing; the vast **majority of secondary cases are due to endotracheal intubation.**

Key diagnostic words—Primarily **inspiratory stridor** beginning shortly after birth, or after the first upper respiratory infection; may present as **recurrent or persistent croup. Stridor does not decrease with switching from the supine to the prone position.**

First step in management/diagnosis—Provide **airway** for severe distress; otherwise, first step is an airway x-ray (subglottic narrowing) and chest x-ray (any associated anomalies).

Most accurate diagnostic step—**Direct laryngoscopy**

Further management—Depending on severity, may need a cricoid split (anterior laryngotracheal decompression) or reconstruction with grafting.

Tracheobronchomalacia

Insufficient cartilage to maintain airway patency (**chondromalacia**); either primary or secondary (due to external compression from vascular rings/slings, masses) or from TEF, or prolonged mechanical ventilation and chronic lung disease.

Key diagnostic words—Infant with a **low-pitched monophonic** (single-tone) **wheeze over central airways**; persistent respiratory congestion; bronchodilators do not help

Diagnostic studies—**Fluoroscopy with spot x-rays** (look for right aortic arch) may show dynamic airway collapse; if inconclusive, then **bronchoscopy** is needed; if there is a right aortic arch and/or if a vascular sling/ring is suspected causing secondary tracheomalacia, then the best study is an **MRI**.

Management—For mildest cases, use **nebulized ipratropium bromide**; for more severe cases, a **tracheotomy with the use of continuous positive airway pressure (CPAP)**, rarely, **surgery** may be required. Airflow typically increases with airway growth, with **most wheezing gone by age 3 years**.

Foreign-body aspiration

Most occur in children **under 3 years of age**, who routinely put objects in their mouths and who have the smallest airways. Most common is the **peanut** (and this always needs to be asked about). **Complete obstruction and asphyxiation will occur with a globular object that is the right size to cause tracheal obstruction (e.g., a hot dog cut into pieces).**

Key diagnostic words—Initially may be **episodes of choking, gagging, and/or coughing** for some period of time, then an **asymptomatic interval** when the object lodges (which may delay the diagnosis if the child appears asymptomatic and the initial history is not clear-cut); then, if foreign body not removed, there are **complications** of obstruction, erosion with bleeding, and/or infection (fever, cough, pneumonia, hemoptysis). Key exam feature is an **asymmetry** in breath sounds and wheezing (the most common finding).

Most important first step in management—Refer for **immediate rigid bronchoscopy** to remove the object (**most accurate test and most effective management**). If not clear-cut, obtain **plain inspiratory and forced expiratory x-rays**. The most common finding is **asymmetric air-trapping** (and possibly **obstructive emphysema**) due to a **ball-valve mechanism** of the obstructing object: intrathoracic airways expand on inspiration and therefore air may still get around the object and fill the distal airway; but the airway gets smaller on expiration, and the object prevents the air from escaping and therefore becomes trapped. If this continues, then there is more and more air-trapping and emphysema will develop. The **mediastinum may be shifted** to the opposite side, and that may result in **atelectasis**.

Lower Airway Disorders

Bronchiolitis

Bronchiolar inflammation, edema, and obstruction with air-trapping and overinflation; ventilation/perfusion inequalities resulting in various degrees of **hypoxemia** and hypercarbia with tiring; more severe with smaller airways and decreased lung function (**prematurity, previous ventilation, chronic lung disease, congenital heart disease, immunodeficiency**); average duration is <2 weeks; most common organism is **respiratory syncytial virus (RSV)**, then parainfluenza, adenovirus, mycoplasma. **Higher incidence of wheezing and asthma in children who have had bronchiolitis.**

Key diagnostic words—Infant exposed to a family member with **URI symptoms** during **cold-weather** months; first URI symptoms with **fever**, then **cough and expiratory wheezing with prolonged expiratory phase, tachypnea, and dyspnea** (to different degrees) with **increased work of breathing** (nasal flaring, chest-wall retractions); may be cyanotic and hypoxemic. In young infants, **apnea** may be prominent early.

Diagnostic evaluation—A **chest x-ray** should be obtained for baseline if the infant is in **acute respiratory distress**. X-ray most likely will show **hyperinflation and patchy atelectasis**; with increased work of breathing and hypoxemia, more likely to see focal infiltrates (also with decreased breath sounds, crackles, and grunting). **Most accurate test is identifying the organism** (rapid immunofluorescence, polymerase chain reaction [PCR]), **not needed unless the diagnosis is not clear or if it needs to be performed for epidemiologic reasons (local or widespread outbreaks).**

Most important first step in management—**Pulse oximeter** placed at the beginning of assessment and **oxygen administered** with low oxygen saturations (<93%). If any signs of **acute respiratory distress, hospitalization** is required, primarily for close observation and supportive care.

Further management—It is appropriate to administer a trial of a short-acting nebulized beta-agonist (albuterol) (there may be a mild, short-term effect in some patients); if there is a positive response, it should be continued. Otherwise, therapy is **supportive with close observation** to respiratory status and hydration. For hospitalized patients: oxygen and monitoring, nasogastric (NG) feeds or IV fluids if respiratory status precludes safe oral feedings, frequent oral and nasal suctioning to clear secretions; steroids are not indicated in a previously healthy infant; **Ribavirin** (aerosolized antiviral) may be administered to patients with underlying conditions who are more likely to have respiratory failure and require mechanical ventilation (research studies show no consistent clinical benefit).

Prevention—**Palivizumab** (Synagis; intramuscular monoclonal antibody to RSV-F protein) should be used **monthly during the RSV season for high-risk infants under 2 years of age** (<34 weeks' gestation at birth, ventilation, chronic lung disease, acyanotic heart disease, and immunodeficiency).

Congenital malformations

Pulmonary hypoplasia—Usually secondary to **intrauterine disorders** (oligohydramnios, diaphragmatic hernia, hydrops with effusions, thoracic deformities); decrease in airways and arterial branching (decreased alveoli and airway generations) → decreased area for gas exchange; may be unilateral or bilateral (**more likely to be fatal**). Severe hypoplasia presents in the newborn period as **respiratory insufficiency**; milder hypoplasia may present later as respiratory distress with a viral infection.

Cystic adenomatoid malformation—Dysplastic lung tissue mixed with normal lung tissue, usually involving one lobe; maldevelopment of terminal bronchial structures; may occur as one or more large cysts (good prognosis), microcysts associated with other congenital anomalies (poor prognosis) or as a solid mass (often fatal). Diagnosis most commonly made with **antenatal ultrasound**. After birth, a **chest x-ray shows a cystic or solid mass, possibly with a shift of the mediastinum**; next diagnostic step: perform **CT for more accurate location, sizing, and anatomy**. Usually presents in the newborn period as respiratory distress. May be excised or aspirated **antenatally** or open **fetal surgery** may be performed; postnatally, **surgery** should be performed on all symptomatic patients by age 1 year (later malignant degeneration); many asymptomatic patients may have resolution over time.

Vascular malformations—Most common is **aberrant innominate artery** presenting as secondary tracheomalacia—expiratory wheezing and cough; also **vascular rings** result from abnormal development of the **aortic arch structures**. Most common vascular ring is a double **aortic arch** (completely encircles the trachea and esophagus); almost all present within the first 3 months of life with **wheezing (worse with feeding and crying; better with neck extension), dyspnea, cough, and dysphagia**. Incomplete structures (**slings**) include a **pulmonary artery sling and an aberrant right subclavian artery,** which is usually asymptomatic. First diagnostic tests should be **plain chest radiography with a barium swallow**. These may show airway and/or esophageal compression, indentation, deviation, or narrowing. Diagnosis may be confirmed with **two-dimensional echocardiography or MRI. Surgery is performed in symptomatic patients with evidence of airway compression.**

Parenchymal Disease

Hydrocarbon aspiration

Only a small number of children have significant pneumonitis, but the risk is increased with >30 mL. The most toxic compounds include **CHAMP: c**amphor, **h**alogenated hydrocarbons, **a**romatic hydrocarbons, **m**etal-associated compounds, **p**esticide-associated compounds.

Key diagnostic words—From 30 minutes to several hours after an aspiration, presents with **acute lung disease**: grunting, retractions, cough, dyspnea, fever, and hypoxemia. **Develops chronic lung disease with pulmonary function abnormalities, possibly for years.**

Diagnostic tests—The **chest x-ray findings peak at 48–72 hours** (earliest at 2–8 hours): focal infiltrates, pneumatoceles, pleural effusions.

Management—**No gastric emptying because the risk of aspiration is greater than systemic toxicities** (unless large quantity aspirated, then with careful placement of a cuffed endotracheal tube first); provide **oxygen, fluids, and mechanical ventilation based on clinical presentation and arterial blood gases.** Patients who are asymptomatic or have a normal chest x-ray still **need to be observed for 6–8 hours**, as symptoms may be delayed.

Pneumonia

Etiology, clinical presentation, diagnostic findings, and treatment

Table 7.2: Pneumonias in Children after the Neonatal Period (based on age and organism)

	Viral (RSV, Influenza, Parainfluenza, Adenovirus)	*Chlamydia trachomatis*	*Streptococcus pneumoniae*	*Staphylococcus aureus*	*Chlamydia or Mycoplasma pneumoniae*
Age	**Most common cause under age 5 years**	**1–3 months** after acquisition from vaginal birth of colonized mother	**Most common cause of focal/lobar pneumonia in child of any age**	Uncommon; may be seen in debilitated, chronically ill, instrumented, or immuno-suppressed child	**Most common cause in children age 5–18 years** (atypical or community-acquired pneumonia)
Key diagnostic features	**URI** symptoms with fever, **tachypnea, dyspnea, crackles, and wheezes**	**Afebrile, no wheezes;** insidious onset; **staccato cough,** tachypnea, rales	Acute onset, shaking chills, and high fever; severe cough, tachypnea, increased work of breathing and signs of distress, tachycardia, cyanosis; early decrease in percussion, scattered rhonchi and rales; then, with consolidation, further **decrease in breath sounds and dullness to percussion**	High fever, progressive respiratory distress, cyanosis and hypoxemia; poor inspiratory effort and pain with **empyema;** exam findings similar to *Strep. pneumoniae*	Both have mild to moderate fever, sore throat, headache, cough, and malaise (no coryza); the **cough worsens over a week** and resolves by 2 weeks; **rales are the most consistent exam finding.**

(continued)

	Viral (RSV, Influenza, Parainfluenza, Adenovirus)	*Chlamydia trachomatis*	*Streptococcus pneumoniae*	*Staphylococcus aureus*	*Chlamydia or Mycoplasma pneumoniae*
Chest x-ray	Hyperinflation with bilateral interstitial infiltrates, peribronchial cuffing, and/or streaky bronchopneumonia	Hyper-inflation with minimal interstitial infiltrates	Confluent lobar consolidation often with pleural effusion/empyema	Unilateral confluent broncho-pneumonia with empyema, pneumatoceles (hemorrhagic necrosis and cavitation), and broncho-pulmonary fistulae	Unilateral (bilateral less so) interstitial (lower-lobe) infiltrates that appear to be worse than the patient
Other findings	WBC count <20,000 with mostly lymphocytes	**Peripheral eosinophilia**	WBC count 15–40,000 with mostly granulocytes	Very high WBC count with mostly granulocytes	Elevated cold agglutinin titers for mycoplasma, but is nonspecific
Treatment	Outpatient treatment with **oral amoxicillin, amoxicillin-clavulanate, or cefuroxime axetil (high rate of superimposed bacterial infection)**; may elect to not treat if diagnosis is certain, patient has no respiratory distress, and there is good follow-up	**Erythro-mycin** orally, 4 times a day for 14 days	Initial empiric inpatient treatment for presumed infection is **IV cefotaxime, cefuroxime, or ceftriaxone**; if positive cultures are obtained, antibiotic may be changed to best sensitivity	Initial empiric treatment with **vancomycin or clindamycin** *plus* a **third-generation cephalosporin**; if positive cultures are obtained, antibiotics may be changed to best sensitivity	**Macrolide** for at least 10 days

Abbreviations: respiratory syncytial virus, RSV; upper respiratory infection, URI; white blood cell, WBC

Additional notes

- *H. influenzae* type B is no longer a common pathogen, except in the very young, under-vaccinated, or immunocompromised.
- Sputum cultures are **rarely useful** in young children; with bacterial pneumonia, **blood culture** is positive in small number; the organism (with sensitivities) may be obtained from aspiration of **pleural fluid/empyema**. **Urine antigen tests** are available for many bacterial pathogens.
- Definitive diagnosis of viral pneumonia is dependent upon isolation of the virus, viral antigen, or genome (**PCR**) in respiratory tract secretions, but rarely needed. Fastest and

easiest way to diagnose *M. pneumoniae* is with **PCR**; there is no commercially available, FDA-approved PCR test for *Chlamydophila pneumoniae*, so the best detection is with tissue culture (but few labs perform this).

- Patients with pneumonia should be hospitalized if <6 months of age, have multilobe involvement, appear toxic, are immunocompromised, have severe distress, require oxygen, are dehydrated, or have no response to outpatient management.
- The most common complications are **pleural effusion, empyema, bronchopleural fistulae, air-leak, pneumatoceles, and bacteremia.**

Cystic Fibrosis

- **Autosomal recessive disorder** most commonly found in **whites (northern Europe, North America, Australia, and New Zealand)** and less in other groups worldwide.
- Abnormality of the **CF transmembrane regulator gene (CFTR)**, expressed mostly in the **epithelial cells of the airways, sweat glands, GI tract, and genitourinary system.**
- Most prevalent mutation is the **ΔF508** (deletion of PHE at amino acid position 508; **major mutation in northern European people with CF**).
- **Over 1,500 known mutations**, but after the ΔF508, no other mutation accounts for more than several percent.
- Depending on the mutation, there is **wide variation in the clinical presentation, and particularly with respect to the severity and progression of lung disease.**
- Abnormal gene leads to absent cyclic AMP (cAMP)-stimulated chloride conductance causing dysfunction of epithelialized surfaces → thickened mucus secretions with increased salt content that is difficult to clear → secretions obstruct airways → chronic, recurrent infections.
- Exocrine pancreatic dysfunction, intestinal malabsorption, and other problems.

Major pathology

- **Pulmonary:** chronic airway infection and progressive dysfunction: first **bronchiolar obstruction**, then larger airways; **persistent bacterial colonization and inflammation** → **bronchiectasis** (cysts, bullae, blebs, fibrosis) and pulmonary artery hypertension; **early obstructive disease and then obstructive + restrictive lung disease**. Most common early infections are due to *Staph. aureus* **and nontypable** *H. influenzae*; most common organism to colonize the airways and cause infection over the life of the patient is *Pseudomonas aeruginosa; Burkholderia cepacia* colonization and infection is associated with severe disease and a rapid deterioration, often to death. Rate of progression of lung disease leading to respiratory failure and cor pulmonale is the main cause of morbidity and mortality.
  - **Sinuses** are filled with secretions and inflammatory products (although recurrent acute sinusitis is not common).
  - Chronic nasal inflammation and edema → **nasal polyps** (CF must be ruled out by sweat test in a child presenting with nasal polyps)
- **Pancreas and intestines: exocrine pancreatic deficiency** (leads to **fat and fat-soluble vitamin malabsorption**) and later-onset **glucose intolerance and diabetes; acute,**

recurrent pancreatitis; problems secondary to severe deficiencies of fat-soluble vitamins: **A**, night blindness; **D**, osteopenia; **E**, peripheral neuropathy and anemia; **K**, bleeding diathesis; **meconium ileus, peritonitis, and meconium plug syndrome in newborn** (see Chapter 1)

- **Hepatobiliary: focal biliary cirrhosis secondary** to obstruction of intrahepatic ducts and cholelithiasis; more common with advancing age; occasional **prolonged neonatal jaundice**
- **Uterine/cervical glands:** distended with mucus, which collects in cervical canal and leads to **endocervicitis; delayed sexual development in girls; decreased fertility, secondary amenorrhea. Azospermia**—failure of development of most of epididymis, vas deferens, and seminal vesicles; **delayed sexual development in boys**
- **Salt loss in sweat: hypochloremic alkalosis; salt depletion easily with gastroenteritis or in hot weather**

Most common presentations

- Infants: **meconium ileus, hypochloremic alkalosis, steatorrhea, and weight loss**
- Young children: **fat malabsorption → steatorrhea** (large, bulky, greasy, foul-smelling, difficult-to-pass stools) or **chronic diarrhea**; weight loss, malnutrition and failure-to-thrive; may have **rectal prolapse** with malnutrition and tissue laxity in the presence of continuing steatorrhea (and straining to pass stool); recurrent and persistent **respiratory infections** (bronchiolitis, pneumonia), sinusitis, nasal polyps, chronic cough (productive of purulent mucus). Later findings also include hemoptysis and pneumothorax (both of which may be life-threatening in the already pulmonary-comprised patient).
- Exam findings: hyperresonance, crackles, expiratory wheeze, **increased anteroposterior diameter, clubbing**, cyanosis

Diagnosis

- **Prenatal:** DNA analysis by amniocentesis or choriovillus sampling to couples with a positive family history or a previous child with CF, or through detection with carrier screening
- **Newborn screening:** measurement of **immunoreactive trypsinogen**: abnormal result is elevated (reflects residual pancreatic function), then sample tested for CF mutations.
- **Sweat chloride test:** pilocarpine-stimulated iontophoresis with collection of sweat and measurement of its chloride content; **two tests on two separate days with chloride concentrations >60 mEq/L plus either a positive newborn screen, presence of typical clinical features, or a sibling with CF is diagnostic. Values of 40–60 mEq/L usually turn out to be positive for CF (may represent certain genotypes). Values <40 mEq/L are considered normal. This is the test that should be performed when CF is suspected. It is recommended after the first 48 hours of life, but sweat may be difficult to obtain in a neonate in the first 2 weeks (so genetic testing would be needed).**
- **Mutational analysis:** used to determine the genotype. Can be used as the primary test if sweat cannot be obtained, or as confirmation if the sweat test is equivocal.

Treatment

- **Best initial treatment** is to reverse nutritional deficiencies with **daily pancreatic enzyme replacement to all meals with vitamin supplementation (high in ADEK)**; generally need more calories for growth (about 130 Kcal/kg/day) with normal to increased amounts of fat.
- **Pulmonary therapy:** daily (multiple times) **nebulized albuterol with 0.9% saline and chest physiotherapy with postural drainage; a single daily dose of nebulized human recombinant DNAse** is used as a mucolytic.
- **Antibiotics:** antibiotics should be started **early with any evidence of a pulmonary infection:** increased cough or sputum production, change in the quality of sputum, change in respiratory baseline of pulmonary function tests, new infiltrates on x-ray, decreased appetite, weight loss
  - **Oral antibiotics** based on demonstration of a pathogen and sensitivity testing; use maximal doses for at least 2 weeks (quinolones are the only consistently effective oral antibiotics for *Pseudomonas* infection, but resistance occurs rapidly).
  - **Aerosolized antibiotics:** significant decrease in *Pseudomonas* density with **aerosolized tobramycin** when given twice daily on alternate months for 6 months in patients with infection or moderate to severe disease.
  - **Intravenous:** if oral or aerosolized therapy is not effective; use for at least 14 days; need two drugs (and three to control for *S. aureus*) for *P. aeruginosa*, e.g., ticarcillin plus tobramycin, ceftazidime, cefepime, or meropenem plus tobramycin; *Burkholderia cepacia* is difficult to treat (meropenem, chloramphenicol).
- **Anti-inflammatory agents:** corticosteroids **only for severe reactive airway disease or bronchopulmonary aspergillosis**; ibuprofen given chronically for 4 years (with particular peak serum levels) has been shown to slow disease progression.
- Treat extrapulmonary complications:
  - **Nasal polyps:** nasal corticosteroids and decongestants; may need surgical removal
  - **Acute/chronic sinusitis:** antibiotics initially; sinus aspiration
  - **Heart failure:** diuretics and digitalis (for left-sided failure); supplemental oxygen; poor prognosis
  - **Rectal prolapse:** improves with enzyme replacement and improved nutrition; also start with stool softeners until malabsorption is controlled; replace prolapsed rectum with gentle pressure; surgery rarely required
  - **Hyperglycemia:** if symptomatic and persistent, start insulin (possibly oral hypoglycemic agents)
  - **Salt depletion:** prompt fluid and electrolyte replacement; free access to salt
  - **Liver dysfunction:** associated with biliary cirrhosis; can improve with ursodeoxycholic acid; sclerotherapy after initial hemorrhage due to portal hypertension

Prognosis

Medium cumulative survival now at >35 years. Lung transplantation has been used for end-stage disease, but repeat transplant is necessary. There is poor outcome with *B. cepacia* infection, poor lung function, and decreased exercise tolerance (and lung transplant would generally not be offered).

Primary Ciliary Dyskinesia (Immotile Cilia Syndrome)

Ciliary ultrastructural changes causing **abnormal beating or immotility of cilia**; absence of normal propulsion of mucus in the airways → **repeated and chronic sinopulmonary infections**; half have **Kartagener syndrome** (chronic sinusitis and otitis, situs inversus, and airway disease leading to bronchiectasis). Most cases are autosomal recessive.

Key diagnostic words

Neonates may present with chronic nasal congestion, rhinitis, and cough; then repeated bouts of acute otitis media or chronic otitis media with effusion (differentiates from CF); nasal polyps, wheezing, and clubbing; hallmark finding is **loose, productive cough with recurrent pneumonia; recurrent infections with dextrocardia on x-ray is virtually diagnostic**; males are usually infertile; females are at increased risk for ectopic pregnancy.

Diagnosis

- **Chest x-ray** shows bronchial thickening, peribronchial infiltrates overinflation, atelectasis, and consolidation; **half will have dextrocardia**; x-rays or CT shows **sinus involvement**.
- Eventually **bronchiectasis** develops (high-resolution CT scan is best test). The **most accurate test is electron microscopy of bronchial biopsies showing ultrastructural abnormalities**.

Management

Mostly **symptomatic** and is similar to pulmonary therapy in CF. Surgery for sinus or middle-ear disease refractory to medical treatment. With good treatment, a **normal life span is possible**.

Pleural and Thoracic Wall Disorders

Pleural fluid—pleural effusion

Accumulation of fluid within the pleural space most commonly caused by infection (**parapneumonic effusion**, possibly resulting in an **empyema**), cancer, lymph (**chylothorax**), or blood (**hemothorax**). It may first be classified as either a **transudate or an exudate**.

Table 7.3: Characteristics of Pleural Effusions

Transudate	Exudate	Chylothorax
• Increased capillary hydrostatic pressure, decrease in pleural space hydrostatic pressure or a decrease in plasma oncotic pressure • Examples: congestive heart failure, nephrotic syndrome, cirrhosis, constrictive pericarditis • Appearance: clear • pH and glucose: normal • Protein: low • LDH: <200 U/L • Pleural/serum LDH <0.6 • Cell count low (<1,000, mostly lymphocytes and monocytes) • Gram stain: negative	• Pleural surface damage with decreased ability to filter pleural fluid or impairment of lymphatic drainage • Examples: infection (most; *Staph. aureus, Strep. pneumoniae, H. influenzae,* TB), toxins, malignancy, connective-tissue disease, thoracic duct injury (postsurgical or post–vaginal delivery of a newborn, chest trauma) • Appearance: cloudy to purulent (empyema) • pH and glucose: low to very low (empyema) • Protein: can be high to very high • LDH: >200 U/L to >1,000 U/L (empyema) • Pleural/serum LDH >0.6 • Cell count high (>1,000 to >5,000 with empyema), mostly granulocytes • Gram stain: may be positive (almost all with empyema unless pretreated)	• Chyle from injury to thoracic duct or lymphatics • Examples: injury during cardio-thoracic surgery, chest trauma, newborn vaginal delivery (rapid increase in venous pressure), metastatic disease (lymphoma) • Appearance: milky (but may be yellow or bloody) or clear in a newborn not yet fed • Cells: T lymphocytes • Triglycerides elevated, chylomicrons present, and pleural fluid/serum triglycerides >1

Abbreviations: lactate dehydrogenase, LDH

Clinical presentation—Fever (if infection), cough, dyspnea, **inspiratory pleuritic pain (not with a chylothorax); decreased chest excursion, breath sounds, and dullness to percussion on ipsilateral side**; early **pleural rub**; trachea and cardiac apex may be displaced (a significant **mediastinal shift** can result in decreased venous return and cardiac output)

Diagnosis

Fluid may be visualized (depending on the volume) on an AP and lateral chest x-ray; but the **best study is a lateral decubitus** (minimal volumes of fluid and determine if there is free flow or if it is loculated) ultrasound is good to visualize small loculated effusions or to determine if there is pleural thickening vs. an effusion. A CT is **best for the underlying lung disease.**

Management—First step in management is to **assure oxygenation and ventilation, hydration (IV fluids), and pain control**. Next step is to **drain the effusion** (if etiology is unclear or patient is symptomatic) by **thoracentesis** with a **chest tube or surgically** (if there is no free flow); a **prolonged course of antibiotics (2–4 weeks) may be needed for infections with empyema. Chylothoraces typically recur** after drainage and repeated drainage may cause significant problems; if there is no cardiorespiratory compromise, feed a low-fat (use **medium-chain triglycerides**) diet high in protein (many problems will slowly resolve); if there is no resolution, **total parenteral nutrition** is generally started; and if this fails, a **thoracic duct ligation** should be considered.

Pneumothorax and pneumomediastinum

Table 7.4: Characteristics of Air Leaks

	Pneumomediastinum	**Pneumothorax**	**Tension Pneumothorax**
Definition	• Alveolar rupture and air dissection through perivascular sheaths to hilum and then the mediastinum	• Leakage of air from the lung to the pleural space causing the lung to collapse	• A continuing leak leads to increasing positive pressure and a shift of the mediastinum with decreased venous return and cardiac output.
Etiology	• From acute or chronic pulmonary disease, aspirated foreign body, penetrating chest trauma, esophageal perforation, or no underlying cause; most common reason in older children and adolescents is an acute asthma attack	• **Primary**: occurs without lung disease or trauma; most common with exertion in teenage boys who are tall and thin (thought to have sub-pleural blebs; often positive family history); also seen in patients with collagen synthesis disorders • **Secondary**: due to an underlying lung disease but not trauma (asthma, CF, infection, abscess or pneumatocele rupture, metastatic disease [rare], and diffuse lung diseases) • **Traumatic**: chest penetration, blunt trauma, or iatrogenic (e.g., mechanical ventilation)	• **Primary**: occurs without lung disease or trauma; most common with exertion in teenage boys who are tall and thin; often positive family history; also seen in patients with collagen synthesis disorders • **Secondary**: due to an underlying lung disease but not trauma (asthma, CF, infection, abscess or pneumatocele rupture, metastatic disease [rare], and diffuse lung diseases) • **Traumatic**: chest penetration, blunt trauma, or iatrogenic (e.g., mechanical ventilation)

(continued)

Table 7.4: Characteristics of Air Leaks *(cont.)*

	Pneumomediastinum	Pneumothorax	Tension Pneumothorax
Symptoms	• Stabbing chest pain (transient), cough, dyspnea	• Abrupt onset of pain, dyspnea, and cyanosis (small to moderate air leaks may cause little to no symptoms)	• With increasing air: distress, decreased breath sounds, tympanic percussion, and mediastinal shift with hemodynamic compromise
Diagnosis	• Difficult to diagnose by exam • Chest X-ray is diagnostic: air dissects into neck and abdomen	• Chest X-ray is diagnostic	• Chest X-ray is diagnostic
Treatment	• Rarely a clinical problem (may be in a newborn); air dissects into the neck and abdomen • Treat underlying problem; if severely symptomatic, can place a drainage catheter	• Small asymptomatic leaks may be observed (many resolve within a week); larger leaks with symptoms (but not tension) may be treated initially with 100% oxygen.	• But with severe distress or tension, do not wait—place a needle in the chest on the side of the suspected leak (can use a transillumination light) • Leaks under tension or large recurrent leaks require a thoracostomy chest tube drainage.

Thoracic deformities

Pectus excavatum (midline narrowing of thoracic cavity; funnel chest)—Usually isolated; occurs with **collagen synthesis disorder and may be secondary to chronic lung disease or neuromuscular disease**; most patients are unaffected (so the management is observation), but with more severe deformities there may be progressive respiratory distress, deterioration of pulmonary function, and cardiac abnormalities (physical therapy in the milder cases or surgery may be needed).

Pectus carinatum (protrusion of the sternum; pigeon breast)—Often **seen in families**; may occur with scoliosis, mitral valve disease, or coarctation of the aorta. Most young children are asymptomatic; older children may have primarily recurrent wheezing, exercise intolerance, and increased respiratory infections. Surgery is not commonly needed.

Kyphoscoliosis

Most are **idiopathic adolescent scoliosis**; with greater degrees of curvature, there is **restrictive lung disease and** some obstructive disease with severe untreated angles of curvature, cor pulmonale may develop.

Neuromuscular disorders

Result in decreasing muscle strength and endurance over time; upper airways tend to collapse, the ability to generate a cough is lessened, and there are recurrent or chronic respiratory infections. Present with repeated bouts of acute respiratory distress and further deterioration of lung function, the end result being **severe restrictive lung disease** (majority of morbidity and mortality in these disorders).

Pulmonary Hypertension and Cor Pulmonale

- **Primary:** no obvious underlying cause (genetic markers with familial occurrence are seen; primarily in newborns and adolescents); **secondary:** due to underlying disease, such as pulmonary venous hypertension (left-sided heart disease), pulmonary hypertension associated with **hypoxemia** (e.g., interstitial lung disease, sleep-disordered breathing, alveolar hypoventilation, chronic thrombo-embolic disease), and other disease (e.g., histiocytosis, pulmonary vessel compression)
- Pathology: pulmonary vascular obstruction secondary to hyperplasia of muscular and elastic tissues and thickened intima of small arteries and arterioles; afterload burden on the right ventricle → right ventricular hypertrophy (cor pulmonale); dilatation of pulmonary artery with or without pulmonary valve insufficiency; late right ventricular dilatation with tricuspid insufficiency and decreased cardiac output
- **Potentially reversible**, depending on the underlying cause, early detection, and treatment instituted. There are a number of drugs which may be used.

Sleep-Related Breathing Disorders

Obstructive sleep apnea (OSA)

Occurs from **benign snoring to severe clinical consequences**, including death; greater obstruction with increased frequency in REM sleep, in the supine position, and with concurrent illnesses; **upper airway collapse** → repetitive arousals and **sleep fragmentation**; represents periods of **hypoxemia** (hypercarbia, acidosis, and hemodynamic changes)

Presenting signs and symptoms

Snoring, **gasping respirations**, unusual posturing during sleep, excessive sweating, restless sleep, **increased nocturnal urination/enuresis**, cyanosis, and increased **daytime sleepiness**

Long-term consequences

- **Repetitive periods of asphyxia** increased **systemic arterial pressure**, hypoxic pulmonary vasoconstriction → **pulmonary artery hypertension** → **right ventricular hypertrophy and failure (cor pulmonale)** + arrhythmias and hypoxic encephalopathy
- Additionally: decreased growth and failure-to-thrive, developmental delay, decreased school performance, hyperactivity, social withdrawal, and aggressive behaviors.

Most important predisposing factors

- **Adenoid/tonsillar hypertrophy** (leading cause)
- Craniofacial abnormalities (e.g., **Down syndrome,** Apert syndrome, Pierre-Robin sequence, Treacher Collins syndrome)
- Cleft palate

- **Obesity** (including Prader-Willi syndrome)
- Chronic nasal obstruction, cerebral palsy, and other neuromuscular disorders
- Mucopolysaccharidoses (structural tissue changes), sickle-cell anemia (adenoid/tonsillar hypertrophy and lymphoid tissue hyperplasia)
- Bronchopulmonary dysplasia
- Due to upper airway obstruction, at significant risk for respiratory distress **postoperatively** due to postoperative airway swelling and obstructive pulmonary edema.

Diagnosis—The **gold standard is polysomnography** to detect the presence and severity of sleep apnea, to assess the relationship of symptoms to OSA, to assess daytime hypersomnolence, and to titrate CPAP.

Management—With evidence of adenoid/tonsillar hypertrophy, an **adenotonsillectomy** should be performed; for cases where this is not warranted, or in children who continue to have problems after surgery, then CPAP may be utilized; for those who fail medical treatment or who have overt airway pathology, other surgical procedures.

Somnolence in adolescence

Most common causes—Inadequate amount of sleep, disturbed sleep (OSA, medical problems, drugs, withdrawal from drugs), **delayed sleep phase**, increased sleep requirements (**narcolepsy**, depression)

- The peak period of onset of narcolepsy is adolescence.
- Narcolepsy is **daytime sleep attacks with cataplexy** (brief periods of muscle weakness, often after an emotional period), sleep paralysis, and hypnagogic hallucinations (vivid auditory and visual hallucinations at sleep onset).
- Presentation with all of these findings together is rare, so the diagnosis should be considered with **true sleepiness**, i.e., after a good night's sleep (adequate number of hours) with episodes of falling asleep during the day.
- High rates of behavioral and emotional disturbances related to narcolepsy.
- Most widely used test for excessive daytime sleepiness is the **multiple sleep latency test** (MLST; measures the time to fall asleep at night and during daytime naps).

Apparent life-threatening events (ALTE)

- An episode that is frightening to the caregiver and presents as a combination of apnea, color change, change in muscle tone, and choking or gagging.
- After appropriate evaluation, only about half are found to have a specific etiology.
- Most appear normal by the time they are seen by a physician.
- Reported symptoms are the most important aspect of making the diagnosis.

Most common causes—Infections (CNS, respiratory), **GER**, GI malformations, **seizures**, breath-holding spells, CNS lesions (mass, vascular, malformation, hemorrhage), **cardiac arrhythmias**, **apnea of prematurity**, central hypoventilation, drug effects, OSA, hypoglycemia, hypocalcemia, fatty-acid metabolism inborn errors, **child abuse**, factitious disorder.

Diagnostic steps—Most important step is a **careful history** including past medical history for any similar events, breathing problems, eating problems, neurodevelopmental abnormalities, and abnormal perinatal events and family history; then a careful physical, including **neurological and funduscopic exam**. If the history and physical are consistent with an ALTE, then:

- **Admit to the hospital for cardiorespiratory monitoring and observation**; CBC; basic chemistries, including Ca, phosphate, Mg, lactate, and ammonia; chest x-ray, electrocardiogram, multichannel cardiorespiratory recording with pulse oximetry
- Other studies based on higher likelihood of certain conditions per the history and physical: infection workup, barium swallow, laryngoscopy, esophageal pH study, brain CT, arterial blood gas, echocardiogram, polysomnogram, Holter monitoring, inborn errors evaluation

Management

Treat the specific etiology. **Home monitoring for apnea and bradycardia** if the etiology is unclear, for apnea of infancy, or if there is the likelihood of subsequent events (use an event recorder: objective recordings of apnea and bradycardia alarms to detect true alarms from false).

Sudden infant death syndrome (SIDS)

Table 7.5: Sudden Infant Death Syndrome (SIDS)

Definition	Unexpected death of an infant unexplained by a thorough review of the medical history, a postmortem examination, and forensic evaluation of the scene of death
Epidemiology/Maternal and antenatal risk factors	Higher incidence with poverty, young maternal age, single mother, low education, higher parity, multiple birth, short birth intervals, poor nutrition, males, low birth weight, prematurity, perinatal hypoxia, maternal smoking during pregnancy (and postnatal exposure to smoke; also cocaine, heroin, and alcohol); higher in African Americans and Native Americans
Infant/Environmental risk factors	Most significant factor—prone sleeping (side sleeping to a lesser degree); highest incidence at 2–4 months of life (most in first 6 months); soft sleeping surface and materials in sleeping area; overheating, recent febrile illness, bed-sharing, and no pacifier use (decreased incidence with pacifiers); higher incidence with previous ALTE
Pathological findings	No specific findings for SIDS; petechial hemorrhages and pulmonary edema; evidence of pre-existing, chronic, low-grade asphyxia
Genetics	Many genes where there are different polymorphisms compared to non-SIDS, which may contribute to abnormal cardiorespiratory and arousal responses; recurrent cases (for which no other cause has been identified) have been documented in families
Pathophysiology	Based on complex gene-environment interactions; impaired ventilation in the prone position with episodes of airway obstruction, and asphyxia to which the infant does not autoresuscitate (as the normal infant does by gasping); may also be predisposed to bradycardia and ventricular arrhythmias
Recommendations per AAP	• Supine-only positioning (unless not warranted due to medical conditions; there are no adverse effects of supine sleep); give tummy time when the infant is awake and observed • Standard infant crib/bassinet in same room as parents; firm mattresses and no soft materials in sleep environment • No overheating or bundling; normal infant sleepwear and room temperature • After breastfeeding is well established, offer pacifier at bedtime/nap time and if pacifier falls out, leave it out • No smoking during pregnancy or secondhand postnatal smoke • Home monitoring not recommended (no evidence that it decreases the incidence of SIDS)

Abbreviations: American Academy of Pediatrics, AAP

ALLERGY AND ASTHMA   8

ALLERGY—GENERAL PRINCIPLES

- **Allergy:** development of immune-mediated adverse reactions; hypersensitivity occurs with re-exposure to a sensitizing allergen, due to release of inflammatory mediators.
- **Atopy:** a genetic predisposition to developing allergies; hyperresponsiveness with asthma, allergic rhinitis, and atopic dermatitis; greater risk for developing allergic diseases (one component increases risk of developing a second).
- Influenced by **genetic susceptibility and environmental factors** and other risk factors (dietary, tobacco-smoke exposure, early antibiotic use, exposure to indoor allergens). **Family history is the single most important factor**.

Allergy Basic Science

IgE-mediated allergic response:

1. **Sensitization:** Antigen-presenting cells are recognized and processed, and interact with T-lymphocytes → cytokines → B cells produce antigen-specific IgE, which is bound by Fcε receptors on mast cells/basophils.

2. **Early-phase, immediate hypersensitivity reaction** (within minutes of exposure): With re-exposure to the allergen, bound IgE is crosslinked → degranulation of mast cells and basophils → release of preformed mediators (histamine, tryptase, heparin) → for newly synthesized mediators (leukotrienes and cytokines) → smooth-muscle contraction and increased mucus and vascular permeability.

3. **Late-phase reaction** (begins 2–4 hours after exposure and can last 24 hours): Newly formed mediators affect capillary endothelial cells → localized edema, adhesion of leukocytes, and tissue infiltration (eosinophils, neutrophils and basophils). Eosinophils produce mediators → tissue damage and chronic allergic reactions; T-helper (TH)-2 lymphocytes release cytokines → further IgE production, attraction of eosinophils, and increased numbers of mast cells.

Allergen exposure

- By inhalation (direct or indirect exposure), ingestion, direct contact, or injection
  - **Common inhaled allergens:** pollens (trees, early to mid spring; grasses, late spring to early summer; weeds, late summer to early fall; or year-round in warmer climates), molds, dust mites, animal dander (mostly from cats), cockroaches, latex particles
  - **Common ingested allergens:** foods, drugs
  - **Common contact allergens:** chemicals, drugs, cosmetics, jewelry, latex products, plants
  - **Common injected allergens:** stinging insects, drugs, blood products

Diagnostic Testing

- **Most important first step is to establish the diagnosis with a careful history** (symptom pattern) **plus a physical examination** (clinical diagnosis).
- General screening tests include a **nasal smear for eosinophils**, plus serum IgE and CBC for peripheral eosinophilia (but AAP states no routine screening test).
- **IgE skin testing of in-vitro assays** (preferred method) **or blood testing** (allergen-specific IgE assay) is recommended when allergic symptoms are persistent and severe enough to impact quality of life, despite management with avoidance and medications and if immunotherapy is being considered as a long-term treatment option.
- Skin tests used for a past reaction with a **drug**. Do not use blood testing for possible **penicillin allergy** as it lacks negative predictive value. Reactions to **radiocontrast agents** are not IgE mediated (mast cell with or without complement activation).
- Blood IgE—specific assays used for severe dermographism, widespread skin disease, risk of prophylaxis, refusal of skin tests, or those in whom stopping antihistamines or antidepressants (interfere with skin tests) would cause problems.

Avoidance Education

Factors that can be changed to prevent/diminish allergic reactions: being aware of allergens, level of exposure to indoor and outdoor allergens, passive exposure to tobacco smoke and air pollutants, timing of introduction of allergenic foods, early exposure to antibiotics.

Immunotherapy

- Consider when there is a (1) **clear relationship between symptoms and exposures** to unavoidable allergens; (2) **allergy symptoms all year or most of the year;** (3) difficulty controlling the allergy with avoidance and medications.
  - Most effective in treating **allergic rhinitis**; allergic disease associated with asthma, insect hypersensitivity, and allergic conjunctivitis.
- Weekly/semi-weekly dosing increments followed by monthly maintenance for **at least 3–5 years. All patients should wait at least 20–30 minutes in the office** after each injection.

- **Not indicated** for patients (1) <3 years of age, (2) on beta-blockers, (3) with severe medical conditions who are likely to die from anaphylaxis, (4) with food hypersensitivities, (5) with latex hypersensitivity, or (6) with atopic dermatitis.

Allergic Rhinitis

- Inflammation of the nasal mucous membranes due to an IgE-mediated response.
- Allergic (**seasonal intermittent or perennial persistent**) or nonallergic (usually no pruritus and negative skin tests: infectious, vasomotor, from topical medications, abnormal anatomy, hormonal and nonallergic eosinophilic rhinitis).
- With **seasonal allergic rhinitis**, IgE-mediated reactions occur with exposure to allergens (periodic, correlating with seasonal aeroallergens).
- With **perennial allergic rhinitis**, symptoms occur to some degree throughout the year (important cause: **indoor inhaled aeroallergens**).

Presenting signs and symptoms

Seasonal allergic rhinitis: watery rhinorrhea; nasal congestion; sneezing; eye, nose, and throat pruritus; and watery eyes. **Perennial:** less rhinorrhea and sneezing; **prominent and severe nasal obstruction, and congestion with postnasal drainage**.

Findings on examination

- **Pale, boggy nasal mucosa with swollen nasal turbinates**
- Inflamed/reddened mucosa
- "**Allergic salute**" (rubbing nose upward with palm)
- **Transverse nasal crease**
- **Allergic shiners** (infraorbital darkening due to venous stasis) with **Dennie-Morgan folds** (creases within allergic shiners)
- **Conjunctival injection with clear discharge**
- **Clear nasal discharge**, usually with **significant numbers of eosinophils**
- Adenotonsillar hypertrophy
- Nasal polyps
- Mouth-breathing

Diagnosis

Most important first step is a **thorough history and physical**: onset, progression, duration, and relationship to seasons; known exposures and associations; history of nasal or facial trauma/surgery, use of medications, any previous testing and response to therapy; and family history. Exam should focus on eyes, ears, nose, throat, chest, and skin for findings supportive of allergic disease.

The **best initial screening test is a nasal smear for eosinophils** (usually positive in symptomatic allergic patients vs. polymorphonuclear neutrophils with infection). **Peripheral blood eosinophilia** is common but not specific; numbers may increase with seasonal exposure and may be suppressed by infections and certain medications. **Serum IgE** may also increase and decrease with allergen exposure and has low sensitivity. Skin tests are used as previously discussed.

Treatment

1. **Avoidance** of factors that cause symptoms
2. **Palliative treatment:** nasal lavage with warm salt water, inhalation of warm mist
3. **Pharmacotherapy** to alleviate and prevent symptoms

   a. Begin with an oral second-generation antihistamine with or without decongestant (or topical nasal antihistamine). May also use nasal cromolyn sodium as a preventive measure before anticipated allergenic exposure.

   b. If prominent eye findings: topical ocular antihistamine with or without vasoconstrictor, topical mast cell stabilizer, and/or topical nonsteroidal anti-inflammatory drug (NSAID).

   c. With increasing severity, add topical nasal corticosteroid (most effective treatment) and consider topical nasal antihistamine and nasal cromolyn, and topical eye treatment as above.

   d. To gain control of severe symptoms, may need a short course (3–10 days) of oral corticosteroids.

Insect-Sting Reactions

- Stinging insects (Hymenoptera order): honeybee, bumblebee, yellow jacket, yellow-faced hornet, white-faced hornet, paper wasp, fire ant, and harvester ant; can cause anaphylaxis
- **Local painful reactions** (transient pain, erythema, swelling, and itching for several hours at the site of sting) in most and large local reactions and/or **systemic reactions (anaphylaxis)** in some (IgE-mediated); **serum sickness** may develop 7–10 days after the sting (urticaria, joint pain, malaise, fever).
- Try to **identify the insect** with history (tables available for description and nesting and behavior patterns of each); cross reactivity may occur among some. Next, perform **skin testing (best diagnostic test)**; use blood test **only** if skin tests cannot be performed, if the reaction is uncertain, or with a negative skin test and a very strong history.

Treatment

If stinger is left in skin, remove it (by flicking) within 20 seconds (otherwise all venom has been released); for immediate local reactions, administer analgesics, ice/cold compresses, oral antihistamines; a short course of prednisone should be considered with extensive/painful swelling. For systemic reactions, **treat anaphylaxis** (see below). Patients then need to:

- Be taught to use an **epinephrine kit** (pen auto-injector), and to have the kit (and antihistamines) always available at home, school, and day care.
- Call 911 after epinephrine administration.

- Wear a medical alert identification.
- **Start venom immunotherapy (best long-term treatment)** after a systemic reaction and a **documented IgE sensitivity** (referral to an allergist).

Drug Reactions

- Any drug or biological agent; skin reactions are the most common form.
- Most **IgE-mediated** (anaphylaxis), **cytotoxic** (IgG or IgM + complement interact with a drug allergen associated with cell membranes → cell destruction), **immune complex disease** (drug combines with antibodies to form immune complexes in the blood, which can cause serum sickness reactions and drug-induced lupus syndromes), or **T cell–mediated** (require specific memory T cells, which become activated and produce an inflammatory response). Other reactions: delayed skin reactions, drug-induced fever, hepatic or pulmonary hypersensitivity, and **nonimmunologic reactions (e.g., radiocontrast, aspirin, or NSAID-induced asthma)**.
- Most common examples of IgE-mediated reactions: **penicillins, blood products, polypeptide hormones, and vaccines.** Most common drugs representing cytotoxic reactions: penicillins, sulfonamides, methyldopa, and quinidine. Immune complex reactions: procainamide, isoniazid, phenytoin, and hydralazine. T cell–mediated reactions: allergic contact dermatitis.
- A **nonimmunologic rash (measles-like) may occur with ampicillin and amoxicillin**, usually with viral infections; no increased risk of future reactions.
- **Most common clinical course—immediate reaction within the first hour after exposure → anaphylaxis**; an accelerated reaction may occur 1–72 hours after exposure → urticaria/angioedema, rash, and fever; a late reaction occurs >72 hours after exposure → rash, serum sickness, and fever.
- **Skin testing has greater sensitivity and specificity for IgE-mediated drug reactions and is preferred**, but only a limited number of drugs can be reliably tested (e.g., penicillin, insulin, streptokinase).
- **Management:** treatment of severe immediate or accelerated reactions with **epinephrine and antihistamines** for pruritus, urticaria/angioedema; may need a course of oral corticosteroids. For severe, progressive, late reactions (rashes, serum sickness), use a course of **oral corticosteroids**. If there is no available substitute for the responsible drug, **desensitization** may be used (administering progressive doses until the full dose is tolerated). Consider avoiding cephalosporins (cross reactivity) in penicillin-sensitive patients.

Food Reactions

- Prevalence greatest in **first few years** of life and is **more likely in atopic children**. Food is the leading cause of anaphylaxis in children.
- 90% of food allergies in children are from **milk (caseins and whey), egg (ovomucoid in egg whites), peanuts, wheat, soy and tree nuts,** fish and shellfish. Allergies **usually outgrown:** eggs, milk, and soy by age 5 years. Allergies **usually not outgrown:** peanuts and tree nuts, fish and shellfish.

- Mechanism may be **IgE-mediated (rapid onset) or non-IgE-mediated and may take hours to days** (enterocolitis/proctocolitis, enteropathy, allergic eosinophilic gastroenteritis, food intolerance). **Cow's-milk sensitivity is the most common cause of food-induced enteropathy** (diarrhea, vomiting, failure-to-thrive).
- **Diet diaries** are helpful in the diagnosis (record everything placed in the mouth and length of time from ingestion to any symptoms).
- A **basic elimination diet** may be initially helpful (10–14 days). Those patients who respond should be referred to an allergist for further testing. The **gold standard** is the double-blind, placebo-controlled food challenge.
- Management: **strict avoidance is the only proven therapy**; less severe, local reactions managed with oral antihistamines, but prophylactic management (cromolyn) has not been proven to be effective or safe.

Urticaria and Angioedema

Acute urticaria: pruritic, papular dermal erythema; blanches with pressure (dilated blood vessels and edema); may occur anywhere and usually resolves in a few days; **most common reasons are foods, drugs, or viral illnesses (URI is the most common reason for urticaria caused by infections)**

Chronic urticaria: lasts >6 weeks (lesions appear quickly and disappear within 24 hours); half go on for >6 months, and smaller numbers for years; the cause is usually not identified. **Most are idiopathic**; autoimmune mechanism suspected; not associated with atopy, so **allergy testing is not warranted**.

Angioedema: similar process, but edema extends into deep dermal and subcutaneous tissue; often involves face, tongue, extremities, and genitalia, with little or no pruritus. Histamine is the major mediator of these reactions.

- Some types of urticaria and angioedema can be brought on by **physical factors** and last 1–2 hours: changes in temperature (**cold-induced, heat-induced**), direct stimulation of the skin (e.g., **dermatographism**, commonly seen with chronic urticaria), **cholinergic** (associated with exercise, hot showers, sweating, anxiety), solar-induced, aquagenic (water contact regardless of temperature).
- Other causes: vasculitis, hereditary angioedema (onset in adolescence and early adulthood), malignancies, systemic lupus erythematosus (SLE), serum sickness, thyroid disease, lymphoma, and Hodgkin disease
- The **history is the most important part of diagnosis. Anything ingested should be considered** as a possible cause; ask about contact allergens, viral illnesses, insect bites and stings, and environmental/physical factors. A thorough physical exam is needed to exclude other similar dermatologic diagnoses. Further tests should be based on the history and physical.
- Management: **avoid causal factors**, use palliative measures to relieve pruritus; **oral H_1 antihistamines are the treatment of choice,** to which an H_2 blocking agent may be added for probable ingested allergens. If control cannot be achieved, and **oral corticosteroids**.

Atopic Dermatitis (Eczema)

Chronic, recurrent atopic inflammatory skin disease; **half begin by age 1 year**, and the majority by age 5 years; **may be the first manifestation of atopy**. Most have **elevated IgE levels and positive skin tests** (mostly **foods** and/or aeroallergens; detection and avoidance may alleviate symptoms); skin abnormalities lead to **transepidermal water loss → dry skin**.

Signs and symptoms—**Intense pruritus and skin reactivity with scratching usually worse at night and with sleep disruption;** often with recurrent skin infections

Table 8.1: Presentation of Atopic Dermatitis

	Acute	**Subacute**	**Chronic**
Presentation	Erythematous **papules and vesicles** over erythematous skin Serous exudates (oozing and weeping); intense **pruritus**	Erythema Excoriation	**Thickened skin plaques** **Fibrotic papules** (lichen simplex chronicus)
Major appearance	**Excoriations** and erosions	**Scaling**	Increased skin markings **(lichenification)**
Population	**Infants and young children**	**Older children and adults**	Older children and adults
Distribution	**Face and extensor surfaces**	**Flexural areas** (neck, antecubital and popliteal fossae, intergluteal creases, wrists and ankles	Same distribution as subacute

Diagnostic tests—Skin tests have **many false-positives;** a **basic elimination diet** may be helpful in assessing food allergy.

Management

- Avoid factors that cause symptoms: **irritants,** cover hands when sleeping, control emotional stress; **food elimination based on testing**
- Skin care: **daily baths with superfatted, unscented soaps, followed by skin hydration with a bland emollient;** for severely affected areas: wet dressings with saline or Domeboro solution; **avoid skin-care products containing perfumes and dyes, and avoid irritating fabrics.**
- **Topical corticosteroids are the key treatment** for acute lesions (only in inflamed areas after bath and before emollient); use the least-potent agent that gives control, and decrease potency when control is achieved (avoid most-potent groups I–III in children <14 years; may use group VII or diluted group VI on face)
  - May use a topical immunomodulator (tacrolimus) as a secondary drug.
- Oral corticosteroids are reserved for extremely severe exacerbations. **Oral antihistamines** to control pruritus, especially at night (older sedating antihistamines). Tar preparations: alternative or adjunct to corticosteroids; shampoos beneficial for scalp treatment and for chronic lichenification. Treat secondary bacterial skin infections with a drug that will treat *Staphylococcus aureus*.

Anaphylaxis

Rapid (seconds to minutes, or delay up to 2 hours) immune-mediated (IgE) systemic reaction to allergens to which the patient has been previously exposed; **most commonly caused by medications, vaccines, latex, blood products, insect stings, allergen extracts, foods, and with exercise**; or idiopathic. Response may be biphasic (abating for several hours then returning) and protracted.

Risk factors—Food allergy, asthma, prior history, beta-blocker use, multiple antibiotic sensitivity, atopy

Most common signs and symptoms

Skin flushing, tingling or pruritus, urticaria/angioedema (and swelling of lip, tongue), throat tightness, difficulty swallowing, nasal congestion, sneezing, rhinorrhea, inspiratory stridor, chest tightness, cough and wheezing, dyspnea; also syncope, arrhythmias, nausea, vomiting

Diagnostic testing—**Best test for emergent care is serum tryptase levels** (differentiates anaphylaxis from a non-IgE anaphylactoid reaction or other events that look similar to anaphylaxis)

Management of anaphylaxis

- Maintain **airway, breathing, and circulation**; administer **oxygen** 8–10 L/min; **treat hypotension** with IV fluids or colloids and consider vasopressors. Place patient in recumbent position and elevate the legs.
- Give **epinephrine (do not delay)** 0.01 mg/kg (max. 0.3 mg or 0.3 mL) of 1:1,000 IM (not subcutaneous); repeat every 15 minutes, up to three doses.
- If reaction from any injection (including insect sting), administer half of the dose into the site.
- Give glucagon to patients on beta-blockers (to counter the danger of epinephrine resistance)
- Give 1–2 mg/kg **diphenhydramine parenterally**; continue with oral diphenhydramine every 4–6 hours as needed.
- Treat bronchospasm with **a short-acting beta-agonist**.
- Give **systemic corticosteroids** if response is inadequate or reaction is very severe.
- **Observe** patient for several hours and **hospitalize** if unresponsive to initial therapy.

Asthma

The following information reflects the most current (2007 revision) NIH National Asthma Education and Prevention Program diagnosis and management guidelines for children with asthma and the tables are summarized from that document.

Definition and pathogenesis

- Reversible chronic airway disorder with **airway hyperresponsiveness, airway obstruction that is at least partially reversible, and airway inflammation**. Most have aeroallergen-induced symptoms, and environmental exposure (e.g., smog, tobacco smoke) is a major inducer of airway inflammation.

- **Interactions of genetics, viral infections, and environmental exposures** → airway inflammation → airway hyperresponsiveness → airflow limitation → signs and symptoms
- **Major triggers** for airway hyperresponsiveness and airflow limitation: respiratory viral infections, passive tobacco smoke, chemicals, pollutants, aeroallergens, changes in weather, exercise, stress, strong emotional responses, medications, foods, hormonal changes
- **Early response** (peaking in 20 minutes)—mast cell–derived mediators → bronchial constriction, airway edema, and mucous plugging.
- **Late response** (4–12 hours later)—infiltration of inflammatory cells into the airway → ongoing inflammatory responses → hypertrophy of smooth muscle and hyperplasia of mucous glands. Bronchial hyperresponsiveness increases with the late-phase response and with viral respiratory infections.
- Long-term changes (**airway remodeling**) in some patients → fibrosis and **irreversible** airway obstruction.

Epidemiology and natural history

Disease onset can occur at any age but appears **most often <6 years**, and may be outgrown (especially by males with no personal or family history of atopy).

- **Least likely to outgrow asthma:** onset <3 years of age with parental history of asthma, an already confirmed history of atopic disease, or sensitization to aeroallergens.
- Largest risk for **increased severity and persistence of asthma:** perinatal exposure to passive cigarette smoke and aeroallergens. Higher risk: males, children with low birth weight and with smaller airways.

Exercise-Induced Bronchospasm

- Begins after 5–6 minutes of exercise and peaks 5–10 minutes after stopping.

- Gradual improvement after 20–30 minutes of rest

- Increased symptoms with poor air quality

- Most patients with asthma have some degree of exercise-induced symptoms, but exercise may be the only trigger.

- Initial treatment—short-acting beta-agonist 5–30 minutes prior to exercise (prevents symptoms for up to 2–3 hours).

- If symptoms occur regularly or more frequently, then use a control medication. May be a sign of poorly controlled asthma.

Presentation

The most common cause of wheezing in infants and young children is **upper respiratory infections** (most end during the preschool years); **strongest predictor for continuation of wheezing is atopic disease**.

- Early severe lower respiratory tract infection (hospitalization)
- Atopic dermatitis
- Allergic rhinitis
- Increased IgE
- Decreased spirometry at 6 years of age

Stepwise approach to the diagnosis and management of asthma

Step 1. Diagnosis

Thorough history and physical exam (focus on respiratory tract, chest, and skin). Must have:

- Episodic symptoms of airflow obstruction
  - Recurrent episodes of **cough with or without wheezing** are almost always caused by may be the only presenting finding (**positive family history**)
  - Chest tightness, shortness of breath, exercise intolerance/wheezing; symptoms **worse at night and may awaken patient from sleep** (exacerbated with **known triggers**)
  - Exam: **expiratory wheezing with prolongation of expiration**, hyperexpansion of thorax, use of accessory muscles, decreased breath sounds, tachypnea, evidence of atopic disease
- Condition at least partially reversible: response to medication
- Other diagnoses excluded (see Chapter 7)

Step 2. Objective measure to confirm diagnosis

- **Spirometry** to confirm diagnosis and assess reversibility in **children >5 years of age**: forced expiratory volume in 1 second (FEV1), forced vital capacity (FVC), and FEV_1/FVC decrease in value to reference/predicted values (standardized norms for age and race) with improvement after use of a bronchodilator.
- Monitor **peak expiratory flow (PEF) variability for 1–2 weeks**; used primarily for monitoring as reference values vary widely and PEF lacks sensitivity for diagnosis. **>20% difference between morning and evening measurements** indicates inadequate control.

Step 3. Classify severity of disease at diagnosis

Assess **impairment** (current) and **risk** (future). See Tables 8.2–8.4 for classification criteria.

- Classify before treatment is started, **but** classification can change over time (reassessed). Classify per the most severe step in which any feature occurs. After treatment is attained, classify according to the level of treatment to maintain **control**.
- Identify **exacerbating factors and comorbidities.**
- Per classification Tables 8.2–8.4: re-evaluate in 2–6 weeks (depending on severity) for level of control; if not significantly improved in 4–6 weeks, adjust therapy or consider another diagnosis or non-treated comorbidity.

Table 8.2: Classification of Asthma Severity in Children <5 Years of Age Not Currently Taking Controller Medication

Components of Severity	Intermittent	Mild Persistent	Moderate Persistent	Severe Persistent
Daytime symptoms	≤2 days/week	>2 days/week but not daily	Daily	Throughout the day
Nighttime awakenings	0	1–2 days/month	3–4 days/month	>1 day/week
Short-acting beta agonist use[1]	≤2 days/week	>2 days/week but not daily	Daily	Several times per day
Interference with normal activity	None	Minor limitation	Some limitation	Extremely limited
Exacerbations requiring oral corticosteroids	0–1 day/year	See Note 2	See Note 2	See Note 2
Therapy initiation step*	Step 1	Step 2	Step 3 ± short-course oral steroids	Step 3 ± short-course oral steroids

Note 1: For symptom use, not for exercise-induced bronchospasm

Note 2: ≥2 exacerbations in 6 months requiring oral corticosteroids or ≥4 wheezing episodes in one year lasting more than one day and with risk factors for persistent asthma

*Therapy initiation step described in Tables 8.7, 8.8, and 8.9.

Table 8.3: Classification of Asthma Severity in Children ≥5–12 Years of Age Not Currently Taking Controller Medications

Components of Severity	Intermittent	Mild Persistent	Moderate Persistent	Severe Persistent
Daytime symptoms	≤2 days/week	>2 days/week but not daily	Daily	Throughout the day
Nighttime awakenings	≤2 days/month	3–4 days/month	>1 day/week but not nightly	Often 7 days/week
Short-acting beta-agonist use	≤2 days/week	>2 days/week but not daily	Daily	Several times per day
Interference with normal activity	None	Minor limitation	Some limitation	Extremely limited
Lung function	-Normal FEV_1 between exacerbations -FEV_1 > 80% predicted -FEV_1/FVC > 85%	-FEV_1 > 80% predicted -FEV_1/FVC > 80%	-FEV_1 60–80% predicted -FEV_1/FVC 75–80%	-FEV_1 < 60% predicted -FEV_1/FVC < 75%
Exacerbations requiring oral corticosteroids	0–1/year	≥2/year	≥2/year	≥2/year
Therapy initiation step	Step 1	Step 2	Step 3, medium dose ICS option ± short-course oral steroids	Step 3, medium dose option or Step 4 ± short-course oral steroids

Abbreviations: forced expiratory volume in 1 second, FEV_1; forced vital capacity, FVC; inhaled corticosteroid, ICS

Table 8.4: Classification of Asthma Severity in Children ≥12 Years of Age Not Currently Taking Controller Medications

Components of Severity	Classification			
	Intermittent	**Mild Persistent**	**Moderate Persistent**	**Severe Persistent**
Daytime symptoms	≤2 days/week	>2 days/week but not daily	Daily	Throughout the day
Nighttime awakenings	≤2 days/month	3–4 days/month	>1 day/week but not nightly	Often 7 days/week
Short-acting beta-agonist use	≤2 days/week	>2 days/week but not daily and not more than once on any day	Daily	Several times per day
Lung function[1]	-Normal FEV_1 between exacerbations -FEV_1 >80% predicted -FEV_1/FVC normal	-FEV_1 >80% predicted -FEV_1/FVC normal	-FEV_1 >60% but <80% predicted -FEV_1/FVC reduced 5%	-FEV_1 <60% predicted -FEV_1/FVC reduced >5%
Exacerbations requiring oral corticosteroids	0–1/year	≥2/year	≥2/year	≥2/year
Therapy initiation step	Step 1	Step 2	Step 3	Step 4 or 5

Abbreviations: forced expiratory volume in 1 second, FEV_1; forced vital capacity, FVC
[1]Normal FEV_1/FVC: age 8–19 years, 85%; 20–39 years, 80%; 40–59 years, 75%; 60–80 years, 70%
Note: For children ≥12 years of age, impairment is also assessed using standardized questionnaires to assess quality of life (Asthma Control Test [ACT], Asthma Control Questionnaire [ACQ], Asthma Therapy Assessment Questionnaire [ATAQ] control index)

Step 4. Assess and monitor response to therapy and control

Goal: maintain control with the least amount of medications and minimal risk for adverse effects.

- Develop a **written action plan** based on **signs/symptoms and/or PEF** for daily management and worsening of symptoms.
- Evaluate and try to **control contributing factors**.
- Prevent frequent use of short-acting beta-agonist for symptoms.
- Maintain near-normal pulmonary function.
- Maintain normal activity levels.
- Minimize need for Emergency Room visits and hospitalizations.
- A monitoring plan should be in place—**based on either PEF measurements or symptom(s)**.
- Routine use at home to determine when to start a short-acting beta-agonist; call the doctor or proceed to the Emergency Room for an acute exacerbation. Can also be used to monitor response to changes in medications and during a short course of oral corticosteroids.

- Establish **a personal best** after diagnosis over 2–3 weeks when asthma is in control. Set zones on PEF: **green**: >80% personal best (no action needed); **yellow**: 50–80% (start beta-agonist and call doctor); **red**: <50% (start beta-agonist, proceed to medical office or ER for acute asthma exacerbation management).
  - **Periodic spirometry assessment if >5 years of age**: at initial visit, after stabilization on treatment, at least yearly, and with any change in therapy.
  - At every visit: provide **ongoing education**; and review medications, use of PEF, symptom monitoring, use of inhalers, and exacerbating factors.

Pharmacotherapy

Table 8.5: Asthma Medications: Quick-Relief

Quick-Relief Medications	Important Points	Adverse Reactions
SABAs (albuterol, levalbuterol [nebulized], bitolterol [age >12 years], metaproterenol, pirbuterol [age >12 years], terbutaline [age 12–15 years, oral; >15 years MDI, as adult])	-For any acute exacerbation for any class of severity -Onset within 5–10 minutes -Preferred delivery by MDI or nebulizer (as opposed to oral) -Drug of choice for exercise-induced bronchospasm -Not for chronic use	-Effects antagonized by beta-blockers -Tachycardia, palpitations, arrhythmias -Tremors -Headache -Hypokalemia -Excessive daily use associated with diminished symptom control and increased mortality -Increased cardiovascular effects with MAOIs, TCAs, and sympathomimetics -May have paradoxical bronchospasm with certain diseases
Anticholinergics (ipratropium bromide)	-Inhaled ipratropium added to beta-agonist may increase duration of bronchodilation -Drug of choice for beta-2 agonist–induced bronchospasm -Used primarily in severe acute exacerbations in combination with SABA	-May see atropine-like side effects -May have increased side effects when used in combination with SABA
Oral/parenteral corticosteroids	-Used as a short course (3–10 days) for acute asthma exacerbations -No tapering necessary -Also long-term with severe asthma not adequately controlled by other medications alone	-Steroid side effects related to dose and length of therapy -No significant side effects on short-course treatment -Decrease side effects with lowest possible long-term dose and alternate-day steroid therapy

Abbreviations: monoamine oxidase inhibitor, MAOI; metered-dose inhaler, MDI; short-acting beta-agonist, SABA; tricyclic antidepressant, TCA

Table 8.6: Asthma Medications: Long-Term Control

Long-Term Control Medications	Important Points	Adverse Reactions
Inhaled corticosteroid (ICS)	-Most potent and effective drug for asthma control -Long-term treatment decreases bronchial inflammation and hyperresponsiveness -Available as MDIs and DPIs -All come in low, medium, and high doses -Interfere with late phase but not immediate response	-Decreased side effects compared to oral -Potential small risk on linear growth but is balanced by efficacy -Most side effects: cough, dysphonia, and oral candidiasis (rinse mouth/throat out after use)
Chromones (cromolyn, nedocromil)	-No longer have a primary use -Alternate drug (not preferred) in mild persistent asthma -Alternate drug to exercise-induced bronchospasm in <5-year-olds -May be used with anticipated exposures to triggers (see previous discussion) -Therapeutic response takes at least 2 weeks -MDI or nebulized (most effective)	-Primary advantage is safety -Cough, nasal congestion, bronchospasm
LABAs (salmeterol, formoterol)	-Slower onset, longer action (use every 12 hours) -Can be administered only as a combined product with inhaled steroid (e.g., fluticasone + salmeterol, Advair®)	-Increase in asthma-related deaths (black-box warning) if used as a sole drug (without a inhaled steroid) -Serevent® (salmeterol) and Foradil® (formoterol) have been removed from the market

(continued)

Long-Term Control Medications	Important Points	Adverse Reactions
LTRAs (montelukast, zafirlukast)	-Montelukast may be used in all patients >2 years old; zafirlukast for those >5 years old -Best used as an add-on medication to an inhaled corticosteroid -Taken orally -May be taken the night before planned exercise as an adjunct to SABA prior to exercise	-Increased hepatic clearance with phenobarbital or rifampin -Elevated liver enzymes, cough, headache, abdominal pain, dizziness, dyspepsia
Leukotriene synthesis inhibitor (zileuton)	-May be used as an add-on alternative therapy for Steps 3 and 4 in children >12 years old	-Similar side effects to the LTRAs
Theophylline	-Mild to moderate bronchodilation -Tablets, capsule, sustained-release capsules -Must follow serum levels: affected by diet, febrile illnesses, and certain other medications -May be used as an add-on medication to achieve control in patients 5–12 years or as an alternative medication for ≥12 years	-Nausea, vomiting, anorexia, abdominal pain, GER -Nervousness, tachycardia, arrhythmias, seizures -Hyperactivity, agitation, changes in school performance
Monoclonal antibody (mAb) (omalizumab)	-Recombinant, DNA-derived, humanized IgG mAb that binds selectively to human IgE receptor on mast cells and basophils -Indicated for moderate to severe persistent asthma in children ≥12 years old with documented perennial allergens whose symptoms are not controlled by other medications alone	-Black-box warning for anaphylaxis

Abbreviations: dry powder inhaler, DPI; gastroesophageal reflux, GER; leukotriene receptor antagonist, LTRA; metered-dose inhaler, MDI; short-acting beta-agonist, SABA

Stepwise approach for managing asthma

Table 8.7: Stepwise Therapy in Children <5 Years of Age

Asthma Classification	Step of Therapy	Preferred Treatment	Alternate Treatment
Intermittent	Step 1	SABA PRN	—
Persistent	Step 2	Low-dose ICS	Montelukast or cromolyn
Step up therapy as needed to gain control *Step down if possible and asthma is well controlled for at least 3 months*	Step 3	Medium-dose ICS	—
	Step 4	Medium-dose ICS	PLUS either: montelukast or LABA
	Step 5	High-dose ICS	PLUS either: montelukast or LABA
	Step 6	High-dose ICS	PLUS either: montelukast or LABA PLUS oral corticosteroid

Abbreviations: inhaled corticosteroid, ICS; long-acting beta-agonist, LABA; short-acting beta-agonist, SABA

Table 8.8: Stepwise Therapy in Children ≥5–12 Years Old

Asthma Classification	Step of Therapy	Preferred Treatment	Alternate Treatment
Intermittent	Step 1	SABA PRN	—
Persistent	Step 2	Low-dose ICS	LTRA, cromolyn, nedocromil or theophylline
Step up therapy as needed to gain control *Step down if possible and asthma is well controlled for at least 3 months*	Step 3	Either: Low-dose ICS + LABA, LTRA, or theophylline OR Medium-dose ICS	—
	Step 4	Medium-dose ICS + LABA	Medium-dose ICS + either LTRA or theophylline
	Step 5	High-dose ICS + LABA	High-dose ICS + either LTRA or theophylline
	Step 6	High-dose ICS + LABA + oral corticosteroid	High-dose ICS + either LTRA or theophylline + oral corticosteroid

Abbreviations: inhaled corticosteroid, ICS; long-acting beta-agonist, LABA; leukotriene receptor antagonist, LTRA; short-acting beta-agonist, SABA

Table 8.9: Stepwise Therapy in Children ≥12 Years Old

Asthma Classification	Step of Therapy	Preferred Treatment	Alternate Treatment
Intermittent	Step 1	SABA PRN	—
Persistent	Step 2	Low-dose ICS	Cromolyn, LTRA, nedocromil, or theophylline
Step up therapy as needed to gain control / *Step down if possible and asthma is well controlled for at least 3 months*	Step 3	Either: Low-dose ICS + LABA OR medium-dose ICS	Low-dose ICS + either LTRA, theophylline or zileuton
	Step 4	Medium-dose ICS + LABA	Medium-dose ICS + either LTRA or theophylline or zileuton
	Step 5	High-dose ICS + LABA AND consider omalizumab (see above)	—
	Step 6	High-dose ICS + LABA + oral corticosteroid AND consider omalizumab	—

Abbreviations: inhaled corticosteroid, ICS; long-acting beta-agonist, LABA; leukotriene receptor antagonist, LTRA; short-acting beta-agonist, SABA

Managing acute exacerbations of asthma

Table 8.10: Severity of Acute Asthma Exacerbations in the ED Setting

Mild	Moderate	Severe	Life-Threatening
Dyspnea only with activity (assess tachypnea, retractions, and oxygen saturations in young infants)	Dyspnea interferes with usual activities	Dyspnea at rest and interferes with conversation	Too dyspneic to speak, and sweating
PEF ≥70% predicted or personal best	PEF 40–69% predicted or personal best	PEF <40% predicted or personal best	PEF <25% predicted or personal best
Usually cared for at home with good relief from a SABA and possible short course of oral corticosteroids	Requires office/ED visit and frequent inhaled SABA + oral corticosteroids; symptoms may last another 1–2 days after start of Rx	ED visit and more likely hospitalization with partial relief from frequent SABA + oral corticosteroids; symptoms may last >3 days after start of Rx	ED/hospitalization and possible PICU; minimal or no relief with frequent SABA + IV corticosteroids

Abbreviations: emergency department, ED; peak expiratory flow, PEF; pediatric intensive care unit, PICU; short-acting beta-agonist, SABA

Assess severity: Less severe signs and symptoms can be initially managed at home with an assessment of response to therapy. Measure PEF: Yellow zone – quick-relief medication and depending on response, contact with MD; Red zone – quick-relief medication + immediate medical care. Initial Rx: up to 2 treatments (2–6 puffs each) 20 minutes apart of SABA by MDI or nebulizer treatments

Good response	**Incomplete response**	**Poor response**
-No wheezing or dyspnea/tachypnea +	-Persistent wheezing and dyspnea/tachypnea	-Marked wheezing and dyspnea/tachypnea
-PEF ≥ 80%	-PEF 50–79%	-PEF < 50%
Contact MD for follow up	*Contact MD urgently*	*If severe and nonresponsive to initial Rx – Call*
Continue SABA every 3–4 hours X 24–48 hours	*Oral corticosteroids*	*MD and proceed to ER (consider 911)*
Consider short course of oral corticosteroids	*Continue inhaled SABA*	*Repeat inhaled SABA immediately*
		Oral corticosteroids

Figure 8.1: Initial Home Assessment and Management of an Acute Asthma Exacerbation

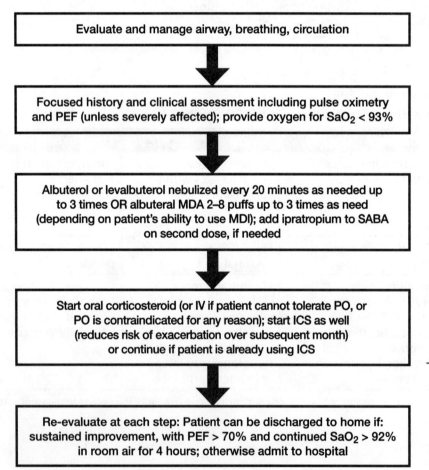

Evaluate and manage airway, breathing, circulation

Focused history and clinical assessment including pulse oximetry and PEF (unless severely affected); provide oxygen for $SaO_2 < 93\%$

Albuterol or levalbuterol nebulized every 20 minutes as needed up to 3 times OR albuteral MDA 2–8 puffs up to 3 times as need (depending on patient's ability to use MDI); add ipratropium to SABA on second dose, if needed

Start oral corticosteroid (or IV if patient cannot tolerate PO, or PO is contraindicated for any reason); start ICS as well (reduces risk of exacerbation over subsequent month) or continue if patient is already using ICS

Re-evaluate at each step: Patient can be discharged to home if: sustained improvement, with PEF > 70% and continued $SaO_2 > 92\%$ in room air for 4 hours; otherwise admit to hospital

Discharge to home on frequent SABA administration (MDI or nebulized) +3 –10 day course of oral corticosteroids and follow up with primary care MD within 24 hours for further management.

Figure 8.2: Emergency Outpatient Management of Acute Asthma Exacerbation

Hospital management of status asthmaticus

1. Supplemental oxygen with pulse oximetry monitoring to maintain $SaO_2 > 92\%$

2. Frequent (every 1–4 hours) or continuously (nebulized; need cardiac monitoring in pediatric intensive care unit [PICU])—administered **short-acting beta-agonist (SABA)**

3. Add **ipratropium** to SABA every 6 hours.

4. Continue **systemic (oral if patient can tolerate) corticosteroids**; every 6–12 hours for 48 hours, then daily.

5. If patient has severe sustained symptoms and high flow oxygen requirements, should be **admitted to PICU; obtain arterial blood gas, chest x-ray** (atelectasis is common, but may be severe; also for possibility of infection and air leak), CBC (infection), and a basic chemistry panel (dehydration; syndrome of inappropriate antidiuretic hormone secretion [SIADH]).

6. For severe case in the PICU: consider IV aminophylline (monitor levels and cardiac status), **IV MgSO$_4$, inhaled heliox,** parenteral epinephrine or terbutaline for life-threatening obstruction not responsive to high-dose SABA (inhaled drug may not reach lower airways).

7. Anticipate need for **ventilation** in advance with pattern of worsening respiratory failure and arterial blood gases so that an **elective rapid-induction intubation** may be performed safely.

8. **No** chest physical therapy, mucolytics, or incentive spirometry during acute exacerbation (can trigger worsening bronchoconstriction).

9. The patient may be **discharged** with same criteria as discharge from the ER on frequent SABA treatments, plus continued short course of oral corticosteroids and follow-up within 24 hours with the primary MD.

IMMUNODEFICIENCIES

When to Suspect an Immunodeficiency

- More than one serious systemic bacterial infection or other serious documented bacterial infections
- Persistent, recurrent bacterial infections (otitis media, sinusitis)
- Inadequate/no response to prolonged antibiotic therapy or the need for parenteral antibiotics for infections usually requiring oral therapy
- Unusual sites of infection (e.g., liver)
- Opportunistic organism infections
- Common childhood organisms resulting in serious infections
- Chronic diarrhea and failure to thrive

Primary Defects in Antibody Production

Most common presenting findings for primary antibody (B-cell) defects

- **Recurrent sinopulmonary infections** (otitis media, sinusitis, pneumonia, much more common than sepsis or meningitis) with **encapsulated bacteria** beginning at **5–7 months of age** (after decrease of maternal transplacental IgG): e.g., streptococcus, staphylococci, *Haemophilus*
- Recurrent/chronic hepatitis and **recurrent central nervous system (CNS) enteroviral infections** (fatal echoviral meningoencephalitis)
- Growth and development usually normal unless recurrent CNS infection or late-stage lung disease
- Later increased incidence (in some defects) **of autoimmune disease, lymphoreticular malignancy, and lymphoma**

Table 9.1: Comparison of the Most Prevalent B-Cell Defects

	Defect	Genetics	Clinical Presentation	Physical Exam	Lab Findings	RX
Bruton Agamma-globulinemia	Defect in B-lymphocyte development → severe hypogamma-globulinemia and absence (<1%) of circulating B cells	Majority are X-linked (gene = Bruton tyrosine kinase); five autosomal recessive defects	Males at age 6–9 months with recurrent infections; also *Mycoplasma*	No tonsils or palpable lymph nodes	Serum IgG, IgA, IgM, and IgE very low for age and sex; low specific antibodies; very low/absent circulating B cells by flow cytometry	Monthly IVIG + antibiotics as needed for documented bacterial infections
Transient Hypogamma-globulinemia of Infancy	Prolonged / increased physiologic hypogamma-globulinemia occurring at 3–6 months of life; usually lasts to age 3–5 years; may have a transient deficiency of T-helper cells	—	Recurrent sinopulmonary infections beginning at ~ age 10 months; ↑ incidence of atopic disease, chronic diarrhea and infections with *Giardia lamblia* and *Clostridium difficile*; no life-threatening infections	No diagnostic findings	Low serum IgG and IgA, normal IgM; may develop selective IgA deficiency; normal antibody production after vaccines and normal blood A and B isohemag-glutinins; B- and T-cell numbers and function are normal; delayed ability to produce antibodies to respiratory viruses	Mostly supportive with appropriate antibiotic use; rarely, short courses of IVIG if not good response to antibiotics

(continued)

	Defect	Genetics	Clinical Presentation	Physical Exam	Lab Findings	RX
Common Variable Immuno-deficiency (CVID)	Phenotypically normal B cells that do not differentiate into Ig-producing cells	Several different known genetic defects; most cases sporadic or autosomal dominant; less autosomal recessive	Later onset (variable) with similar infections to Bruton, but rarely echoviral meningoen-cephalitis; equal sex distribution; many associated autoantibody disease and large increased incidence of lymphoma later in life	Normal to increased tonsillar size and lymph nodes ± splenomegaly	Low IgG; low to undetectable levels of IgA and IgM; poor specific antibody responses; no Ig production to mitogen stimulation	Same as Bruton but must screen periodically for anti-IgA antibodies (then remove IgA from Ig)
Selective IgA Deficiency	Isolated absence or almost complete absence of serum and secretory IgA; most common immuno-deficiency; deficit is unknown (there are phenotypically normal B cells)	Seems to be autosomal dominant with variable expression	Mostly recurrent respiratory, gastrointestinal and urogenital infections; high incidence of intestinal giardiasis; increased autoantibody disease and malignancy later in life.	No diagnostic findings	Very low or absent IgA; other immunoglobulins are normal and IgM may be increased	Treat documented infections aggressively; *do not* give IVIG (many patients have IgE class antibodies to IgA and may develop anaphylaxis); also, most make IgG normally (and IVIG is 99% IgG)

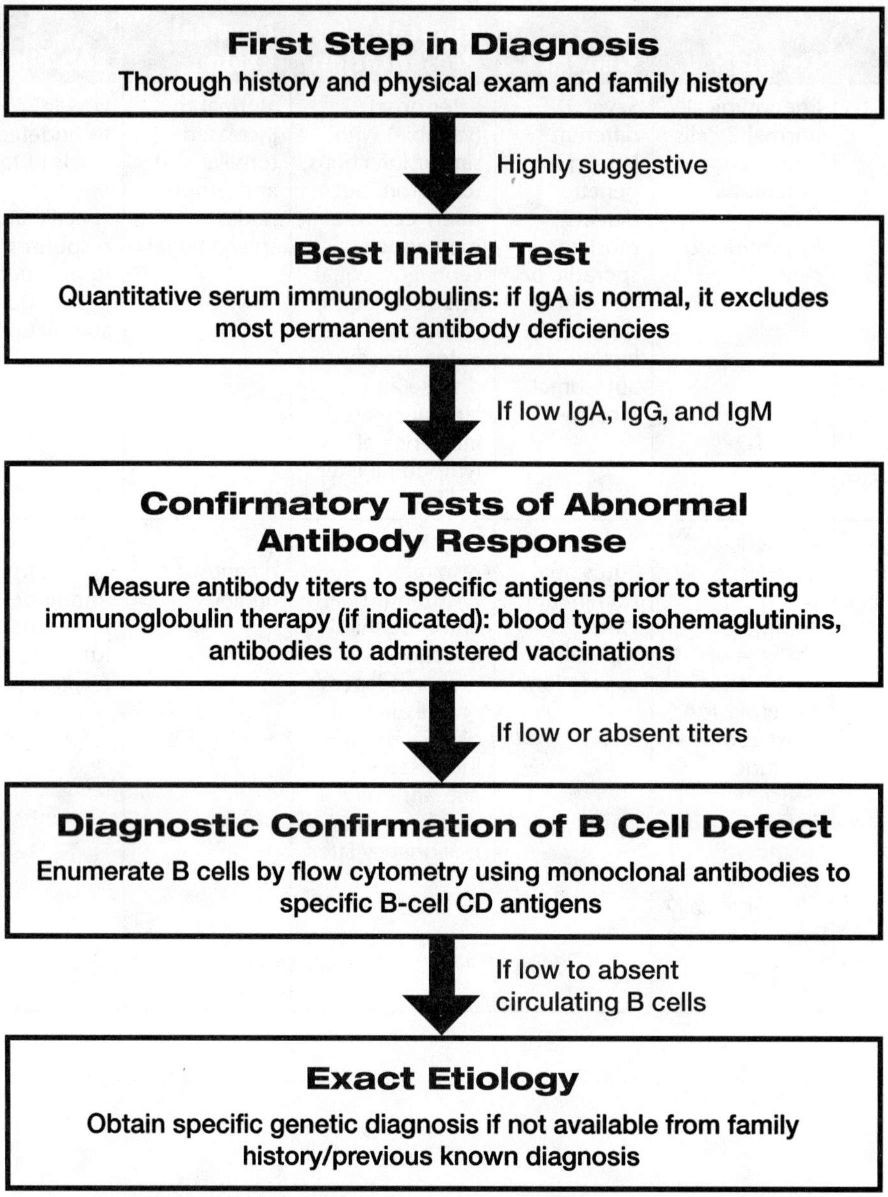

```
┌────────────────────────────────────────────────────────┐
│                  First Step in Diagnosis                 │
│     Thorough history and physical exam and family history│
└────────────────────────────────────────────────────────┘
                          │
                          ▼  Highly suggestive
┌────────────────────────────────────────────────────────┐
│                   Best Initial Test                      │
│  Quantitative serum immunoglobulins: if IgA is normal,   │
│  it excludes most permanent antibody deficiencies        │
└────────────────────────────────────────────────────────┘
                          │
                          ▼  If low IgA, IgG, and IgM
┌────────────────────────────────────────────────────────┐
│            Confirmatory Tests of Abnormal                │
│                  Antibody Response                       │
│    Measure antibody titers to specific antigens prior to │
│    starting immunoglobulin therapy (if indicated): blood │
│    type isohemaglutinins, antibodies to adminstered      │
│    vaccinations                                          │
└────────────────────────────────────────────────────────┘
                          │
                          ▼  If low or absent titers
┌────────────────────────────────────────────────────────┐
│          Diagnostic Confirmation of B Cell Defect        │
│  Enumerate B cells by flow cytometry using monoclonal    │
│  antibodies to specific B-cell CD antigens               │
└────────────────────────────────────────────────────────┘
                          │
                          ▼  If low to absent
                             circulating B cells
┌────────────────────────────────────────────────────────┐
│                    Exact Etiology                        │
│  Obtain specific genetic diagnosis if not available from │
│  family history/previous known diagnosis                 │
└────────────────────────────────────────────────────────┘
```

Figure 9.1: Diagnostic workup for suspected B-cell defect

Primary T-Cell Defects

Most common presenting findings with T-cell defects: Opportunistic infections (*Mycobacteria,* Epstein-Barr virus (EBV), cytomegalovirus (CMV), other viruses, *Candida albicans, Pneumocystis carinii)* in the first months of life with chronic diarrhea and failure-to-thrive

DiGeorge syndrome

Etiology and genetics—Microdeletion at 22q11.2 (DiGeorge chromosomal region); **CATCH 22 association**: **C,** cardiac defects; **A,** abnormal facies; **T,** thymic hypoplasia; **C,** cleft palate; **H,** hypocalcemia (another example is the velocardiofacial syndrome). Leads to **dysmorphogenesis of the 3rd and 4th pharyngeal pouches →**

- **Thymic** hypoplasia/dysplasia
- **Parathyroid** hypoplasia/aplasia
- Anomalies of **the great vessels** (e.g., right-sided aortic arch, interrupted aortic arch)
- **Congenital heart disease** (conotruncal, atrial septal defect [ASD], ventral septal defect [VSD])
- Esophageal atresia
- Bifid uvula
- Characteristic pattern of **facial dysmorphism**

There are two forms: **partial DiGeorge syndrome** (variable hypoplasia of thymus and parathyroid [much more common]), and **complete DiGeorge syndrome** (aplasia); one-third of the complete forms also have the **CHARGE association** (see Chapter 2).

Clinical presentation—The most common is **neonatal hypocalcemic seizures**; with the partial form, children have minimal problems with infection and tend to grow normally; the complete form is severe: recurrent/persistent infections with opportunistic organisms and hypocalcemia with or without congenital heart disease and findings consistent with the CHARGE association. May have a graft-versus-host disease (GVHD; acute = skin rash, anorexia, vomiting, diarrhea, and liver dysfunction) if transfused with non-irradiated blood components (i.e., containing immunocompetent T-cells).

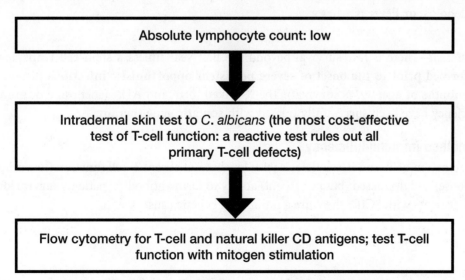

Figure 9.2: Diagnostic workup for suspected T-cell defect

Laboratory findings—Immunoglobulins are, for the most part, normal (but may have a decreased IgA with an increased IgE); **moderate to severe decrease in absolute lymphocyte count** and decreased to absent response to mitogens (proportional to the degree of thymic hypoplasia); **moderate to severe decrease in serum calcium concentration**.

Treatment—Thymic transplant or major histocompatibility complex (MHC)-compatible sibling or half-matched parental stem-cell transplant

Combined T- and B-Cell Defects

Severe combined immunodeficiency disease (SCID)

May occur with a number of different genetic mutations (with respect to any of 12 genes which are needed for lymphoid cell development), causing **absence of all immune function and also lack of natural killer (NK) cells and function** in most severe form. **X-linked**: most common form in the United States; very low percentage of T-cells and NK-cells with increased percentage of B cells. **Autosomal recessive**: autosomal chromosome mutations → 11 identified.

Clinical findings/presentation
- **Recurrent/persistent diarrhea with growth failure beginning in first few months of life**
- Initially, **recurrent/persistent bacterial then opportunistic infections**
- May have **early GVHD** from maternal T cells crossing placenta
- No T cells from birth → **severe lymphopenia and no response to mitogens**
- **Severe decrease to absent serum immunoglobulins and no antibody responses after vaccination**
- Very small thymus and spleen depleted of lymphocytes; **no lymph nodes, tonsils, adenoids, or Peyer patches**

Treatment—There is rare survival beyond the first year unless a **stem-cell transplant is performed prior to the onset of severe persistent opportunistic infections (usually by 3.5 months of age; >95% survival)**. The X-linked form and ADA (adenosine deaminase) deficiency have been successfully treated with **somatic gene therapy**.

Combined immunodeficiency

Combination of T- and B-cell defects with low but not absent T-cell function (low mitogen response) and decreased (but not absent) ability to form antibodies; patients survive longer than patients with SCID; there are a number of genetic causes.

Wiskott-Aldrich syndrome

Genetics—**X-linked recessive**; abnormal gene at X-11.22-11.23 (Wiskott-Aldrich syndrome protein, WASP)

Findings
- **Atopic dermatitis** (eczema)
- **Thrombocytopenic purpura** (small, defective platelets with normal-appearing megakaryocytes)
- **Recurrent infections**

Most common clinical presentation—**Early prolonged bleeding** (e.g., after a circumcision); eczema and recurrent sinopulmonary infections, **sepsis, and meningitis with encapsulated bacteria in the first year of life**; later, increased incidence of *Pneumocystis carinii* and herpesvirus infections; rarely live past adolescence without definitive treatment. Most causes of death are from overwhelming infection, hemorrhage, and **malignancy associated with EBV (Epstein-Barr virus)**.

Laboratory findings—**Moderate decrease in T-cells** and decreased mitogen response; **variable difference in immunoglobulin concentrations** (most with low IgM, increased IgA and IgE, and normal or slightly low IgG)

Management—Supportive care: **monthly IVIG**, skin care for dermatitis, control bleeding (platelet transfusions splenectomy), and replace blood volume; **bone marrow or cord blood transplantation**

Ataxia-telangiectasia

Genetics—Ataxia-telangiectasia mutation (ATM) at 11q22-23 → **thymic hypoplasia and moderate decreased response to T- and B-cell mitogens**; moderate decrease in CD3 and CD4 percentages with normal to increased CD8

Most common clinical presentation—**Progressive cerebellar ataxia after onset of walking**, ending up in a wheelchair in late childhood; then **onset of chronic sinopulmonary disease**; **oculocutaneous telangiectasias** first seen between age 3–6 years; **high incidence of lymphoreticular malignancies and adenocarcinoma.**

Laboratory findings—**Variable B- and T-cell deficiencies**; most have a **selective absence of IgA** with a low IgE and at times a decrease in IgG; specific antibody titers may be normal to low.

Management—Primarily supportive; there is no known treatment of the CNS pathology; immune reconstitution (bone marrow, stem-cell transplant) is difficult and has not been very successful.

Abnormalities of Phagocytic Function

Most common presenting findings for phagocytic defects

Very **similar in appearance to primary antibody defects**; should be considered if initial screening tests for other immunodeficiencies are normal in a patient with **recurrent or unusual bacterial infections**.

Workup for suspected phagocytic defects

Initial CBC for total neutrophils and monocytes; then flow cytometric assessment of the **respiratory burst** using a rhodamine dye; specific diagnoses may be made using flow cytometry assays of lymphocytes or neutrophils with monoclonal antibodies for **specific CD antigens**. Final diagnosis is **molecular analysis for exact diagnosis**.

Leukocyte adhesion deficiency

Genetics/etiology—Autosomal recessive; two types; **inability of neutrophils to adhere firmly to surfaces and undergo transepithelial migration**

Key diagnostic words—Infants with recurrent/persistent bacterial (*Staphylococcus aureus* and Gram-negatives) and fungal infections; large, chronic skin ulcers; delayed separation of umbilical cord and omphalitis; severe gingivitis and loss of primary and secondary teeth; absence of typical signs of inflammation and no pus at sites of infection (low amount of neutrophils in tissue but increased neutrophils seen in peripheral blood)

Laboratory findings—Finding of specific CD abnormalities using flow cytometry; abnormal neutrophil and monocyte function; very high neutrophil counts during infection, and higher-than-normal neutrophils in peripheral blood in absence of infection

Management—Supportive plus other therapy dependent on phenotype; early allogenic **stem-cell transplant**

Chediak-Higashi syndrome

Genetics/etiology—Autosomal recessive; mutated gene at 1q2-q44; **oversized and abnormal lysosomes, storage granules, or vesicular structures (increased fusion of cytoplasmic granules)** → generalized cellular dysfunction → deficiency in proteolytic enzymes → **decreased neutrophil chemotaxis, degranulation, and bactericidal function, and therefore impaired killing**; also, abnormal melanocytes and compromised delivery to keratinocytes and hair follicles.

Key diagnostic words—Light skin/silvery hair (**partial oculocutaneous albinism**); impaired platelet aggregation → increased bleeding time and a **mild bleeding diathesis**; **recurrent mucocutaneous and respiratory infections with Gram-positive and Gram-negative bacteria**; sensory or motor **neuropathy** beginning in adolescence and **becoming the most prominent finding** over time; inability to control EBV infections; development of **life-threatening lymphoma-like syndromes**

Laboratory finding—The key to the diagnosis is **finding large inclusions in all nucleated blood cells**.

Management—Supportive; only cure is **a stem-cell transplant**.

Myeloperoxidase (MPO) deficiency

Autosomal recessive disorder causing decreased production of MPO (green heme protein in lysosomes of neutrophils and monocytes; **gives green color to pus**) → decreased production of hypochlorous acid → early depression of Gram-positive and Gram-negative bacteria in vitro but killing rates shortly return to normal due to other mechanisms; is **usually clinically silent**, but may **rarely present with disseminated candidiasis** (especially with diabetes). The treatment is that of treating fungal infections, if present.

Chronic granulomatous disease

- **X-linked** (more common) or autosomal recessive (three autosomal chromosomes); often seen with a positive family history (mostly **males** affected). Most common inherited disorder of phagocytosis.
- **Neutrophils and monocytes can ingest but not kill catalase-positive organisms.** Normal neutrophils stimulate phagosomal hydrogen peroxide; MPO is delivered to the phagosome (degranulation). Hydrogen peroxide is a substrate for MPO → oxidation of halide → hypochlorous acid/chloramines → microbial killing. Many aerobic micro organisms produce **catalase → metabolizes hydrogen peroxide**; the amount of hydrogen peroxide produced is more than the ability of catalase to metabolize it. Therefore, since the **patient does not produce hydrogen peroxide**, the organisms entering the neutrophils will not be destroyed by it, and the hydrogen peroxide that is made by the microorganism is metabolized by its own catalase → **survival of catalase-positive organisms.** Catalase-negative organisms (e.g., streptococci) will generate enough hydrogen peroxide and be killed.

Findings—Recurrent infections with catalase-positive organisms causing pneumonia, skin infections, lymphadenitis, abscesses (liver and elsewhere), and osteomyelitis at more than one site; from early infancy to early adulthood. **Granuloma formation** may be the present finding and leads to obstruction depending on the site; e.g., intestinal or rectal fistulae, pyloric obstruction, bladder obstruction. The most common organism is *Staphylococcus aureus*. Then a number of **Gram-negative enterics:** *Aspergillus, Candida,* and *Nocardia*.

Diagnosis—The nitroblue tetrazolium has been replaced by the **more accurate flow cytometric assay using 123 dihydrorhodamine dye**, which detects production of oxidants and increases fluorescence when oxidized by hydrogen peroxide (i.e., the normal condition).

Management—Supportive therapy and prophylactic antibiotics for bacterial and fungal infections; interferon decreases the number of serious infections; only cure is a **stem-cell transplant**.

Complement System Disorders

Complement is a system of interacting proteins (classical, lectin, and alternative pathways) functioning as a cascade system; important for aiding in a number of immune functions. The screening test is a decrease in **total hemolytic complement (CH_{50})**, which tests for deficiencies of the 11 components of the classical pathway and membrane attack complex (not any others). For most of the disorders there are **recurrent pyogenic infections**, especially pneumococcal and meningococcal, and autoimmune disease (especially systemic lupus erythematosus [SLE] and glomerulonephritis). Deficiency of C1 is responsible for hereditary angioedema. Treatment is supportive; there is **no available long-term therapy** for complement deficiencies.

COLLAGEN VASCULAR DISORDERS

10

Juvenile Rheumatoid Arthritis (JRA)

Autoimmune disease resulting in **chronic inflammation of the joints**; may lead to **joint destruction and severe disability**. Genetic predisposition (family history of autoimmune disease) and increased immune reactivity with an environmental triggering event. Patients with **certain HLA types appear to be more susceptible**.

Criteria for diagnosis

American College of Rheumatology diagnostic criteria:

- **Onset at <16 years** of age
- Evidence of **arthritis in at least one joint**
- Duration of signs and symptoms for **at least 6 weeks**
- **Pauciarticular, polyarticular, or systemic disease** in the first 6 months of involvement
- **Exclusion of other causes** of arthritis

Laboratory findings are supportive and not necessary for the diagnosis.

- **Elevated acute-phase reactants**
- **Microcytic anemia**
- Positive **antinuclear antibody (ANA)**
- **Positive rheumatoid factor (RF)**
- Arthrocentesis: **exclude septic arthritis with monoarticular swelling**

Management

- **First-line medication—NSAIDs** (most with pauciarticular and some with polyarticular disease will respond) ± intra-articular corticosteroids; use oral corticosteroids for severe inflammation and for bridging therapy
- If **insufficient response**—add an **immunosuppressive agent** (**methotrexate** oral or subcutaneous) or alternative (**sulfasalazine** or leflunomide)
- For those **unresponsive to conventional therapy**—add a tumor necrosis factor inhibitor (etanercept) or an immunomodulator (azathioprine, cyclophosphamide)

- Plus: physical and occupational therapy; psychosocial evaluation/therapy; annual ophthalmologic evaluation; diet (good nutrition plus calcium-rich foods and/or calcium supplementation); physical activity with self-limitation for pain.

Diagnostic and prognostic findings based on classification of JRA

Pauciarticular Disease

- ≤ **4 affected joints** at onset: large joints of **lower extremity (not the hip)**
- Most likely to have **positive ANA;** marker for the development of **chronic anterior uveitis** (iridocyclitis), especially with presentation of disease in **young girls** (may develop **significant visual problems**)
- Less likely to have **positive RF;** but if present, looks more like polyarticular disease (**long-term severe joint involvement and poorer prognosis**)

versus

Polyarticular Disease

- ≥ **5 joints involved** at onset – large and small joints
- Looks more like **adult rheumatoid arthritis – severe hand and wrist involvement**
- **Rheumatoid nodules – more severe**
- Early cervical spine and hip involvement
- May have positive ANA – if younger females, tend to have less severe joint involvement and a better long-term prognosis
- More likely to have **positive RF; marker for adult-type RA with poor prognosis**

versus

Systemic Disease

- Systemic/visceral involvement at onset: daily **spiking fevers + evanescent salmon-colored polymorphous rash** on trunk and extremities; lymphadenopathy, hepatosplenomegaly and serositis (pleural, pericardial, peritoneal)
- Presents with arthraligia and without findings of arthritis, **but will develop pauciarticular or polyarticular disease.**
- Systemic problems at onset may be severe and difficult to control, but tends to regress after first few years
- **Prognosis worse with greater and more severe joint involvement**
- More common to have negative serology

Figure 10.1: Classification of JRA with Diagnostic and Prognostic Features

Systemic Lupus Erythematosus (SLE)

Autoantibody disease that can affect **any organ** with organ damage through the production of antibodies against specific antigens (**against DNA and other nuclear antigens, ribosomes, blood cells, and many tissue-specific antigens**) and immune complex deposition. **Renal disease may occur at any time and is a common complication.** Greater prevalence in non-white Americans (largest number in African Americans) with female preponderance. Almost one-quarter of cases present by age 20 years.

Table 10.1: Autoantibodies in SLE

Antibody	Clinical Significance
Antinuclear antibody (ANA)	Present in **most with SLE**, but is not specific (also with: JRA, scleroderma, drug-induced lupus, dermatomyositis chronic active hepatitis, some vasculitis, and infectious mononucleosis); **best screen**
Anti-double stranded DNA (anti-ds-DNA)	**More specific for SLE; reflects disease activity**
Anti-Smith antibody (anti-Sm)	**Specific for SLE; does not reflect disease activity**
Anti-ribosomal P antibody	Marker for **lupus cerebritis**
Anti-Ro and Anti-La	SLE in children with Sjögren syndrome (rare)
Anti-Ro/SSA or Anti-La/SSB	**IgG maternal antibodies crossing the placenta → neonatal lupus**
Antiphospholipid antibodies (APL)	Antiphospholipid syndrome: thrombosis, livedo reticularis, Raynaud phenomenon, thrombocytopenia, positive lupus coagulant, recurrent fetal loss
Lupus anticoagulant	In most patients with SLE; **associated with APL antibodies;** increased incidence of **deep venous thrombosis** and neurological complications; may give a **false-positive serological test for syphilis and an increased PTT**
Coombs-positive	Hemolytic anemia
Antiplatelet antibodies	Thrombocytopenia
Antithyroid antibodies	Hypothyroidism
Antihistone antibodies	May be found after exposure to **certain drugs** (sulfonamides, certain antiarrhythmic agents, certain anticonvulsants) → drug-induced lupus (cross reactivity)

Abbreviations: antinuclear antibody, ANA; antiphospholipid antibodies, APL; juvenile rheumatoid arthritis, JRA; partial thromboplastin time, PTT; systemic lupus erythematosus, SLE

Diagnosis and clinical presentation—American College of Rheumatology diagnostic criteria—**presence of 4 of 11 criteria** (serially or simultaneously). The LE cell preparation is no longer one of the criteria, which has been replaced with a false-positive syphilis serological test.

Table 10.2: Diagnostic Criteria for SLE (need 4 of 11)

1	Malar rash
2	Discoid rash
3	Photosensitive rash
4	Oral or nasopharyngeal ulcers, usually painless
5	Non-erosive peripheral arthritis in at least two joints
6	Serositis: pleuritic or pericarditis
7	Renal disease (persistent proteinuria or cellular casts)
8	Neurological disease: seizures or psychosis (without cause from drugs or metabolic problems)
9	Hematological disorder: hemolytic anemia or thrombocytopenia or leukopenia/lymphopenia on at least two occasions
10	Antibodies: abnormal titer anti-ds-DNA, positive anti-Sm, APL (abnormal anticardiolipin antibodies, lupus anticoagulant, or false-positive serologic test for syphilis)
11	Abnormal titer of ANA at any time (and in absence of evidence of drug-induced lupus)

Table 10.3: Most Common and Less Common Presenting Symptoms in Childhood SLE

Most Common	Less Common
Fever, anorexia, weight loss	Pulmonary (hemorrhage, evidence of pleuritis, infection, fibrosis)
Arthralgia/arthritis	Neurologic (seizures, thromboembolism, psychosis, peripheral neuritis, behavioral and cognitive changes)
Rash (as above plus livedo reticularis and vasculitic)	Cardiovascular (thromboembolic phenomena, pericarditis, myocarditis, endocarditis, heart failure, arrhythmias)
Lymphadenopathy	Peritonitis
Hepatosplenomegaly/hepatitis	Bowel infarction
Abdominal pain, diarrhea, melena	Endocrine disorders (thyroid, glucose, adrenal)
Hematological (anemia of chronic disease or hemolytic anemia, thrombocytopenia, leukopenia)	
Renal (hypertension, glomerulonephritis, nephrosis, acute renal failure; from minimal mesangial changes to advanced sclerosing nephritis)	
Laboratory findings: elevated acute-phase reactants (ESR, CRP, platelets); anemia, elevated WBCs or leukopenia/lymphopenia; **depressed** CH_{50}, **C3, C4**; positive ANA; positive anti-ds-DNA; positive anti-Sm	

Abbreviations: antinuclear antibody, ANA; anti-double stranded DNA, anti-ds-DNA; anti-Smith antibody, anti-Sm; C-reactive protein, CRP; erythrocyte sedimentation rate, ESR; white blood cells, WBC

Management

Multidisciplinary management frequently:

- Thorough interim history and physical
- Lab studies for possible complications
- Normal activities and exercise
- Diet—no added salt, low fat, calcium-rich foods

Table 10.4: Pharmacologic Treatment of SLE

Medication	Clinical Considerations
NSAIDs	First medications for **mild disease** without nephritis; particularly for **arthralgia/arthritis**; possible **hepatic and renal toxicities**
Hydroxychloroquine	**Additional drug for milder symptoms**; long-term use may be **steroid-sparing**, decreases risk of thromboembolism. Most side effects: eye changes (retinal), diarrhea, and neurobehavioral changes
Corticosteroids	With **more severe systemic disease**, especially with **renal disease** and persistently low complement levels; monitor for usual short- and long-term steroid side effects
Low molecular-weight heparin	Drug of choice for **thrombosis, APL, lupus anticoagulant**; may use warfarin
Cyclophosphamide, azathioprine, mycophenolate (alternative drug for certain types of nephritis); newer investigative drugs and procedures per research evaluation	Severe disease, especially with proliferative glomerulonephritis, continued vasculitis, pulmonary hemorrhage, severe persistent CNS disease

Abbreviations: antiphospholipid antibodies, APL; central nervous system, CNS; nonsteroidal anti-inflammatory drugs, NSAIDs

Neonatal lupus

Maternal transfer of IgG antibodies across placenta; may manifest with any findings of lupus, although most common presentation is that one organ is involved (**usually rash on face and scalp** after exposure to ultraviolet radiation). Symptoms may be delayed in presentation; most of the findings resolve (over several months); with the exception of **congenital heart block** (from prolonged PR interval to hemodynamically significant third-degree block), which is **permanent**. (If the patient has a hemodynamically significant block, pacing is required.)

Spondyloarthropathies

Juvenile ankylosing spondylitis

- Inflammation of **peripheral and axial skeleton** plus **enthesitis** (inflammation of sites of attachments of tissues to bone, e.g., tendons, ligaments, fascia) plus a **negative RF**
- Familial, with majority HLA-B27–positive; mostly in males in late childhood, adolescence, or young adulthood
- Most common presentation: nonspecific constitutional symptoms plus **arthritis mostly in leg joints** (hips may be involved; difference from JRA) plus enthesitis (especially at the tendons of the knees and feet), plus seronegativity (negative RF and ANA); later development of axial skeletal joint problems, especially sacroiliac; highly variable course with long periods of disease activity and remission; possible complications: **anterior uveitis**, aortic valve regurgitation, atlanto-axial subluxation. May have progressive disease with **spinal/sacroiliac joint fusion and severe disability**.
- Laboratory findings: increase in acute-phase reactants, **negative ANA and RF; positive HLA-B27**; characteristic x-ray changes at affected locations

- Management: nonsteroidal anti-inflammatory drugs (NSAIDs) for inflammation and pain with or without intra-articular corticosteroids; add **sulfasalazine** if poor response, and then **methotrexate** if needed. Regular exercise to maintain joint mobility.

Arthritis associated with inflammatory bowel disease (IBD)

- Most common presentation: **polyarthritis of small and large joints proportional to degree of intestinal inflammatory activity;** no spinal joint involvement and HLA-B27 is negative.
- Less common: **similar to ankylosing spondylitis**; severity is not dependent upon bowel inflammatory activity; most are HLA-B27–positive.

Arthritis associated with psoriasis

Positive family history of psoriasis or early nail changes in patient with onset of oligoarthritis: asymmetric involvement of large and small joints; or symmetrical involvement of distal interphalangeal joints; or, rarely, as an HLA-B27–positive sacroiliitis

Reactive and post-infectious arthritis

- **Post-infectious arthritis is a sterile synovitis** after treatment of a suppurative arthritis.
- **Reactive arthritis** (with or without **urethritis and conjunctivitis**): onset of a severe **oligoarthritis, usually of the lower extremities or of an HLA-B27–positive sacroiliitis with enthesitis**, most commonly following a gastrointestinal (*Salmonella, Shigella, Campylobacter jejuni, Yersinia enterocolitica, Cryptosporidium parvum, Giardia intestinalis*) or genitourinary (*Chlamydia trachomatis, Ureaplasma*) tract infection; possible autoimmune reaction due to similarity between self antigens and bacterial antigens; may be predisposed by certain HLA types, especially HLA-B27.
- Usually clinical presentation: **one or more joints involved plus enthesitis, with or without urethritis and conjunctivitis; days to weeks after infection** and usually lasting less than 6 weeks; may evolve to a chronic arthritis. Diagnosis is by exclusion and often only after resolution. Treatment is pain management and control of inflammation (NSAIDs).

Juvenile Dermatomyositis

- **Inflammatory myopathy**
- Most with class II HLA antigen DQA1*0501
- Genetic predisposition plus interaction with antigenic stimulation and environmental factors (**most children have an illness in the 3 months prior to disease onset**: upper respiratory infection [URI], gastroenteritis, group A streptococcal)
- Most are white, female, with average age of 7 years
- First symptoms nonspecific constitutional symptoms and musculoskeletal complaints
- Then insidious development of proximal muscle weakness (sparing the eyes and facial muscles) → easy fatigability
- Half develop characteristic rash on sun-exposed areas, called a heliotrope: violaceous erythema around the eyes; may or may not cross the nasal bridge (masklike)
- Accompanied by periorbital, scalp, and generalized edema.

- Rash may be the first finding, with later development of the myositis (weakness and tender muscles).
  - Erythematous, palpable rash also over extensor joint surfaces, especially **metacarpals and interphalangeal joints**.
  - A **diffuse, severe vasculopathy** develops (skin, oral, and GI infarction → possible progressive bowel infarction and death)
  - **Upper airway dysfunction** with dysphagia and aspiration.
  - **Pathological calcifications** in children who have a longer time to diagnosis and decreased early aggressive immunosuppression (subcutaneous and fascial); may become infected with *Staph. aureus* → septicemia and death.

Laboratory findings—**Elevated muscle enzymes** (creatinine kinase, aldolase, lactate dehydrogenase [LDH]); **positive ANA with speckled pattern**; negative tests for other antibodies except for **antibody to the Pm/Scl antigen** (polymyositis/scleroderma; positive in some → fingers look similar to scleroderma and may have cardiac findings plus interstitial lung disease); **normal ESR**; Coombs-negative anemia; **best diagnostic test: MRI-directed electromyogram (myopathy) and muscle biopsy** (characteristic pathological findings at active sites of disease).

Management—**Hydroxychloroquine and daily prednisone** for milder disease; if extensive vasculopathy: intermittent **high-dose intravenous methylprednisolone**; with persistent disease: **cyclophosphamide or mycophenolate**. Less than 1% mortality in children; many stabilize and improve.

Scleroderma

Autoimmune disease **with antinuclear antibody to topoisomerase 1 (anti-Scl 70) and centromeres** leading to **dermal fibrosis and arterial fibrosis** of kidneys, lungs, and GI tract.

Clinical presentation—Often, first sign is **Raynaud phenomenon** (arterial spasm → blanching, then cyanosis, and then hyperemia, often with pain/paresthesias; mostly fingers and toes).

Patterns

- With **localized disease**, only the skin is typically involved; rarely progresses to the systemic form: thickness, tightening, and non-pitting induration of the skin proximal to the metacarpophalangeal or metatarsophalangeal joints; or sclerodermatous skin changes limited to the digits with digital pitting scars and bibasilar pulmonary fibrosis; **morphea** is a localized form: early inflammatory lesions anywhere, but especially on the face (become indurated, hypopigmented, and atrophic); or **linear form**: essentially same appearance but in short to longer lines, more on extremities.
- Major complications: **loss of muscle mass** due to fibrosis extending from the dermis to the muscle; leg-length discrepancy; joint flexion **contractures**; facial and scalp deformations with scarring, loss of hair

Laboratory studies—May have a **positive anti-Scl plus anticentromere antibodies and/or a positive ANA with a speckled or nucleolar pattern;** anemia with or without eosinophilia

Management—**Immunosuppressives**, physical/occupational therapy, local therapy and medications (calcium channel blockers, angiotensin-converting enzyme [ACE] inhibitors) for Raynaud phenomenon

Outcome—Highly variable; most stabilize after initial findings without progression; or rapid progression with cardiac, pulmonary, or renovascular disease

Sarcoidosis

Chronic multisystem granulomatous **(non-caseating granulomas) disease** of unknown cause; more common in young adults (25–35 years) than in childhood; presence of certain class I and II major histocompatibility complex (MHC) alleles influence age of onset and severity of illness; both sexes and all ethnic groups worldwide may be affected but more common in African Americans; often a positive family history

Clinical presentation—Constitutional symptoms plus bone/joint pain plus anemia; then cough, chest pain, and dyspnea (representing lung involvement); all have lung (infiltrates, node enlargement, military nodules; restrictive lung disease) and thoracic lymph node involvement at some time with variable occurrence at other sites; granulomas usually heal, but may become **fibrotic** and lead to **irreversible organ damage.**

Diagnosis—The best test is **biopsy** of skin or lung to find **non-caseating epithelioid granulomas**; other findings: increased ESR, increased total protein, hypercalcemia, and hypercalciuria.

Management—Mostly **symptomatic and supportive** (corticosteroids, methotrexate, and other immune-modulators); disease may be progressive or self-limited, but half have some permanent degree of organ dysfunction.

Kawasaki Disease (KD)

KD is an **acute vasculitis, mostly involving medium-sized vessels especially coronary arteries**; the cause is still unknown. It occurs worldwide, with the highest incidence in **Asians**. Most in children between **3 months to 5 years of age** (few cases in older children, adolescents, and even young adults).

Table 10.5: Diagnostic Criteria and Features of Classic and Atypical/Incomplete Kawasaki Disease

Classic KD Requirements	Incomplete KD Requirements	Other Findings
Fever ≥5 days (high, recurrent, and unresponsive to treatment; lasts 1–2 weeks without treatment, or possibly longer) PLUS four of the following five criteria:	Persistence of fever but only two or three clinical features present	**Carditis:** myocarditis (and pericarditis) in acute phase (tachycardia out of proportion to fever, small effusion, ST/T wave changes)
• **Bilateral bulbar injection** without exudate	• Draw blood for CRP (at least 3 mg/dL) and/or ESR (at least 40 mm/hour), then:	**Coronary artery aneurysm** in up to 25% in week 2–3; may have giant aneurysm, multiple aneurysms, thrombosis/stenosis, and myocardial ischemia and infarction
• **Oral/pharyngeal erythema**, strawberry tongue, dry/cracked lips	• If at least three other laboratory criteria are present (anemia, low serum albumin, pyuria, elevated WBC count, elevated liver enzymes, and platelets after 7 days ≥450,000/mm³), treat and perform echocardiography (specific characteristics diagnostic of coronary artery abnormalities).	**Arthralgia/arthritis:** may occur during acute phase but is not a diagnostic criterion
• **Hand/foot erythema and edema** (may have periungual **desquamation** over entire hand/foot at the 2nd–3rd week of illness)	• If less than three other lab criteria are initially present, perform echocardiography and base decision to treat on results and the persistence or abatement of fever.	Abdominal pain, diarrhea, vomiting, mild hepatitis; **hydrops of gallbladder**
• Non-suppurative **cervical adenopathy** (usually single, unilateral node >1.5 cm)	• It the initial ESR and CRP are low; follow the patient for persistence of fever and the presence of typical desquamation. With resolution of fever and onset of desquamation, an echocardiogram should be performed (not needed with fever resolution and no desquamation).	Extreme irritability in all
• Any type of **body rash** (except vesicular); in diapered infants, is more in groin/perineal area and may have desquamation in acute phase	• If the fever continues, the patient is reassessed and alternate diagnoses should be considered.	Aseptic meningitis; otitis media; sterile pyuria

Abbreviations: C-reactive protein, CRP; erythrocyte sedimentation rate, ESR; white blood cells, WBC

Clinical course and management—The typical course is **6–8 weeks from onset with an acute, subacute, and convalescent phase** (see Figure 10.2).

Other notes on course and management

- Addition of IVIG to the high-dose aspirin leads to the finding of a more rapid decrease of fever and resolution of clinical findings, and a decrease in the prevalence of coronary artery disease; half of aneurysms resolve within 2 years; longer time and higher morbidity and mortality with multiple or giant aneurysms
- KD **may recur** in a very small number of patients
- All patients should have an **influenza vaccine** if course is during the influenza season; and need to check on status susceptibility of varicella (relationship of aspirin, influenza, and varicella to **Reye syndrome**).
- Patients with thrombotic events, multiple aneurysms, or giant aneurysms are treated with additional drugs and procedures, e.g., abciximab, clopidogrel, dipyridamole, warfarin, catheter ablation, stent placement, or even coronary artery grafting.

Acute Phase
1–2 weeks (depending on time of diagnosis/treatment)

Fever and acute inflammatory findings	– Admit, place IV and hydrate; labs: CBC, differential and **platelets**; chemistries (including liver); ESR, CRP; urinalysis, **ECG** (myocarditis), **baseline 2D-echocardiogram** – Administer **IVIG** per protocol and **start high-dose aspirin** (anti-inflammatory); consider second course of IVIG (and then IV methylprednisolone) if poor response.

Subacute Phase
2–4 weeks after onset of findings

Fever and **acute findings resolve** (but may still have anorexia, irritability and conjunctival injection); presence of **desquamation; onset of coronary aneurysm; platelets continue to increase** often to greater that $1 \times 10^6 \rightarrow$ thrombosis, myocardial infarction	– Follow platelets (they will continue to rise) and ESR and/or CRP; **second echocardiogram** for coronary artery abnormalities (if positive, need to follow carefully with further echocardiograms and possibly angiography). – Switch to **low-dose aspirin** (anti-thrombotic) when afebrile for at least 3 days or on the 14th day from onset.

Convalescent Phase
4–6 (or to 8) weeks after onset of findings

All clinical signs have resolved; ESR and CRP return to normal in most by end of this period.	– **Final echocardiogram** if previous was normal (none further needed if no aneuysm by 8 weeks and with ESR/CRP return to normal; if no aneurysm within 2 months of onset, no long-term sequelae). – Continue low-dose aspirin **until no evidence of aneurysm by 8 weeks and normal ESR/CRP**; otherwise continue indefinitely per cardiologist.

Figure 10.2: Clinical Course and Management of Kawasaki Disease

Henoch-Schönlein Purpura (HSP)

IgA-mediated small vessel vasculitis of primarily the **skin, joints, glomeruli, and GI tract**; the etiology is unknown; it often follows a URI in the winter, with most at age 2–8 years, with a male preponderance.

Clinical presentation

- Acute or insidious onset of **low-grade fever and constitutional signs with arthralgia and arthritis in most** (serous effusions, mostly of the **knees and ankles**; resolves spontaneously).
- Characteristic rash and edema, mostly on **dependent areas**: buttocks and legs, and also backs of arms (less so on other areas); lesions come in **crops**, beginning with **pink maculopapules that blanch with pressure**; these develop into **petechiae/palpable purpura that start as red-purple and become brown;** the crops occur in periods of 3–10 days and may go on for only a few days to several months, **most resolving in 1–4 weeks**.
- Some will have **GI involvement**. The most common complaint is **colicky abdominal pain** and pain on palpation; may be diarrhea and hemorrhage (hematemesis, **heme-positive stools**) and **intussusception** (with perforation, peritonitis, sepsis, and death).
- Up to half of patients will develop **renal vasculitis** and present with a nephritic or nephrotic syndrome; acute renal failure may develop and lead to chronic renal failure, hypertension, and end-stage renal disease (in a very small number).
- Less common findings: hepatosplenomegaly, lymphadenopathy and neurological problems, thrombotic events

Laboratory findings—Moderate increase in acute-phase reactants (ESR, CRP, WBCs, platelets), anemia (blood loss), azotemia, hematuria, proteinuria, urine sediment casts; the **best test** is to biopsy a lesion but only if the diagnosis is unclear or there is an atypical presentation; for progressive renal disease (perform renal biopsy).

Management

- Most present with constitutional, joint, and skin findings—**symptomatic treatment**: pain control with acetaminophen or NSAIDs, bland diet, adequate hydration, and rest.
- **Oral or IV corticosteroids are indicated with any evidence of GI involvement →** rapid improvement of GI vasculitis. Treat orally (outpatient) or IV (inpatient). Treatment depends on the severity of findings, presence of bleeding, and ability to tolerate oral fluids and medications. Stool for occult blood should be obtained at the time of diagnosis.
- Renal findings managed the same as for acute glomerulonephritis; some evidence that early treatment with corticosteroids may prevent progression of renal disease; patients should be hospitalized if they have severe hypertension, renal insufficiency, oliguria, or electrolyte abnormalities. Patients should have a urinalysis at the time of diagnosis, and this should be followed carefully.

Disorders of the Eyes, Ears, Nose, and Throat

EYE DISORDERS

Table 11.1: Most Common Disorders of the Eyes Seen in Primary Care

Strabismus	-Eye deviation only under certain conditions (heterophoria) or constant (heterotropia); the most significant condition is **esotropia** (medial deviation of one or both eyes); the most serious type is **unilateral esotropia**, as the non-deviated eye becomes the preferred eye and **amblyopia** (see below) develops. The most common form of exotropia is intermittent, occurring under conditions of fatigue or stress, with maintenance of normal vision.
	-**Diagnosis:** Best initial test is the Hirschberg corneal light reflex: with normal alignment, shining a light in the midline gives a symmetric light reflex seen on the nasal side of each pupil; with esotropia, the light reflex will be displaced. Best test to determine heterophorias from heterotropias is the cover test (or alternating cover/uncover test); cover each eye, and if there is no movement of the non-covered eye, there is no strabismus.
	° Differentiate true strabismus from pseudostrabismus (appearance of esotropia usually due to a broad nasal bridge, or epicanthal folds); reassurance may be provided that this will correct with further growth. **Management:** Best initial therapy—eliminate as much of the misalignment as early as possible with patching of the good eye to treat the amblyopia; definitive therapy is then surgery to realign the eye(s).
Amblyopia	-Decrease in visual acuity from absence of a good retinal image during the early, critical period of visual development (prior to completion of development of visual cortical pathways); examples: strabismus, cataract, tumor, significant refractive errors

(continued on next page)

Table 11.1: Most Common Disorders of the Eyes Seen in Primary Care (*cont.*)

Nystagmus	-Rhythmic oscillation of one or both eyes -*Congenital sensory:* associated with intrinsic eye abnormalities such as aniridia, cataracts, optic atrophy; leads to decreased vision; may also be an isolated genetic trait; treat the underlying problem -*Congenital idiopathic motor:* horizontal, jerky oscillations (more jerking in the direction of gaze); no intrinsic eye problems and vision is normal; best treatment is surgical -*Acquired:* cerebral, cerebellar, or brain-stem disease; brain imaging necessary for diagnosis of underlying problem
Red eye	-Most common causes of unilateral or bilateral red eye in childhood: infective conjunctivitis, allergic conjunctivitis, foreign body, chemical conjunctivitis, corneal abrasion, dacryocystitis, keratitis (corneal infection; most with adenovirus or *Herpes simplex*), anterior uveitis (iridocyclitis), posterior uveitis (chorioretinitis), periorbital and orbital cellulitis
Ptosis	-Most are congenital and due to abnormality of the levator muscles; may occur unilaterally or bilaterally; may be familial; amblyopia may occur. May occur with other eye or with systemic disorders (e.g., myasthenia gravis, muscular dystrophy, botulism, third-nerve palsy). Ptosis requires a complete ophthalmologic and full physical/neurological exam; various types of surgery are available.
Congenital nasolacrimal duct obstruction	-At birth or shortly thereafter: excessive tearing and mucoid material from the lacrimal sac, erythema, and skin maceration; may develop acute inflammation and infection -**Best initial treatment:** nasolacrimal massage 2-3 times per day and cleansing with warm water; if there is mucopurulent discharge, antibiotics; best long-term therapy: duct probing for those that do not resolve (most are gone by age 1 year)
Lid infections	-**Hordeolum:** tender, local swelling with erythema of the glands of the lid due to *Staph. aureus*; involvement of the meibomian glands = internal hordeolum (large abscess pointed to the skin or conjunctiva) or involvement of the glands of Zeis or Moll (external hordeolum = stye; smaller and more superficial, pointed toward the lid margin); treatment = frequent warm compresses with or without topical antibiotics; excision for those that do not resolve -**Chalazion:** granulomatous inflammation of the meibomian glands; firm, nontender nodule in the upper or lower lid; chronic and be large enough to decrease vision; needs surgical removal

(continued)

Conjunctivitis in the newborn	**Ophthalmia neonatorum**
	-Infection of the conjunctivae in the first 4 weeks of life; **most common cause in the United States is now** *Chlamydia trachomatis; Neisseria gonorrhea* **is uncommon** due to prenatal recognition and treatment and neonatal eye prophylaxis; can also see **chemical conjunctivitis (silver nitrate is used** as the eye prophylaxis); (6–12 hours after instillation; **conjunctival injection with clear discharge** and resolved by 24–48 hours).
	-**Presentation: redness and chemosis of the conjunctiva, eyelid edema and purulent discharge;** *N. gonorrhea* has the shorter incubation period (2–5 days) and is seen at birth or after 5 days (due to partial suppression from eye prophylaxis); *C. trachomatis* has an incubation period of 5–14 days and may take more than 2 weeks for signs and symptoms to appear (generally a **cobblestone appearance of the tarsal conjunctiva with relative sparing of the bulbar conjunctiva**).
	-**Diagnosis:** Swab for **Gram stain and culture/sensitivity and send conjunctival scrapings for the best test** for *C. trachomatis* is **PCR.**
	-**Management:** Repeated and **frequent saline irrigation** of eyes until pus clears; treat *N. gonorrhea* (based on early results of Gram stain) with **ceftriaxone IM one time;** treat suspicion of *C. trachomatis* (based on appearance, timing) with **erythromycin orally for 2 weeks.**
Conjunctivitis in the older child	-**Viral:** most commonly seen with upper respiratory illnesses (common with adenovirus) or systemic viral illnesses (e.g., measles, enterovirus); **bilateral conjunctival injection with watery discharge;** no treatment.
	-**Bacterial:** most common causes are non-typable *Haemophilus influenzae, Strep. pneumococcus,* staphylococci, and other streptococci; produces an **acute (usually unilateral) purulent discharge with conjunctival injection and chemosis; eyelids are stuck together in the morning with crusted material.** No diagnostic tests needed; management with frequent warm water/compresses and **topical optic antibiotics** (e.g., optic ciprofloxacin); consider sexually transmitted organisms as a possibility in the adolescent (treat as in neonate).
Foreign body	-Most can be seen under good light and magnification or with ophthalmoscope; also need to evert lids (object embedded under lids may cause corneal abrasions); x-ray may be needed for an intraocular foreign body.
	-**Best initial management: eye irrigation or gentle swabbing** with a moistened cotton-tip applicator; next step in management: check for corneal abrasion and follow up carefully; patient with any embedded object that cannot be removed easily needs to be referred immediately to an ophthalmologist.
Hyphema	-**Blood in the anterior chamber** after blunt or penetrating trauma (is painful); appears as red fluid level between the cornea and iris or diffuse darkening of the aqueous
	-**Best initial management:** should be evaluated by ophthalmologist; needs specific therapy to prevent re-bleeding; bed rest with head of bed elevated, plus sedation (may need hospitalization)

(continued on next page)

Table 11.1: Most Common Disorders of the Eyes Seen in Primary Care (*cont.*)

Corneal abrasion	-Superficial to deep/large abrasion of the corneal epithelium; **acute intense pain, excessive tearing, photophobia, and decreased visual acuity** -**First step in management**: careful ocular exam (for foreign bodies, gross damage, and vision screen) after instillation of a **topical anesthetic (only for exam; delays epithelial healing)**; next step (diagnosis of corneal abrasion): **fluorescein dye plus blue-light examination** -**Treatment: topical antibiotics** to prevent infection during healing; with larger, deeper abrasions, refer to ophthalmologist (possibility of ulceration and scarring); may need a topical cycloplegic for relief of severe pain
Orbital fracture	-Indirect orbital floor fracture (**blowout fracture**) common when objects larger than the orbit strike the eye, especially at the inferior, lateral aspect -**Findings:** limitation of upward gaze, lower-lid ecchymoses, epistaxis, decreased sensation of ipsilateral cheek and upper lip (disruption of infraorbital nerve) -**Best initial test:** plain x-ray (Waters view is best for orbital floor and maxillary sinus) and CT scan -**Management:** prophylactic antibiotics, topical nasal decongestants, ice packs; possible surgery; ophthalmology consult
Cataracts	-Any **opacity of the lens** which may affect vision; may be isolated or be a part of a systemic disease process -**Most common causes: prematurity** (opacities may disappear spontaneously), isolated genetic trait (most autosomal dominant), with congenital infections (TORCH; most with **rubella**), with metabolic/endocrine disease (e.g., **galactosemia, diabetes**), with chromosomal abnormalities (e.g., trisomies, Turner syndrome), **drug-induced**, with **trauma, radiation**-induced, or as part of syndromes
Congenital glaucoma	-**Increased pressure** in the eye → **optic nerve damage and visual loss**; most cases are **congenital** (presenting in the first 3 years of life) and **primary**, caused by **obstruction of fluid drainage**; secondary causes include trauma, hemorrhage, inflammation, tumor, chromosomal defects, congenital rubella, **Sturge Weber syndrome**, Marfan syndrome, and many others -**Triad of symptoms: excess tearing, photophobia, and blepharospasm** (each due to corneal irritation); corneal edema and cloudiness, ocular enlargement and conjunctival injection -Management in children is always **surgical**.
Anterior uveitis	-Inflammation from **ciliary body to iris**; presents as **pain, lacrimation, photophobia, decreased vision;** also conjunctival injection (patient may complain of seeing "floaters and flashers") -**Initial diagnosis: slit-lamp exam** (inflammatory cells in aqueous) -Most common causes: **JRA**, Kawasaki disease, sarcoidosis, Reiter syndrome, ankylosing spondylitis, ulcerative colitis, post-infectious arthritis, Stevens-Johnson syndrome, and with early disseminated Lyme disease -Primary treatment—**treat the underlying cause**; eye treatment includes **topical steroids** and immunomodulators and cycloplegic agents; always **refer to an ophthalmologist.**

(continued)

Papilledema	-Swelling of the optic nerve head secondary to **increased intracranial pressure**
	-**Exam:** blurring of the disc margin, elevation of the nerve head, congestion or hyperemia of the disc head, or venous engorgement
	-Acute papilledema: vision is usually normal; with **chronic papilledema: visual loss with permanent atrophy**
	-**Most etiologies:** tumors, obstructive hydrocephalus, intracranial hemorrhage, cerebral edema from trauma, infection, toxins and drugs, metabolic causes
	-**Papilledema is a medical emergency: first step in diagnosis is neuroimaging; if negative → lumbar puncture**
Retinoblastoma	-**Most common malignant intraocular tumor in childhood**
	-**Hereditary types:** bilateral and multifocal and present earlier (average age 15 months); **nonhereditary types:** unilateral and unifocal and present later (average age 25 months)
	-Most common presentation: **leukocoria** (white pupillary reflex); second most common finding: **strabismus**; a white mass can be seen with retinoscopic examination.
	-**First step in diagnosis:** ultrasound or CT scan; cannot biopsy due to easy spread
	-**Management:** combination of cryotherapy, chemotherapy, irradiation, and **possible enucleation** if tumor has spread into the orbit or optic nerve (significant decrease in survival)
Retinopathy of prematurity	-Disease of developing retinal vasculature in **preterm infants;** mild/transient to severe proliferative **neovascularization with scarring, retinal detachment, and blindness**
	-Major factors: **hyperoxia** and the production of **free radicals;** with an increase in vascular endothelial growth factors → **abnormal fibrovascular growth**
	-**Management: systematic, serial ophthalmologic exams needed (beginning at 4–6 weeks after birth) in infants born at <32 weeks' gestation or <1,500 grams birth weight** or with any more mature/larger birth-weight infant with an unstable course at risk for severe therapy of choice is **laser photocoagulation.**

Abbreviations: juvenile rheumatoid arthritis, JRA; polymerase chain reaction, PCR

Periorbital and Orbital Cellulitis

Table 11.2: Comparison of Periorbital and Orbital Cellulitis

Periorbital (preseptal)	Orbital
Inflammation of the **lid and soft periorbital tissue** (facial cellulitis)	Inflammation of the **tissues of the orbit**
Most common associations: contiguous infection (lid, periorbital region), trauma, or bacteremia	**Most common associations: most commonly from ethmoid sinusitis;** also direct extension or venous spread from contiguous site of infection, direct infection from a wound or from bacteremia
Most common organisms: Group A streptococci, non-typable *Haemophilus influenzae*, **Staphylococcus aureus**, *H. influenzae* type B (now uncommon)	**Most common organisms:** *Streptococcus pneumoniae*, Group A streptococci, **Staph. aureus**, nontypeable *H. influenzae*, and anaerobes
Findings: erythema, warmth, and swelling **around the eyes; no evidence of orbital involvement**, low-grade fever, non-toxic appearing	**Findings:** Severe chemosis and swelling of the eyelids (often the eye is swollen shut) with **ophthalmoplegia, proptosis, and abnormal pupil function; decreased visual acuity;** child is **toxic-appearing with high fever**
Diagnosis: clinical diagnosis unless question as to whether or not there is orbital involvement, then a CT with contrast	**Diagnosis:** Most important diagnostic step is a **CT with contrast** (contrast for possible **subperiosteal abscesses** or intracranial extension); CBC shows leukocytosis with a left shift; blood culture may be positive.
Treatment: oral beta-lactamase (e.g., first-generation cephalosporin, amoxicillin-clavulanate, or cloxacillin)–with careful monitoring	**Treatment:** hospitalization with **IV broad-spectrum (and beta-lactamase) antibiotics** (e.g., ampicillin/sulbactam); if no improvement, may need **sinus drainage and/or drainage of any abscesses**

EAR DISORDERS

External Ear

Malformations and deformations

- Most common: **preauricular pits and tags**, pinna malformations, anomalies of pinna size, absence of pinna (microtia), and congenital stenosis/atresia of the external auditory canal
- Associations: craniofacial anomalies, other abnormalities of the ear and temporal bone, **hearing loss, renal defects (need to perform hearing testing and renal ultrasound)**

Otitis externa

- External ear infected from excessive **wetness**, dryness, skin pathology, and trauma; normal flora: coagulase-negative staphylococci, *Staphylococcus aureus*, micrococcus, diphtheroids, streptococcus viridans and *Pseudomonas aeruginosa*
- **Swimmer's ear:** most from *P. aeruginosa* (less so from other organisms, including *P. mirabilis*, *Klebsiella pneumoniae*, *Candida* and *Aspergillus* spp.)

- **Findings: acute ear pain (manipulation of pinna/tragus)**; canal edema and erythema with thick, white otorrhea (usually difficult to visualize the tympanic membrane); conductive hearing loss, preauricular adenopathy and facial paralysis; may spread to temporal bone and even skull base
- **Treatment: Clear canal** so that topical antibiotics can be effective (may need several days of **antibiotic-soaked cotton wicks placed** in the canal, then cleansing is easier due to decreased pain) plus **oral analgesia; topical otic antibiotics** (neomycin plus colistin or polymyxin; or ofloxacin or otic ciprofloxacin/dexamethasone) will treat Gram-positives and -negatives and *P. aeruginosa.*
- **Prevention:** drying of ear canals after being in water, use of earplugs and instillation of dilute alcohol **or 2% acetic acid** (available over-the-counter)

Acute suppurative otitis media (AOM)

Higher prevalence—Children 6–20 **months old (decreases after age 2 years);** earlier in life—more severe, recurrent, and chronic otitis; children with craniofacial anomalies **(cleft palate and children with Down syndrome);** more common in males, Native Americans, whites > blacks; + family history; decreased socioeconomic status (SES), **tobacco smoke, bottle-propping;** infants fed **formula rather than breast milk;** during cold weather and exposure to other young children (**day care**)

Pathogenesis—Occurs mostly with **viral upper respiratory infections (URIs); obstruction of the eustachian tube** and a shorter, more horizontal tube in young children → impaired mucociliary clearance → reflux of material into middle ear cavity → **effusion and inflammation**

Microbiology—Bacterial in up to three-quarters of cases: most are *Strep. pneumococcus,* **then non-typable** *H. influenza,* **then** *Moraxella catarrhalis.*

Clinical findings—**Fever, ear pain, irritability, disruption of sleeping, depressed appetite, and signs and symptoms of a viral URI;** but **may be afebrile and have little or no signs and symptoms** (especially in young infants, who may just present with irritability and a change in behavior); may also present with a ruptured tympanic membrane (TM).

Diagnosis—**Best initial test is pneumatic otoscopy (best exam for determination of middle-ear effusion,** which is the hallmark of AOM); need to have: (*1*) acute onset of signs and symptoms, (*2*) the presence of a middle-ear effusion (bulging TM, decreased movement on insufflation, otorrhea, or air–fluid levels), and (*3*) the presence of inflammation of the TM (distinct erythema or distinct otalgia, which is clearly from the ear and disrupts daily activities); cannot use TM erythema alone as diagnostic, as this may be caused from crying or fever.

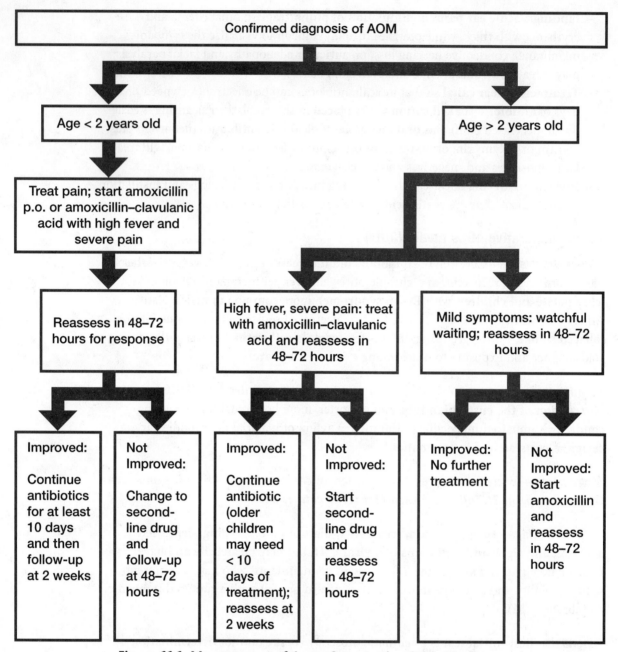

Figure 11.1: Management of Acute Suppurative Otitis Media

Management—The American Academy of Pediatrics (AAP) Consensus Guidelines of an **initial no-treatment option** (watchful waiting) in **some milder cases in older children or unconfirmed, milder cases**, based on the fact that most cases (especially due to *H. influenza* and *M. catarrhalis*) resolve spontaneously.

Further notes on above management algorithm:

- **Preferred first drug of choice: high-dose (80–90 mg/kg/day) amoxicillin** as opposed to more traditional dose of 20–40 mg/kg/day; more effective against penicillin-intermediate and some resistant strains; resistance is from beta-lactamase production with non-typable *H. influenzae* and *M. catarrhalis* and from alteration in penicillin-binding proteins with *Strep. pneumoniae*.

- **If diagnosed with AOM and already on antibiotics or with a recent AOM which did not respond to amoxicillin:** then initial drug should be either amoxicillin-clavulanate (high-dose amoxicillin component) or the drug to which the patient previously responded.
- **Preferred first-line drug for penicillin allergy:** if previous reaction was urticarial or anaphylactic, with concern about cephalosporin cross reactivity, then **azithromycin** (or clarithromycin); if previous reaction was a rash (non-urticarial) with little concern about cephalosporin cross reactivity, then **cefdinir, cefuroxime-axetil, or cefpodoxime.**
- **Initial treatment failures with a first-line drug** (still with significant signs and symptoms after reassessment at 48–72 hours), acceptable drugs are (best for beta-lactamase resistance and against resistant *Strep. pneumococcus*): **amoxicillin-clavulanate (high-dose amoxicillin component), cefuroxime-axetil, cefdinir, or cefpodoxime.**
- **Cannot tolerate or refuse oral medications:** IM ceftriaxone with possible 1–2 more doses at 2–3-day intervals
- Must be **reassessed** at each step after 48–72 hours (either with no initial therapy, with initial antibiotic therapy, or with a change in antibiotic therapy) and at the end of treatment (2 weeks).
- **Third-line treatment:** if no response to second-line drug, next step in management **perform a tympanocentesis** (or myringotomy). Tympanocentesis/myringotomy is also indicated:
  - For **severe refractory pain or hyperpyrexia**
  - With **complications** such as mastoiditis
  - For an AOM in a patient with **immunocompromise**
  - As part of a sepsis workup in **a neonate with AOM** and systemic findings (fever)

Recurrent otitis media

- Early recurrence (within several days) usually due to **incomplete eradication, resistance, or re-infection with the same or different organism**; treat with antibiotics to relieve the symptoms. If AOM recurrent despite medical therapy (three or four courses of antibiotics in a 6-month period, or five to six courses in a year), consider **tympanostomy tubes (decrease rate of recurrent AOM).**
- If **infection with tympanostomy tubes in place**, there will be **tube otorrhea** with or without fever and pain; first line of treatment is **cleaning the canal and topical ofloxacin or otic ciprofloxacin with dexamethasone** (FDA-approved drugs for the **middle ear without ototoxicity**); will treat most resistant, *Staph. aureus* and *P. aeruginosa*. With systemic findings, if topical therapy is not tolerated or if does not result in improvement, then oral antibiotics are added; if still poor response → hospitalization with IV broad-spectrum antibiotics.
- Adenoidectomy: primary indication—**continuation of episodes of AOM after tubes have fallen out**; otherwise is not indicated unless **at the time of tube insertion there is a history of significant nasal obstruction or recurrent sinusitis.**

Otitis media with effusion (OME)

Etiology—**Continued effusion after one or more AOMs**; most episodes subside within weeks of an AOM; persistent effusions are more common in children who have **recurrent acute infections, particularly if they are spaced close together**; for diagnosis, need evidence of a **middle-ear effusion without evidence of acute inflammation**

Morbidities with OME—Most common is **hearing loss, with the possibility of secondary speech and language delay**; predisposes to recurring AOM, discomfort, problem with balance, and long-term problems:

- Retraction pockets
- TM atelectasis (high retraction or prolapse from long-standing negative pressure or chronic inflammation)
- Adhesions (may impair ossicular movement, or lead to a cholesteatoma or hearing loss)
- Tympanosclerosis (white plaques in the TM and middle-ear nodules from deposits of calcium and phosphate crystals; most common cause in tube insertion)
- Cholesteatoma (see below)

Diagnosis—With **pneumatic otoscopy**, if uncertain or to follow the course of an effusion, a **tympanogram** is helpful (graph of middle ear's ability to transmit sound energy as a function of varying the air pressure in the external canal; a probe is placed that varies air pressure with presentation of a tone and sound pressure levels are then measured, with volume on the y-axis and pressure on the x-axis); but cannot distinguish between effusion of AOM and OME.

Management
- Follow effusions **monthly**; if present for **at least 3 months, next step is to refer to audiology for a hearing test**.
- Antibiotics are not effective (only if there is good evidence of a current bacterial infection); antihistamines and decongestants are not effective; there is a greater risk vs. benefit of short course of corticosteroids.
- The **most effective treatment is placement of tympanostomy tubes** if there is a persistent bilateral effusion (more than 3–4 months) with any degree of bilateral hearing loss (otherwise **most children resolve effusions, have normal hearing, and have no speech and language delay at age 3 years**).
- Tubes last an average of 12 months, but in this amount of time most effusions and hearing loss are reversed and the incidence of recurrent AOM is decreased. The vast majority of children do not require tube reinsertion after extrusion. **Potential problems after tube extrusion**: residual perforation, tympanosclerosis, scarring, residual conductive hearing loss, cholesteatoma.

Complications of otitis media
Intratemporal
- **Tympanic membrane perforation:** (AOM or OME) usually heals spontaneously but a small number are chronic and require surgery

- **Chronic suppurative otitis media:** persistent middle-ear infection with discharge from a perforated TM, originating with an AOM with TM rupture; mastoid air cells always involved; most common organisms are *Staph. aureus* and *P. aeruginosa*; needs cleansing and IV antibiotics and, possibly, tympanomastoidectomy
- **Acute mastoiditis:** all cases of AOM cause early inflammation of the mastoid air cells, usually responsive to therapy (or self-resolves with mild cases); it may spread over the periosteum (**acute mastoiditis with periosteitis**), → usually signs and symptoms (**postauricular inflammation and inferior/anterior displacement of the pinna**); may progress to bony destruction (**acute mastoid osteitis**) with signs and symptoms of acute mastoiditis. Most common organisms are *Strep. pneumococcus*, **non-typable** *H. influenzae*, and *P. aeruginosa*.
  - **First step in diagnosis: immediate ear, nose, and throat (ENT) referral for tympanocentesis/myringotomy** to drain effusion and culture/sensitivity; then **CT scan** of temporal bone and surrounding area for evidence of bony destruction in intracranial spread
  - **Treatment:** IV broad-spectrum antibiotics (with beta-lactamase coverage and for *P. aeruginosa)* and mastoidectomy if evidence of trabecular bone involvement

- **Acquired cholesteatoma:** cystlike growth (keratinized, stratified squamous epithelium with desquamated epithelium or keratin) in middle ear or pneumatized portion of temporal bone; **discrete white opacity** or polyp-appearing mass protruding into the canal; most are from long-standing chronic OM, deep retraction pockets, traumatic perforation of TM, or insertion of a tympanostomy tube; **expands progressively to cause bony resorption and intracranial involvement** (life-threatening). **Next step in management: obtain CT scan of temporal bone and surrounding area and consult ENT** immediately for surgery; start prophylactic broad-spectrum antibiotics.
- **Labyrinthitis:** uncommon complication usually secondary to cholesteatoma or chronic suppurative OM; signs and symptoms: **vertigo, nystagmus, tinnitus, nausea, vomiting, hearing loss**

Intracranial

Focal encephalitis, meningitis, abscess (epidural, subdural, cerebral), lateral sinus thrombosis from direct extension, hematological spread or acute thrombophlebitis; if any suspected, **first step in diagnosis is a CT scan and if no mass effect, then a lumbar puncture**; also need tympanocentesis/myringotomy for culture and sensitivity and IV antibiotics; any abscesses need to be drained

DISORDERS OF THE NASOPHARYNX

Table 11.3: Most Common Disorders of the Nasopharynx Seen in Primary Care

Choanal atresia	-Unilateral or bilateral membranous or bony septum separating anterior nares from nasopharynx; most with other abnormalities (CHARGE association) -Bilateral: presents at birth with alternating episodes of cyanosis as baby tries to breathe through nose (initially obligate nose-breathers), with pinking-up associated with crying -Unilateral: persistent nasal stuffiness/noisy breather or nasal obstruction and distress with first URI (diagnosed later) -Diagnosis: cannot pass a catheter more than 3–4 cm; then direct visualization with fiberoptic rhinoscopy (ENT), then CT scan -Treatment: initial oral airway or intubation in neonate with bilateral atresia; surgery with stent placement to assure continued patency (may be delayed with unilateral atresia)
Epistaxis	-Most common bleeding in anterior septum (Kiesselbach plexus), mostly from digital trauma, dry air, irritation with URI, allergy, or topical medication. Also consider foreign body or nasal polyp. -More serious/prolonged bleeding from vascular anomalies or bleeding disorders -First step in management: compress nares, use cold compress, and tilt head forward; with continued bleeding: use topical oxymetazoline or Neo-Synephrine; next step: anterior nasal packing, then posterior nasal packing, then silver nitrate cauterization (ENT) -Best prevention: no fingers in nose; use humidifier during dry, cold months; saline nose drops or petrolatum in anterior nares for lubrication
Nasal trauma	-Nasal trauma can cause a septal hematoma; if treatment is delayed (drainage of the hematoma) it may lead to necrosis of the septal cartilage and eventual saddle nose deformity. -Any small foreign body can be placed in the nose of a small child; initial presentation is unilateral obstruction with sneezing and discomfort; if not removed: nonsuppurative, malodorous nasal drainage with inflammation (nasal speculum in good light); most can be removed with suction or alligator forceps; if not: patient should be sent to ENT for removal, possibly under general anesthesia.
Rhinosinusitis (common cold)	-Most causes: rhinoviruses, coronavirus, adenovirus, RSV, and parainfluenza from early fall to late spring; spread by small-particle aerosols and direct contact -Young children may have six to eight infections per year (more if in day care); decreases with age to two or three by adulthood; typical course is 1–2 weeks -Signs and symptoms: nasal congestion, sneezing, rhinorrhea, sore throat, cough; little or no systemic findings (common with influenza) -A change in color and consistency of secretions is common and by itself does not represent a superimposed bacterial infection.

(continued)

	-No studies have shown a significant effect on symptoms with OTC medications; first-generation antihistamines may be of benefit for severe rhinorrhea due to **cholinergic effects;** FDA has recently recommended no OTC cold preparations for children <2 years and even for children <6 years. Topical decongestants are the best therapy for severe nasal congestion, but should not be used in the very young and for not more than 2–3 days due to rebound effects; guaifenesin, codeine, and dextromethorphan are not effective antitussive medications for the common cold. With longer, chronic coughs, consider bronchospasm (and treated with bronchodilators or a short course of steroids).
Acute and chronic sinusitis	-Acute sinusitis—bacterial complication of 2% of URIs in children; organisms are the same as those causing AOM; inflammation and edema may block sinus drainage and impair clearance of mucus. -Sinus development: ethmoids are present and pneumatized at birth; maxillaries are present at birth but not pneumatized until age 4–5 years; frontal sinuses do not start to form until age 7–8 years and are not complete and pneumatized until early adolescence. -Signs and symptoms: nonspecific until at least adolescence (may be more like adult presentation with headache, sinus pressure/pain, tenderness to palpation); may have purulent discharge, congestion, fever, cough, bad breath, decreased sense of smell, periorbital edema, maxillary tooth discomfort -Exam: erythema, edema of nasal mucosa, opaque sinuses (or fluid level) on transillumination -Diagnosis: based only on history: persistent URI symptoms without improvement for at least 10 days or severe symptoms (fever >102°F [38.8°C]) with purulent nasal discharge for at least 3 consecutive days; **x-rays are nonspecific** (do not distinguish between viral and bacterial etiologies); **only accurate diagnostic test** is sinus aspirate for culture (only in cases that are persistent and do not respond to medical therapy) -Chronic sinusitis—persistent respiratory symptoms for >90 days; may be due to repeat episodes of acute sinusitis or secondary to allergy, cigarette smoke, immunodeficiency, cystic fibrosis, ciliary dysfunction, nasal polyps, gastroesophageal reflux, foreign body, and/or anatomical abnormalities; most organisms: *H. influenzae*, alpha- and beta-hemolytic streptococci, *Strep. pneumonia, M. catarrhalis*, and coagulase-negative *Staph. epidermidis*; **best diagnostic test:** sinus CT scan; if failure of antibiotic therapy, will need sinus aspiration and drainage by ENT -Treatment (AAP Guidelines): treat initially with amoxicillin; if lack of response, use a second-line drug (same antibiotic therapy as in AOM) but treat for 7 days longer after resolution of symptoms; no evidence of benefit for corticosteroids, mucolytics, decongestants, or antihistamines -Complications: periorbital/orbital cellulitis, meningitis, epidural abscess, cavernous sinus thrombosis, subdural empyema, brain abscess, osteomyelitis of frontal bone from frontal sinusitis (Pott puffy tumor)

Abbreviations: American Academy of Pediatrics, AAP; acute suppurative otitis media, AOM; over-the-counter, OTC; respiratory syncytial virus, RSV; upper respiratory infection, URI

DISORDERS OF THE MOUTH AND OROPHARYNX

Table 11.4: Most Common Disorders of the Mouth/Oropharynx Seen in Primary Care

Delayed tooth development	-Most causes: hypothyroidism, hypopituitarism, chromosomal disorders and syndromes (Pierre-Robin, Treacher Collins), familial, rickets, ectodermal dysplasia, Albright osteodystrophy
Dental caries/ infections	-Dietary carbohydrate (**sucrose** is most cariogenic) interacting with organic acids from bacterial fermentation (mutans streptococci) → decreased dental plaque → decreased pH → demineralization → cavitation → colonization with lactobacilli → further demineralization -**Bottle-propping:** leads to continuous exposure to sugar during sleep; most commonly with caries in an infant or toddler -Untreated → gingivitis (rarely progresses in healthy prepubertal children), pulpitis, necrosis, dental abscesses (poor periodontal hygiene), and periodontitis (associated with anaerobic infections); may present as swelling below the jaw (mandibular abscess) -If at risk, refer to dentist at age 1 year; counsel regarding decreased dietary sugar, bottle-propping, daily supervised brushing, use of fluoride when appropriate.
Dental trauma	-If tooth becomes avulsed, replacement in the socket within 20 minutes may lead to replantation (poor outcome if >2 hours); counsel to find tooth, rinse it in tap water holding the crown, insert it into the socket (or cold milk), and go to the dentist with the child holding the tooth in place.
Ankyloglossia ("tongue-tie")	-Abnormally short frenulum, which may hinder tongue movement; rarely interferes with feeding or speech; may increase in length with age; if severe: surgery
Oral lesions	-**Hand-foot-mouth disease:** most caused by **coxsackie A16** and enterovirus 71; low-grade fever, red throat with **painful scattered vesicles** anywhere in the oral cavity (and may ulcerate); maculopapular, then vesicular and pustular rash on hands (mostly dorsum), feet, buttocks, and groin; resolve within a week; major issue is dehydration from refusal to drink (may need IV fluids and analgesia) -Herpangina: most caused by **coxsackie A;** sudden onset of sore throat with small vesicles/ulcers (that enlarge), surrounded by erythema, in posterior pharynx; temperature may be normal to very high; resolves in 3–7 days -Acute lymphonodular pharyngitis: coxsackie; yellow/white nodules on posterior pharynx -Aphthous ulcer (canker sore): distinct lesion with white necrotic base surrounded by red halo; unknown cause; lasts 10–14 days and tends to be recurrent; treat with over-the-counter (OTC) palliative therapy -Herpetic gingivostomatitis: fever/malaise with red gingiva and clusters of small vesicles through the mouth; heals in about 2 weeks; oral acyclovir helpful to decrease symptoms

(continued)

Cleft lip and palate	-**Cleft lip with or without cleft palate** is more common than isolated cleft palate; may see **autosomal dominant** transmission of any form in some families; higher prevalence in Asians and Native Americans; increased incidence of other malformations, especially with isolated cleft palate
	-**Cleft lip**: from a vermillion border notch to complete separation to the bone; may be unilateral or bilateral and may involve the alveolar ridge and lead to problems with tooth development
	-**Isolated cleft palate**: mostly midline from uvula alone to complete defect through soft and large palate
	-Cleft lip with cleft palate: may expose nasal cavities
	-Submucosal cleft palate: bifid uvula, partial separation of muscle or a notch in the posterior palate
	-Any form of cleft palate is associated with middle-ear effusions and recurrent or chronic AOM; also associated with hearing loss, malposition of teeth, and speech and language problems
	-Management: Immediate problem is feeding: feed using with a soft nipple with a large opening and a squeezable bottle; the lip is surgically closed at age **3 months and is revised at age 4–5 years;** nose corrective surgery is delayed until later childhood or adolescence; palatal surgery is based on the severity, but best to **correct at <1 year** because delay past 3 years associated with major speech problems.

Abbreviations: acute suppurative otitis media, AOM; Epstein-Barr virus, EBV; over-the-counter, OTC

PHARYNGOTONSILLITIS AND COMPLICATIONS

Group A Beta-Hemolytic Streptococcal (GABHS) Pharyngitis

Mostly seen in **younger school-age children** (uncommon <3 years of age) and in the **winter-spring** months; spread is by direct contact; presents as acute infection, but also as **asymptomatic carriage.**

Clinical presentation—Rapid onset, often with **fever, painful throat/dysphagia, headache, abdominal pain,** vomiting, and at times diarrhea

Exam

- Pharyngeal erythema
- Enlarged tonsils with pits
- Exudate (also may be in posterior pharynx)
- Posterior pharyngeal and palatal petechiae
- Bad breath
- Strawberry tongue (red papillae protruding through white covering)
- Increased, tender anterior cervical nodes
- **Scarlet fever** (caused by erythrogenic toxin A, B, or C; immunity is toxin-specific, so can have scarlet fever three times):
  - Findings as above plus **circumoral pallor**

- Characteristic rash: diffuse erythema with fine papules that give the feel of **sandpaper**
- Rash is **typically heavier/brighter in skin creases**, i.e. pastia lines (neck, inguinal area, antecubital fossa), and less on the face
- Rash begins to fade after 3–4 days and then **desquamates** from the head down.

Diagnosis—**Best initial test:** rapid strep (from throat swab); if positive, no need to perform a throat culture and **next step in management** is to treat; if the rapid strep test is negative (15% false negative), **next step is to perform a throat culture and start treatment** until the culture results are obtained in 48 hours.

Treatment—Early antibiotic treatment increases recovery by no more than a day; main reason to treat (within 9 days of onset) is to **prevent acute rheumatic fever** (acute glomerulonephritis may or may not be prevented) and suppurative complications; drug of choice is oral penicillin V for 10 days (amoxicillin is acceptable) or single administration of IM benzathine or benzathine/procaine penicillin. In allergic patient, drug of choice is a macrolide.

Streptococcal carriage—Some patients will **remain culture-positive** after a complete course of treatment; if still symptomatic, reculture and re-treat; the best way to **eradicate continued carriage** (asymptomatic) is with 10 days of **clindamycin**.

Suppurative complications

- **Peritonsillar abscess** (GABHS + mixed oral anaerobes)
  - Most common in an adolescent with a recent history of acute pharyngitis
  - Bacteria invade through the capsule of the tonsil
  - Presents as **sore throat/dysphagia with trismus**
  - Diagnostic finding on exam is an **asymmetric tonsillar bulge with uvular displacement** (may be difficult to see with trismus, in which case a CT scan is helpful)
  - Management: **parenteral antibiotics** (most resolve)
  - If does not resolve, then **needle aspiration or incision and drainage**
  - If still no resolution → **tonsillectomy**
- **Retropharyngeal and lateral pharyngeal abscess** (polymicrobial: most with GABHS, anaerobes, *Staph. aureus, H. influenzae*)
  - Present in **deep nodes** between the pharynx and cervical vertebrae and in the deep tissues of the lateral neck (Usually involute by age 5 years)
  - Infection from extension of a localized oropharyngeal infection in children <3–4 years of age with recurrent ear, nose, or throat infections
  - Presents as fever, sore throat, **neck pain, torticollis, muffled voice, and stridor** (must differentiate from meningitis and epiglottitis)
  - May or may not see bulging of the posterior pharyngeal or lateral pharyngeal wall
  - A **soft-tissue plain radiograph with the neck extended** is the first diagnostic step, followed by a **CT scan with contrast** for localization and extension

- **Management:** initial parenteral broad-spectrum antibiotics (ampicillin/sulbactam + clindamycin + third-generation cephalosporin); if poor response, need surgical drainage
- **Complications:** upper airway obstruction, rupture with aspiration, erosion of carotid artery sheath, mediastinal extension.

CERVICAL ADENITIS

Most Common Causes

- Enlarged, swollen, red, and tender node, unilateral = **adenitis.**
  - Associated with a pharyngitis (within 1 week).
    - Positive throat culture: due to **GABHS.**
    - Negative throat culture: possible **Epstein-Barr virus (EBV)**, mumps, enterovirus, adenovirus, herpes.
  - Acute onset, suppurative or abscess: probable **Staph. aureus** or **GABHS** (less common: tularemia, diphtheria, actinomycosis); treat with **beta-lactamase–resistant antibiotic**; either spontaneous suppuration or needle aspiration (or incision and drainage) when fluctuant.
- Subacute, chronic presentation (1 week): place **PPD.**
  - **PPD positive:** *Mycobacterium tuberculosis* or atypical mycobacterium; obtain chest x-ray.
  - **PPD negative:** bacterial or viral causes as above, or careful history and physical for suggestion of **cat-scratch disease or Kawasaki disease.**
- Generalized
  - Fixed or matted nodes, progressive, painless enlargement, constitutional symptoms → consider malignancy (Hodgkin and non-Hodgkin lymphoma, leukemia, neuroblastoma, rhabdomyosarcoma).
  - Signs and symptoms do not suggest malignancy → consider mycobacterial infection, EBV, cytomegalovirus (CMV), HIV, toxoplasmosis, syphilis.

Table 11.5: Etiology of Neck Masses

Congenital	-**Hemangioma**: soft, red/purple; may increase with crying; does not transilluminate; may have a bruit; can diagnose with ultrasound if needed. Can occur anywhere on neck.
	-**Thyroglossal duct cyst**: usually anterior and midline, near to hyoid bone; moves with tongue protrusion; painless; ultrasound will diagnose and then thyroid scan for ectopic thyroid tissue
	-**Goiter**: congenital hypothyroidism (or maternal medication) or from maternal Graves disease; anterior, midline
	-**Branchial cleft cyst, sinus, fistula**: most from the second branchial arch along the anterior border of the sternocleidomastoid; CT, MRI will confirm
	-**Cystic hygroma**: cystic mass formed by dilated lymphatics; soft, nontender, and compressible; may increase with crying; most transilluminate; diagnosis by ultrasound
Acquired	-Midline and moves with swallowing: **thyroid disease** (goiter, lymphocytic thyroiditis, Graves disease, adenoma, carcinoma)
	-Lateral neck: **salivary gland** enlargement (see above) or **lymph node** involvement (see above)

TONSILLECTOMY AND ADENOIDECTOMY

Guidelines for Tonsillectomy

American Academy of Otolaryngology: three or more infections of tonsils/adenoids per year despite adequate medical treatment (but recommendations vary widely and none are uniformly accepted; other guidelines are more conservative than this)

Guidelines to Adenoidectomy

- Chronic adenoiditis
- Chronic sinusitis that has failed medical treatment
- **Recurrent AOM with otorrhea in children with tympanostomy tubes** or in conjunction with tube placement for those with chronic nasal obstruction or recurrent sinusitis
- Upper airway obstruction causing craniofacial/occlusive abnormalities
- With chronic nasal congestion, mouth breathing, loud snoring, and hyponasal speech

Guidelines for Tonsillectomy and Adenoidectomy

- For recurrent infections, same for tonsillectomy alone (vary widely)
- **Adenotonsillar hypertrophy resulting in sleep-disordered breathing** and upper airway obstruction with other chronic problems
- Peritonsillar abscess unresponsive to parenteral antibiotics and incision and drainage
- Tonsillar malignancy

CARDIOVASCULAR DISEASE

SIGNS AND SYMPTOMS REFERABLE TO THE HEART

Table 12.1: Evaluation of Heart Murmurs in Children

Type of Murmur	Characteristics
PPS or pulmonary flow murmurs	-Most common newborn murmur -Ejection of blood through pulmonary branches -Grade 1–2 SEM at LUSB or RUSB to both axillae and back, or along the left sternal border
Benign ejection murmurs	**Still murmur** grade I–II short systolic ejection murmur along left sternal border with minimal radiation; heard most in preschool children; louder in supine, diminishes in sitting or standing and with Valsalva; increases with fever and exercise **Pulmonary flow murmur:** ejection of blood into pulmonary artery; heard more in older children and adolescents; same characteristics as Still murmur but best heard at LUSB and radiates into neck **Aortic outflow murmur:** adolescent athletes; same characteristics but at RUSB; murmur decreases with Valsalva (differentiates from IHSS) **Supraclavicular systolic murmur:** short systolic murmur heard above the clavicles, radiating to neck; disappears with raising the head and pushing the shoulders backward
Venous hum	Turbulence from internal jugular and subclavian veins entering the superior vena cava; continuous murmur at RUSB or LUSB and radiating to neck; murmur disappears in supine position and with head turned to opposite side of murmur

(continued on next page)

Table 12.1: Evaluation of Heart Murmurs in Children *(cont.)*

Type of Murmur	Characteristics
Carotid bruits	Most in adolescents; localized, early to mid-systolic murmur over neck vessels or right supraclavicular area but not the aortic area
Pathological murmurs	-With cardiorespiratory symptoms -Any diastolic murmur -Any pansystolic murmur -Continuous murmur -Late systolic murmur ± thrill (grade 4–6) -Murmur associated with abnormal heart sounds (clicks, abnormal splitting of S2) -With cyanosis -With abnormal pulse quality

Abbreviations: hypertrophic obstructive cardiomyopathy, HOCM; left upper sternal border, LUSB; peripheral pulmonic stenosis, PPS; right upper sternal border, RUSB; systolic ejection murmur, SEM

Table 12.2: Evaluation of Chest Pain in Children

Major presentation:	First Diagnostic Steps	Differential Diagnosis
Chest wall tenderness ± history of trauma or vigorous exercise	With localized symptoms: a good history and physical should give the diagnosis without any laboratory studies unless concern about significant chest wall trauma, then obtain chest x-ray	-**Costochondritis:** pain at costal cartilages (usually unilateral; 4th–6th costochondral junctions); radiates to back and abdomen; increased with movement; can last for months -**Musculoskeletal chest wall pain:** with overuse, exertion, severe cough; tender muscles; pain increased with truncal movement -**Pleurodynia: sharp pain** in spasms for minutes in chest or upper abdomen ± fever (few days to 2 weeks); most due to **coxsackie** and **echovirus** -**Slipping rib syndrome: trauma** to the **8th–10th ribs**; lower costal margin sudden pain and slipping sensation with click felt (tip of lower ribs overriding the one above); increased with straining or movement; may last for hours with **residual tenderness** -**Rib fractures**
Chest pain with no chest wall tenderness	A good history and physical should elicit the diagnosis **without any laboratory studies**	-**Precordial catch syndrome** (benign): **brief bouts** (<1 minute) of **sharp pain** near cardiac apex or left sternal border; **increased** with **deep inspiration**; greater occurrence with poor posture and improves with correction of posture

(continued)

Major presentation:	First Diagnostic Steps	Differential Diagnosis
With heart murmur (not functional)	Most cost-effective next step is to **refer to cardiology**	-Mitral valve prolapse: most **do not** complain of chest pain -Coronary artery disease: rare in childhood (see below) -Obstructive cardiomyopathy -Pulmonic stenosis, aortic stenosis
Respiratory distress, ± systemic findings/ fever	-**Important historical features:** recent symptoms preceding the pain, exposures, activity, possible foreign-body aspiration, past medical history of known disease -Best initial test: **chest x-ray**	-**Pneumonia, asthma,** pulmonary vascular disease (pulmonary hypertension, embolism) -**Pleuritis:** most from bacterial pneumonia; pain worse on inspiration -**Pneumothorax** -**Myocarditis** (see later discussion) -**Pericarditis** (see later discussion) -Acute chest syndrome in sickle-cell anemia
With prominent cough	-**Important historical features:** other symptoms related to cough, any previous diagnoses of respiratory disease, known exposures, medications, foreign-body aspiration -Best initial test: **chest x-ray** -Rule out asthma (see Chapter 8); consider sweat test to rule out cystic fibrosis	-**Asthma** -**Cystic fibrosis** -**Infection** of airways or pulmonary parenchyma -Foreign body -Malignancy: lymphoma, Hodgkin disease, rhabdosarcoma
With palpitations	-**Focus history on issues related to:** anemia, thyroid disease, medication use, history of drug use, anxiety-related disorders, structural heart disease, primary dysrhythmias -Screening tests: **CBC, thyroid studies** -Then **drug screen, chest x-ray, and ECG; refer for cardiology; consult/ echocardiogram as needed**	-**Anemia** -**Hyperthyroidism** -**Medications, drug use/abuse** -Anxiety/hyperventilation -Structural heart disease -**Arrhythmias** (see later discussion)

(continued on next page)

Table 12.2: Evaluation of Chest Pain in Children *(cont.)*

Major presentation:	First Diagnostic Steps	Differential Diagnosis
Related to eating or position	If reflux/esophagitis is suggested, may **treat empirically** (H2-blocker or proton pump inhibitor) and follow up for response -If lack of significant response, may need **barium swallow and upper GI endoscopy**	-**GER/esophagitis** -Hiatal hernia -Peptic ulcer disease -Other esophageal abnormalities (achalasia, esophageal spasm)

Abbreviations: gastroesophageal reflux, GER

Evaluation of Most Common Causes of Syncope in Children

Syncope: Loss of consciousness, postural tone, and falling secondary to decreased cerebral perfusion to the reticular activating system and cerebral cortex, is not due to a seizure, usually due to **idiopathic or familial fainting episodes.** Physical exam is usually normal. The most helpful and best initial test (after a thorough history and physical) is an **ECG.**

Table 12.3: Evaluation of Most Common Causes of Syncope in Children

Type	Mechanism	Causes	Features	Management
Neurogenic syncope (previously called vasovagal)	Sudden fall in blood pressure → decrease in brain oxygenation → presyncope (dizziness) → loss of consciousness	Frightening experience; unpleasant stimulus (pain); in prolonged hot, humid environments; after **prolonged standing with little movement**; extreme fatigue; with fasting; psychological factors	Most during standing; prodrome (dizziness, weakness, nausea, sweating, blurring of vision) → faint from seconds to minutes with **no postsyncopal confusional state**; secondary clonic movements if prolonged unconsciousness	If episodes are recurrent, a **tilt-table evaluation** may be helpful; treatment: prevention through avoidance of aggravating factors, increased water and salt intake; psychobehavioral therapy if factors indicate; if recurrent, **beta-blocker** may be helpful
Orthostatic	**Hypotension** as a result of movement to an upright position→ shifts in blood volume and failure of peripheral vasoconstriction	Prolonged bed rest, decreased intravascular volume, certain medications (decreased venous return), anemia	**No prodrome other than lightheadedness**	Measure changes in blood pressure in the supine and then standing positions; maintain fluid and salt intake; discontinue (if possible) causative medications (diuretics, antihypertensives, phenothiazines); correct anemia; rise slowly from supine.

(continued)

Type	Mechanism	Causes	Features	Management
Cough syncope	Severe cough paroxysms → increased intrathoracic pressure → decreased venous return	Most commonly with **asthma**; but with any prolonged coughing paroxysm (e.g., pertussis)	Coughing → lightheadedness and alteration of consciousness	Treat underlying problem causing the severe coughing.
Neurological disorder	Multiple physiological mechanisms	Seizures, CNS mass lesion	**Compared with syncopal episode:** seizure lasts longer, may occur in supine, associated with a rigid posture, has a postictal period, has a longer period of unconsciousness	EEG, neurology consult; if evidence of focality, neuroimaging for possible mass lesion
Cardiac causes	Multiple physiological mechanisms	Coronary artery anomaly; pulmonary artery hypertension; pulmonic stenosis, aortic stenosis, **HOCM**; mitral valve prolapse, arrhythmias; heart block; **long QT syndrome**, cardiac tumor, myocarditis	Syncope with exertion, palpitations, precordial pain; possible **positive family history for HOCM**	With signs and symptoms of cardiac disease or abnormal ECG, refer to cardiology for Holter monitoring, electrophysiological studies, exercise testing, echocardiography
Psychological causes	Multiple physiological mechanisms	Hysteria, panic disorder, anxiety disorders, hyperventilation, conversion reaction	See Chapter 5	See Chapter 5

Abbreviations: central nervous system, CNS; hypertrophic obstructive cardiomyopathy, HOCM

ECG AND THE MOST COMMON CHILDHOOD ARRHYTHMIAS

Developmental Changes in the ECG

Birth—Due to the high pulmonary vascular resistance (PVR) in utero and physiological right ventricular hypertrophy in the first days of life, there is **right axis deviation** (RAD) with a mean QRS axis of +110 to +180 and large R waves with **upright T waves in the right precordial leads** (V_1, V_3R, V_4R).

The first days of life—With a decrease in PVR, the **right precordial T waves become negative (most within the first 48 hours); the T wave in V_1 is never positive in a child <6 years of age and may remain negative into adolescence; persistence of an upright T after 1 week of age is indicative of right ventricular hypertrophy (RVH).**

Infancy–early childhood—The right ventricular wall remains relatively thick and the R/S in V_5 and V_6 is <1; as the **right ventricle gradually thins, the right ventricular forces gradually regress and the QRS axis gradually shifts to the left;** prominent R waves are present in the right precordial leads (until as long as 8 years of age), after which is seen the adult pattern of left ventricular dominance.

Sinus Arrhythmias and Extrasystoles

Sinus arrhythmia

- Increase in heart rate with inspiration and decrease with expiration
- **Normal finding**—with significant slowing, there may be an AV junctional escape beat
- Increased with fever and digitalis and decreased with exercise

Sinus tachycardia

- Rate of sinus node discharge higher than normal for age
- **Normal physiological response** to need for increased cardiac output or oxygen delivery
- P waves are present and normal; heart rate varies with activity (variable R-R); constant PR interval
- Increased heart rate with fever, hypoxemia, hypovolemia, pain, anxiety, drugs
- Treat underlying problem.

Sinus bradycardia

- Heart rate that is slow compared with age-related rates (<90/min in neonates and <60/min in older children)
- Clinically significant with heart rate <60/min and poor systemic perfusion; **most common pre-arrest rhythm in children**
- Slow rhythm with normal P waves and a constant PR interval, rate may vary

- Hypoxemia, hypotension, acidosis, hypothermia, heart block, drugs and toxins, increased vagal tone

Extrasystoles

- **Common in children and usually of no clinical significance**. Premature atrial complexes (PACs) are common in the absence of any structural abnormality. ECG shows a premature P wave preceding the QRS that appears to be different from other P waves; Premature ventricular contractions (PVCs) are clinically significant if there are **two or more in a row, if they are multifocal, if they increase with exercise, or if there is any known underlying heart disease.** Can arise from any area of the ventricle.
- QRS can be normal in appearance, widened or absent; there is **no compensatory pause.**
- ECG shows **widened, abnormal-appearing QRS complexes not preceded by a P wave and often with a compensatory pause;** unifocal or multifocal. If occurring regularly, they may take on a definite rhythm, e.g., bigeminy. Treat underlying problem; treat clinically significant PVCs first with a **lidocaine** bolus and then an infusion; if refractory, use **amiodarone.**

Supraventricular Arrhythmias

Supraventricular tachycardia

- Involves the conduction system **at or above the bundle of His**—most caused by re-entry with an accessory pathway or AV nodal re-entry **abrupt onset and cessation** (usually from minutes to hours) may be recurrent
- **Most common tachyarrhythmia that produces cardiovascular compromise during infancy**; most are well-tolerated but if prolonged may lead to heart failure and shock.
- **P waves absent or abnormal; heart rate does not vary with activity (rate of 220–300/ min in most infants; usually >180/min in older children); abrupt rate changes; majority with a narrow QRS (<0.08).**

AV re-entrant tachycardia

- Utilizes a bypass tract that may be able to conduct anterograde, i.e., **Wolff-Parkinson-White syndrome (WPW);** if rapid, patient at **risk for atrial fibrillation and then ventricular fibrillation.** In WPW, there is a **short PR interval with a delta wave (slow upstroke of the QRS).** It may be seen with congenital heart disease (**Ebstein anomaly**) or with a normal heart.
- With poor perfusion, respiratory distress, unconsciousness, hypotension: **synchronized DC cardioversion** is the treatment of choice (or rapid IV push of adenosine if can be given immediately).
- **With adequate perfusion:** First, evaluate 12-lead ECG, then try **vagal maneuvers** (face in icy saline for older children, or ice bag to face for infants) while establishing IV access; if vagal maneuvers are unsuccessful, **adenosine is the drug of choice** (rapid

IV push and repeat with doubled dose if needed); if resistant, cardiology consultation should be obtained for the administration of other possible drugs (procainamide, digoxin, beta-blockers, amiodarone).

Atrial flutter

- Regular or regularly-irregular tachycardia with an atrial beat of 250–400/min due to a circus rhythm from an atrial ectopic focus
- More common in **older children with underlying congenital heart disease**, particularly any that leads to chronic stretching of the atria (Ebstein anomaly, tricuspid regurgitation) **or after intra-atrial surgery**
- Characteristic is the **rapid atrial sawtooth flutter wave**; all of the rapid beats cannot be transmitted so there is **some degree of AV block present.**
- Treatment of choice for an acute episode is **DC cardioversion** (prolonged flutter may lead to heart failure); with chronic atrial flutter, the patient is at **risk for thromboembolism** and anticoagulation is needed prior to cardioversion; then **digitalize the patient followed with a Class I antiarrhythmic** (inhibits sodium channel, e.g., procainamide, quinidine) to maintain control. Some may require radiofrequency ablation.

Atrial fibrillation

- Chaotic atrial excitation with an irregularly-irregular ventricular response and pulse
- Most result from **chronically stretched atria in older children with rheumatic mitral disease, or from intra-atrial surgery, WPW, or atrial flutter;** may occur in a child without heart disease due to thyrotoxicosis, pericarditis, or pulmonary embolism.
- Atrial rate is 300–700/min with absence of P waves, **fibrillatory waves**, and an irregularly irregular ventricular rate (changing R-R).
- Best initial treatment is **digitalization,** which restores the ventricular rate to normal; **then need quinidine, procainamide, amiodarone, or DC cardioversion**; chronic atrial fibrillation requires anticoagulation (risk of thromboembolism).

Ventricular Arrhythmias

Ventricular tachycardia

- **At least 3 PVCs at >120 beats/min**, and may be paroxysmal or continuous
- Uncommon in children—have **underlying structural heart disease, prolonged QT syndrome, WPW, or myocarditis, or occurs with drug use (antiarrhythmic, cocaine, amphetamines) or after intraventricular surgery**
- Ventricular rate at least 120/min and **regular; QRS >0.08 sec; P waves often not seen;** if they are seen, they may not be related to the QRS (unless the ventricular rate is slower); T waves opposite in polarity to QRS.
- **Torsade de pointes:** form of ventricular tachycardia with **QRS complexes that change in amplitude and polarity**; seen in conditions with **long QT segments**

(congenital long QT syndromes), electrolyte abnormalities, tricyclic antidepressants, type IA antiarrhythmics (quinidine, procainamide, disopyramide) and type III antiarrhythmics (amiodarone, sotalol).

- **Defibrillation without delay** is the treatment of choice for ventricular tachycardia (VT) **without palpable pulses**; but if VT is present **with pulses and poor perfusion**, the treatment of choice is **immediate synchronized cardioversion**; support the ABCs of resuscitation and use continuous ECG monitoring and establish IV access (provide sedation/analgesia); attempt to identify the underlying cause; if refractory: consider **amiodarone, procainamide, or lidocaine** (do not use amiodarone and procainamide together as they both prolong the QT interval and may precipitate torsades des pointes). The treatment of choice for torsades des pointes is **magnesium sulfate by rapid IV infusion.**

Ventricular fibrillation

- Chaotic, disorganized series of depolarizations leading to a **quivering myocardium** that cannot produce blood flow
- Uncommon terminal event in children. Possible causes: hypoxemia, hypovolemia, hypothermia, metabolic disorders (hypo or hyperkalemia), toxins, drugs, pulmonary embolism, tension pneumothorax, tamponade
- Fine ventricular fibrillation (VFib) is a low-amplitude, fine undulating wave; coarse VFib is a chaotic series of high-amplitude waveforms that vary in size, shape, and rhythm with no identifiable P, QRS, or T waves.
- **Prompt defibrillation for VFib and pulseless VT**; continue oxygenation, chest compressions, ventilations (correction of hypoxemia and acidosis); fine low-amplitude VFib may be converted to coarser, higher-amplitude VFib which is more responsive to defibrillation. Establish vascular access as soon as possible; **defibrillate three times** and if this fails, administer **epinephrine, continue cardiopulmonary resuscitation (CPR), and defibrillate again within 30–60 seconds**. May repeat drug-CPR-shock two more times; if still fails, start **amiodarone, lidocaine, or magnesium sulfate for torsades des pointes and attempt defibrillation again**. Identify and treat causes.

Long QT syndrome

- Abnormal prolongation of the QT interval
- Half are **familial abnormalities** of ventricular repolarization; the rest are sporadic; may lead to torsades des pointes (see above) and result in syncope and sudden death; may present with presyncope, seizures, palpitations, or cardiac arrest.
- **QTc (correct for heart rate) >0.47 is highly indicative; QTc >0.44 is suggestive (especially with a positive family history)**; other findings: notched T waves, alternating T waves, low heart rate for age
- **Beta-blocker in doses that do not allow the increased heart rate to exercise**; if drug-induced profound bradycardia, may need a **pacemaker**; if no response or if there has been a cardiac arrest, the patient needs an **implantable defibrillator.**

Atrioventricular (AV) block

- **Congenital complete heart block** is most commonly produced by **autoimmune injury from maternal IgG antibodies in systemic lupus erythematosus (SLE) or Sjögren syndrome**; also seen with complex congenital heart disease, myocarditis, cardiac tumors, and myocardial abscesses secondary to endocarditis, and postoperatively with suturing near the AV valve.
- **Types**
  - **First-degree block:** long PR interval with conduction of all impulses
  - **Second-degree block:** some impulses are not conducted

    Mobitz I (Wenckeback): successive increase in PR interval until there is a dropped beat

    Mobitz II: no change in PR interval but there is an occasional dropped atrial impulse

  - **Third-degree block:** no conduction of atrial impulses; **no constant relation between P waves and QRS complexes**; QRS may be normal or wide; may be asymptomatic or present with syncope, dizziness, exercise intolerance, heart failure, or sudden death. **Cardiac pacing** is the treatment of choice in neonates with: **heart rates <50/min**, congenital heart disease, wide QRS complexes, and heart failure; older children require a pacemaker if heart rate is **<40/min**, with prolonged pauses, or progressive heart enlargement. Temporizing drugs to increase heart rate include epinephrine, atropine, and isoproterenol.

DISEASES OF THE PERICARDIUM, MYOCARDIUM, AND ENDOCARDIUM

Pericarditis

- Inflammation of the visceral and/or parietal layers of the pericardium resulting in a **pericardial effusion** (serous, purulent, fibrinous, or hemorrhagic) of varying volumes and rapidness of fluid production. With significant fluid (especially with rapid accumulation) → decrease in cardiac chamber capacity → decreased venous return and cardiac output (**cardiac tamponade**). Slow accumulation of fluid may lead to a large effusion prior to the onset of symptoms.

Most etiologies

- **Viral** (most common cause is **coxsackie B**; others: **adenovirus, echovirus**, influenza, Epstein-Barr virus (EBV), cytomegalovirus (CMV), mumps, varicella, and others)
- **Bacterial** (most in children <4 years old as a **direct extension from an adjacent pneumonia or empyema** or as a distant hematogenous spread; also secondary to trauma or within the first few months after cardiac or esophageal surgery, from **Staph. aureus**, *Haemophilus influenzae*, *Neisseria meningitidis*, and *Strep.*

pneumococcus; also *Pseudomonas aeroginosa,* salmonella, *Francisella tularensis,* listeria, mycoplasma, and mycobacteria)
- Fungal, parasitic, metabolic/endocrine causes (**uremia**, hypothyroidism), malignancy (primary or metastatic), connective tissue disease (**juvenile rheumatoid arthritis (JRA), sarcoidosis, SLE, rheumatic fever**)
- Other: **radiation,** pancreatitis, trauma, and **postpericardiotomy syndrome** (from cardiac surgery; hypersensitivity reaction to pericardial trauma during surgery, with effusion occurring at least 1–2 weeks after heart surgery)

Clinical presentation—Symptoms dependent on the underlying cause:
- **Viral causes:** fever and preceding systemic features of the specific virus; then sharp precordial chest pain radiating to the left shoulder and back, aggravated in the supine position and relieved to some extent in sitting and leaning forward.
- **Purulent pericarditis** (bacterial and other etiologies): signs and symptoms of specific infection or disease precede onset of pericarditis; acute, onset with fever, respiratory distress, tachycardia out of proportion to the fever, abdominal pain, and precordial chest pain.
- **Constrictive pericarditis:** obliteration of the pericardial space secondary to inflammation, thickening and fusion of the pericardial layers; venous return decreases → decreased right ventricular filling → right-sided heart failure → deceased cardiac output; very rare in children; **most common cause worldwide is tuberculosis (TB).**

Physical exam—Related to amount of pericardial effusion present; with small effusion, may hear a **friction rub** (heard during ventricular contraction, ventricular filling, and atrial contraction) larger effusions, the heart sounds may be **distant (muffled)**. Signs of a large effusion/**tamponade:** distended neck veins, hepatomegaly, tachycardia, pulsus paradoxus, decreased pulse pressure with weak pulses and hypotension.

ECG findings—**Low QRS voltages**; mild elevation of ST segments (from myocardial pressure) and T-wave inversion (myocardial inflammation); **electrical alternans** (changes in P, QRS, and T-wave voltages from the heart swinging in a large effusion)

Chest x-ray—With a large effusion, there will be **cardiomegaly and the classic "water-bottle configuration"** of the mediastinum and heart without an increase in pulmonary markings.

Echocardiogram—This is the **definitive test** for the presence and size of effusion and for any myocardial dysfunction.

Management—With evidence of a viral etiology, the pericarditis is mild and **symptomatic treatment** is indicated (bed rest, analgesia, and nonsteroidal anti-inflammatory drugs [NSAIDs]); pericarditis associated with connective tissue disease is usually very responsive to corticosteroids. For bacterial infections, need **IV antibiotics** (empiric, broad-spectrum, and then based on culture and sensitivity; usually for 3–4 weeks) and an initial **needle pericardiocentesis** (for fluid removal and evaluation) and then **open drainage and removal of adhesions** (or tamponade recurs). For effusions that are more transudative, a pericardial drain may be effective.

Myocarditis

Inflammation of the myocardium with necrosis of cardiac muscle cells due to many infective and noninfective etiologies. There is a decrease in myocardial function with **cardiac enlargement**. The heart is unable to increase its contractility due to muscle damage, → increased left ventricular end-diastolic volume → pulmonary venous congestion and **heart failure** (pulmonary edema and increased hydrostatic arterial forces); may also lead to arrhythmias or sudden death. Chronic inflammation and fibroblast replacement of muscle cells during healing may lead to a **dilated cardiomyopathy with chronic heart failure.**

Most etiologies

- **Most common cause is a viral infection (coxsackie B, adenovirus, echovirus,** influenza, EBV, CMV, and others less commonly).
- Nonviral causes: other infective organisms (bacteria, rickettsia, fungi, parasitic [*Trypanosoma cruzi* in South America → Chagas disease]), toxins (venoms, diphtheria, irradiation), drugs (sulfonamides, chloroquine, chloramphenicol, cyclophosphamide), autoimmune (connective-tissue disease, ulcerative colitis, rheumatic fever, Kawasaki disease), and idiopathic

Clinical presentation

- **Acute viral myocarditis: neonates have a fulminant course with fever or hypothermia, lethargy, respiratory distress and cyanosis, and evidence of severe heart failure and shock**
- Physical findings include **tachycardia out of proportion to the fever, distant heart sounds**, a gallop rhythm, rales, hepatomegaly, peripheral edema, poor perfusion and pulses, hypotension, acidosis, atrioventricular valve regurgitation (mitral), and arrhythmias
- Older infants and children: signs and symptoms develop more gradually after an acute infection
- Lethargy, irritability, abdominal pain, anorexia, poor feeding, exercise intolerance, and eventual heart failure (dilated cardiomyopathy) or the appearance of an arrhythmia

Chest x-ray—Usually a **very large heart with pulmonary edema**

ECG—**Low-voltage QRS complexes**, T-wave changes, Q waves in the left precordial leads, left ventricular hypertrophy (LVH), prolonged PR and QT, **sinus tachycardia** (most common finding), arrhythmias (including ventricular tachycardia)

Echocardiography—This is the **most cost-effective study to demonstrate abnormal cardiac function, AV valve regurgitation, and pericardial effusion in the absence of any underlying structural anomalies.**

Other laboratory studies—Elevated creatinine phosphokinase [CPK], lactate dehydrogenase [LDH], and troponin as are acute-phase reactants; a blood culture should be performed to rule out bacterial infection; the **best test is myocardial biopsy (by cardiac catheterization) with polymerase chain reaction (PCR)** to identify the viral genome or to detect other causes.

Management—Maintain tissue perfusion with adequate oxygenation and treat heart failure (inotropes, afterload reduction) and arrhythmias; there has been success in some patients with IVIG and corticosteroids; with refractory failure, **heart transplant** is the treatment of choice. For other causes of myocarditis, treatment is also aimed specifically at the underlying cause.

Cardiomyopathy

Table 12.4: Cardiomyopathies in Childhood

Dilated	Hypertrophic	Restrictive
Definition: dilatation of ventricles (especially the left)	**Definition:** varying degrees of abnormal ventricular hypertrophy; in HOCM, there is asymmetric septal hypertrophy leading to left ventricular outflow tract obstruction with decreased distensibility of the cardiac muscle → decreased left ventricular filling	**Definition:** poor ventricular compliance with decreased ventricular filling; looks like **constrictive pericarditis**
Etiologies: most are familial (**different** genetic inheritances), idiopathic, or secondary to viral myocarditis; associated with some inborn errors of **metabolism, neuromuscular disease,** autoimmune disease, thyroid disease, nutritional deficiencies, severe anemia, coronary artery anomalies, and cardiotoxic drugs (e.g., doxorubicin)	**Etiologies:** primary genetic disease (**familial hypertrophic cardiomyopathy; most autosomal dominant**); or secondary to **obstructive structural lesions** of the heart; also some inborn errors of metabolism	**Etiologies:** primary (idiopathic) or secondary to **mucopolysaccharidoses,** amyloidosis, **sarcoidosis, radiation**, malignancy, scleroderma, or Löffler syndrome

(continued on next page)

Table 12.4: Cardiomyopathies in Childhood *(cont.)*

Dilated	Hypertrophic	Restrictive
Presentation: principal manifestation is heart failure.	**Symptoms:** respiratory distress, chest pain, palpitations, syncope, sudden death **Signs:** systolic ejection murmur heard best at left sternal border and apex and increases in intensity with Valsalva and standing; normal heart sounds and no ejection click (differ from aortic stenosis); left ventricular lift and brisk pulse	**Presentation:** signs and symptoms of right and left heart failure with pulmonary artery hypertension (high left atrial pressures); usually with rapid deterioration and **poor prognosis**
CXR: cardiomegaly and pulmonary congestion	**CXR:** mild heart enlargement (left ventricle)	**CXR:** mild to moderate cardiac enlargement
ECG: left (and right) ventricular hypertrophy, atrial enlargement, and nonspecific T-wave changes	**ECG: LVH** with ST-T wave changes; may see intraventricular conduction defects	**ECG:** large P waves with normal QRS complexes and ST-T wave changes
Echocardiogram: diagnostic for chamber dilatation and poor contractility	**Echocardiogram:** demonstrates the pattern of hypertrophy and Doppler studies show flow gradients and diastolic dysfunction	**Echocardiogram:** significant atrial enlargement with normal-size ventricles; Doppler flow shows decreased ventricular filling
Rx: treat congestive heart failure and arrhythmias until no longer responsive (usual progressive deterioration), then heart transplant	**Rx: no vigorous exercise— increased risk of sudden death; no inotropes—increases LV outflow obstruction;** primary medication to decrease outflow obstruction are **beta-blockers or calcium channel blockers**, but they do not change the long-term prognosis; an **implantable defibrillator** should be used for syncope or arrhythmias. **Surgery** may be used with LV outflow tract obstruction and severe symptoms, but does not reduce risk of sudden death.	**Rx:** treat heart failure and arrhythmias; cardiac transplant

Abbreviations: chest x-ray, CXR; hypertrophic obstructive cardiomyopathy, HOCM; left ventricular, LV; polymerase chain reaction, PCR

Infective Endocarditis

- High-velocity flow across an abnormal valve or shunt (but can occur without cardiac abnormalities) damages the endothelium → platelet and fibrin adherence → small thrombotic lesion; inflammatory cells and organisms adhere to this and grow → **infected vegetation** which may then **embolize to any organ**
- The vast majority of children have a pre-existing abnormality or **identifiable predisposing factor for infection** (surgical procedure, invasive diagnostic procedure, dental procedure or poor dental hygiene, bacteremia).

Risk—Increased with: **prosthetic valve left-sided lesions, cyanotic congenital heart disease, systemic to pulmonary shunts and previous endocarditis, indwelling intravascular catheter, IV drug abuse**

Organisms

- **Most common are alpha-hemolytic streptococci** (viridans; common after **dental procedures**; also with **prosthetic valve**) and *Staph. aureus* (most have **no underlying heart disease** or **prosthetic valve**)
- **Group D streptococcus** (enteroccocus): more common with **gastrointestinal (GI) or genitourinary (GU) procedures/surgery**; usually highly resistant
- *Strep. pneumoniae, H. influenza, N. gonorrhea*
- **Coagulase-negative staphylococci**: more common with **central venous catheters and prosthetic valves**
- *Pseudomonas aeruginosa, Serratia marcescens*—more common in **IV drug abusers; also with prosthetic valve**
- **HACEK**: Haemophilus (*H. paraphrophilus, H. parainfluenza, H. aphrophilus*), *Actinobacillus actinomycetemcomitans, Cardiobacterium hominis, Eikenella corrodens,* and *Kingella* spp.—more common in neonates and immune-compromised
- Fungi (*Candida* spp., *Aspergillus* spp., *Histoplasma capsulatum*)
- Other (may be **culture-negative**; need special media with longer culture time and serology): *Coxiella burnetii* (**Q fever**), *Bartonella* spp., *Brucella* spp., *Legionella* spp., *Chlamydia* spp.

Symptoms

- **Acute bacterial endocarditis:** acute onset; with high, spiking fevers with rigors and toxic appearance persistently for at least 2 weeks; most common cause is *Staph. aureus*.
- **Subacute bacterial endocarditis:** more insidious with constitutional (flulike) symptoms: low-grade fever, headache, malaise, chills, sweats, myalgia, arthralgia, anorexia for at least 2 weeks; **more common with underlying heart disease**

Physical findings

- **New or changing heart murmur, tachycardia,** heart failure, arrhythmia; **petechiae; splenomegaly**

- Septic emboli: pulmonary findings (more common with fungi), neurological findings (more with *Staph. aureus* and occur late), myocardial abscesses (more with *Staph. aureus*), renal failure
- Late, uncommon findings with early treatment (vasculitis from circulating immune complexes):
  - **Splinter hemorrhages:** dark-red lines under fingernails and toenails
  - **Osler nodes:** small, tender intradermal nodules in the pads of the fingers and toes
  - **Janeway lesions:** small, painless, hemorrhagic lesions on palms and soles
  - **Roth spots:** small, hemorrhagic retinal spots with central white areas
  - Immune complex glomerulonephritis

Diagnosis

- **Most important laboratory study is a positive blood culture:** need **multiple blood cultures from three separate venous samples within a 24-hour period for aerobes and anaerobes and grown for at least a week**; if initial cultures are negative, need two more plus special media cultures and serology.
- **Two-dimensional and Doppler echocardiography is the primary diagnosis for cardiac lesions** or pathology (but vegetations may not be seen and this does not rule out the diagnosis); may need sequential echocardiograms.
- Ancillary supportive studies: elevated erythrocyte sedimentation rate (ESR), C-reactive protein (CRP), leukocytes, anemia (normochromic/normocytic), positive rheumatoid factor, immune complexes, decreased total hemolytic complement, proteinuria, microcytic hematuria
- **Modified Duke criteria** (diagnostic criteria); need **two major criteria, one major plus three minor criteria, or five minor criteria**; see Table 12.5

Table 12.5: Duke Criteria for Diagnosis of Infective Endocarditis

Major Criteria	Minor Criteria
1. **Two separate positive blood cultures for usual organisms, and at least two for less-common organisms**	1. Predisposition (heart disease, IV drug use)
2. **Echocardiographic demonstration of an intracardiac mass/vegetation, a paravalvular abscess, or dehiscence of a prosthetic valve and/or new valvular regurgitation**	2. Fever >100.4°F (38°C)
	3. Vascular phenomenon (arterial emboli, pulmonary infarcts, intracranial hemorrhage, Janeway lesions)
	4. Immune complex phenomenon (glomerulonephritis, Roth spots, Osler nodes, positive rheumatoid factor)
	5. A single positive blood culture or positive serology
	6. Echocardiographic signs not meeting the major criteria

Management

- **Immediate IV antibiotics with high serum bactericidal levels for 4–6 weeks.** Treatment protocols are available for the various organisms, and based on resistance and the presence of prosthetic valves.
- Treat heart failure with salt restriction, inotropes, and diuretics; treat arrhythmias.
- **Surgery** for progressive cardiac failure from severe mitral or aortic valve involvement, valve or patch dehiscence, mycotic aneurysm, worsening of vegetations while on therapy, myocardial abscess, and/or recurrent emboli

Guidelines regarding prevention of infective endocarditis

Table 12.6: Use of Prophylactic Antibiotics

Based on evidence showing that for most people, the risks of antibiotic prophylaxis for certain procedures outweigh the benefit; patients at greatest risk of bad outcomes from infective endocarditis and in whom prophylactic antibiotics *should* be used are listed below.
Patients with artificial heart valves
Patients who have history of previous infective endocarditis
Patients with certain congenital heart disease **only**: unrepaired or incompletely repaired cyanotic heart disease, including those with palliative shunts/conduits; a completely repaired defect with prosthetic material that was placed during the first 6 months after the procedure; or any repaired congenital defect with a residual defect at the site or adjacent to the site of prosthetic material
Patients who had a cardiac transplant which then develops a problem in a heart valve

Updated 2007: Prevention of infective endocarditis: Guidelines from the American Heart Association; Committee on Rheumatic Fever, Endocarditis and Kawasaki Disease. *Circulation,* e-published April 19, 2007

Dental procedures for which prophylaxis is recommended: any manipulation of gingival tissue or the periapical area of the teeth, or perforation of the oral mucosa; for children, a single dose of the following 30 minutes before the procedure:

- Oral amoxicillin or parenteral ampicillin
- If unable to take oral: cefazolin or ceftriaxone parenterally
- Allergic to aminopenicillins, oral regimen: cephalexin, clindamycin, azithromycin, or clarithromycin
- Allergic to aminopenicillins and unable to take oral: cefazolin, ceftriaxone, or clindamycin parenterally

GI/GU procedures: Prophylaxis is **no longer** recommended **even** in those listed above with the highest risk.

Other procedures: Prophylaxis for procedures of the respiratory tract, infected skin, tissues just under the skin, or musculoskeletal tissue is recommended **only** with the high-risk conditions listed in Table 12.6.

Endocardial Fibroelastosis (EFE)

- Either primary (no cause identified; resulting in a dilated left ventricle) or secondary to severe left-sided obstructive disease (resulting in a small left ventricle)
- **White, fibroelastic thickening of the left ventricle that may involve the mitral and aortic valves**
- Usually presents in neonates or young infants with the onset of severe congestive heart failure that continues to worsen and results in death
- Chest x-ray **enlarged heart** ECG—**left atrial enlargement, left ventricular hypertrophy**
- Echocardiogram shows a **bright endocardial surface with poor left ventricular function**
- **Endocardial biopsy**—definitive diagnosis
- Survival is dependent upon **heart transplantation**.

Acute Rheumatic Fever and Rheumatic Heart Disease

- **Acute rheumatic fever (ARF)** is now rare in the United States (widespread antibiotic use and possible changes in organism virulence), but is still the leading cause of acquired heart disease on a worldwide basis.
- Primarily a disease of childhood, with an average age of 10 years for the first acute attack
- Occurs **3–4 weeks after pharyngitis** with particular strains of group A beta-hemolytic streptococci (GABHS). Appropriate treatment of streptococcal pharyngitis within 9 days of symptom onset has been found to prevent ARF.
- Valvular disease results from carditis associated with ARF, with worsening as a result of recurrences. Acute carditis—**pancarditis** with **enlargement of the left ventricle and mitral regurgitation with congestive heart failure**.
- In small number—**chronic mitral regurgitation** is severe with the development of possible arrhythmias.
- **Isolated aortic regurgitation** is uncommon, and generally occurs in **combination with mitral disease**.
- **Tricuspid valve disease is rare** and usually is a result of right-sided heart failure; pulmonary valve disease is a late complication of pulmonary artery hypertension.

Diagnosis—Need **two major or one major plus two minor criteria** of the revised **Jones criteria (1992; see Table 12.7) plus absolute microbiologic or serologic evidence of a recent GABHS infection.**

Table 12.7: Jones Criteria for Diagnosis of Acute Rheumatic Fever and Characteristics of the Major Findings

Major Criteria	Clinical Characteristics	Minor Criteria
1. Polyarthritis	-Most common and earliest symptom -Migratory polyarthritis, mostly of large joints (red, hot, painful); responds dramatically to salicylates	Fever
2. Carditis	-Second most common finding -Pancarditis, from mild to severe findings, mostly involving mitral valve or mitral plus aortic valve -New murmur, tachycardia, evidence of pericarditis, heart failure, and arrhythmia	Arthralgia: cannot use polyarthritis as a major criterion
3. Sydenham chorea	-Next most common finding; may occur alone with a latent period often of months prior to onset; improvement within 1–2 weeks of onset and return to normal within a few months -Purposeless movements of arms and legs, involuntary grimacing, weakness, speech impairment, difficulty writing, and emotional lability -May be the sole diagnostic feature without another major criterion	Prolonged PR interval
4. Erythema marginatum	-Uncommon finding -Erythematous nonpruritic circles with slightly raised serpiginous borders and central clearing; on trunk and proximal limbs; never on face -Occurs early and may remain after resolution of other findings	Increased acute-phase reactants on ESR and CRP
5. Subcutaneous nodules	-Rare -Firm, nontender nodules on extensor surfaces of elbows, knees, ankles, fingers, scalp, and thoracolumbar vertebrate -Occurs several weeks after onset of symptoms and resolves after a month -Presence is a marker for severe carditis	

Abbreviations: C-reactive protein, CRP; erythrocyte sedimentation rate, ESR

Laboratory studies—If there is no microbiologic evidence of a recent GABHS infection, then **serological evidence** is needed: **antistreptolysin O, antihyaluronidase, anti-DNAse B**. Clinical features begin at the peak of antibody titers (in the first month, then titers plateau for 3–6 months and return to baseline in 6–12 months). Acute-phase reactants are elevated and may be used to follow the clinical course for resolution and for recurrences. If there is heart failure, chest x-ray may show an enlarged heart and pulmonary edema; ECG: AV block of various degrees, evidence of pericarditis; 2-D and Doppler echocardiography for valvular involvement and cardiac function.

Management

- First **treat with oral penicillin or erythromycin (if allergic) for 10 days or IM benzathine penicillin to eradicate GABHS**; then start on **long-term antibiotic prophylaxis** (see below).
- **Bed rest** until inflammation subsides.
- Drug of choice is **oral salicylates** in anti-inflammatory doses (for >4 weeks); patients with cardiac enlargement or heart failure receive **corticosteroids**.
  - **Do not start salicylates if it is not clear as to whether arthritis is polymigratory**, as the arthritis may be significantly decreased because of the response to the salicylates; acetaminophen may be used tentatively for pain control.
- Inotropes, diuretics, salt restriction for heart failure
- **Antibiotic prophylaxis to prevent recurrent episodes: IM benzathine penicillin once every 4 weeks is the treatment of choice;** twice-per-day penicillin V and once-per-day sulfadiazine are equally effective (twice-per-day erythromycin if allergic to both).
- Length of treatment is dependent on absence of carditis:
  - 5 years or until age 21, whichever is longer
  - Presence of carditis without residual valvular disease (10 years or well into adulthood, whichever is longer)
  - Presence of carditis with residual valvular disease (at least 10 years since last episode and at least until 40 years of age; consider lifelong treatment)

Congestive Heart Failure

Cardiac output is insufficient to meet metabolic functions and oxygen requirements.

- ↑ neurochemical acidity
- Peripheral vasoconstriction
- Salt and water retention

Most common causes

- **Increased preload (volume overload):** left-to-right shunts, valvular regurgitant lesions and various types of complex heart disease (large mixing defects), and fluid overload (renal failure, iatrogenic)
- **Increased afterload:** obstruction to the right or left ventricular outflow tracts, systemic hypertension, pulmonary hypertension with resultant cor pulmonale
- **Myocardial dysfunction:** myocarditis, dilated cardiomyopathy, cardiac ischemia (all with dysfunction or failure of systolic contraction); hypertrophic or restrictive cardiomyopathy, constrictive pericarditis or tamponade, arrhythmias (all with dysfunction or failure of diastolic filling)
- **High-output failure:** thyrotoxicosis, severe anemia, arteriovenous fistulas, septic shock

Clinical presentations

- First response is chronotropic, i.e., **tachycardia**
- Then venous congestion—**left-sided**—**pulmonary venous congestion** (pulmonary edema → respiratory distress, rales, wheezing, difficulty feeding with sweating); **right-sided** with **systemic venous congestion** (peripheral edema, jugular venous distension, hepatomegaly, ascites).
- Ongoing heart failure → decreased cardiac output (weight loss, anorexia, malaise, lethargy, syncope, exercise intolerance, cool extremities, pallor, decreased pulses, blood pressure, and urine output).

Diagnostic studies

- Chest x-ray: **cardiomegaly** (unless associated with a condition leading to a small heart, e.g., restrictive cardiomyopathy) with variable lung findings (pulmonary edema, pulmonary venous congestion)
- ECG: chamber enlargement, ST-T wave changes (inflammation, ischemia), and arrhythmias (best use of the ECG)
- Echocardiogram: cardiac anatomy and ventricular function (**fractional shortening**); Doppler studies to estimate cardiac output
- Blood studies: CBC (anemia, infection) and chemistries (hyponatremia, hyperkalemia, hypocalcemia, renal function, liver enzymes) are the most important.

Therapy—Should be individualized per the etiology and hemodynamics. Eliminate underlying cause, control failure then any surgery if needed.

Acute heart failure—Manage airway, breathing, and circulation first; give oxygen and monitor with pulse oximetry; IV access for fluids and medications (see Table 12.8); draw blood and correct electrolyte abnormalities (glucose, calcium, potassium); correct hemodynamically significant anemia; treat arrhythmias; obtain chest x-ray, ECG, and echocardiogram; prostaglandin E1 (PGE1) if possible ductal-dependent lesion in a neonate.

Chronic heart failure—Allow for an adequate amount of rest and sleep, provide a good nutritious diet with increased calories, decreased salt intake, and no excess total daily fluids; correct anemia with iron supplementation or transfusion; use medications (see Table 12.8) as needed based on underlying cause and hemodynamic picture.

Table 12.8: Pharmacological Treatment of CHF in Children

Drug class	Drugs	Clinical Effects/Use
Inotropes (increases contractility)	**Digoxin**	-May be used in **combination with ACE inhibitors and diuretics** -Rate of excretion dependent upon **renal function (dose must be adjusted)** -**Rapidly digitalize intravenously** (monitor carefully for longer PR interval, arrhythmias; also follow serum electrolytes [hypokalemia, hypercalcemia]) -Give oral maintenance doses when feedings are established -Check digoxin levels **only** if accidental ingestion, if toxicity is suspected, with impaired renal function, with possible drug interactions, and for possible noncompliance (routine digoxin levels are **not** helpful). -Increased risk of toxicity: **hypokalemia, hypercalcemia, hypomagnesemia, myocarditis, and prematurity**
	Dopamine (beta-adrenergic agonist with alpha effects at higher doses)	-At 2–10 mcg/kg/min: results in **increased contractility with selective renal vasodilatation** -**With further increases → is more peripheral vasoconstriction.** -IV in an ICU setting for acute failure with close monitoring
	Dobutamine (direct inotropic effects with a moderate reduction in peripheral vascular resistance)	-May **use together with dopamine** (IV in ICU setting) so that the dopamine does not have to be increased to the extent that vasoconstriction is produced
	Isoproterenol (pure beta-adrenergic agonist with a prominent chronotropic effect)	-Use with **slow heart rates** (IV in ICU setting) -More **arrhythmogenic** than either dopamine or dobutamine
	Epinephrine (mixed alpha- and beta-adrenergic agonist)	-Significant increase of systemic vascular resistance → increased blood pressure -Usually for **cardiogenic shock**; often in conjunction with other inotropes
	Milrinone, amrinone (phosphodiesterase inhibitor → prevents degradation of intracellular AMP)	-Especially useful for low cardiac output after heart surgery or in patients refractory to other drugs (adjunct to dopamine and dobutamine; IV infusion) -Positive inotrope and peripheral vasodilator (afterload reduction → may cause hypotension) -Amrinone may cause thrombocytopenia (reversed with discontinuation of drug)

(continued)

Drug class	Drugs	Clinical Effects/Use
Beta-blockers	**Metoprolol** (beta$_1$ selective antagonist) and **carvedilol** (alpha- and beta-blocker and free-radical scavenger)	-Gradual introduction for **chronic failure** (not given during acute failure)
Diuretics (reduction of ventricular filling and pulmonary overload)	Furosemide	-**Acute diuresis with IV dosing** -Chronic oral therapy; follow electrolytes (**hypochloremia, hypokalemia, metabolic alkalosis, and hyponatremia, especially with severe heart failure**) -Requires **increased dietary potassium or supplemental potassium**
	Spironolactone (aldosterone inhibitor)	-Usually in combination with another diuretic because of its **potassium-sparing effect** -Oral administration for chronic diuresis
	Chlorothiazide/ hydrochlorothiazide (decreases proximal tubular reabsorption)	-Less potent; use for **milder CHF orally** -May need **potassium supplementation** unless concurrent use with spironolactone
Afterload-reducing agents (decreases peripheral vascular resistance to increase myocardial performance); some may decrease venous tone → decreased preload; particularly useful with cardiomyopathy, mitral regurgitation, aortic regurgitation, and left-to-right shunts; not used for left ventricular outflow tract obstructions	Nitroprusside	-IV titration for critically ill in the ICU -**Peripheral arterial vasodilatation with afterload reduction and also venodilatation with preload reduction** -May cause **significant hypotension** and is contraindicated if low blood pressure is already present -If used for a long period, must monitor **thiocyanate** levels for toxicity (cyanide is a metabolite which is detoxified in the liver and excreted in the urine)
	Hydralazine	-Direct effect on vascular smooth muscle of **arterial-resistance vessels** with little effect on venous dilatation; decreased peripheral vascular resistance → increased cardiac output and renal and cerebral blood flow -Significant sympathetic reflexes that may counteract hyptotensive effect increased heart rate and stroke volume -Contraindicated in coronary artery disease, rheumatic mitral valve disease; and already-existing tachycardia
	ACE inhibitors: captopril, enalapril (blocks production of angiotensin II → afterload reduction) with some venodilatation and preload reduction; effect on aldosterone production → control of salt and water retention	**Captopril:** oral; side effects: chronic cough, maculopapular pruritic rash that disappears spontaneously, renal toxicity, neutropenia, hyperkalemia, and hypotension -**Enalapril:** longer-acting

Abbreviations: angiotensin-converting enzyme, ACE; adenosine monophosphate, AMP; congestive heart failure, CHF; intensive care unit, ICU

Cardiogenic Shock

- Shock caused by severe cardiac dysfunction (low cardiac output, hypotension, and poor systemic perfusion and oxygenation), often with sudden onset. There is initial significant tachycardia with decreased ventricular filling; further compensation is not possible unless filling pressure (preload) is increased in order to increase stroke volume; if fluid administration does not result in improvement, then the problem is with intrinsic cardiac contractility and/or a high afterload.
- Most common causes: Myocarditis, cardiomyopathies, severe cardiac dysfunction related to congenital heart disease (before or after surgery); myocardial ischemia due to severe hypoxemia, myocardial infarction (rare), and continuing arrhythmias

Management

- Institute treatment of **underlying cause.**
- Intravascular catheters should be placed and **echocardiography** utilized to follow central venous pressure (CVP), pulmonary capillary wedge pressure (PCWP) or left atrial pressure (LAP), contractility, cardiac output, systemic vascular resistance (SVR), systemic blood pressure, and mixed venous oxygen saturations.
- Provide adequate oxygen and ventilation and monitor carefully; correct acidosis and electrolyte abnormalities.
- Trial **fluid bolus** (crystalloid, colloid, or blood, if indicated) with monitoring of perfusion and above parameters for improvement
- If cardiac contractility is the primary problem, then **beta-adrenergic agents** are indicated (**do not use digoxin for cardiogenic shock**—longer time of action, toxicities) in combination with a **phosphodiesterase inhibitor.**
- If high afterload is the problem, then an **afterload-reducing agent** (nitroprusside, angiotensin-converting enzyme [ACE] inhibitor, hydralazine) is indicated and in combination with an inotrope (as above) if there is also evidence of poor contractility (dobutamine also results in decreased SVR).

Cardiac Ischemia and Myocardial Infarction

- Myocardial infarction (MI) is rare in childhood. Children with myocardial ischemia may present with typical angina pain as in adults. In addition, there may be a number of other presenting signs and symptoms: respiratory distress, syncope, depressed sensorium, confusion, signs of poor perfusion, palpitations; tachycardia, bradycardia, or arrhythmia; signs of heart failure, abnormal heart sounds, murmurs, rales, rhonchi, and rubs.
- Most common causes of acute MI are **Kawasaki disease** (ruptured coronary aneurysm or coronary artery thrombosis) and **anomalous left coronary artery from the pulmonary artery (ALCAPA**; irritable, anxious infants with apparent pain on exertion [i.e., crying and extreme irritability while feeding]). The ECG will show ischemic changes (deep Q waves, peaked T waves, and ST wave changes).

CONGENITAL HEART DISEASE

Acyanotic Lesions—Left-to-Right Shunts (Volume Overload)

Ventricular septal defect (VSD)

- **Most common congenital heart lesion**
- Most occur in the membranous septum
- The size of the VSD and gradient of the systemic and pulmonary vascular resistances determine the hemodynamics and clinical significance.
- Many small defects **likely to close spontaneously** (more common in muscular defects).
- Moderate to large defects may become smaller over time but are less likely to close, and more likely to be symptomatic.

Hemodynamic explanation of findings—Systemic venous return from the right atrium (RA) fills the right ventricle (RV) during diastole. The end diastolic volume (EDV) of the RV early is normal. With systemic vascular resistance (SVR) greater than pulmonary vascular resistance (PVR), blood is shunted across the defect from the left ventricle (LV) during systolic ventricular contraction (directly into the right ventricular outflow tract). As the ventricles empty, the amount of shunted blood from the LV combines with the EDV of the RV and is ejected into the right ventricular outflow tract (RVOT) across the pulmonary valve and into the pulmonary artery (PA). Therefore, the **blood flow through the pulmonary circulation is greater than what it would be under normal conditions** (where it would simply be equivalent to the venous return). The amount of the shunt may be quantified by comparing the pulmonary blood flow (Qp) to the systemic (Qs), which gives the **shunt fraction (Qp:Qs)**. It is the combination of the shunted blood across the defect combining with the RV output (resulting in this larger volume across the RVOT) that produces the classic **holosystolic (pansystolic) VSD murmur**. In addition, since there is a larger volume to be ejected from the RV, the **right ventricular ejection time is longer, thus the closure of the pulmonary valve is delayed further.** This causes a **wider splitting of the second heart sound**, but the splitting **still** varies with respiration (i.e., it is **not** fixed). The increased pulmonary volume returns to the left atrium (LA) via the pulmonary veins, and if the Qp:Qs is large, there will be left atrial enlargement over time. There is an increased volume flowing across the mitral valve during diastolic ventricular filling and this may produce a **low-pitched mid-diastolic flow rumble**. The EDV of the LV is greater than normal, which may lead to left ventricular dilatation (**hypertrophy as read on the ECG**). With systolic contraction, the amount of blood shunted across the VSD must be regulated so that the remaining blood flowing across the aortic valve and into the aorta (cardiac output) is equal to the venous return. The **VSD murmur may not be heard in the first days to weeks after birth** due to the significant increase in pulmonary vascular resistance (PVR; and hence pressure) and right ventricular pressure after birth (from the normal in-utero physiology). As **PVR and RV pressures decrease over the first weeks of life**, there will be increased left-to-right shunting and the murmur may then be heard. In addition, if there is a significantly large enough shunt, it may result in heart failure that may then be clinically evident. With large, continued, unrestricted shunts (usually >2:1), **pulmonary vascular remodeling** will occur, PVR (and pulmonary artery pressure) increases, and the shunt may become right-to left, leading to cyanosis (**Eisenmenger physiology**). In this case, right ventricular hypertrophy (RVH) also develops.

Table 12.9: VSD Clinical Findings

Auscultation/Other Findings	Chest X-ray	Electrocardiogram
-S2 more widely split, but continues to vary with respiration -Holosystolic murmur heard best at lower left sternal border with or without thrill (at least grade IV/VI); a smaller hole may present with a harsher murmur (that may sound more ejection in quality) than a larger hole (which may be more blowing). -Low-pitched, mid-diastolic flow rumble (heard best with the bell) at the apex with larger shunts (2:1) -May see and feel a left parasternal lift/apical thrust	-Depending on the size and direction of the shunt, with continued large left-right shunt will see cardiomegaly and pulmonary edema	-With a hemodynamically significant shunt, LVH and LA enlargement -With continued large left-to-right shunts over time, also RVH from both LV failure and ↑ PA pressure

Abbreviations: biventricular hypertrophy, BVH; left atrium, LA; left ventricular hypertrophy, LVH; pulmonary artery, PA; right ventricular hypertrophy, RVH

Clinical presentation
- Small restricted VSDs usually result in no symptoms, and the diagnosis is made by hearing the murmur.
- Larger defects present with dyspnea, tachypnea, poor feeding, decreased growth, and eventually signs and symptoms of heart failure.

Management—Medical management to **control heart failure first**; then surgery (patching the VSD in first year of life to **prevent Eisenmenger**).

Atrial septal defect (ASD)
- Hole in the atrial septum and may be an isolated **secundum defect**, an **ostium primum defect,** or a **sinus venosus defect**. Ovale (PFO) is very common and is not classified as an ASD.
- **Ostium secundum defect is the most common** and may consist of a single hole or multiple holes.

Hemodynamic explanation of findings—The normal venous return to the RA immediately combines with the shunted blood from the LA across the defect. Thus, there is an **increase in right atrial volume and pressure**. This added volume now flows across the tricuspid valve (TV) during diastolic filling of the RV, and with a large enough shunt, may produce a **low-pitched diastolic flow rumble heard best at the lower sternum**. Because of the increase in the EDV in the RV, the **right ventricular ejection time is longer** and **pulmonic valve closure is delayed**, producing a **wider splitting of the second heart sound**. This time the wider splitting is **fixed with respect to respiration** (i.e., it does **not** increase with inspiration, as is the case with the normal physiology) because the increased right atrial volume and pressure limits the further increase in venous return that would otherwise occur with inspiration. In addition, the increased volume flowing into the RVOT and across the pulmonary valve creates a **medium-pitched systolic ejection murmur** (SEM) heard best at the left mid to upper sternal border (the murmur is **not** created by the low-pressure flow across the ASD). This creates increased pulmonary blood flow (increased Qp:Qs) that returns to the LA. At this point, the volume of blood must be regulated to flow across the shunt so that the volume of blood that flows across the mitral valve into the LV and to the aorta (cardiac output) is equivalent to the venous return.

Table 12.10: ASD Clinical Findings

Auscultation/Other Findings	Chest X-ray	Electrocardiogram
-Wide, fixed splitting of S2 -SEM at left mid to upper sternal border -With a large shunt, a mid-diastolic low-pitched rumble across the tricuspid valve heard best at the lower sternum -Right ventricular systolic lift at the lower left sternal border	-Usually normal until patient becomes symptomatic, in which case there is a variable degree of cardiomegaly (increased RA, RV, and PA) and pulmonary edema	-RV volume overload (right-axis deviation with minor right ventricular conduction delay; rsR pattern in right precordial leads = diastolic overload pattern)

Abbreviations: pulmonary artery, PA; right atrium, RA; right ventricle, RV; systolic ejection murmur, SEM

Clinical presentation—Most defects are associated with few symptoms. PVR remains low through most of childhood and lesion is usually found during a routine exam due to the typical auscultory findings. Older children, adolescents, and adults may present with exercise intolerance and dyspnea on exertion, CHF and pulmonary artery hypertension are not common.

Management
- Small lesions (and shunts) do not require closure and should just be followed.
- ASD should be closed when the patient becomes symptomatic or if there is greater than a 2:1 shunt. The greatest risk for surgery is in adulthood.

Atrioventricular defects

- The ostium primum defect occurs in the lower atrial septum overlying the tricuspid and mitral valves; there may be a cleft in the anterior leaflet of the mitral valve.
- It presents as a large left-to-right shunt with mitral regurgitation. The **AV canal** is also known as the **endocardial cushion defect (ECD).** This is a **continuous defect across the atrial and ventricular septum** and is associated with **abnormalities in the AV valves** (may be a single AV valve).
- **Shunting at both atrial and ventricular levels** and, due to the large open area, there may be **mixing of blood** from both sides of the heart → **mild desaturation and mild intermittent cyanosis.**
- **Tricuspid and mitral regurgitation** leads to further volume overload on the ventricles.
- Large, continuous pulmonary volume overload early with resultant **heart failure and Eisenmenger physiology** if not corrected.

Hemodynamic explanation of findings—Venous return in the RA combines with the atrial level shunt and flows across the abnormal tricuspid valve during diastole, then combines with the ventricular level shunt during systolic contraction. This results in a greater Qp:Qs than what is seen in either an isolated ASD or VSD. A large volume of blood returns to the LA, where part of this volume is shunted at the atrial level and the remaining increased volume flows across the abnormal mitral valve during diastolic filling of the LV. Since there may be some right- and left-side mixing, the blood flowing into the aorta may be **mildly desaturated, resulting in mild, intermittent cyanosis.** Because of the large volume of blood that must be ejected from the RV, there is both a **wide, fixed S2** (same physiology as the ASD) and a **loud SEM often accompanied by a thrill** and heard loudly from the lower to upper sternal border, radiating to the pulmonary area (2nd left intercostal space). There is also most commonly a **low-pitched mid-diastolic rumble** (increased diastolic flow across a single AV valve in the complete form) and the **murmur of mitral regurgitation** (harsh holosystolic murmur at the apex). If there are still two separate but abnormal AV valves, there may be **bilateral diastolic rumbles with the murmurs of bilateral AV valve regurgitation** (heard at the lower sternum and at the apex).

Table 12.11: AV Canal (Endocardial Cushion Defect) Clinical Findings

Auscultation/Other Findings	Chest X-ray	Electrocardiogram
-Very wide, fixed splitting of S2 -Loud, harsh SEM with thrill (at least a grade IV/VI) along the sternal border and radiating to the pulmonic area -Single or bilateral (tricuspid and mitral) low-pitched mid-diastolic flow rumbles -Single or bilateral holosystolic murmur of tricuspid/mitral regurgitation (lower sternum, apex) -Precordial lift	-Moderate to huge cardiomegaly (all four chambers with prominent PA) with significant pulmonary edema	-Superior QRS axis and left axis deviation -Biventricular hypertrophy -Right ventricular conduction delay -Right atrial and left atrial enlargement

Abbreviations: pulmonary artery, PA; systolic ejection murmur, SEM

Clinical presentation—Infant with signs of symptoms of **heart failure, recurrent pulmonary infection, poor growth, and intermittent mild cyanosis; early pulmonary artery hypertension with Eisenmenger physiology** (6–12 months of age) if not repaired

Management—First, control heart failure with medications (and possible pulmonary artery banding), then **early surgical repair** (patch defect and reconstruct valves) before the onset of increased pulmonary artery pressure.

Patent ductus arteriosus (PDA)

- True congenital heart lesion occurs in the **term infant** in which the ductus does not close spontaneously within the first few weeks of life (and at that point rarely closes).
- PDA present in **preterm infants** is a normal developmental occurrence.
- The incidence, size of the ductus, and magnitude of the shunt are related to the degree of prematurity and to the degree of illness (hypoxia and acidosis) in the low birth-weight, extremely premature infant.
- It is important to attempt to close the PDA in the preterm infant, starting first with **indomethacin**; then surgical closure in the infant with a continued hemodynamically significant shunt despite medical therapy.

Hemodynamic explanation of findings—With systolic contraction of the LV, blood is shunted into the PDA and directly to the pulmonary circulation. There is also **runoff of blood from both sides of the ductus at the aortic insertion into the pulmonary artery during diastole.** This results in **diastolic hypotension with a resultant increase in pulse pressure**. Because of the shunt essentially occurring in both phases of the cardiac cycle, the classic murmur of the PDA is a **continuous murmur, beginning just after the first heart sound and across S2 into early to mid-diastole.** The murmur is often described as a **"machinery" murmur** and may be accompanied by a thrill. It is heard best in the 2nd left intercostal space and radiates to the left clavicle, down the left sternal border and to the apex. It is the **increase in pulse pressure** that produces the other findings: **bounding pulses and a hyperdynamic precordium** (prominent apical impulse or heave). The increased pulmonary blood flow returns to the LA, and with increased diastolic filling there may be a **low-pitched, mid-diastolic rumble across the mitral valve** heard best at the apex. There will, therefore, be an increase in EDV of the LV, resulting in **left ventricular dilatation** (LVH on the ECG).

Table 12.12: PDA Clinical Findings

Auscultation/Other Findings	Chest X-ray	Electrocardiogram
-Continuous "machinery" murmur with or without thrill, heard maximally in the pulmonic area and radiating widely -Diastolic hypotension with increased pulse pressure -Bounding pulses -Hyperdynamic precordium	With a significant shunt, cardiomegaly (left atrial and ventricular enlargement) to various degrees with pulmonary edema	-LVH or BVH -LA enlargement

Abbreviations: biventricular hypertrophy, BVH; left atrium, LA; left ventricular hypertrophy, LVH

Clinical presentation—Respiratory distress and heart failure in a neonate or young infant

Management—The term infant, regardless of age, requires medical treatment of heart failure and then surgery or catheter closure (in the cardiac catheterization lab).

Obstructive Lesions

Coarctation of the Aorta

Occurs in two forms: as a small narrowing around the insertion of the ductus arteriosus (**juxtaductal coarctation**), or as a long segment of **tubular hypoplasia** (from severe narrowing to complete interruption of the aortic arch) beginning at head or neck vessels and extending to just before the ductus arteriosus.

Hemodynamic explanation of findings—With a **juxtaductal coarctation**, blood is generally still able to flow across the coarctation, but at the expense of the left ventricle, i.e., there is **left ventricular hypertrophy**. With an open ductus arteriosus, there is usually left-to-right shunting of blood from the aorta to the pulmonary artery. With **more significant constriction** from a juxtaductal coarctation or with tubular hypoplasia of the aortic arch, **right ventricular blood supplies the descending aorta** across the ductus arteriosus (right-to-left shunting), resulting in **differential cyanosis** with the upper part of the body remaining pink (from normal aortic blood flow through head and neck vessels proximal to the narrowed segment) and the bottom half of the body blue from venous right ventricular blood. With the **closure of the ductus arteriosus**, perfusion to the lower body worsens and the patient may then present with **shock** due to failure and severe hypoxemia and acidosis to the lower body. **Increased blood pressure will be found in vessels proximal to the obstruction** with decreased blood pressure and pulse intensity and pulse lag distal to the obstruction. Over time, neurochemical changes add to the hypertension. In addition, with an undiagnosed juxtaductal coarctation there will be the development of **collateral circulation involving branches of the subclavian, superior intercostal, and internal mammary arteries**. These collaterals become enlarged and tortuous and may **erode the inferior margin of the ribs**; this is seen as **rib-notching** on chest x-ray.

Table 12.13: Coarctation Clinical Findings

Auscultation/Other Findings	Chest X-ray	Electrocardiogram
-Usually normal heart sounds and normal precordial impulse -There may be a short systolic murmur best heard in the left 3rd–4th intercostal space radiating to below the left scapula and to the neck. -With differential cyanosis, there will be a decrease in postductal oxygen saturation with pulse oximetry compared to preductal. -Upper-extremity hypertension with a decrease in blood pressure in the lower extremities (the normal systolic pressure in the legs is 10–20 mm Hg greater than the arms) -Upper-extremity bounding pulse (radial) with weak pulses in lower extremities (femoral) and a radial-femoral pulse delay; if there is a decrease in pressure in the left arm compared to the right, the left subclavian artery is involved.	-Infants with severe juxtaductal coarctation or tubular hypoplasia have cardiac enlargement and pulmonary venous congestion; after prolongation of a juxtaductal coarctation into childhood (after first 10 years without diagnosis) there will be some cardiomegaly (LVH), and possibly post-stenotic dilatation of the descending aorta; in addition, rib-notching may be seen.	-Normal or with LVH, depending on severity of obstruction

Abbreviations: left ventricular hypertrophy, LVH

Clinical presentation
- Neonates presenting with a severe juxtaductal coarctation or tubular hypoplasia will have **differential cyanosis, heart failure, and cardiogenic shock with closure of the ductus arteriosus**.
- Older children are generally asymptomatic and the diagnosis is picked up on routine physical examination with **blood-pressure and pulse findings**.

Management
- Neonates stabilized with oxygenation and ventilation, correction of acidosis, maintenance of blood pressure, a prostaglandin infusion to maintain ductal patency (**PGE$_1$**), and then surgical correction (excision with primary anastamosis, or a patch aortoplasty).
- Older children should have any heart failure treated and then be sent to surgery without any delay.
- Younger children (in the first year) generally need a **later revision**. There is also the possibility of **re-coarctation** (these are usually treated with balloon angioplasty) or aortic aneurysm. Delay of surgery beyond age 20 years may lead to premature cardiovascular disease.

Less Common Lesions

Pulmonic stenosis (PS)

Deformation of the valve cusps so that during systolic ejection, they open incompletely to varying degrees. PS due to valvular dysplasia occurs in **Noonan syndrome**. With increasing stenosis, there is **greater right ventricular hypertrophy (RVH)** with normal to decreased pulmonary artery pressures. **Isolated PS does not cause cyanosis unless there is an associated intracardiac shunt.** Critical PS occurs when there is valvular obstruction in the neonate with right-to-left shunting across a patent foramen ovale. When PS is severe, there is **right ventricular failure**, as the right ventricle cannot hypertrophy any further.

Clinical findings and presentation—Patients with mild to moderate degrees of stenosis are asymptomatic or minimally symptomatic with dyspnea on exertion. Respiratory distress and cardiac failure occur with severe stenosis, e.g., critical PS in a neonate. Sharp **ejection click (varies with respiration), followed by the low-medium pitched systolic ejection murmur heard best in the pulmonic area (2nd left intercostal space)** with minimal radiation to both lungs. There may be a **right ventricular lift**. Chest x-ray shows cardiac enlargement due to **RVH** (main finding on the ECG) in addition to post-stenotic dilatation of the pulmonary artery and **decreased pulmonary vascularity**, all proportional to increasing severity of stenosis. With further RVH and right ventricular dysfunction, there is ventricular dilatation and tricuspid regurgitation.

Management—Mild PS is followed carefully with respect to any change of the gradient across the valve. With moderate to severe obstruction, a **balloon valvuloplasty** is performed as the initial procedure in most patients. If the valve is thick and very stenotic, surgery is needed.

Aortic stenosis (AS)

Occurs at the valve (**bicuspid aortic valve**, which is almost never symptomatic in childhood), as subvalvular stenosis (**obstructive cardiomyopathy**), or as a supravalvular stenosis (as in **Williams syndrome**).

Clinical findings and presentation

- With any significant degree of obstruction (e.g., critical AS in the neonate), there will be **LVH and possible left ventricular failure with decreased cardiac output (weak pulses, decreased blood pressure, poor peripheral perfusion).**
- Can result in **syncope and sudden death.**
- Early **ejection click (which does not vary with respiration) occurs after S2**, heard best at the apex and the aortic auscultation area (2nd right intercostal space).
- With increasing stenosis, **S1 may be softer, along with the aortic component of S2.**
- An **S4** may also be present (atrial kick against a noncompliant ventricle).
- With increasing stenosis the **systolic ejection murmur** increases in duration and becomes louder and harsher. It is best heard in the **2nd right intercostal space** radiating to the neck and the mid-sternal border.
- Chest x-ray may show a normal to enlarged heart (LVH) with post-stenotic dilatation (prominent ascending aorta).

- ECG shows **LVH**.
- Both serial echocardiography and exercise testing in older children may be used to determine any worsening of the gradient across the valve.

Management—For moderate to severe AS, a **balloon aortoplasty** is performed first with surgery used for valves that are particularly thick and for obstruction above or below the valve. Calcification or re-stenosis may occur years later.

Regurgitant Lesions

Mitral valve prolapse (MVP)

The chordae tendinae do not support the mitral valve cusps during the **end of systolic contraction** when the volume of the LV is low and so they **billow into the LA; mitral regurgitation** may or may not be present. MVP occurs as an autosomal dominant trait with variable expression and is more common in females.

Clinical findings and presentation—Most children are **asymptomatic**, and MVP often is not recognized until later in childhood or adolescence. Some present with **chest pain, palpitations, or arrhythmias** (mostly premature ventricular contractions). The diagnostic finding is a **mid to late systolic click, best heard at the apex with the patient's left side down**. The click may be **followed by a late systolic murmur (regurgitation)**. The chest x-ray is normal and the ECG may show T-wave abnormalities that can vary in the patient. **Echocardiogram is diagnostic**. MVP is **not progressive** and no treatment is indicated.

Mitral regurgitation (MR)

- Congenital MR is rare and is found more often with other congenital defects or dilated cardiomyopathy, or is acquired from rheumatic fever.
- Mitral valve annulus is dilated.
- With increasing severity, there is LA enlargement and the LV becomes dilated and hypertrophied, leading to pulmonary venous congestion, pulmonary artery hypertension, and RVH.
- **Apical, high-pitched holosystolic murmur** and, with more severe regurgitation, a low-pitched diastolic rumble from increased flow across the mitral valve.
- Chest x-ray shows cardiomegaly, primarily due to a large LA and prominent LV with pulmonary venous congestion.
- With moderate to severe disease, a valvuloplasty or prosthetic valve replacement is needed.

Cyanotic Lesions—With Decreased Pulmonary Blood Flow (PBF)

Tetralogy of Fallot (TOF)

Underlying malformation is anterior deviation of the infundibulum which results in **(1) pulmonic valvular and infundibular obstruction (hypertrophic infundibular muscle), (2) a large unrestricted ventricular septal defect (VSD) with (3) RVH, and**

(4) an overriding aorta (the aortic annulus sits over the VSD). In the worst form, there is pulmonary atresia with a VSD. The timing and severity of cyanosis and symptoms are **directly related to the degree of pulmonary obstruction**. TOF is a **conotruncal lesion** and is associated with the **CATCH 22 syndrome**.

Hemodynamic explanation of findings—With systolic ventricular contraction, blood from the right ventricular outflow tract is obstructed proportionally to the degree of stenosis. To compensate, the right ventricle becomes **hypertrophied** so that a volume of blood is pumped past the obstruction and into the pulmonary circulation, but the rest of the right ventricular volume is pumped **right-to-left across the VSD and into the aorta**, where it meets with the oxygenated blood that has returned from the lungs to the left atrium and the left ventricle → **aortic blood is desaturated** because of the mixing with venous right ventricular blood. The worse the obstruction, the greater the RVH (until no further hypertrophy is possible and right ventricular failure ensues) and the greater is the shunting and the degree of desaturation. After tissue oxygen extraction, blood returning to the right atrium is desaturated (low mixed venous saturation). The auscultory findings will be that of the pulmonic stenosis.

Table 12.14: TOF Clinical Findings

Auscultation/Other Findings	Chest X-ray	Electrocardiogram
-Loud, harsh systolic ejection-type murmur heard at the upper sternal border and pulmonary auscultation area; radiates to lungs -Murmur may be accompanied by a thrill. -Murmur may be preceded by a pulmonary click. -S2 may be soft (softer pulmonary component) or single (with severe stenosis). -Substernal right ventricular impulse/bulge	-Decreased lung markings due to decreased pulmonary blood flow proportional to the degree of obstruction -With significant obstruction and RVH, the apex is lifted off the diaphragm, giving the appearance of a boot-shaped heart.	-Right-axis deviation -RVH -Tall, peaked P waves (atrial enlargement)

Abbreviations: right ventricular hypertrophy, RVH

Clinical presentation—With mild to moderate disease, the patient may initially be asymptomatic, with cyanosis evident at the **closing of the ductus** or later (weeks to months). More significant obstruction presents after birth and worsens with ductal closure. The patient is **cyanotic and dyspneic**. If definitive repair is delayed, the patient may experience **paroxysmal hypercyanotic attacks (tet spells)**, which are seen as dyspnea on exertion or with stress and sudden increase in appearance of cyanosis (increase in infundibular obstruction with greater right-to-left shunting). If not relieved, it may result in unconsciousness and a seizure. This may be relieved by placing the child in the **knee-chest position (or squatting**; this increases systemic vascular resistance to decrease the right-to-left shunting). Complications of unrepaired TOF include cerebral thrombosis, brain abscess, and endocarditis.

Management—Neonates who are cyanotic should be placed on an IV infusion of **prostaglandin E₁ (PGE₁)** to maintain ductal patency. Corrective surgery (valvulotomy, removal of muscle bundles, and patching of the VSD) is now performed early in infancy or even in the neonatal period; if there is a delay in surgery with a significant obstruction to pulmonary blood flow, a **palliative systemic to pulmonary shunt is placed (modified Blalock-Tausig shunt)** to improve pulmonary blood flow. This is taken down at the time of definitive repair.

Tricuspid atresia

No tricuspid valve forms; therefore, there is no usual outlet for the venous return in the right atrium. The **right ventricle is hypoplastic**. For survival, a **patent foramen ovale or an ASD must be present**. Initially, pulmonary blood flow will occur through the **ductus arteriosus** and will be improved in those patients with a **VSD.**

Hemodynamic explanation of findings—Venous return entering the right atrium cannot take its usual course across the tricuspid valve because there is no communication to the right ventricle. Blood is therefore **shunted right-to-left across a foramen ovale (minimal shunting; more likely to result in death) or an ASD (better with larger-size ASD)**. This is the reason for **cyanosis**, as this venous blood will combine with the pulmonary venous blood in the left atrium, enter the left ventricle, and exit the aorta as severely desaturated blood. At this point, prior to the ductus arteriosus, there is still no pulmonary blood flow unless there is also a **VSD. Without a VSD, the right ventricle is usually completely hypoplastic in conjunction with pulmonary atresia** (high mortality rate). With a large VSD, there may be pulmonary overcirculation and heart failure. The most common situation is a small to moderate VSD with some degree of pulmonary stenosis so that pulmonary blood flow is decreased.

Table 12.15: Tricuspid Atresia Clinical Findings

Auscultation/Other Findings	Chest X-ray	Electrocardiogram
-Increased left ventricular impulse (right ventricle is hypoplastic) -Single S2 -Holosystolic murmur along the left sternal border (VSD)	-Decreased pulmonary blood flow in most (unless large VSD with minimal pulmonary stenosis or with transposed great vessels)	-Left-axis deviation and left ventricular hypertrophy (exactly opposite the normal neonatal ECG and the **key** to the diagnosis)

Abbreviations: ventral septal defect, VSD

Clinical presentation—The majority will present in the immediate newborn period with **severe cyanosis and respiratory distress**.

Management—PGE₁ for newborn (ductal-dependent lesion); systemic-to-pulmonary shunt to increase pulmonary blood flow (unless there is pulmonary overcirculation in the condition stated above); definitive surgical procedures (at age 4–8 months, take down Blalock-Tausig shunt and place bidirectional Glenn shunt with the later modified Fontan procedure).

Ebstein anomaly

Tricuspid leaflets displaced into the right ventricle to varying degrees during cardiac development, results in **abnormal development of the right side of the heart**. There is a **smaller, decreased-functioning right ventricle** (to the extent of the severity of the downward displacement of the valve leaflets) and a **huge, thin-walled right atrium** that encompasses the space of the normal right atrium plus that part of the right ventricle within the confines of the tricuspid leaflets (this is called **atrialization of the right ventricle**). The tricuspid valve is regurgitant.

Hemodynamic explanation of findings—In the more severe form, there is **decreased forward blood flow** to the right ventricle due to its smaller size and decreased contractility; there may be a significant amount of **tricuspid regurgitation**. Blood is therefore shunted **right-to-left across a foramen ovale or ASD** (as was the case in tricuspid atresia). This results in the **cyanosis** which will be present to the degree of the shunting, which is dependent upon the severity of the lesion. Milder degrees of valve displacement may be asymptomatic until later in childhood, adolescence, or even adulthood (and may present in another manner—see the following sections).

Table 12.16: Ebstein Anomaly Clinical Findings

Auscultation/Other Findings	Chest X-ray	Electrocardiogram
-Most have the holosystolic murmur of tricuspid regurgitation heard widely over the left anterior chest -Gallop rhythm with multiple clicks (from the abnormal valve) over the lower left sternal border	-In the severe form, presenting in the neonatal period, the heart is huge (due to the large right atrium); often called box-shaped heart -Pulmonary vessels decreased (may be normal in less severe forms)	-Right bundle branch block -Very tall and broad P waves (right atrial enlargement) -Prolonged PR interval -Episodes of SVT -Underlying WPW

Abbreviations: supraventricular tachycardia, SVT; Wolff-Parkinson-White syndrome, WPW

Clinical presentation—Patients with severe tricuspid displacement will present in the neonatal period with **cyanosis, respiratory distress, and heart failure;** cyanosis worsens with ductal closing. Patients with **mild forms** of the lesion may remain asymptomatic for years and present initially with an **unexplained episode of supraventricular tachycardia (SVT)**. After resolution of the SVT, a 12-lead ECG may disclose the underlying diagnosis of **Wolff-Parkinson-White syndrome (WPW)**.

Management—For neonates: PGE_1, then a Blalock-Tausig shunt alone or with patch closure of the tricuspid valve and atrial septectomy. A later Glenn shunt may be needed to decrease the volume load on the right ventricle if there is significant associated tricuspid regurgitation after the previous procedure. In older patients (adolescents or adults), treating the SVT is the first step with possible surgical correction.

Cyanotic Lesions—With Increased PBF

Dextro-transposition of the great arteries (D-TGA)

The normal anatomy of the great vessels is that the aorta is posterior and to the right of the pulmonary artery, whereas in dextro-transposition of the great arteries (d-TGA), the **aorta is anterior and to the right**. The **ventricles remain physiological** but now the **aorta arises from the right ventricle and the pulmonary artery from the left**. The heart has therefore been converted from a series circuit into **two parallel circuits. Mixing occurs across the foramen ovale and the ductus arteriosus.** There is better mixing in those patients who also have a **VSD** (about half). In L-TGA, called **corrected transposition**, the aorta arises to the left of the pulmonary artery (they are usually side-by-side) and there is also a double inversion—i.e., a physiological right atrium is connected to a left ventricle, which is connected to the pulmonary artery; and the physiological left atrium is connected to the right ventricle, which is connected to the aorta. If there are no other defects, then the patient appears normal (no cyanosis); but most do have **other abnormalities** which result in symptoms and allow for diagnosis (VSD, pulmonary stenosis, conduction defects). In another variety, both aorta and pulmonary artery arise from the right ventricle (double outlet) and there is also transposition. The only left ventricular outlet is a VSD. In this lesion without the transposition, the appearance is that of a left-to-right shunt with mild desaturation. With the transposition there is also a VSD, and this results in heart failure and cyanosis early in infancy. TGA is another conotruncal lesion seen in **CATCH 22** syndromes and has a higher incident in **infants of diabetic mothers**.

Hemodynamic explanation of findings—In simple d-TGA (intact ventricular septum), blood returning to the right atrium flows into the right ventricle and directly into the aorta and systemic circulation. At this point, the only mixing comes from blood that has returned from the lungs (and is therefore oxygenated) to the left atrium and is shunted left-to-right across a foramen ovale to step up the saturations of the blood flowing into the aorta. Oxygenated blood returning to the left atrium flows to the left ventricle and directly back to the pulmonary circulation; as long as the ductus is still patent, this also results in mixing at this level. However, as the ductus closes, further cyanosis and symptoms result. The only way that the situation is improved is if there is an ASD present to then allow for greater atrial mixing and in those who have a VSD, where mixing at this level may allow for a significant increase in systemic saturations.

Table 12.17: D-TGA Clinical Findings

Auscultation/Other Findings	Chest X-ray	Electrocardiogram
-Parasternal heave -Single, loud S2 -Most with no murmur or a nonspecific systolic murmur at the left sternal border -If there is a small VSD, there is also a harsh systolic murmur at the lower sternal border; and if the VSD is large, there will be the classic holosystolic murmur.	-Mild increase in heart size with a straight, narrow mediastinum (because of the relationship of the great vessels), called an "egg-on-a-string" appearance -Normal to increased pulmonary blood flow that may increase further (because of left-to-right shunting) with decreasing pulmonary vascular resistance after birth	-Normal neonatal ECG with right-axis deviation (unless there is a large VSD, in which case there will be prominent P waves with either RVH or bilateral ventricular hypertrophy)

Abbreviations: right ventricular hypertrophy, RVH; ventral septal defect, VSD

Clinical presentation—This is the **most common lesion that most consistently presents with cyanosis in the immediate newborn period** (but the most common cyanotic lesion overall is TOF); cyanosis and tachypnea increase as the ductus closes. If there is a small VSD the findings are more subtle, and with a large VSD the cyanosis may not be visible (or may again be subtle) but the patient will present with early heart failure.

Management—PGE₁ after birth for ductal patency in the cyanotic infant; if there is a significantly low PaO₂ despite the PGE₁, or if there is any significant delay in corrective surgery, then a **Rashkind balloon atrial septostomy** is performed (for better mixing). The definitive procedure is the **Jatene arterial switch in the first 2 weeks of life**. After birth, there will be a decrease in left ventricular pressure with the fall in pulmonary vascular resistance (since the pulmonary artery is connected to the left ventricle) and if there is a delay in surgery, the left ventricle will not be able to sustain enough pressure to then support the systemic circulation.

Truncus arteriosus

There is **failure of conotruncal development** such that a **single common trunk** arises from the heart and **sits directly on top of a large VSD**. The pulmonary artery arises distally from the common trunk.

Hemodynamic explanation of findings—Because there is a large VSD below their outlet, i.e., the common arterial trunk, both **ventricles are at systemic pressure**. There is **complete mixing of blood** going into the common trunk (and across a **single valve**). As pulmonary vascular resistance falls after birth, there is **more and more pulmonary blood flow** until it typically becomes torrential and results in **heart failure with minimal cyanosis**. If this condition continued, it would typically result in **Eisenmenger physiology** with worsening of cyanosis. There is also **runoff of blood from the truncus to the pulmonary artery during diastole** (as in a PDA), resulting in a **wide pulse pressure**. There may also be varying degrees of **truncal valve insufficiency**.

Table 12.18: Truncus Arteriosus Clinical Findings

Auscultation/Other Findings	Chest X-ray	Electrocardiogram
-Hyperdynamic precordium -Loud, single S2 -Loud systolic ejection murmur with thrill at the lower left sternal border, radiating upward; it may be preceded by an ejection click -If there is truncal insufficiency, there is a high-pitched early diastolic decrescendo murmur at the mid-left sternal border. -Apical mid-diastolic low-pitched rumble (increased flow in diastole across the mitral valve) -Bounding pulses	-Significant cardiomegaly and pulmonary edema	-Bilateral ventricular hypertrophy

Clinical presentation—Neonates will present with **minimal cyanosis and the auscultory findings**, and an older infant (i.e., with decreased PVR) will present with **heart failure and minimal cyanosis**.

Management—First, control the **heart failure medically** (this may also require **initial pulmonary artery banding**), then definitive surgery (separation of pulmonary artery from the truncus, closing of the VSD, and creation of a conduit between the RV and pulmonary artery).

Total anomalous pulmonary venous return (TAPVR)

There is **no pulmonary venous return to the left atrium**. Instead it returns either **above the diaphragm** (into the right atrium directly, into a coronary sinus, or into the superior vena cava via a vertical vein and then into the right atrium) or **below the diaphragm** (into a descending vein and then into the inferior vena cava [IVC] or another vessel that joins the IVC, e.g., the ductus venosus). There is **total mixing of systemic venous and pulmonary venous blood**, which leads to **cyanosis**. There may be some element of **obstruction** (more common below the diaphragm) and the presentation is dependent on how much obstruction there is.

Hemodynamic explanation of findings—Whatever the anatomy of the pulmonary venous return, there is mixing of the venous and pulmonary circulations **prior to or at the level of the right atrium**. Blood from this point may take its usual course to the right ventricle and pulmonary artery or it may flow **right-to-left across an ASD** into the left atrium, resulting in further cyanosis. Without obstruction, there is then **enlargement of the right atrium, right ventricle, and pulmonary artery**. If there is severe obstruction to pulmonary venous return, then there will be **severe pulmonary venous congestion and pulmonary hypertension**. This leads to rapid deterioration.

Table 12.19: TAPVR Clinical Findings

Auscultation/Other Findings	Chest X-ray	Electrocardiogram
-Auscultation findings depend on the presence and degree of obstruction. With severe obstruction, there are generally no murmurs. With decreasing degrees of obstruction, one may hear a gallop rhythm and systolic murmurs along the left sternal border.	-If the veins enter just above the right atrium, there will be a large supracardiac shadow with a normal heart, which gives the appearance of a snowman. -Without obstruction, there is a large heart with a prominent RA, RV, and pulmonary artery, and increased pulmonary markings. -With obstruction, there is a small heart and pulmonary venous congestion.	-RVH with tall, spiked P waves (right atrial enlargement), unless severe obstruction is present

Abbreviations: right atrium, RA; right ventricle, RV; right ventricular hypertrophy, RVH

Clinical presentation—**Severe obstruction** will present in the **immediate neonatal period** as a **seriously ill and cyanotic infant who has no response to PGE₁**, requires an echocardiographic diagnosis and surgery as soon as possible. If there is a mild to moderate degree of obstruction, then there will be early heart failure and the development of pulmonary venous hypertension (from the obstruction) and pulmonary artery hypertension. Cyanosis is mild in this case. If there is **no obstruction** at all, then there may be **little or no symptoms until the patient develops heart failure** (and may have **mild cyanosis with no pulmonary artery hypertension**).

Management—If surgery cannot be done emergently, the patient may be stabilized on extracorporeal membrane oxygenation (ECMO). The surgery is to anastamose the common pulmonary venous trunk to the left atrium and close the ASD. There is generally recurrent stenosis in the long term, and a heart/lung transplant may offer the only means to survival.

Hypoplastic left heart (HLH)

The **left side of the heart from the mitral valve through the ascending aorta is hypoplastic with a left ventricle (LV) that is small or totally atretic and therefore has poor function**. The LV cannot supply the systemic circulation in utero and this is done by the **right ventricle (RV),** which also has to supply the pulmonary circulation. A VSD is usually not associated with this lesion. It may be accompanied by **extracardiac anomalies** (especially renal and central nervous system [CNS]) that may not be compatible with life. In addition, there may be a **chromosomal abnormality** (particularly associated with trisomy 18).

Hemodynamic explanation of findings—Blood returning from the lungs enters the left atrium. Because of the hypoplasia and poor function of the left ventricle, **forward flow of blood into the systemic circulation is diminished** and results in the primary finding of **poor systemic perfusion**. A significant portion of left atrial blood is therefore shunted left-to-right across a foramen ovale (restricted flow will lead to pulmonary venous congestion and pulmonary hypertension) or ASD with pulmonary overload into the right atrium and into the pulmonary circulation. Blood from the right ventricle may cross the ductus arteriosus to supply the descending aorta, which can account for some degree of **cyanosis**.

As the ductus closes, systemic blood flow decreases further and the patient **presents with shock**.

Table 12.20: Hypoplastic Left Heart Clinical Findings

Auscultation/Other Findings	Chest X-ray	Electrocardiography
-Right ventricular parasternal lift -Nondescript systolic murmur -Hypotension, tachycardia, cool extremities, absent pulses, acidosis -Extracardiac anomalies	-Usually an increased heart size and increased pulmonary vascularity (from the more common shunting through a moderate to large ASD)	-RVH -Tall P waves in right precordial leads (large right atrium) -Low left ventricular voltage

Abbreviations: atrial septal defect, ASD; right ventricular hypertrophy, RVH

Clinical presentation—Newborns will present with a **variable amount of cyanosis and poor perfusion** resulting in a **gray to blue skin color**. This will be more evident with **ductal closure**, and at that time the infant develops **respiratory distress and signs and symptoms of heart failure and shock**.

Management
- **PGE$_1$ infusion in order to continue to support the systemic circulation**.
- In order to **decrease the amount of pulmonary blood flow**, the patient should be in **room air or in decreased oxygen** (blended with nitrogen).
- If there is a delay in surgery, a balloon septostomy is performed if there is an inadequate intra-atrial communication.
- Prior to any definitive surgery, a **thorough evaluation of life-threatening associations needs to be undertaken**. If there are such lesions, or a chromosomal constitution that is not compatible with life, the appropriate management is to remove the infant from life support (after appropriate discussion with the family, and at a time and in a manner that is ethical).
- If correction is to be performed, the most common procedure is the **Norwood procedure**, which occurs in three steps over a period of years.
- Cardiac transplantation is generally no longer recommended, as the success with surgery has improved significantly.

CHOLESTEROL SCREENING IN CHILDREN (NATIONAL CHOLESTEROL EDUCATION PROGRAM)

- There is no current consensus for universal screening of all children.
- Screening is based on: children who have parents and grandparents who have coronary artery disease documented in grandparents < age 55 years or who have a parent with

a documented cholesterol level >240 mg/dL, or if the family history is unobtainable (especially with other risk factors).

- A fasting lipid profile should be obtained (minimum age 2 years for institution of safe dietary therapy; but no later than age 10 years). A second blood sample should be obtained and the two values averaged:
  - <110 mg/dL is acceptable and should be repeated in 5 years; educate family to decrease risk factors.
  - At 110–129 mg/dL (borderline) a Step One Diet should be instituted (see below) and other risk factors addressed; re-evaluation should occur in 1 year.
  - At ≥130 mg/dL (high), evaluation for secondary causes should be undertaken plus evaluation of other family members. Institute a Step Two Diet and set low-density lipoprotein (LDL) goal at a minimum <103 mg/dL and ideally at <100 mg/dL. Re-evaluate every 3–6 months.

- American heart Association (AHA) Step One Diet: ≤30% of total daily calories as fat, ≤10% of calories as saturated fat, and total cholesterol intake <300 mg/dL/day.
- AHA Step Two Diet: Same as Step One, except restrict saturated fat to <7–8% and cholesterol to <200 mg/dL. No restrictions for children <2 years of age (rapid growth and development and CNS development).
- Drug treatment: at least age 8 years (statins are equally effective in children, and the same type of monitoring should be done as with adults)
  - With no risk factors and LDL persistently >190 mg/dL despite diet therapy
  - With risk factors (obesity, hypertension, cigarette smoking, positive family history) and LDL persistently >160 mg/dL despite diet therapy
  - With diabetes mellitus and LDL persistently ≥130 mg/dL
    - Initial goal with any of the above is to decrease the LDL to <160 mg/dL and ideally to <130 (and even <110) mg/dL with any of the risk factors.

GASTROINTESTINAL DISORDERS

ACUTE ABDOMINAL PAIN

Appendicitis

- Luminal obstruction, ischemia, and bacterial invasion; major complication is gangrene with perforation, peritonitis, and sepsis
- Peak incidence is in **adolescence**; most common cause of need for acute surgery in children
- Presentation is dependent on the **location of the appendix** and the presence of a localized abscess contained by the omentum.

Key diagnostic words—Initial slow-onset **colicky periumbilical pain** with nausea, vomiting, and decreased appetite; then low-grade fever with **right lower quadrant pain** that is increasing in intensity, exacerbated by movement over 1–2 days. If **perforation** occurs, then peritonitis ensues → **diffuse severe abdominal pain** and toxicity. With a **retrocecal appendix**, pain develops **more slowly over days and is lateral and posterior**.

Findings on examination—Early findings: normal to increased bowel sounds and **localized abdominal tenderness**, maximal at **McBurney's point** (or in almost any other location); rigidity over the rectus muscles and **rebound tenderness**; **rectal exam** is very painful (and **should be avoided**, as it provides no other information); there may be pain on movement of the hip and thigh in the supine position.

Diagnosis—Plain radiographs are not sensitive enough and should not be ordered. If not certain after a history and physical (or with serial exams and observation over 12–24 hours), **best test is a CT scan with contrast**. The appendix may not be seen with ultrasound (good in girls for pelvic organ disease). **Supporting studies:** increased white blood cell (WBC) count, urine with few WBCs and red blood cells (RBCs); increase in serum amyloid A protein.

Management—**Preoperative management:** fever and pain control, fluid administration, correction of electrolyte abnormalities and acidosis, blood pressure, renal insufficiency, antibiotics; **no emergency surgery** unless there is evidence of diffuse peritonitis, then surgery should occur after initial stabilization.

Cholecystitis and Cholelithiasis

- Cholecystitis (inflammation of the biliary tree) without the development of stones (**acalculous**): usually caused by **infection** (Gram-positive, Gram-negative, parasitic).
- Cholecystitis with stones (**calculous**): most often secondary to abdominal trauma, severe burns, or vasculitis. Acute presentation: gallstone obstructs cystic duct → inflammation and infection.
- **Cholelithiasis** is rare in children unless there is an **underlying disorder** or condition (**hemolytic anemia**, prolonged total parenteral nutrition, prematurity, **cystic fibrosis**, chronic liver/biliary disease).

Key diagnostic words

- **Cholecystitis: right upper quadrant or epigastric pain**, nausea, vomiting, **fever**, jaundice.
- **Cholelithiasis: recurrent colicky right upper quadrant abdominal pain radiating to the right scapula**, jaundice, and intolerance for fatty foods in a child with the underlying problems listed above.

Diagnosis

- **Initial best test**—ultrasound (for either cholecystitis or cholelithiasis).
- If gallbladder cannot be visualized, perform **hepatobiliary scintigraphy**.
- Other supportive evidence: ↑ WBCs, ↑ serum alkaline phosphatase, ↑ direct bilirubin (if obstruction).

Management

- **Cholecystitis:** broad-spectrum parenteral antibiotics, follow with serial ultrasounds; if no improvement, then surgery.
- **Cholelithiasis:** cholecystectomy with operative cholangiography to look for stones in the common bile duct (or endoscopic retrograde cholangiopancreatography [ERCP] in older children).

Acute Pancreatitis

- **Most common pancreatic disorder in children.**
- From stasis with continued pancreatic enzyme synthesis and activity → **autodigestion** and release of cytokines → **diffuse inflammation**.
- Most common causes—**infectious** (**mumps**, rubella, hepatitis, coxsackie, Epstein-Barr virus [EBV], ascaris, and others), drug-induced (**valproate** most common, plus

alcohol, **corticosteroids, chemotherapy drugs**, and others), obstruction (tumors, malformations, cholelithiasis), trauma and systemic diseases (**cystic fibrosis**, Crohn disease, **hypercalcemia**, and others). Chronic or recurrent pancreatitis most likely due to **cystic fibrosis, hyperparathyroidism, hyperlipidemias**, congenital duct anomalies, and hereditary pancreatitis.

Key diagnostic words—Severe, constant epigastric (or either upper quadrant) pain with persistent vomiting and fever

Findings on examination—Toxic appearance with a **distended, very tender abdomen**; a mass may be palpated in the epigastrium/upper abdomen; the patient is generally dehydrated and may have electrolyte abnormalities.

Diagnosis—**Increased pancreatic amylase isoenzyme and lipase** (more specific; peaks at 24–48 hours and is increased longer than amylase). The **best diagnostic study is a CT scan** (better than ultrasound); **plain films** are nonspecific; ↑ WBCs, ↑ bilirubin, ↑ γ-glutamyl transpeptidase (GGTP), ↑ glucose, and ↓ serum calcium. The **best test** for **recurrent pancreatitis**—ERCP or magnetic resonance cholangiopancreatography (**MRCP**).

Management—**Control pain**, nothing by mouth (NPO), nasogastric (NG) suction, IV fluids, correct electrolyte abnormalities; most recover within a week.

Intussusception

- **Telescoping** of a proximal segment of bowel distally, dragging the mesentery with it → **bowel ischemia** (with **sloughing of the mucosa**) and **venous obstruction** with bleeding (dark blood). Most common is **ileocolic**, then cecocolic, then ileal-ileal. Age range is 3 months to 6 years (**most <2 years**).
- Previous (within a week) nonspecific illness (upper respiratory infection [URI], otitis media, gastroenteritis) or unrecognized underlying **anatomic lead point** (Meckel diverticulum, polyp, neurofibroma, or hemangioma)

Key diagnostic words—Sudden onset of **severe, paroxysmal abdominal pain with vomiting** (early in course), **straining, and progressive lethargy**; decreased stooling after initial onset; most pass bloody stool in the first 12 hours (classic **"currant-jelly" stool**), but **bleeding may be delayed or there may be no bleeding**. Without diagnosis → perforation, shock, and death.

Examination findings—Abdominal tenderness and guarding; **right upper quadrant, tender, sausage-shaped mass with axis in the cephalocaudal direction**; rectal exam yields bloody mucus

Diagnosis and Treatment

- **Best initial test to confirm diagnosis**—ultrasound (tubular mass in long-axis view and doughnut appearance in transverse).
- If positive or equivocal, perform **air-contrast enema** (negligible risk of perforation compared to barium), which will be **diagnostic** (filling defect plus a **coiled spring sign**) **and possibly therapeutic** in terms of **hydrostatic reduction.**
- **Should not be performed if any suggestion of perforation**
- Rate of successful reduction is increased if done **within the first 48 hours** of symptoms
- If hydrostatic reduction is not successful, the patient requires **surgical reduction** (resection only if there is necrotic bowel)
- Most recurrences can be treated successfully with repeat hydrostatic reduction
- Recurrence rate after surgical reduction is low and does not occur after surgical resection.

Obstruction

For congenital bowel obstruction, see Chapter 1.

- May occur anywhere along the intestinal tract from: congenital **atresias and stenosis**, external compression, strictures, inflammatory lesions, or trauma (see above).
- **Ileus** absent peristalsis not due to an anatomic obstruction; caused by many conditions (infection, medications, metabolic imbalances, surgery, and trauma).
- **Adhesions** are caused by fibrous bands that occur most commonly **after abdominal surgery.**

Key diagnostic words—Increasing pain and abdominal distension with vomiting, then decreased to absent bowel sounds and constipation

Diagnosis—The **best initial test** is a plain radiograph, which may show **multiple air-fluid levels without air in the distal bowel.**

Management—Place **NG tube**, provide IV fluids, and correct any electrolyte abnormalities; if the cause is identified as medical, **treat the underlying problem**; otherwise broad-spectrum antibiotics, then **surgery.**

CHRONIC ABDOMINAL PAIN

Functional/Recurrent Abdominal Pain

- **Nonorganic pain** (the **majority of recurrent abdominal pain** in children and adolescents); cannot be accounted for by history, exam, and lab studies. Episodes monthly for **at least 3 months** which disrupt normal routines.
- **Periumbilical pain, paroxysmal, not occurring with meals, in children older than 6 years**. May also occur as epigastric pain with nausea and bloating after eating. If the evaluation is negative, this is **non-ulcer dyspepsia**. Pain below the umbilicus with cramping, abdominal distension, and a change in bowel pattern is consistent with **irritable bowel syndrome**.
- **Organic causes** more common in children <6 years with systemic findings, weight loss, and pain away from the umbilicus; may awaken the child from sleep; may present with vomiting, diarrhea, hematochezia, and abnormal positive physical findings.
- Laboratory studies for recurrent abdominal pain should **only be performed as suggested by the history and physical**. Screening studies: CBC, urinalysis (UA), erythrocyte sedimentation rate (ESR), stool for parasites, and at most an ultrasound of the abdomen and/or pelvis.
- Management is reassurance and avoidance of reinforcing behaviors. Medications do not help.

Irritable Bowel Syndrome (IBS)

- **Abdominal pain or discomfort for 12 weeks in the past 12 months, plus two of the following three findings**: abdominal pain is **better with stooling**; onset of pain occurs with a **change of stool frequency** (>3 stools per day or <3 per week) or pain occurs with a **change in stool form**; presence of **mucus, bloating, straining, urgency, or incomplete evacuations**.
- Recurrent/chronic abdominal pain (including IBS) related to anxiety and depression, personality, and reinforcement from the family (see Chapter 6).
- With loose stool, additional dietary fiber is helpful; anticholinergic agents or tricyclic antidepressants may be beneficial (but should certainly not be used routinely).

Acid-Peptic Disorders (Peptic Ulcer Disease)

- Presents with varying degrees of **gastritis or ulceration**.
- **Peptic ulcers:** deep duodenal mucosal lesions (majority in the duodenal bulb) or the stomach (most in the lesser curvature)
- **Primary** peptic ulcers: more common in the **duodenum** and present with **chronic symptoms**. Most often associated with *Helicobacter pylori* (acquired mostly from the fecal-oral route; chronic colonization increases the risk of duodenal ulcer, gastric cancer, and lymphomas) or are idiopathic.

- **Secondary** ulcers are **more acute** and more commonly **gastric** (erosions). Seen with **stress**, sepsis, shock, with central nervous system (CNS) lesions, **nonsteroidal anti-inflammatory drugs (NSAIDs), and aspirin**, and in hypersecretory states (**Zollinger-Ellison syndrome**: autonomous secretion of gastrin by a neuroendocrine tumor resulting in severe peptic ulcer disease).

Key diagnostic words—**Epigastric dull ache or periumbilical pain** for short periods to hours with exacerbations; may be **relieved by food or antacids**; younger children with irritability, poor feeding, vomiting; may also have hematemesis or melena.

Diagnosis—The **procedure of choice is endoscopy with biopsy** (for histology and *H. pylori*). A stool antigen test for *H. pylori* and serological tests are available (need biopsy for active infection and to follow success of treatment).

Management

- If *H. pylori* is present on biopsy—**eradication therapy (two of the following antibiotics** for 14 days—amoxicillin, clarithromycin, metronidazole—plus a **proton pump inhibitor** for 1 month [omeprazole, lansoprazole, rabeprazole, or pantoprazole]).
- Idiopathic ulcers treated with **acid suppression alone** (H2 receptor antagonist [cimetidine, ranitidine, famotidine, or nizatidine] or a proton pump inhibitor). **Stress ulcers** found most commonly in critically ill children in intensive care unit (ICU); prophylactic gastric acid inhibitors are often used as part of overall therapy.

Inflammatory Bowel Disease (IBD)

- **Bowel inflammation plus extraintestinal manifestations** (slightly greater in Crohn disease).
- Most common childhood presentation is at **10–20 years of age** (but may occur earlier).
- Both ulcerative colitis and Crohn disease have genetic predispositions plus environmental influences.

Table 13.1: Comparison of the Features, Diagnosis, and Management of Ulcerative Colitis and Crohn Disease

Antibody	Ulcerative Colitis	Crohn Disease
Intestinal location	**Colon only**, beginning in rectum and extending proximally to various extents	Anywhere from the **mouth to the anus**; segmental (**skip lesions**) and **transmural involvement**; initially most present with **ileocolitis**
Clinical findings	Insidious to acute; **diarrhea, blood in stool, crampy abdominal pain, urgency, nocturnal bowel movements**; fever and leukocytosis (colitis associated with Crohn disease looks the same initially); with **chronic symptoms** → anorexia, weight loss, anemia, and low albumin	**Systemic findings** more common (fever, fatigue, malaise), **growth failures**, and lack of sexual development. Small-bowel disease most commonly presents with **right lower quadrant pain and obstruction and colonic disease** (in up to 75% of patients) **presents most commonly with signs of ulcerative. colitis. Classic presentation is not common:** **diarrhea, weight loss, and abdominal pain with or without bleeding.**
Other intestinal features	No abdominal mass palpable; perianal disease very uncommon; mouth ulcerations rare; ileal disease does not occur unless there is **backwash ileitis**; strictures and fistulas are uncommon and fissures do not occur.	An **abdominal mass** (RLQ) often palpable; **perianal disease** (skin tags, drainage, fistulas) common but **rectal disease occurs much less commonly**; **mouth ulcerations** common; **ileal disease** common but not stomach or esophageal; **strictures, fissures, and fistulas** common (between segments of bowel; between bowel and bladder, bowel and vagina, or bowel and skin).
Most common extraintestinal manifestations	-Joint (sacroiliitis, ankylosing spondylitis) -Skin (**pyoderma gangrenosum**) -Hepatobiliary (**sclerosing cholangitis**, chronic active hepatitis) -Eye (**anterior uveitis**)	In general, **more common**: especially **erythema nodosum**, oral aphthous ulcers, arthritis, renal stones, gallstones, episcleritis, and clubbing
Clinical course	Periods of **remissions and relapses**; increased **risk of colon cancer after 10 years** of disease (needs colonoscopy and biopsy every 1–2 years); risk of toxic megacolon	Symptoms **recur despite treatment**, and **bowel involvement increases with time**, but extensive small-bowel involvement causing short bowel syndrome is less common; **complications also increase with time**, and surgery is common; with ileal disease (or surgical resection) → bile acid malabsorption with diarrhea, B12 deficiency, and possibly cholelithiasis.

(continued on next page)

Table 13.1: Comparison of the Features, Diagnosis, and Management of Ulcerative Colitis and Crohn Disease *(cont.)*

Antibody	Ulcerative Colitis	Crohn Disease
Diagnosis	-Symptoms present for **at least 2 weeks and infective colitis ruled out** (stool culture, O and P, amoeba serology, *Clostridium difficile* toxin). -**Supportive lab studies**: increased WBCs, anemia, increased ESR, hypoalbuminemia; presence of **p-ANCA** -Barium enema not diagnostic. -**Most accurate test**: colonoscopy and histological examination (not during fulminant colitis): **friable** mucosa, often a **cutoff line** (unless there is total colonic involvement), **linear ulceration**, inflammation and edema; biopsy shows **crypt abscesses**; transmural involvement uncommon.	-**Supportive**: Fe-deficiency anemia and anemia of chronic disease, elevated ESR, increased platelets, mildly increased WBCs, hypoalbuminemia, **anti-***Saccharomyces cerevisiae*; **increased stool alpha-1-antitrypsin, fecal calprotectin, and lactoferrin** -**Initial best study** depends on suspicion of disease location: upper GI contrast study with small-bowel follow-through for small-bowel disease (characteristic pathology; most with terminal ileum involvement; skip lesions; strictures, fistulas); may also use ultrasound, CT, or MRI for better examination of localized involvement and complications; colonoscopy with biopsy for suspected colitis (most characteristic finding is **non-caseating granulomas**) plus ileal intubation
Management	-For **mild disease** and for remission, **first-line drug is sulfasalazine** (sulfur-5-aminosalicylate; major side effect is sulfur hypersensitivity); may also be given as an enema for proctitis. -**Moderate to severe**: start with **prednisone**, gradually taper to alternate day therapy over 1–3 months and then discontinue; if unresponsive, use azathioprine, 6-mercaptopurine, cyclosporine, or infliximab. -**Surgery (total colectomy)** used for intractable disease, unresponsive to immunomodulators, or with any complications of therapy; also if significant dysplasia.	-**Mild terminal ileal disease or colitis**: initially start with **mesalamine** (releases the active 5-ASA in the ileum and colon; sulfasalazine may be used for mild colitis but not for small-bowel disease; also for mild ileal or ileocecal disease, may use budesonide (corticosteroid). -**More extensive disease**: start with **prednisone** and taper with improvement to alternate-day therapy (maintenance not effective for preventing relapses). -**Unresponsive**: immunomodulators as per ulcerative colitis -**Perirectal fistulae**: short-term metronidazole -Nutritional therapy with **enteral nutrition** (NG supplementation of high caloric supplements) -**Surgery** is the treatment of choice for local disease unresponsive to treatment, perforation, stricture, abscesses, or intractable bleeding.

Abbreviations: acetylsalicylic acid, ASA; erythrocyte sedimentation rate, ESR; gastrointestinal, GI; nasogastric, NG; ova and parasites, O and P; perinuclear antineutrophil antibodies, p-ANCA; right lower quadrant, RLQ; white blood cells, WBCs

OTHER GASTROINTESTINAL BLEEDING

- Most common causes of gastrointestinal (GI) bleeding in children: causes of **erosion to some part of the GI tract,** portal hypertension, vascular anomalies
- Bleeding from the upper GI tract (through the duodenum) presents with **hematemesis** (darkens; appearance of coffee grounds; large blood loss is generally still red).
- Blood in the stool (**hematochezia**) from the distal intestine: red or dark-red; bleeding from above the ileum = **melena**

Most Common Etiologies

Table 13.2: Most Common Etiologies of GI Bleeding

Upper GI Tract	Small Intestine	Colon	Anorectal
Esophagitis	Bacterial enteritis	Colitis (infection, IBD)	Anal fissure
Mallory-Weiss tear	Necrotizing enterocolitis	Hemolytic-uremic syndrome	Polyp
Swallowed blood	Intussusception	Polyp	Hemorrhoids
Varices	Volvulus	Coagulopathy	
Gastritis	Meckel diverticulum		
Peptic ulcer disease	Henoch-Schönlein purpura		
Milk-protein allergy	IBD		
Foreign body			

Abbreviations: inflammatory bowel disease, IBD

Meckel Diverticulum

- Gestation: 5–7 weeks; embryonic yolk sac develops a **lining similar to the stomach (acid-secreting mucosa),** then attenuates and separates. Failure of this process leaves a **remnant on the antimesenteric side of the small intestine.**
- Meckel diverticulum is the **most frequent GI anomaly**—Rule of 2's: **2%** of the population; on the average **2 inches** in length; located about **2 feet** from the ileocecal valve (on average; depends on the age of presentation); average age of presentation **2 years.**

Key diagnostic words

- **Intermittent, painless, brick-red blood per rectum** (acid secretion causes ulceration of adjacent normal ileal mucosa); bleeding is generally mild and self-limited.
- Less common presentations occur with a **complication:** partial or complete bowel obstruction and intussusception; may also present like an acute appendicitis if there is inflammation of the diverticulum, and may perforate and cause acute peritonitis. With no complications, there are no positive physical findings.

Diagnosis and Management

Best test is the Meckel scan, which is a technetium-pertechnetate scan (the mucus-secreting cells of the ectopic gastric mucosa take up the label). Plain radiography and contrast studies are non-diagnostic. When confirmed with a Meckel scan, **surgery is indicated**.

Polyps and Hemangiomas

- Most common tumor in children—**juvenile colonic polyp:** anywhere through the colon; usually a solitary lesion, but more than one may be present.
- **Multiple juvenile polyps** occur as an **autosomal dominant condition (juvenile polyposis).** Other congenital anomalies are often seen with this. May be involvement of the **entire GI tract,** → abdominal pain, anemia, malabsorption, and poor growth. With at least 3 polyps and a positive family history of GI malignancy, there is a **significant risk for cancer,** and this must be screened for relatively frequently (upper and lower endoscopy and upper-GI contrast study with small-bowel follow-through). A polyp may also act as a **leading point for an intussusception**.
- In **familial adenomatous polyposis (autosomal dominant),** may be **hundreds of polyps** throughout the colon (diagnosis with at least 5 and a positive family history); presents most commonly with recurrent abdominal cramps and hematochezia. Most with a **malignancy by age 40 years** (some as young as 10 years). All with positive family history need a **colonoscopy and genetic analysis.** Management is **proctocolectomy**.
- **Peutz-Jeghers syndrome:** autosomal dominant condition with **abnormal pigmentation of the lips, gingiva, and buccal mucosa;** may be evident from birth or early infancy; also **hamartomas of the GI tract** → intestinal cramps, bleeding, and intestinal obstruction. **Intestinal malignancy** occurs in about half.
- **Hemangiomas** may occur anywhere throughout the GI tract (half in the colon). Cause **bleeding, which can be severe and cause death;** may also have cutaneous hemangiomas and telangiectasia.

Hemorrhoids and Anal Fissures

- **Hemorrhoids** are usually benign in children (associated with obesity and constipation) but may be secondary to portal hypertension from hepatobiliary disease.
  - Findings: **rectal bleeding,** pruritus, and discomfort, particularly sitting
  - Complication: **thrombosis** of an external hemorrhoid acute onset of severe pain. The hemorrhoid needs to be surgically excised.
  - Hemorrhoids generally treated conservatively; with relief of any fecal impaction and treatment of **constipation.** Recurrence may need surgery.

- **Anal fissure: laceration** of the junction between the anal mucosa and skin. Most in **infants less than 1 year of age** due to the passage of **hard stool** (may be a history of constipation).
  - **Bright-red blood on the surface of the stool**
  - Constipation should be treated and simple measures used for healing of the fissure, (sitz baths and the application of topical glyceryl trinitrate).

CONSTIPATION

- Relates to hardness, decreased frequency, and difficulty in passing stool; may be caused by any one of a number of etiologies related to **decreased filling (due to a decrease in peristalsis) or emptying of the rectal vault. Stool retention** is also voluntary—**functional or nonorganic (retentive) constipation** and may have associated **overflow** (see Chapter 6).

Most Common Organic Etiologies

- Primary intestinal disorders (**IBS**)
- Anorectal malformations (**imperforate anus**)
- Abnormal abdominal muscles (**prune belly syndrome**)
- Spinal cord/neurological disorders
- Metabolic disorders (**hypokalemia, hypocalcemia, hypomagnesemia**)
- Endocrine disorders (hypothyroidism)
- Drugs/poisons (anticholinergic agents, narcotics, **lead**)
- Psychiatric disorders
- Most important diagnoses to consider with true **constipation beginning in the neonatal period** are congenital hypothyroidism, **Hirschsprung disease** (see Chapter 1), and chronic intestinal pseudo-obstruction (abnormal muscle and/or neural activity → obstruction without evidence of an anatomic obstruction; may be primary or secondary to another disease and be transient or permanent).
- In the child diagnosed with chronic constipation, the diagnosis of **Hirschsprung disease** (see Chapter 1) should be considered.
  - With Hirschsprung disease, there will be some evidence of problems with stool passage since birth
  - Chronic functional constipation—begins **after age 2 years**. On exam, the patient with Hirschsprung disease may develop **abdominal distension**, but does not happen in functional constipation.
    ○ More likely to feel **hard stool in the rectum** with functional constipation and no stool with Hirschsprung disease. Not finding hard stool does not rule out the diagnosis of functional constipation; obtain a **plain radiograph**, where clumps of stool may be seen.

  - If the diagnosis is considered, a **contrast study might show the line of demarcation of normal to aganglionic bowel segment with proximal dilatation in Hirschsprung disease**; whereas in functional constipation, there are clumps of stool in the large bowel without any line of demarcation.

VOMITING

The congenital obstructions and tracheoesophageal fistula are presented in Chapter 1.

- Obstruction below the second part of the duodenum: **bile-stained vomiting**
- Vomiting also from **nonobstructive causes**: metabolic; CNS lesions; upper intestinal disease (reflux, infection); disease of the liver, biliary system, and pancreas; renal disease; poisoning and systemic infections
- **Cyclic vomiting:** episodes of vomiting over 2–3 days with normal intervals; often prodromal symptoms and a precipitating event or cause; starts at age 2–5 years; may also represent **abdominal migraine**.

Esophageal Disorders Causing Obstruction or Dysmotility (other than tracheoesophageal fistula and esophageal atresia)

- **Esophageal obstruction** may occur from **narrowing of the lumen** from strictures, inflammation, and anatomic abnormalities; or from **external compression** from duplication cysts (this is the most frequent intestinal duplication), enlarged mediastinal lymph nodes, or vascular anomalies (most of which also compress the airway and present with respiratory distress).
- **Esophageal dysmotility with swallowing dysfunction:** may be the primary problem (more often related to a CNS abnormality, e.g., spinal-cord dysraphism, hydrocephalus, cranial nerve defects), neurological disorder (anterior horn cell, myopathy), infectious etiology, connective tissue disorder, or certain medications.
- **Achalasia:** functional obstruction due to **decreased lower esophageal sphincter (LES) relaxation** (abnormalities causing high LES pressure) familial or secondary to other causes in school-age children; presents as **dysphagia for both liquids and solids** and may lead to esophagitis
  - **X-ray** may show dilated esophagus, and a barium swallow shows the tapered end of the esophagus above a closed LES ("bird's-beak" appearance); the **definitive test is esophageal manometry** (high-pressure LES during swallowing). Treatment is **endoscopic esophageal dilatation or surgical myotomy**.

- **Hiatal hernia:** herniation of the stomach through the esophageal hiatus in the diaphragm causing a **sliding hernia** (the gastroesophageal junction slides into the thoracic cavity) presenting problem is **reflux**; or a part of the stomach is herniated through the hiatus next to the lower esophagus, and presents as fullness and pain.

Gastroesophageal Reflux (GER)

- GER is very common in infants due to **low LES tone and increased episodes of transient LES relaxations**. Usually has episodes of **regurgitation** (spitting-up) **with feedings** and no other symptoms or weight loss, within the first months of life and **resolves by age 1 year**. This is a **clinical diagnosis** and **no tests** should be performed. Treatment: normalizing feeding volumes and techniques, keeping the infant upright after a feed, raising the angle of the bed somewhat, and thickening of formula feeds with cooked rice cereal. GER is pathologic (GER disease; GERD) if associated with reflux, weight loss, failure-to-thrive, and/or extraintestinal symptoms.

- The **older child** with GER has a genetic predisposition to it; often has recurrent symptoms similar to the adult with GER; symptoms less likely to resolve; earlier presentation is regurgitation; and later pain. May also be **respiratory symptoms that may be increased with asthma**. Initial therapy similar to that for an adult: decreasing acidic foods, carbonated beverages, and caffeine; weight loss; decreasing cigarette-smoke exposure; and using with antireflux medications.

- **Regurgitation/vomiting associated with dysphagia or respiratory symptoms** (pneumonia, recurrent wheezing, sinusitis, otitis), the **best initial test is a barium swallow** to rule out **esophageal dysmotility problems or anatomic disorders** (TE fistula, strictures, achalasia, hiatal hernia, or lower obstruction). Other studies depending on these results: radionuclide scintigraphy for aspiration and laryngoscopy/bronchoscopy for airway pathology related to recurrent aspiration (including bronchoalveolar lavage to detect lipid-laden macrophages).

- If the history and physical suggest **reflux esophagitis** (irritability during feeds and when placed in the supine position, feeding refusal/aversion, and **back-arching** during feeds), then the **most cost-effective initial management is antireflux therapy with an H_2-receptor blocker first and then a proton pump inhibitor,** if needed. If any significant lack of improvement, the **next test is endoscopy with biopsy** to confirm the diagnosis and severity. Prokinetic agents (metoclopramide) have not been found to be effective in children, and generally the doses that would be necessary are associated with too many side effects.

- Infants with **reflux and obstructive apnea** (due to laryngeal spasm) should be admitted for **pH monitoring** with a **pneumogram** in order to document severity of GER and to correlate episodes to obstructive apnea. This is the **best use of pH monitoring** (also for evaluation of atypical GERD and for the effectiveness of antireflux therapy).

- If medical therapy for all GER and GERD fail and significant problems persist or worsen, then **surgical fundoplication**.

- Complications similar to those seen in an adult: strictures, Barrett esophagus, and adenocarcinoma, and increase with age if the disease continues.

Ingestions

- **Esophageal foreign bodies**—mostly in children up to age 3 years and mostly consist of **coins or small objects** (toys) and food which lodge mostly at either the **upper or lower esophageal sphincter**; present as **acute choking and coughing and then pain, dysphagia, and increased salivation**. The **first step in evaluation** should be plain anterior and lateral radiographs. If negative, **endoscopy** should be performed immediately. If the patient is asymptomatic, observe for 12–24 hours to determine whether a blunt object will pass into the stomach. If not, it needs to be endoscopically removed.

- **Caustic ingestions:** the most significant problem is ingestion of a **liquid alkali** (which is tasteless and so increased volumes may be ingested). Will cause **esophagitis, stricture, and perforation.** Presents with **vomiting, drooling, dysphagia, and pain.** Acids tend to cause fewer problems (taste bitter, so smaller volumes are generally swallowed); May cause **severe gastritis and, if aspirated, respiratory distress. Endoscopy** should be performed as soon as possible if a caustic ingestion is suspected. Therapy is primarily supportive; initial therapy—**dilute the substance with water or milk but to not induce vomiting.** Further endoscopies are needed to determine the complications and to then treat accordingly (e.g., dilatation for strictures).

Hypertrophic Pyloric Stenosis

- Most common cause of gastric outlet obstruction in children (others are rare).
- Not present at birth; presents mostly in infants age **3–6 weeks** (but may present over the first 4–5 months) **first-born, white male of northern European ancestry.**
- **Progressive, projectile vomiting with feeds; after vomiting, the infant wants to feed again.** On exam, an **"olive" is palpated as a firm, moveable mass in the epigastric area** (easier to palpate after the infant has vomited).
- **Best diagnostic test**—ultrasound which shows a **target lesion** (the small lumen appears as white surrounded by a thick black circle, representing the hypertrophied pylorus); if non-diagnostic → upper GI contrast study → shows the very narrow pylorus (string sign).
- Electrolytes: **hypokalemic, hypochloremic, metabolic alkalosis** associated with mild to moderate dehydration
- Management: **IV hydration with 0.45–0.9% NaCl with KCl** to rehydrate and correct the electrolyte imbalance (usually within 24 hours) and then **surgical pylorotomy**; feeding can be re-started within 12–24 hours of surgery and advanced quickly to full volume and full strength; discharged within 48 hours of surgery.

ACUTE DIARRHEA

Viral

- Most common cause of acute diarrhea in all ages
- Most common pathogens: **noroviruses**, rotavirus, adenoviruses, astroviruses, hepatitis A
- Spread by **fecal-oral route or directly from contaminated foods or water** (which may be contaminated directly by food-handlers)
- Produces a **noninflammatory diarrhea** (some with enterotoxin; otherwise interruption of normal intestinal villi with decreased surface for absorption)
- Symptoms: nausea, vomiting, abdominal cramps, watery diarrhea, fever, and other systemic findings

Bacterial dysentery

- Presents as **inflammatory diarrhea** (mucosal invasion and cytokine production) → increased motility, decreased colonic reabsorption.
- Most: ***Salmonella, Campylobacter,*** *Shigella, Cryptosporidium, Escherichia coli 0157:H7, Yersinia, Listeria.* Also: *Staphylococcus aureus, Bacillus cereus,* and *Clostridium botulinum* (all with **preformed enterotoxins**); *Vibrio cholerae* and *C. perfringens* (both produce **toxins**), enterotoxigenic *E. coli* (this and other *E. coli* are the major causes of **traveler's diarrhea**). Infection from **contaminated foods** (not cooked long enough, not refrigerated properly, unpasteurized dairy products, improper canning, shellfish), or **water**.
- Symptoms: acute-onset nausea, vomiting, **fever, abdominal pain, bloody diarrhea with mucus and fecal leukocytes**; often with severe systemic findings; variable presentation.

Parasitic

- Generally longer incubation periods and long or recurrent illness
- Most common in United States: ***Giardia lamblia,*** *Cryptosporidium, Cyclospora, Entamoeba histolytica* (these first four are the most commonly seen parasitic etiologies of traveler's diarrhea), *Toxoplasma gondii, Trichinella.*
- **Raw or undercooked contaminated meat, drinking water**, food contaminated by a food-handler, contaminated fresh produce, raw or undercooked shellfish, and other sources.
- Symptoms: nausea, cramps, **watery diarrhea** (may contain blood, e.g., *E. histolytica),* vomiting, weight loss, and various systemic findings depending on the organism

Antibiotic-Associated

- **Any antibiotic**, but most common with ampicillin, cephalosporins, and clindamycin
- Produces altered bowel flora → relative increase in ***Clostridia difficile*** (spore-forming, Gram-positive, anaerobic bacillus); binding of toxin to receptors causes inflammation and formation of **pseudomembranes.**
- Test for *C. difficile* toxin in stool.
- Symptoms: mild to large amount of watery diarrhea with blood to **pseudomembranous colitis** (fever, pain, nausea, vomiting, and **bloody diarrhea**)
- If symptoms persist after stopping the antibiotic, then preferred therapy is oral **metronidazole.**

Non-Infectious Causes

Many possible from heavy metals (in foods or contamination from containers), mushroom toxins, fish and shellfish toxins, contaminating pesticides, and others; some produce severe systemic findings, including death.

Risk factors and complications

- Morbidity and mortality increase with **poor hygiene**, especially in **malnourished children** with nutrient deficiencies (**vitamin A and zinc**)
- Worse with younger children, with immunocompromise and decreased breastfeeding.
- Most important complications are—**dehydration and electrolyte abnormalities**; with prolonged diarrhea—**weight loss and malnutrition with nutrient deficiencies and secondary infections**.
- Number of the organisms associated with systemic manifestations that may not be related to the acute presentation of the diarrheal illness (e.g., arthritis, glomerulonephritis, hemolytic uremic syndrome, focal infections).

Evaluation

The most important **first step in management is to assess the degree of dehydration and to correct shock with IV fluids**; initiate oral rehydration with ongoing replacement of losses (see Chapter 3). Based on the history of exposure, travel, and intake of food and water, and the description of symptoms, the most likely etiology may be determined, i.e., the presence of a bacterial pathogen that may need to be treated.

For the **acute-onset watery diarrhea**, stool evaluation does not need to be performed at initial presentation. Initial lab studies—**UA** (specific gravity plus any evidence of urinary tract infection) with possible culture (depending on the results of the UA) and a **basic chemistry panel** (if evidence of moderate to severe dehydration) to assess acidosis and electrolyte imbalance. If findings suggestive of **dysentery,** examine stool for **blood, leukocytes, and mucus**; if positive, a **stool culture and sensitivity** should be performed to determine antibiotic treatment (no indiscriminate use of antibiotics).

Management

- The **first step** is to determine if the child is **severely dehydrated**, and resuscitation should be instituted with **intravenous rehydration** as described in Chapter 3. In addition, IV hydration may be used initially in those children who have persistent vomiting and cannot tolerate even small volumes of fluids.
- Otherwise, **oral rehydration** with an appropriate **oral rehydrating solution** (see Chapter 3) is preferred. Fluids are started with very small volumes (5 mL for those with vomiting) and increased slowly.
- When rehydration is complete, reintroduce solids (avoid foods high in fat and simple sugars) with the continuation of oral rehydration to **replace ongoing losses**. Breastfeeding or formula should be reintroduced.
- The addition of **zinc** during and after the diarrheal illness in children at risk (particularly those in developing countries) leads to decreased incidence of protracted diarrhea and morbidities.
- If the stool culture is positive for a particular organism, and an antibiotic is indicated (for the particular species and based on the age and presentation of the illness), then that antibiotic should be started.

- A **probiotic** may be used to decrease the duration of diarrhea (*Lactobacilli, Bifidobacteria,* and *Saccharomyces boulardii*).
- **Antimotility agents are contraindicated** and antiemetics are generally not very effective, except for a single oral dissolvable tablet of ondansetron with persistent vomiting for the introduction of oral rehydration therapy.

CHRONIC DIARRHEA

Diarrhea lasting >2 weeks

Pathologic Causes

- **Osmotic diarrhea:** solute which is not absorbed → water secreted into the intestinal tract; diarrhea stops if the substance is removed; examples: **infant or toddler taking in large amounts of fruit juices or carbonated beverages**, disaccharidase deficiencies, laxatives (magnesium hydroxide, lactulose); stool is **acidotic** (pH <5) and is **positive for reducing substances**.
- **Secretory diarrhea:** inhibition of NaCl absorption from toxic injury; examples: diarrhea produced from **C. difficile enterotoxin,** *E. coli, Yersinia enterocolitica, Shigella, Salmonella,* and *Campylobacter,* and from tumors that produce certain hormones (e.g., vasoactive intestinal peptide), neurotransmitters (serotonin), or paracrine agents (bradykinin); also congenital defects resulting in diarrhea from birth; usually **large-volume stool with large sodium losses, stool pH >6 and does not contain reducing substances**; still continues when NPO.
- **Abnormal intestinal motility:** most common is malnutrition and diabetes.
- **Less absorptive surface:** short-bowel syndrome due to surgical resection; also celiac disease

Most Common Etiologies

- **Pancreatic insufficiency: cystic fibrosis** (most common), Shwachman-Diamond syndrome
- **Intestinal disorders:** osmotic diarrheas: **laxatives, carbohydrate disorders** (primary and secondary deficiencies); undiagnosed/continuing infections, **post-gastroenteritis malabsorption, celiac disease, IBD**, IBS, food allergy, immunodeficiencies, short-bowel syndrome, tumors (see above), malrotation with recurrent incomplete bowel obstruction, enterocolitis associated with Hirschsprung disease, rare enzyme defects
- **Bile acid disorders:** most are secondary to **disorders of chronic cholestasis and disease/resection of the terminal ileum.**

Diagnosis

Most important and cost-effective first step
• Thorough Hand P, and assessment of hydration and nutritional status (weight, height, weight/height BMI) • Stool studies: stool culture, 0 and P, C. difficile toxin, blood, mucus, fecal leukocytes, pH, osmolality, reducing substances, and fecal fat (Sudan stain, qualitative) • CBC, ESR, chemistry panel, UA

More specific tests for fat or carbohydrate malabsorption
• Quantitative 72 hour fecal fat collection • Sweat chloride (if negative, consider other diagnoses for fat malabsoprtion) • If no fat and stool pH < 5 with reducing substances → breath hydrogen test* • If no fat and high stool osmolality, consider laxative abuse (test for magnesium sulfate, phosphates, and phenolphthalien)

More invasive tests
• Barium studies of the small and large bowel • Endoscopy/colonoscopy with biopsies • Hormonal studies (uncommon causes; see above)

*If the nutritional status is normal and there is no fat in the stool (and the stool is acidic and contains reducing substances), the most common diagnosis is **chronic nonspecific diarrhea of infancy due to excessive intake of fruit juices and/or carbonated beverages (simple sugars).** The treatment is to decrease the intake of these drinks. Less commonly, this could be due to a diet that is very low in fat (but stool pH > 5 and no reducing substances). The treatment is to add more fat to the diet.

Figure 13.1: Evaluation of Chronic Diarrhea

MALABSORPTION

Chronic **diarrhea with weight loss, poor growth, loss of subcutaneous fat, muscle wasting, and loose skin** (and eventually decreased brain growth with neurological signs and symptoms); may be caused by biochemical defects leading to carbohydrate malabsorption, fat malabsorption, amino-acid and protein malabsorption (protein-losing enteropathies), or mineral and vitamin malabsorption; underlying problem may be secondary to defects of the intestinal mucosa, infection, immunodeficiency, autoimmune pathophysiology, drugs, or short bowel.

Specific Malabsorption Syndromes (most common)

Intestinal Infections

Bacterial overgrowth (from alteration of gastric pH or small-bowel motility): premature infants, malnutrition, immunodeficiency disorders, diabetes mellitus, partial bowel obstruction, with intestinal duplications, and in short-bowel syndrome; results in **steatorrhea** (brush border damage); diagnosis: aspirate duodenal fluid and check culture; **treat the underlying problem and cycle antibiotics** (metronidazole, ciprofloxacin, azithromycin, trimethoprim-sulfamethoxazole) usually for months.

Giardia lamblia: seen with **poor sanitation**, in developing countries, **most common parasitic disease in the United States** (contaminated food and water and directly from infected individuals, especially in child-care centers); infects **duodenum and small intestine**; may be **asymptomatic**, or present with signs and symptoms of **acute infection** or **chronic infection with malabsorption** (chronic watery, **non-bloody diarrhea**; abdominal cramps and bloating; weight loss; and failure-to-thrive). **Best initial test** is stool for *Giardia* antigens (direct fluorescent antibody tests or enzyme immunoassay); if negative results → **duodenal aspiration/biopsy** (trophozoites). Treatment: preferred is either **tinidazole (single dose) or nitazoxanide (suspension)**.

Short-bowel syndrome—May be caused by **congenital lesions** affecting bowel length or significant **bowel resection**; amount of bowel (>50%) resected and location are important (worst with **ileal and ileocecal valve** resection with loss of sodium and water, malabsorption of vitamin B12 and bile salts); management: **total parenteral nutrition** for fluid and electrolyte losses, then gradual reintroduction of continuous enteral feeds (protein hydrolysate and medium chain triglycerides) with management of specific micronutrient and vitamin deficiencies, treatment of infections; with improvement, volumes may be consolidated and administered bolus and/or orally.

Food-induced enteropathy—Celiac disease: **immune-mediated** enteropathy from genetic (HLA associations) and environmental factors; **permanent sensitivity to gluten (gliadin fraction; after introduction of wheat, rye, barley).**

- Gliadin fraction induces sensitization of lymphocytes of the lamina propria (interacts with **transglutaminase** → small-bowel surface damage and crypt hyperplasia mostly in the **proximal small bowel and extending a variable distance** → decreased absorptive area and digestion and secondary pancreatic dysfunction). Increased in patients with **Down syndrome, Turner syndrome**, Williams syndrome, **type I diabetes mellitus (DM)**, thyroiditis, and IgA deficiency.

- Diarrhea—most consistent finding; toddler (after the introduction of gluten) presenting with **diarrhea, abdominal distension, and failure-to-thrive with or without abdominal pain**; with continued exposure to gluten, → increasing irritability with **muscle wasting, gross motor delay, and ataxia**; may present later in childhood or adolescence with a less-obvious clinical spectrum (abdominal pain, bloating, anemia, fatigue).

- The **best initial test**—blood for anti-tissue transglutaminase (IgA antibody) measured in conjunction with serum IgA (false positive if IgA deficiency); then **definitive test** is a small intestinal biopsy showing characteristic histological features, and a **positive response to gluten elimination**.

- Only treatment is **lifelong elimination of gluten** (improvement is seen in 1 week).

- Increased risk of **intestinal lymphoma, small intestine adenocarcinoma**, and other adenocarcinomas (prevent with early diagnosis and strict gluten avoidance).

Fat malabsorption—pancreatic exocrine dysfunction

- **Screening tests (best initial tests):** fecal elastase-1 (pancreas-specific endoprotease), serum trypsinogen (elevated early in life with cystic fibrosis and decreased with Shwachman syndrome); can also measure serum levels of fat-soluble vitamins (ADEK)

- **Most accurate test:** secretin/cholecystokinin stimulation test → duodenal aspirate for lipase, trypsinogen, and bicarbonate

Cystic fibrosis: See Chapter 7.

Shwachman-Diamond syndrome: autosomal recessive pancreatic **insufficiency** (characteristic fat malabsorption stools) **plus neutropenia, neutrophil chemotactic defects** (recurrent pyogenic infections; may cause death), **metaphyseal dysostosis, failure-to-thrive, short stature**; majority with thrombocytopenia and half with anemia; may develop acute myeloblastic leukemia (about 25%)

Liver and biliary disorders: any condition leading to a **decreased duodenal bile acid concentration** will lead to fat and fat-soluble vitamin malabsorption; pancreatic exocrine dysfunction may be present. Specific findings with respect to the vitamin deficiencies may occur.

Abetalipoproteinemia: rare, autosomal recessive condition; results in **lack of lipoproteins**; presents with **severe fat malabsorption from birth** with abdominal distension, failure-to-thrive, and findings of fat-soluble vitamin deficiencies; GI symptoms during most of early childhood, then **neurological findings** (ataxia, intention tremors, loss of position and vibration sense). The diagnosis may be made by *1)* seeing **acanthocytes** in the peripheral blood smear; and *2)* **low to absent levels of triglycerides, cholesterol, chylomicrons, low-density lipoproteins (LDL), and very low-density lipoproteins (VLDL) in the blood**. Treatment is supportive, i.e., decreasing long-chain fatty acids in the diet (supplement with medium-chain triglycerides), and supplementing with vitamins ADEK.

Carbohydrate malabsorption

Lactose malabsorption: carbohydrate malabsorption with ingestion of **lactose-containing foods** (osmotic diarrhea with watery diarrhea, abdominal distension, flatulence, pain); **congenital lactase deficiency** (malabsorption since birth with breast milk or lactose-containing formula) **is very rare**; most cases in children are **transient secondary lactose intolerance post-gastroenteritis** (healing occurs; may need a short-term withdrawal of dietary lactose); **primary lactose intolerance—physiological decrease in lactase with age, beginning at age 3 years,** and varies among ethnic groups. Diagnosis is made with a **hydrogen breath test** or by the child showing improvement in symptoms with withdrawal of lactose from the diet; definitive diagnosis is with measuring lactase on a small intestinal mucosal biopsy.

Sucrase-isomaltase deficiency: rare, autosomal recessive condition → **complete absence of sucrose and a decrease in maltase activity; symptoms** (diarrhea, abdominal pain, weight loss) begin if a non-lactose infant formula is used or with the addition of solid foods (**fruits, other sweet foods**). **Diagnosis**—need to first hydrolyze stool sample because sucrose is not a reducing substance (and then will find positive reducing substances in the stool); **breath hydrogen test** or **mucosal biopsy** shows specific defect; **treatment** is lifelong dietary restriction of sucrose.

Glucose-galactose malabsorption: rare, autosomal recessive disorder caused by **mutations in the Na+/glucose co-transport** gene → **malabsorption of glucose and galactose** → **osmotic diarrhea; begins at birth** with introduction of any milk feedings containing glucose; leads to **severe dehydration and acidosis; Diagnosis**—finding a small amount of **glucosuria with a low blood sugar, and acidic stool containing reducing substances;** confirmation—**breath hydration test** or **mucosal biopsy;** only safe dietary carbohydrate is **fructose.**

Protein-losing enteropathy

Protein-losing enteropathy—Lymphangiectasia: obstruction of lymphatic drainage leading to leakage of lymph containing protein and lymphocytes into the intestine → protein-losing enteropathy and lymphopenia

Primary lymphangiectasia caused by congenital defects and is associated with other lymphatic abnormalities (e.g., in **Turner or Noonan syndromes**)

Secondary lymphangiectasia caused by congestive heart failure, malignancies, abdominal tuberculosis, sarcoidosis, constrictive pericarditis, or malrotation

Presentation—**fat and fat-soluble vitamin malabsorption** (as above) **with edema** (↓ albumin and gammaglobulins) **and chylous ascites; diagnosis—increased stool alpha-1-antitrypsin;** confirmed—biopsy showing **distorted villi and dilated lacteals; treatment—decrease dietary long-chain fatty acids** (formula with protein and medium-chain triglycerides)

Mineral and vitamin malabsorption

- **Congenital chloride diarrhea:** defective chloride/bicarbonate transport in the distal ileum and colon → severe watery diarrhea from birth with resultant hypokalemic, hypochloremic metabolic acidosis and dehydration; stool Cl– is greater than the sum of the stool Na and K; treat with IV rehydration and oral solution replacement; if done early in infancy, growth and development are normal, but this does not alter the diarrhea.

- **Acrodermatitis enteropathica:** autosomal recessive; **inability to absorb enough zinc** for the metabolic pathways in which it is needed; presents with **chronic diarrhea, stomatitis, and glossitis with failure-to-thrive first seen when weaning from breast milk or formula**; different **skin eruptions**, especially around the **mouth**, on the **perineum**, and on the **hands and feet**; also eye pathology and decreased lymphocyte function → bacterial and fungal infection. Diagnosis: clinical findings and low plasma zinc concentration; with appropriate **oral zinc therapy**, patient improves.

LIVER DISEASE

Findings Suggestive of Liver Disease

Pruritus (cholestasis), spider **angiomas**, **palmar erythema**, **xanthomas** (increased cholesterol), **ascites** (portal hypertension and hepatic insufficiency), **bleeding varices** (porto-systemic collaterals; increased pressure gradient in portal drainage; main complication of cirrhosis), **digital clubbing, ascending cholangitis, encephalopathy, hepatorenal syndrome, endocrine abnormalities** from abnormal hormone synthesis or metabolism in the liver

Examples of Intrinsic Liver Disease and Systemic Disease Manifesting as Liver Problems

Bacterial sepsis (endotoxins interfere with bile secretion), **cardiac disease** (passive congestion, decreased cardiac output resulting in ischemia and necrosis: congestive heart failure, cyanotic heart disease, pericarditis, tamponade), **hepatic vein obstruction** (hepatomegaly due to increased hepatic vascular space), **obesity (non-alcoholic liver disease)**, **prolonged total parenteral nutrition** (especially in sick premature infants), **cystic fibrosis** (impaired secretory function), **infiltration** (tumors, cysts, leukemia, other masses), extrahepatic biliary obstruction (**biliary atresia**, choledochal cyst), **intrahepatic biliary fibrosis**, storage disease (lipid, glycogen, Wilson disease), **hepatic infection** (viral, bacterial, parasitic, fungal), **inflammation** (toxic, drug, autoimmune, IBD, sarcoidosis, collagen vascular disease), **sickle-cell disease** and other hemolytic anemias (cholelithiasis, ischemic necrosis, hemosiderosis)

Indirect Hyperbilirubinemia

See Chapter 1.

Neonatal Cholestasis

- Increased **conjugated hyperbilirubinemia** in the first 2 weeks of life from either **mechanical obstruction** or **bile duct/hepatocellular injury causing decreased hepatic excretion**

- Findings of cholestasis: **jaundice, dark urine, acholic stools, hepatomegaly**, decreased liver function (bleeding, hypoproteinemia)
- Initial consideration is for **infection** (sepsis, TORCH), **anatomic obstruction** (biliary atresia, choledochal cyst), **metabolic disease** (galactosemia, tyrosinemia, hypothyroidism, alpha-1-antitrypsin deficiency, cystic fibrosis), **idiopathic** (neonatal hepatitis), and **genetic** (Alagille syndrome, trisomy 21, and others).

Intrahepatic Obstruction

- **Idiopathic neonatal hepatitis:** Unknown cause of **familial or sporadic cholestasis → severe diffuse hepatocellular disease**; few cases due to specific causes (hepatitis B, cytomegalovirus [CMV], enterovirus, herpes simplex); **liver biopsy** is necessary for diagnosis.
- **Alagille syndrome (arteriohepatic dysplasia): most common syndrome with intrahepatic bile-duct paucity; normal-size portal vein and hepatic arterioles;** may present with other variable findings (facial dysmorphic features, heart defects, kidney disease, and vertebral defects); **cholestasis** (jaundice, pruritus), **increased cholesterol** (xanthomas), **neurological findings** (vitamin E deficiency); treatment is symptomatic but prognosis is good.
- **Others: Zellweger syndrome** (progressive degeneration of the liver and kidneys; fatal in first year of life), cystic fibrosis (decreased canalicular secretion due to abnormal ion transport), familial intrahepatic cholestasis (defects in bile acid transport), inborn errors of bile acid synthesis and conjugation

Extrahepatic Obstruction

Biliary atresia (progressive obliterative cholangiopathy): mostly seen as **obliteration of the entire extrahepatic biliary tree to the porta hepatis**; may present at birth (severe, fetal onset) or later; clinically **looks like idiopathic neonatal hepatitis;** the **fetal-onset form of biliary atresia** is frequently accompanied by **other abnormalities**, such as polysplenia, malrotation, abdominal situs inversus, and vascular anomalies; persistently acholic stools and an abnormal size and consistency of the liver (not so with neonatal hepatitis).

Evaluation

- **Best initial test:** ultrasound: may see a **triangular cord** (fibrotic mass) and any associated anomalies, including a **small or absent gallbladder**
- **Most accurate test:** percutaneous liver biopsy: see bile ductular proliferation, bile plugs, portal or perilobular edema and fibrosis
- **Next step:** exploratory laparotomy and direct cholangiography for presence and site of obstruction, and size and patency of residual ducts and whether there is a correctable lesion; if **no drainage** possible, perform **hepatoportoenterostomy (Kasai procedure)**, i.e., jejunum is anastomosed to the surface of the transected porta hepatis in order to allow drainage (tiny bile ductules communicating with extrahepatic ductules); if there is no drainage, there will be **progressive obliteration and cirrhosis;** there is generally **ongoing inflammation of the intrahepatic biliary tree** so the Kasai procedure only slows the cirrhosis and allows for growth until a **liver transplant** may be performed.

Management of cholestasis

- Supplement with medium-chain triglycerides and decrease long-chain fatty acids. Replace fat-soluble vitamins, micronutrients (Ca, P, Zn), and water-soluble vitamins. Use **ursodeoxycholic acid** for retention of cholesterol and bile acids (xanthomas, pruritus). **Decrease dietary Na**, use **spironolactone** and monitor and treat any infection with respect to ascites. **Endoscopy** and **sclerotherapy** for bleeding varices.

- **Cholestasis in older children:** Most due to **acute viral hepatitis and drugs**; in adolescents: acute and chronic hepatitis, alpha-1-antitrypsin deficiency, Wilson disease, IBD, autoimmune hepatitis, and the familial direct hyperbilirubinemias (Rotor and Dubin-Johnson syndromes); obstruction from cholelithiasis, abdominal tumors, increased lymph nodes, and hepatic inflammation from drug use.

Metabolic Liver Disease

See Chapter 2 for discussion of inborn errors of metabolism resulting in liver disease.

Alpha-1-antitrypsin deficiency (α1AT)—**Major serum protease inhibitor (protects lung alveolar tissues from destruction by neutrophil elastase)**; the most common allele is M and the normal phenotype is PiMM; the Z allele represents clinical deficiency and most of the severe liver disease (with very low enzyme levels) is PiZZ.

- Liver damage is **highly variable** (exact mechanism not known); in neonates, looks the same as idiopathic neonatal hepatitis and biliary atresia; older children with **hepatomegaly, chronic liver disease, or portal hypertension and cirrhosis**. Lung disease rare in children and usually occurs by the third to fourth decade (emphysema). Liver disease may resolve, persist, or develop into cirrhosis.
- Diagnosis: **low serum alpha-1-antitrypsin** (by serum immune-electrophoresis) and then **polymerase chain reaction (PCR) for the genotype**
- Management: **liver transplant** if severely progressive; otherwise, weekly **enzyme replacement** from pooled human plasma, with supportive care

Wilson disease

- Hepatolenticular degeneration: **degenerative changes in the liver, kidney, brain, and cornea**
- Autosomal recessive; gene codes for **copper transporting ATPase** critical for **biliary copper excretion** → **progressive diffuse accumulation of copper in hepatocytes** (eventually leads to fibrosis) → spills into other tissues.
- Most are compound heterozygotes; **if there is no gene function, disease begins at about age 2–3 years; milder mutations are associated with a later onset (even into adulthood).**
- **Younger children present mostly with liver signs and symptoms**—hepatosplenomegaly, hepatitis (usually subacute or chronic), fulminant hepatic failure, or other hepatic dysfunction (**think of the diagnosis in any child with unexplained liver disease**).

- **Older patients: neurological symptoms predominate:** intention tremors, decreased coordination, abnormalities of tone, speech problems, behavioral and psychological changes, decreased school performance; **Kaiser-Fleischer rings (golden rings in Descemet's membrane of the cornea) are always present with neurological changes,** (may be seen with a slit-lamp examination).
- Coombs-negative hemolytic anemia, renal Fanconi syndrome, and progressive renal failure
- **Best initial test:** serum ceruloplasmin (decreased because of failure of Cu to be incorporated into it, so there is a decreased production) → increased serum Cu and increased urinary Cu excretion; also **screen family members**
- **Most accurate test:** liver biopsy for liver Cu content; may also obtain a genetic diagnosis
- Treatment: decrease Cu intake (liver, shellfish, chocolate, nuts); **D-penicillamine to chelate Cu;** also give vitamin B6 supplement (penicillamine is an antimetabolite of B6); **liver transplant with progressive disease**

Viral Hepatitis

Table 13.3: Viral Hepatitis in Children

	Hepatitis A (HAV)	Hepatitis B (HBV)	Hepatitis C (HCV)	Hepatitis D (HDV)	Hepatitis E (HEV)
Epidemiology	Most prevalent in the world	Worldwide disease; decreased in United States since vaccine chronic carrier state/chronic liver disease	Mostly due to previously named transfusion-related non-A, non-B hepatitis; most common cause of chronic liver disease in adults	Defective virus; needs co-infection or superinfection with HBV	Epidemic form of previously named non-A, non-B hepatitis
Disease acquisition and spread	Fecal-oral, person-to-person contact; contaminated water, foods; not sexually or perinatally transmitted	Most important is perinatal acquisition (decreased >95% with appropriate treatment of the infant); no greater risk with breastfeeding; also transmitted in blood, exudates, saliva, semen, vaginal fluid; no fecal-oral spread	Illegal drug use and blood from HCV-infected persons; also from sexual transmission with multiple sex partners; in children, most from perinatal acquisition (especially with HIV-positive mother)	Transmission is intra-familial or intimate contact in high-prevalence areas; in low-prevalence areas (United States), parenteral route more common; uncommon in children in United States	Fecal-oral (water); present in United States only from persons who have visited or emigrated from endemic areas
Contagion	Incubation 15–19 days; fecal excretion 2 weeks prior to symptoms and until 1 week after symptoms (end of viral shedding)	Mean incubation: 120 days	Incubation period: 2 weeks to just less than 6 months	Incubation period: 3–6 weeks	Incubation: 3–9 weeks
Most common symptoms	Fever, anorexia, nausea, vomiting, diarrhea, malaise, jaundice for 7–14 days	Similar to HAV, but more severe with involvement of skin and joints; hepatosplenomegaly, lymphadenopathy, encephalopathy (with acute liver failure)	Mild (acute illness least severe of all), insidious onset; most likely to cause chronic infection (remains clinically silent until there is a complication)	Acute hepatitis more common in co-infection with HBV; chronic infection more common in superinfection with HBV and highest risk of acute liver failure	Similar to HAV but more severe; no chronic illness

(continued)

	Hepatitis A (HAV)	Hepatitis B (HBV)	Hepatitis C (HCV)	Hepatitis D (HDV)	Hepatitis E (HEV)
Other less-common symptoms	Lymphadeno-pathy, splenomegaly, bone marrow suppression	Extrahepatic illness: aplastic anemia, polyarteritis, glomerulonephritis	Small vessel vasculitis	—	—
Serology	Total anti-HAV = IgM + IgG: anti-HAV-IgM at onset of symptoms until 4–6 months; anti-HAV-IgG within 2 months of onset (denotes recovery)	-First marker to increase is HBeAg (marker of acute infection); represents active disease; anti-HBe is a marker of improvement. -HBsAg (surface antigen) increases at symptom onset and decreases prior to symptom resolution. -Anti-HBc-IgM (core antibody) is the best marker for acute infection; it is positive almost as early as HBsAg and continues to be positive after HBsAg has disappeared; is then replaced by anti-HBc-IgG which persists for years. -Anti-HBs marks recovery and protection (only antibody present with immunization).	-Anti-HCV is present simultaneously with the virus and does not produce immunity (most commonly used serological test, but false positives and negatives). -Most common virologic test is PCR for the viral RNA; qualitative test detects disease within days of infection and quantitative test aids in management.	No circulating antigen is identified (virus has not been isolated); IgM-HDV is present 2–4 weeks after co-infection and 10 weeks after superinfection.	Virus cloned, not isolated; IgM antibody to viral antigen becomes positive after 1 week of illness; IgG is positive in resolved infection.

(continued on next page)

Table 13.3: Viral Hepatitis in Children *(cont.)*

	Hepatitis A (HAV)	**Hepatitis B (HBV)**	**Hepatitis C (HCV)**	**Hepatitis D (HDV)**	**Hepatitis E (HEV)**
Laboratory abnormalities and symptom onset	Increase in liver enzymes (nonspecific) before symptoms, and peaks at onset of symptoms (with increased bilirubin)	Increased liver enzymes; then onset of lethargy, anorexia, and malaise about 6 weeks after exposure; then jaundice in another week	Liver enzymes tend to increase and decrease, and do not correlate with chronic liver disease (confirmed with liver biopsy); ALT peaks after onset of jaundice and other symptoms.	More severe symptoms than the other hepatitis viruses	Similar to HAV
Complications	Fulminant liver disease is uncommon (unless underlying liver disease or immunocompromise); no chronic disease; prolonged cholestasis (resolves)	Acute liver failure (increased risk if co-infected with HDV); chronic carrier state, chronic liver failure, and end-stage liver disease; hepatocellular carcinoma	Chronic liver disease, cirrhosis, and liver failure over 20–30 years	Acute and chronic liver failure	Increased in pregnant women; acute liver failure with increased mortality
Management	Supportive	Acute: mostly symptomatic; chronic: interferon-α–2b (goal is to seroconvert HBeAg → stops active viral replication)	Only Interferon α–2b is FDA-approved for children >3 years; response rate dependent on genotype and quantitative PCR-RNA	Symptomatic; control and treat concurrent HBV infection	Symptomatic

Abbreviations: alanine aminotransferase, ALT; polymerase chain reaction, PCR

GENITOURINARY DISORDERS

PART ONE: DISORDERS OF THE URINARY TRACT

Congenital Anomalies

Renal agenesis

Bilateral agenesis presents as the **Potter sequence** with possible death due to pulmonary hypoplasia (see Chapter 2). **Unilateral agenesis** is often found with other anomalies (as part of the **VACTERL** association, **single umbilical artery**). The **best initial exam** for renal anatomy is an **ultrasound** and if agenesis is found, a **renal scan** (for an ectopic kidney). The American Academy of Pediatrics states that an individual assessment should be made in children with one kidney with respect to participation in sports and play that involves contact and collision.

Multicystic dysplastic kidney

Bilateral dysplastic kidneys present with oligohydramnios and the **Potter sequence**. **Unilateral multicystic dysplastic kidney is the most common cause of an abdominal mass in the newborn** (familial). There are non-communicating cysts of variable sizes and the kidneys are also variable in size. Most are discovered during **prenatal ultrasound**. The **best initial test** after birth to confirm the diagnosis is ultrasound. A **radionuclide renal scan** will demonstrate a non-functioning kidney. A **voiding cystourethrogram (VCUG)** assesses possible **obstruction and reflux** in the other kidney. Complications: decreased renal function in the contralateral kidney, increased risk for future hypertension and **Wilms tumor**.

Polycystic kidney disease

Autosomal recessive polycystic kidney disease (ARPCKD, infantile type; abnormal gene): both kidneys are **enlarged** with many **microcysts, (cortex and medulla)**. The most severe cases present in the neonatal period as **bilateral flank masses, the Potter sequence (various degrees of pulmonary hypoplasia), and severe hypertension**. Over time, there is progressive fibrosis and atrophy; there is also involvement of the **liver** leading to **fibrosis and liver failure**. The **best initial test** is ultrasonography showing enlarged, hyperechoic kidneys with discrete cysts (**diagnostic with bilateral flank masses, decreased renal**

function, and no kidney disease in the parents). Treatment is supportive, with dialysis. More than half will have end-stage renal disease in the first decade.

Autosomal dominant polycystic kidney disease (ADPCKD, adult type; three chromosomal anomalies): **the most common inherited kidney disease.** Both **kidneys are enlarged with multiple bilateral macrocysts** in the cortex and medulla. Most common presentation is between age 30–50 years, but may be seen in neonates or in older children and may be asymptomatic. The **best initial test** is an ultrasound, which shows bilateral macrocysts. **Parenteral ultrasound** should also be performed (if no diagnosis yet made). Extrarenal disease (**ruptured berry aneurysm, hepatic cysts**, renal stones, pancreatic cysts) are common in adults. The most important part of management is **blood pressure (BP) control**; otherwise treatment is supportive (dialysis and transplantation).

Hydronephrosis

Represents **obstruction** of the urinary tract; in the neonatal period, seen as a **palpable abdominal mass** and may have been detected on **routine prenatal ultrasound**. The most common etiology is unilateral partial obstruction of the ureter (intrinsic or extrinsic obstruction) at the **ureteral-pelvic junction (UPJ obstruction)**. The **best initial test** is an ultrasound, which will show an **enlarged kidney without enlargement of the ureter (hydroureter)**. Use VCUG to look for vesicoureteral reflux (VUR). Renal function may be decreased (renal radionuclide scan). Older children may present with flank pain, UTI, and/or hematuria. Surgery is needed in most after the diagnosis is made.

Ureterocele

Cystic dilatation of the end of the ureter (above the bladder; may be bilateral); represents **obstruction** due to a very small opening of the ureter into the bladder; seen more commonly in girls; usually detected with prenatal ultrasound or a UTI in a young child. Almost all occur with **ureteral duplication**. An **ultrasound is the best initial test**; then perform a VCUG to look for VUR, then a renal radionuclide scan to assess function.

Hydroureter/megaureter

May be unilateral or bilateral, and primary or secondary to obstruction, and may be associated with **VUR**; may be seen on prenatal ultrasound or may present later in childhood as abdominal pain, hematuria, or UTI. The **best initial test** is an ultrasound, then VCUG to assess for reflux, then a radionuclide scan to assess renal function (and assessment of upper tract drainage). Surgery is reserved for those with decreased renal function, decreased upper tract obstruction, or UTIs.

Posterior urethral valves (PUVs)

Most common cause of obstructive uropathy in males; secondary to abnormal leaflets in the prostatic urethra → obstruction; presentation—**neonate with a palpable bladder (enlarged, hypertrophied) with or without hydronephrosis and a weak to absent urinary stream**; may present as the **Potter sequence**, or less severe and present later in childhood as urinary incontinence and UTIs. The diagnosis is often with prenatal ultrasonography.

The **best initial test** (and therapy) is to **pass a feeding tube into the urethra** (after starting broad-spectrum antibiotics) to allow for bladder drainage and to perform a **VCUG**. The corrective surgery is **endoscopic ablation of the valves. Electrolyte abnormalities due to postobstructive diuresis** need to be corrected. After correction, there is generally still some degree of hydronephrosis and incontinence; some will develop end-stage renal disease (ESRD).

Vesicoureteral reflux (VUR)

Most causes are **congenital** (autosomal dominant trait; primary VUR; may be associated with other abnormalities) due to **abnormal entry of the ureter into the bladder** (submucosal tunnel), → to retrograde flow to the ureter(s) and kidney(s). This predisposes to recurrent infection and ultimately reflux nephropathy (decreased renal function, renin-mediated hypertension, renal scarring, and poor kidney growth with the possibility of ESRD); may also be secondary to bladder outlet obstruction, neurogenic bladder, inflammatory conditions, or surgery. VUR is graded from grade I (reflux into the ureter with no dilatation) through grade V (significant intrarenal reflux with grossly dilated ureter and calyces). Most present with a **UTI early in childhood** (see later discussion). **The best initial test** is a VCUG to document and grade the reflux, followed by a **renal radionuclide scan for detection of renal size and scars**. All grades of reflux (except grade 5) **generally resolve over the first years of life**. Treat all UTIs aggressively. Follow renal function growth, scarring, and VCUG for gradual improvement. **Surgery is indicated for any breakthrough UTI, new scars, failure to resolve, or persistent grade IV–V reflux.**

Alport syndrome

X-linked hereditary nephritis (also cases of autosomal dominant and recessive); defect of type IV collagen; **males have more severe disease**; most common presentation is **microscopic hematuria** (a first-degree relative may be affected); any time in childhood, adolescence, or young adulthood; the most common extrarenal problems are **sensorineural hearing loss** (**not congenital**; worse in males) and ocular abnormalities (many pathologies; displacement of the lens into the anterior chamber is diagnostic). **The renal disease is progressive** and most (hemizygous boys) have ESRD by age 30 years. Treatment is supportive for renal function (dialysis, transplantation).

Urinary Tract Infections (UTIs)

Cystitis: infection of the bladder; **pyelonephritis:** infection of the kidneys. **Asymptomatic bacteriuria:** positive urine culture without signs or symptoms; benign condition seen mostly in preschool girls.

Etiology

Ascending infection from fecal organisms that colonize the perineum; most common in girls is *Escherichia coli*, then *Klebsiella* spp., *Proteus* spp., and *Enterococcus* spp. In boys older than 1 year, most are *E. coli*, then *Proteus* spp., *Staph. saprophyticus*, and *Enterococcus* spp.

Epidemiology

More common in boys in the **first 1–2 years** of life (greater in uncircumcised), then **much greater incidence in girls** (peaks in infancy and during toilet training). Also increased risk with urinary tract anomalies and reflux, voiding dysfunction, wiping back to front in girls, and chronic constipation.

Key diagnostic words

Cystitis: discomfort/pain/burning on voiding, urinary frequency, urgency, suprapubic pain, malodorous urine, no fever. **Pyelonephritis: fever with abdominal or flank pain** with or without nausea, vomiting, and diarrhea; may result in **scarring and renal dysfunction** (greatest in infants and young children; greater risk with increased number of occurrences); associated with **VUR**.

Diagnosis

- May present in any child age 2 months to 2 years with **unexplained fever with no localizing findings** and in any child with the above signs and symptoms.
- Toilet-trained children can usually provide a good **midstream urine** sample.
- In younger children, a bag specimen is good if there is no growth on urine culture or if there is one organism with >50,000 colony-forming units and signs and symptoms are present. Otherwise, a **catheterized or suprapubic urine sample** (the best method) is needed.
- Obtain urine analysis and culture prior to starting antibiotics, and consider a **blood culture** if pyelonephritis is suspected (sepsis is common).
- **Urine analysis findings suggestive of UTI:** pyuria (not specific for UTI), microscopic hematuria, positive for nitrites and leukocyte esterase

Clinical evaluation

- Assess toxicity, dehydration, and ability to retain oral fluids.
- For children with recurrent **UTI and UTIs with complications** (pyelonephritis), **obtain ultrasound** for underlying structural abnormality and to rule out hydronephrosis (does not detect VUR); then **obtain VCUG** for evaluating a primary or secondary VUR.

Treatment

Pyelonephritis: if neonate or young infant is toxic, dehydrated, or unable to take oral fluids/medications: admit for **parenteral antibiotics** (ampicillin or ticarcillin plus an aminoglycoside, or a third-generation cephalosporin) until improved and able to take oral antibiotics (10–14 days of antibiotics); otherwise, **oral cefixime** (use also after parenteral antibiotics to complete the course). **Cystitis:** trimethoprim-sulfamethoxazole, nitrofurantoin (not for a febrile UTI), or amoxicillin for 10–14 days. Obtain **another urine culture to document resolution after treatment.**

Hematuria

At least 5 red blood cells (RBCs)/microliter of urine (if dipstick is positive for blood, need at least 10–15 mL of fresh centrifuged urine for microscopic analysis)

Red urine with negative dipstick for RBCs

Hemoglobin (from hemolysis), **myoglobin** (rhabdomyolysis), red/dark urine that is hemoglobin-negative: **drugs** (ibuprofen, salicylates, nitrofurantoin, metronidazole, rifampin), certain **foods and food dyes, urinary metabolites**

Causes of hematuria

Table 14.1: Evaluation of Gross and Microscopic Hematuria

Location	Urine Characteristics	Most Common Causes
Glomerular	-Brown to dark-red urine -RBC casts -Some proteinuria	-Postinfectious glomerulonephritis -Other (idiopathic) glomerulonephritis pathologies -Alport syndrome -IgA nephropathy -Hemolytic uremic syndrome -Henoch-Schönlein purpura -Lupus nephritis -Sickle-cell disease
Tubular	-Renal tubular epithelial or WBC casts	-Pyelonephritis -Interstitial nephritis -Acute tubular necrosis -Anatomic/vascular abnormalities -Hemoglobinopathies -Nephrocalcinosis -Crystals
Renal pelvis, calyces, ureter, bladder, urethra	-Gross hematuria or hematuria at the end of urinary stream -May contain clots -RBC morphology is normal -Small amount of proteinuria	-Infection (cystitis, urethritis) -Urolithiasis -Trauma -Coagulopathy -Heavy exercise -Tumor -Hypercalciuria

Abbreviations: red blood cell, RBC; white blood cell, WBC

Evaluation

Isolated microscopic hematuria (otherwise asymptomatic) → two more urine analyses over next 1–2 weeks; if still positive = persistent asymptomatic isolated microscopic hematuria:

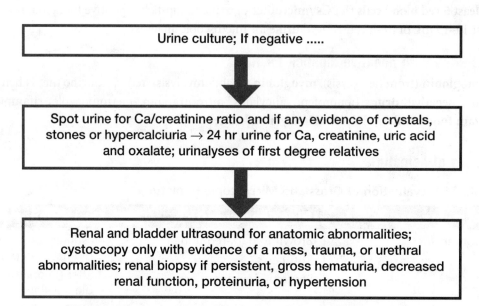

Urine culture; If negative .....

Spot urine for Ca/creatinine ratio and if any evidence of crystals, stones or hypercalciuria → 24 hr urine for Ca, creatinine, uric acid and oxalate; urinalyses of first degree relatives

Renal and bladder ultrasound for anatomic abnormalities; cystoscopy only with evidence of a mass, trauma, or urethral abnormalities; renal biopsy if persistent, gross hematuria, decreased renal function, proteinuria, or hypertension

Figure 14.1: Evaluation of Isolated Microscopic Hematuria

IgA Nephropathy (Berger nephropathy)

Abnormality in the IgA immune system → **IgA within mesangial deposits of glomeruli**; most common cause of **chronic glomerular disease** in the world; familial clusters

Clinical presentation—Most present with **gross hematuria, commonly after a respiratory or gastrointestinal (GI) infection**; may have mild to moderate **hypertension**; if proteinuria is present, it is usually a small amount; C3 is normal (compare to poststreptococcal glomerulonephritis).

Outcome—In most, **does not lead to significant renal disease**; but in some, disease progresses into adulthood.

Management—Main treatment is **blood-pressure control; angiotensin-converting enzyme (ACE) inhibitors and receptor-blockers** control BP and decrease proteinuria progression. In more severe cases, corticosteroids are used and renal transplantation may be necessary (but disease may still recur).

Acute poststreptococcal glomerulonephritis (GN)

Caused by **nephritogenic strains of streptococcus causing throat and skin infections**; probably **immune-mediated** disorder with activation of the **alternative complement pathway** and **depression of C3.**

Clinical presentation—Sudden onset of **gross hematuria, edema, hypertension, and renal insufficiency 1–2 weeks after a throat infection and 3–6 weeks after a skin infection**, but may present from microscopic hematuria to acute renal failure; also constitutional signs and symptoms with or without fever; acute phase generally lasts 6–8 weeks; highest incidence between 5–12 years of age.

Diagnosis—**Best initial step** obtain a urinalysis which may show **RBCs, RBC casts, mild to moderate proteinuria, and white blood cells (WBCs)**; CBC generally shows a mild anemia (dilution and hemolysis); obtain blood for **C3 level: depressed** during the acute phase; need evidence of a recent streptococcal infection with either a **positive throat culture** or increasing antibody titers: **antistreptolysin O** (ASO, rarely increased after skin infection), **anti-DNAse B** (best for recent skin infection), **streptozyme** (slide agglutination test that detects antibodies for streptolysin O, DNAse B, hyaluronidase, streptokinase, and NADase). **Biopsy** performed if persistence for at least 2 months, absence of evidence of streptococcal infection, acute renal failure, or normal complement levels.

Other causes of acute GN—Include membranoproliferative GN (most common cause of chronic GN in older children and adults), lupus nephritis, rapidly progressing GN (rapid progression to ESRD), and Henoch-Schonlein purpura (HSP) nephritis (same renal pathology as IgA nephropathy, but with systemic findings).

Management—Treat with a **10-day course of penicillin** (or amoxicillin) for streptococcal infection (does not alter course); symptomatic treatment of renal insufficiency—decreased sodium intake, diuretics (furosemide), and blood-pressure control (ACE inhibitors, calcium channel blockers, vasodilators); **patients with oliguria and electrolyte abnormalities should be admitted** for monitoring of fluid input and output, correction of electrolyte abnormalities, and BP control (see below for management of acute renal failure). Almost all recover completely.

Hemolytic-uremic syndrome (HUS)

Most common cause of acute renal failure in young children; most cases secondary to **verocytotoxin-producing *E. coli* 0157:H7** (intestinal tract of domestic animals; most cases from **undercooked meat or unpasteurized milk**); less commonly with *Shigella*, other bacteria, viruses, drugs toxins, and systemic illnesses; initial infection → **endothelial cell injury** with glomerular changes (subendothelial and mesangial deposition of amorphous material → fibrin thrombi in the kidney → sclerosis, ischemia and vascular occlusion) with **complement activation** (decreased C3) after injury. RBCs are destroyed while passing through disrupted vessels (**microangiopathic hemolytic anemia**) and there is intrarenal and systemic **platelet damage**.

Clinical presentation—**Bloody diarrhea** first (most are <4 years of age), then 5–10 days later: nonspecific constitutional symptoms, **sudden pallor (hemolysis), petechiae, decreased urine output, edema**

Diagnosis—Clinical findings as above plus microangiopathy **(schistocytes, burr cells, helmet cells), thrombocytopenia, and uremia** [increased BUN and creatinine and oliguria to anuria] and other evidence of hemolysis (Coombs-negative): decreased haptoglobin, increased reticulocyte count. WBCs are usually elevated. Urinalysis shows **microscopic hematuria and proteinuria.**

Complications—**Acute renal failure** (edema, electrolyte abnormalities, hypertension), heart failure, **seizures, coma**, GI ischemia, myocardial dysfunction, pericarditis; long-term: hypertension and chronic renal failure; worse outcome with central nervous system (CNS) symptoms and prolonged anuria (>1 week)

Management—Supportive treatment (attention to fluid balance, electrolyte correction, hypertension), early nutritional support (total parenteral nutrition, TPN), **early dialysis; avoid platelet transfusions** (platelets will be destroyed and renal insufficiency can worsen); support BP with colloids and cardiopressor agents and transfuse for low hemoglobin (Hgb) when tissue oxygenation may be affected. **No antibiotic treatment for *E. coli* 0157:H7** (leads to higher incidence of HUS). No role for antithrombotic therapy. Plasmapheresis for some cases only.

Proteinuria

Positive if **dipstick is at least 1+ (30 mg/dL) with a urine specific gravity of ≤1.015 or at least 2+ (100 mg/dL if urine specific gravity is >1.015)**; most commonly used quantitative method now (replaced the 24-hour urine) is a spot urine protein/creatinine ratio on the first morning void; normal ratio is <0.5 in a child under 2 years of age and <0.2 in a child ≥2 years. The nephrotic range is >2. This corresponds to a 24-hour excretion >40 mg/m^2/hr as the nephrotic range.

Etiology

Transient

- Single dipstick protein ≤ 2+ and subsequently normal
- Seen with: **fever, exercise**, dehydration, cold exposure, stress

---

Orthostatic

- Normal urine protein in **supine** and **significant increase upright; most common cause of asymptomatic persistent proteinuria**
- **Diagnosis:** obtain 1st AM void for UA and spot protein/creatinine for 3 consecutive days; if normal for protein and protein/creatinine < 0.2, no further tests are needed.

Fixed

- Indicates **renal disease;** 1st AM void for 3 consecutive days with > 1+ protein on urine dipstick or **protein/creatinine > 0.2.**
- **Glomerular:** 1st AM void urine **protein/creatinine > 1** or with hematuria, hypertension, edema, or renal dysfunction; glomerular pathologies
- **Tubular:** injury to proximal tubule; **urine protein/creatinine < 1;** usually seen with other proximal tubular defects (see below)

Figure 14.2: Evaluation of Proteinuria

Nephrotic syndrome

(*1*) >40 mg/m^2/hr proteinuria or spot urine protein/creatinine > 2; (*2*) hypoalbuminemia; (*3*) edema; and (*4*) hyperlipidemia (with hypoalbuminemia, there is general hepatic protein synthesis [lipoprotein] and also decreased lipoprotein lipase)

Etiology—Most cases are **steroid-sensitive minimal change disease** (effacement of the epithelial cell foot processes seen on **electron microscopy**) followed by mesangial proliferation and focal segmental glomerulosclerosis, and then by other pathologies secondary to systemic diseases. There is increased permeability of the glomerular capillary wall → decreased serum protein → decreased plasma oncotic pressure → transudation of fluid to the interstitial spaces.

Clinical presentation—Most occur between 2–6 years of age and often **after a minor infection or allergic reaction**; begins with constitutional symptoms and **mild dependent edema** (periorbital or pretibial) and may progress to generalized edema (**anasarca, effusions); hematuria and hypertension are uncommon.**

Diagnosis—**First diagnostic test** is a urinalysis which shows **3–4+ protein** (and perhaps a small amount of microscopic hematuria); next step is to obtain a **spot urine protein/creatinine which will be >2** (>40 mg/m^2/hr), a **serum albumin** (usually <2.5 g/dL), and a lipid panel (**increased serum cholesterol and triglycerides**). The serum creatinine, C3, and C4 are normal. Significant hematuria and hypertension should suggest another pathology.

Management

- Mild to moderate edema can be managed on an outpatient basis, while those with a large amount of edema or effusions (ascites, pleural, pericardial) should be admitted to the hospital.
- **Edema fluid may be mobilized with use of intravenous 25% albumin followed by furosemide** (with careful monitoring of fluid and electrolytes).
- Start all patients on **prednisone in daily divided doses for 4–6 weeks** (the vast majority will respond); taper dose **over 2–3 months.**
- Many have **at least one relapse → re-treat with the full prednisone dose until there is no proteinuria for 3 consecutive days and then taper over 1–2 months.**
- **Steroid-resistant nephrotic syndrome** = continued proteinuria after 8 weeks of treatment;
- **Steroid-dependent nephrotic syndrome** = relapse within 28 days of discontinuing the prednisone.
- Both should have a **renal biopsy** (also for those <1 year of age with hypertension, hematuria, renal insufficiency, or decreased complement levels) and may need treatment with other immunosuppressive drugs or certain corticosteroid protocols (high-dose pulse methylprednisolone).

Complications—**Infection** due to loss of immunoglobulin and properdin factor B plus immunosuppressive therapy with ascites → **spontaneous bacterial peritonitis** (most common with *Strep. pneumoniae* and then Gram-negatives); **thromboembolism** (avoid overly aggressive diuresis and indwelling catheters); hyperlipidemia (if very high, may need an HMG-CoA-reductase inhibitor).

Outcome—With minimal change disease, relapses become less common with age and the outcome is generally good with unlikely development of chronic renal insufficiency; but **with steroid-resistant nephrotic syndrome** (most cases are focal segmental glomerulosclerosis), **renal insufficiency and ESRD** are more likely.

Tubulointerstitial Disorders

Nephrogenic diabetes insipidus (DI)

Renal tubular acidosis

- **Inability to concentrate the urine** in the presence of antidiuretic hormone (ADH). Most are **X-linked recessive** (primary disease) or secondary due to **resistance of ADH** (kidney cystic disease, interstitial nephritis, nephrocalcinosis, hypokalemia, hypercalcemia, lithium, amphotericin B).
- Clinical presentation: **newborn with polyuria, volume depletion, hypernatremia** and increased temperature, failure-to-thrive, developmental delay, and mental retardation (if not diagnosed and treated early); secondary causes generally present later in life.
- Diagnosis: male infant with polyuria, hypernatremia (**serum osmolality >290 mOsm/kg), and dilute urine (<290 mOsm/kg)**; if these are the findings a water deprivation test is not needed, but need to determine if it is **central DI**, so **administer IV vasopressin and check hourly serum and urine osmolality for 4 hours** (no change if nephrogenic, vs. decrease in serum osmolality and increase in urine osmolality if central DI); a **water deprivation test** is needed if the initial serum osmolality is <290 mOsm/kg (partial defect) → measure urine and serum osmolality until serum osmolality is >290 mOsm/kg and then give IV vasopressin and measure for effect.
- Treatment: (*1*) always have **access to water**; (*2*) **low-Na, low-osmolality diet** (breast milk or PM 60/40); (*3*) **thiazides** → promote Na loss and stimulate proximal tubular reabsorption of water; (*4*) if response is inadequate, add **indomethacin** (decreased water excretion in some).

Table 14.2: Renal Tubular Acidosis

	Proximal (Type II)	Distal (Type I)	Hyperkalemia (Type IV)	Type III
Defect/diagnosis	Impaired proximal tubular bicarbonate reabsorption with normal anion gap acidosis and urine pH <5.5 (intact distal acidification) Dx: non-anion gap metabolic acidosis plus urine pH <5.5 and a negative urine anion gap [urine Na⁺ + urine K⁺] − urine Cl−	Impaired distal hydrogen ion secretion; cannot decrease urine pH to <5.5 despite severe metabolic acidosis (normal anion gap); loss of NaHCO₃ → hyperchloremia and hypokalemia; also hypercalciuria Dx: non-anion gap metabolic acidosis plus urine pH >6 plus a positive urine anion gap (represents deficiency of ammonia genesis)	Occurs as a result of hypoaldosteronism or pseudohypoaldosteronism (decreased tissue responsiveness) → decreased excretion of hydrogen ion, potassium, and NH₄⁺, and increased sodium excretion Dx: non-anion gap metabolic acidosis plus hyperkalemia	Combined proximal and distal RTA Dx: urine pH <5.5, other proximal tubular dysfunction, hyperchloremia, hypokalemia, hypercalciuria
Occurrence	Most cases as part of Fanconi syndrome (glycosuria, phosphaturia, amino aciduria and proximal RTA)	Inherited or acquired disease of distal tubule	Adrenal gland disorders	Mostly in infants
Clinical presentation	Growth failure in first year plus nonspecific symptoms plus rickets and findings of Fanconi syndrome	Growth failure, severe acidosis, vomiting, and polyuria; hypercalciuria; and in older children, nephrolithiasis and metabolic bone disease	Growth failure, polyuria, dehydration (sodium loss), hyperkalemia, and non-anion gap acidosis; increased urinary sodium and decreased urinary potassium	Presents as either type I or II with severe non-anion gap metabolic acidosis

(continued)

	Proximal (Type II)	Distal (Type I)	Hyperkalemia (Type IV)	Type III
Primary causes	Isolated (uncommon): autosomal dominant and recessive forms	Isolated: genetic (autosomal recessive form with sensorineural hearing loss) or idiopathic	Aldosterone deficiency (Addison disease, congenital adrenal hyperplasia, familial, and others) or aldosterone resistance (types 1 and 2 pseudohypoaldosteronism, drugs, lupus nephritis)	Inherited deficiency
Secondary causes	Secondary to: cystinosis (defect in metabolism of cystine), Lowe syndrome (oculocerebrorenal syndrome), cystic kidney disease, renal transplantation, multiple inborn errors, hyperparathyroidism, vitamin D deficiency, and others	Secondary to: disorders of collagen synthesis, a number of inborn errors, some connective tissue disease, cystic kidney disease, some hepatobiliary disease, hyperparathyroidism, thyroiditis, Wilson disease, some drugs and others	May occur transiently with pyelonephritis, or chronically in children with a history of obstructive uropathy	—
Rx	Sodium bicarbonate or citrate salts at 10–20 mEq/kg/day; may also enhance proximal bicarbonate reabsorption with sodium restriction or hydrochlorothiazide; also supplement with K, P, and vitamin D for Fanconi	Sodium bicarbonate or citrate salts at 2–3 mEq/kg/day (also corrects K-wasting); if low urinary citrate: supplement with citrate to decrease risk of nephrolithiasis	Correct volume depletion, decrease dietary potassium with bicarbonate or citrate supplementation	Sodium bicarbonate or citrate salts at 2–10 mEq/kg/day

Abbreviations: renal tubular acidosis, RTA

Bartter syndrome

- Renal tubular defect leading to **chronic hypokalemic, hypochloremic metabolic alkalosis** (defective chloride reabsorption in the ascending limb of the Loop of Henle). Later: interstitial nephritis and **chronic renal failure** (especially if untreated).
- Clinical presentation: usually in infant **with polyuria, dehydration, failure-to-thrive, decreased appetite, and hypoventilation**; in older children, mostly **muscle weakness due to hypokalemia**; BP is normal to slightly low.
- Labs: **low serum chloride, and potassium; low to normal sodium and elevated bicarbonate**; elevated plasma renin and aldosterone concentrations (loss of fluids and electrolytes → increased production); **urine is dilute (with increased chloride and potassium) and cannot be concentrated after administration of vasopressin.**
- Treatment: up to 10 mEq/kg/24 hours of **potassium chloride combined with a potassium-sparing diuretic and indomethacin if response is not adequate.**

Urinary Tract Stones (Urolithiasis)

For **renal calculi**, crystals in the calyx form a calculus; **bladder stones** are formed in the bladder or travel down the ureters from the kidneys. Calculi are more common with **metabolic abnormalities, neuropathic bladder, or urinary reconstruction**. The majority are **calcified** to some degree (**radiopaque**).

Clinical presentation

Gross or microscopic hematuria; if in the pelvis, calyx, or ureter, presents with **obstruction and severe intermittent renal colic** (radiating to the scrotum or labia); if in the distal ureter, there is dysuria, urgency, and frequency of voiding; bladder stones are asymptomatic; urethral stones present with dysuria and difficulty voiding.

Diagnosis

- **Best initial test** when stones are suspected: Non-enhanced spiral CT of the abdomen and pelvis for the number of stones and the obstruction; if the **CT positive** for stones → ultrasound or plain films.
- **Any passed stone should be sent for analysis.**
- All children should have a **metabolic evaluation**: blood studies—serum electrolytes, calcium, phosphorus, uric acid, creatinine, and alkaline phosphatase; a urinalysis and culture should be obtained, plus a spot urine for cystine and a 24-hour urine for creatinine clearance, calcium, phosphorus, oxalate, citrate, uric acid, and dibasic amino acids (if spot urine is positive for cystine).

Table 14.3: Most Common Urinary Calculi

Calcium Oxalate and Calcium Phosphate Stones	Oxalate Stones	Struvite Stones	Cystine Stones	Uric Acid Stones
Most from hypercalciuria (calcium oxalate more common) without hypercalcemia (idiopathic); may be familial; also less commonly secondary to other causes (hyperparathyroidism, hyperthyroidism, corticosteroids, renal disease, malignancy, sarcoidosis, JRA, Wilson disease, vitamin D, furosemide, and others)	Hyperoxaluria. Genetic: multiple stones and nephrocalcinosis (infants) with deterioration of renal function and deposition of oxalate in other organs Enteric: secondary to fat malabsorption (fatty acids chelate intestinal calcium to form soaps; with less calcium available to bind intestinal oxalate, it is absorbed and excreted in the urine)	Staghorn stones composed of magnesium ammonium phosphate and carbonate apatite from recurrent infections with urea-splitting organisms (*Proteus, Klebsiella, E. coli,* and *Pseudomonas*) → alkaline urine rich in ammonium and phosphate ions; especially with underlying anatomic abnormality	Cystinuria: autosomal recessive; prevents absorption of dibasic amino acids cystine, ornithine, lysine, and arginine; large excretion of cystine → radiopaque hexagonal cystine stones (only known complication)	Hyperuricosuria and/or low urine pH; seen with Lesch-Nyhan syndrome, malignancies, and during treatment with pancreatic enzymes

Abbreviations: juvenile rheumatoid arthritis, JRA

Management

- Small stones may pass spontaneously with **IV hydration, analgesia, and smooth-muscle relaxants**.
- Symptomatic stones removed by **endoscopic lithotripsy or extracorporeal shock-wave lithotripsy**.
- Medical treatment (stopping growth of stones and preventing new stone formation): most important is **high fluid intake** and specific medications depending on the nature of the stones (e.g., allopurinol for hyperuricosuria; thiazide diuretics to decrease renal calcium excretion; potassium citrate inhibits stone formation).
- Dietary changes depending on the underlying problem and cause of the stones

Renal Failure

Acute renal failure

- **Sudden deterioration in renal function with inability to maintain normal fluid and electrolyte balance; pre-renal azotemia** is due to a decreased circulating volume with decreased renal perfusion and decreased glomerular filtration rate (GFR); most likely causes are dehydration, blood loss, sepsis, severe hypoproteinemia, and heart failure.
- **Intrinsic renal failure** is due to renal parenchymal damage (e.g., glomerulonephritis, acute tubular necrosis, HUS); **postrenal failure** is due to obstruction (both kidneys affected).

Clinical evaluation—The history and physical will point to the underlying problem, and laboratory studies should then be geared to confirming the most likely diagnosis (e.g., hemolytic anemia, thrombocytopenia, and uremia in HUS; urinalysis with hematuria, RBC casts, and proteinuria point to intrinsic renal azotemia).

Table 14.4: Evaluation of Pre-Renal, Intrinsic Renal, and Post-Renal Azotemia

Pre-Renal	Intrinsic Renal	Post-Renal
Urine SG >1.020	SG <1.010	SG <1.010
Urine osmolality >500 mOsm/kg	Urine osmolality <350 mOsm/kg	Urine osmolality <350 mOsm/kg
Urine Na <20 mEq/L	Urine sodium >40 mEq/L	Urine Na <20 mEq/L acutely, then >40 mEq/L with diuresis
FENa <1% (<2.5% in neonates)*	FENa >2% (>10% in neonates)	FENa <1% acutely, then >1% with diuresis

* FENa (%) = [(Urine Na × Plasma creatinine)/(Plasma Na × Urine creatinine)] × 100
Abbreviations: fractional excretion of sodium, FENa; specific gravity, SG

Management

1. Attempt intravascular volume expansion if clinically not fluid-overloaded: give 20 mL/kg normal saline over 30 minutes and repeat if insufficient improvement; if no urine output within 2 hours → intrinsic or postrenal acute renal failure.

2. Give a diuretic only with a normal circulating blood volume (furosemide, mannitol) and if no improvement, give a continuous diuretic infusion and a low-dose dopamine infusion; if no response, need fluid restriction

3. Then see Table 14.5 for specific management.

Table 14.5: Clinical and Laboratory Abnormalities and Management in Acute Intrinsic Renal Failure

Clinical/Laboratory Abnormalities	Management
Fluid overload and hyponatremia	400 mL/m^2/24 hr (insensible losses) + urine output + replacement of other losses volume for volume; hypertonic saline only for those with serum Na <120 mEq/L or symptomatic
Hyperkalemia (K >6 mEq/L)	Discontinue all K sources; give Na polystyrene sulfonate resin (Kayexalate) PO or by enema every 2 hour; follow protocol outlined for emergency treatment of hyperkalemia in Chapter 3.
Metabolic acidosis (severe; pH <7.15, HCO$_3$ <8 mEq/L or if contributing to hyperkalemia); retention of H$^+$, phosphate, and sulfate	Give NaHCO$_3$ to raise pH to 7.20; the PO NaHCO$_3$ after serum Ca and P have been normalized (rapid correction of acidosis → hypocalcemic tetany).
Hypocalcemia → hyperphosphatemia	Lower serum P with phosphate-binders (calcium carbonate, calcium acetate); no IV calcium except for tetany (aluminum binders no longer used due to aluminum toxicity)
Hypertension (hyperreninemia and/or expansion of extracellular fluid volume)	Salt and fluid restriction; rapid reduction in BP with isradipine (calcium channel blocker); see further discussion below
GI bleeding (platelet dysfunction, stress)	Oral or IV H$_2$-blocker
Seizures	Administer IV diazepam and correct underlying cause.
Anemia (mostly from volume expansion and is mild)	Fresh washed, packed RBCs with a slow transfusion for Hgb <7 g/dL or with a deterioration of hemodynamic status
Nutrition	Restrict K, P, Na with moderate protein restriction; maximize calories; if prolonged NPO, use TPN.

Abbreviations: blood pressure, BP; gastrointestinal, GI; hemoglobin, Hgb; nothing by mouth, NPO; by mouth, PO; red blood cells, RBCs; total parenteral nutrition, TPN

Dialysis

- **Types: Peritoneal**: standard therapy for infants and children. Infuse hyperosmolar dialysate through a peritoneal catheter → dwells in peritoneal cavity for 45–60 minutes → drain; the process is repeated as needed. **Intermittent hemodialysis**: through a large central venous catheter with a pump-driven extracorporeal circuit three to seven times per week. **Continuous renal replacement therapy**: continuous removal of fluid and solutes from the blood (double-lumen large-vein catheter using a pump-driven machine); usually for patients who are unstable or in the ICU.
- **Indications**: persistent hyperkalemia, volume overload refractory to treatment, severe resistant metabolic acidosis, altered mental status or seizures, BUN >150 mg/dL or rising rapidly, hypocalcemic tetany resistant to drug treatment, or need for severe decrease in fluids with inadequate nutrition

Chronic kidney disease (CKD) and end-stage renal disease (ESRD)

Persistent proteinuria and /or GFR <60 mL/min/1.73 m^2 for at least 3 months from any cause; may progress; standardized staging system from 1 to 5 based on GFR (stage 1 = damage with normal or increased GFR, >90 mL/min/1.73 m^2; stage 5 = renal failure with GFR <15 mL/min/1.73 m^2 or on dialysis)

Clinical findings—Based on underlying cause of CKD; generally pale (normochromic, normocytic anemia), short stature (poor growth), bony changes (renal osteodystrophy), edema, and hypertension. Laboratory findings—**increased BUN and creatinine, hyponatremia** (with volume expansion), **hyperkalemia, acidosis, hypocalcemia, hyperphosphatemia, increased uric acid**, hypoalbuminemia (if proteinuria), hyperlipidemia, and urinalysis with hematuria and/or proteinuria

End-stage renal disease: despite maximal medical therapy, renal function can no longer support life without dialysis or transplantation. Most patients need dialysis prior to transplantation and early enough to prevent severe complications.

Table 14.6: Findings in CKD and Management

Clinical/Laboratory Finding	Reason	Management
Fluid overload and Na retention	Oliguria, increased renin	Na restriction and diuretics if edema, increased BP, heart failure
Na wasting and urinary concentrating defect	Tubular damage, solute diuresis, decreased renin → decreased aldosterone	Increased volume with Na supplementation if polyuria and increased urinary Na loss
Acidosis	Decreased acid excretion, NH$_3$ synthesis, and HCO$_3$ reabsorption	Bicitra (Na citrate) or NaHCO$_3$ to maintain HCO$_3$ >22 mEq/L

(continued)

Clinical/Laboratory Finding	Reason	Management
Hyperkalemia	Decreased GFR, deceased renin → decreased aldosterone, metabolic acidosis	Most with normal-range K until severe deterioration, leading to dialysis; restrict dietary K, administer oral alkali, and treat as per above discussion
Anemia	Decreased erythropoietin, Fe, and B12 deficiency	Recombinant human erythropoietin (rHuEpo) decreases need for transfusion; start when Hgb <10 g/dL one to three times/week subcutaneously (or longer-acting darbepoetin-alfa); Fe supplementation
Hypertension	Volume expansion, increased renin	Low Na intake, thiazide diuretic first, then loop diuretic as GFR declines; ACE inhibitor or blocker is the drug of choice for proteinuria (decreases progression to ESRD); if lack of control, use calcium channel blocker, beta-blocker, or centrally acting agent
Decreased growth	Growth hormone resistance, renal osteodystrophy, anemia, metabolic acidosis	If poor growth despite maximal medical management, use recombinant human growth hormone (rHuGH) to attain normal height velocity (significant improvement in growth); maintain good nutrition with RDAs and high biological-value protein; add supplements as needed for increased calories, water-soluble vitamins
Renal osteodystrophy	Decreased $1,25(OH)_2$ vitamin D → decreased intestinal absorption of Ca → increased PTH → increased bone resorption plus inadequate P excretion (late with significant decline in GFR)→ decreased Ca → increased PTH; osteitis fibrosa cystica (fractures with minor trauma, rachitic changes, bone pain, long-bone deformities); decreased serum Ca, increased P, increased alkaline phosphatase, and normal to increased PTH	Decrease dietary P, use phosphate-binders (newer non-calcium binders such as sevelamer) + vitamin D (ergocalciferol if decreased serum 25-OH vitamin D and calcitriol with increased PTH); maintain PTH, Ca, and P within normal range for age

Abbreviations: angiotensin-converting enzyme, ACE; blood pressure, BP; chronic kidney disease, CKD; end-stage renal disease, ESRD; glomerular filtration rate, GFR; hemoglobin, Hgb; parathyroid hormone, PTH; recommended daily amounts, RDAs

Renal Transplantation

- Optimal with a **living related donor renal transplant**; also good success with non-related or cadaveric donor (less function by 5 years); **may need many grafts;** half have graft failure from **acute or chronic rejection** and more from less common reasons (thrombosis, disease recurrence).

- Criteria: ESRD from any cause; appropriate age and weight for an adult-size kidney; free of acute infection; without severe mental retardation or psychosocial or behavioral problems; without GI or heart disease or massive obesity; HIV and metastatic malignancy are contraindications to transplant.

- **HLA-A, HLA-B, and HLA-DR** most important (class I and II proteins) for transplantation; the best match is when HLA-A, -B, -C and -DR are **identical with a major histocompatibility complex (MHC)-sibling donor**; second best is a sibling or parent with one haplotype match

- **Graft rejection:** tenderness, swelling, hypertension, fever, oliguria, increased serum creatinine; renal scan shows decreased blood flow; and biopsy (needed to differentiate between acute tubular necrosis [ATN], disease recurrence, drug toxicity) shows signs of rejection.

- **Increased risk for graft loss:** age <2 years old, donor cadaveric transplant <6 years old, previous renal transplantation, delayed graft function

- **Immunosuppression** is needed to avoid graft loss; **new corticosteroid and calcineurin inhibitor–sparing drugs** avoid many nephrotoxic and steroid-related complications.

- **Complications:** most common cause of death in first year is **infection**. Infections commonly from **Epstein-Barr virus (EBV) and cytomegalovirus (CMV)**; also from polyoma bradykinin (BK) virus, varicella zoster, herpes simplex, and hepatitis; may lead to graft loss; prophylactic trimethoprim-sulfamethoxazole is used to prevent infection with *Pneumocystis carinii*. Also malignancy: immunosuppression leads to increased EBV replication—**post-transplant lymphoproliferative disorder** (fever, lymphadenopathy, mediastinal mass, GI findings [mass, bleeding, obstruction, ascites] and CNS abnormalities).

Hypertension

Per the Task Force on Blood Pressure Control in Children, National Heart, Lung and Blood Institute (NHLBI), National Institutes of Health:

- **Prehypertension**: average BP in a child >90% (percentile curves for age and sex; normative data for systolic and diastolic BP with corrections for height and weight) but <95%; an **adolescent with BP >120/80 mm Hg** is also prehypertensive.
- **Stage I hypertension:** BP ≥95% but ≤99% + 5 mm Hg.
- **Stage II hypertension:** BP >99% + 5 mm Hg. (Full table of normative values for BPs is available from NHLBI.)

Measurement

- BP should be measured **yearly during well-child care visits beginning at age 3 years**, with the auscultatory method (sphygmomanometer). **Multiple measurements** over time are needed for abnormal results.
- The length of the BP bladder should cover **80–100% of the arm circumference**, and the width at least 40% and midway between the olecranon and acromion process.
- Inflate the cuff to 20 mm Hg greater than the disappearance of the radial pulse, and deflate at 2–3 mm Hg/sec.
- The disappearance of the pulse sound defines the **first Korotkoff sound, and this is the systolic pressure**. Disappearance of all sounds is the **fifth Korotkoff sound, and this is the diastolic pressure**.
- If there is evidence of increased BP in the arms, take **four extremity measurements**.

Initial evaluation

Plot all BPs (average of multiple measurements) on the appropriate percentile chart.

- **Pertinent history includes:** birth history (gestational age, size, problems, **umbilical artery catheterization**, chronic problems after discharge), weight gain and dietary history (including any supplements given), trauma, medications, evidence of **renal disease** (including pyelonephritis), **family history**, sleep history (any evidence of obstructive sleep apnea), and drug use (including alcohol and tobacco).
- **Important physical findings include:** growth retardation, specific dysmorphic features (suggestive of a syndrome associated with hypertension), neurocutaneous lesions, retinal vessel changes, abnormal heart sounds, leg BP greater than arm BP; decreased pulse and pulse lag in femoral compared to brachial artery; bruits, goiter, abnormal pulmonary exam, abdominal mass, neurological deficits, and ambiguous genitalia.
- **Prehypertension:** monitor at 6-month intervals and institute appropriate **diet modification and exercise program**.
- **Stage I:** repeat BP over three visits (in next 1–2 weeks); if BP remains ≥95%, a diagnostic workup should be pursued (see below); identify signs of secondary hypertension (metabolic syndrome, heart disease, endocrinopathy, genetic syndrome, malignancy, neurological disease).
- **Stage II:** re-evaluate in 1 week, or sooner if symptomatic, and begin diagnostic workup; identify signs of secondary hypertension.

Most likely etiologies

- Hypertension more likely **secondary** (to a particular disease process) with higher BPs in younger children. In adolescence, hypertension more likely to be **primary (essential;** normal, low, or high renin hypertension).
- Most common cause of hypertension in a young child (preadolescent)—**renal parenchymal problem** (congenital anomaly, infection, GN, hydronephrosis, reflux nephropathy, renal tumors). The rest are mostly due to **renal artery lesions** (stenosis, thrombosis, vasculitis); then to **coarctation** and to **endocrine** (thyroid, parathyroid, diabetic nephropathy, adrenal, pheochromocytoma, neuroblastoma), and **CNS lesions** (post-traumatic, hemorrhage, mass lesion).

Evaluation of secondary causes

- After measurement of **four extremity BPs,** the most important initial test is a **urinalysis**. Hematuria indicates nephritis (multiple possible causes), renal vein thrombosis, tumor, urinary tract calculi, nephrocalcinosis and white cells indicate infection (with possible underlying anomaly), reflux nephropathy, or tubulointerstitial disease. Renal disease should be evaluated as previously discussed in this chapter.
- Normal urinalysis—**nonrenal diagnosis, including essential hypertension:** a **urine culture** should be performed for the possibility of chronic/recurrent infection.
- Other **screening tests**: CBC (anemia, infection), electrolytes (hypo- or hyperkalemia, acid-base status, hyponatremia), BUN and creatinine (renal function), calcium (parathyroid disease, nephrocalcinosis), and uric acid (urolithiasis).
- A **lipid panel**—obtain in an obese child, evidence of the metabolic syndrome and/or a positive family history.
- **Echocardiogram** is used to evaluate possible heart disease and left ventricular hypertrophy (effect of chronic hypertension).
- A **peripheral plasma renin** level—screen for renovascular or renal parenchymal disease (low value suggests excess mineralocorticoid, while elevated value suggests renal or renovascular disease).
- Renal artery stenosis is best diagnosed with **renal Doppler studies and angiography** (with renal vein and inferior vena cava renin sampling).
- **Urinary catecholamine levels** may be measured to screen for neuroblastoma or pheochromocytoma (unless a mass is evident, in which case an ultrasound should be the best initial test).

Management

- BP should be lowered to <95%; begin with **weight reduction in obese children, healthy diet, exercise program, sodium restriction, elimination of tobacco and alcohol**. If there is diabetes, chronic renal disease, or end-organ damage, BP should be lowered to <90%.
- If BP cannot be controlled, if noncompliant, and for most secondary hypertension, medication is required.
- Drug therapy per the underlying problem (most commonly used drugs):
  - **ACE inhibitors** (captopril, enalapril, lisinopril): for high renin hypertension secondary to renovascular or renal parenchymal disease and high renin essential hypertension; may cause hyperkalemia
  - **Beta-blocker** (propranolol, atenolol, metoprolol): suppression of renin release; also for high cardiac output hypertension; drug of choice for hypertension with migraine; nonselective agents (propranolol) contraindicated in heart failure and asthma; causes bradycardia
  - **Alpha-adrenergic blocker** (phentolamine, phenoxybenzamine) **plus beta-blocker** (for heart rate control): with high levels of catecholamines (or can use dual blocker, labetalol)

- **Diuretics:** volume-dependent hypertension; add calcium channel blocker if inadequate control; loop diuretics (furosemide, bumetanide) are less effective than thiazides in patients with normal renal function (useful in treating hypertension with renal insufficiency); potassium-sparing diuretics (spironolactone, amiloride) may cause hyperkalemia, especially with renal insufficiency or if used with ACE inhibitors; monitor electrolytes.
  - **Calcium channel blockers** (amlodipine, isradipine, nifedipine, nicardipine): decrease peripheral vascular resistance; short-acting drugs may cause tachycardia, and long-acting drugs may cause bradycardia.
  - **Angioplasty, stent, or surgery** for renal artery stenosis
- **Hypertensive crisis:** most with acute or chronic renal disease and renal failure, heart failure, cerebral edema, and seizures; drugs of choice are **IV labetalol** (alpha- and beta-blocker) or **nitroprusside** (dilatation of arterioles and venules) or **nicardipine** (calcium channel blocker); also attention to fluid balance and diuresis (furosemide)

PART TWO: GENITAL DISORDERS

Male Congenital Disorders

Hypospadias—**Ventral urethral opening** anywhere from glans to the perineum; most severe with bifid scrotum; prepuce absent ventrally = **dorsal hood**; ventral curvature during erection = **chordee**; mostly isolated, but most common anomaly is **cryptorchidism** (consider possibility of virilized female; **obtain karyotype with midpenile to proximal hypospadias with cryptorchidism**). Optimal repair at **age 6–12 months** (do not perform circumcision; foreskin used in repair).

Epispadius—Simplest form of the **exstrophy sequence; prepuce is ventral and urethral meatus is dorsal**; repair at **age 6–12 months**; more severe forms require significant surgical reconstruction and may have urinary incontinence.

Hydrocele/inguinal hernia—Accumulation of fluid in the **tunica vaginalis**; if **noncommunicating** (processus vaginalis obliterated), fluid is reabsorbed over first year; if the **processus vaginalis is patent**, the hydrocele persists; hydrocele may also occur in older boys secondary to an **inflammatory condition; communicating hydrocele** may present with inguinal hernia; smooth and nontender with **positive transillumination**. Large, tense hydroceles should be treated with surgery, as well as those persisting beyond a year. Most hernias in children are **congenital indirect inguinal hernias** due to a patent processus vaginalis, and is increased in preterm infants.

Varicocele—Abnormal **dilation of the pampiniform plexus** (valvular incompetence of the spermatic vein); becomes **distended with increased blood flow of puberty** and may result in **subfertility** (surgically correctable); **painless paratesticular mass = "bag of worms,"** becoming evident while standing; surgical repair is generally indicated.

Cryptorchidism

- Majority of undescended testes will descend **within the first 3 months of life**
- Undescended **by 4 months**, they will not
- Most are **in or just distal to the inguinal canal** (but may be abdominal or ectopic)
- **If bilateral and nonpalpable, consider female virilization and obtain karyotype**
- Imaging to determine if testes are present (**CT scan is best**, simplest test)
- Consider **retractile testes** in boys >1 year of age, due to a brisk cremasteric reflex (need careful exam in frog-leg position) vs. acquired undescended testes (ascending due to tension on spermatic cord).
- Surgery (orchiopexy) best performed at **age 6 months** (and no later than 15 months)
- Hormone therapy is not effective; most immediate complications are associated **inguinal hernia** and torsion
- Long-term complications are **infertility** (more with bilateral) and malignancy (significant increase over the general population, and greater if bilateral); most are seminomas (peak at 15–45 years of age; uncommon if orchiopexy <2 years of age).

Phimosis—**Inability to retract prepuce; physiological at birth;** adhesions that lyse usually by age 3 years; with persistent physiologic or pathological (inflammation, scarring) phimosis, use a **corticosteroid cream** for 1 month (most will improve); **circumcision** if corticosteroid treatment is ineffective

Micropenis—**Stretched penile length** (under the pubic symphysis to the tip of the glans) **<1.9 cm** (<2.5 SD below the mean) in a term infant; most commonly from **insufficient gonadotropin-releasing hormone** (hypogonadotropic hypogonadism) and may occur with growth-hormone deficiency; others from primary testicular failure (hypergonadotropic hypogonadism) or idiopathic; evaluate with a **karyotype, anterior pituitary hormones, testicular hormones, and MRI of the brain**.

Circumcision—UTIs are greatly increased through age 5 years in the uncircumcised; also with circumcision, decreased incidence of sexually transmitted disease, penile cancer (but rare with good hygiene), phimosis, and balanitis; must use either a dorsal nerve block or eutectic mixture of lidocaine anesthetic (EMLA) cream during the procedure; most common complications include insufficient foreskin removal, prolonged bleeding, infection, and meatal stenosis.

Male Acquired Disorders

Testicular trauma—From blunt trauma during athletics with **rupture of the tunica albuginea** and subsequent hemorrhage; can be seen with **ultrasound; prompt surgery** is required to save the testis.

Testicular torsion—**Most common cause of testicular pain >12 years of age** (and uncommon <10 years) **sudden-onset pain and swelling;** testis is **tender, enlarged, and high-riding, and has a transverse lie; referred pain** to the groin or abdomen with absent **cremasteric reflex; color Doppler flow study plus Tc-pertechnetate testicular flow scan**

(ischemia vs. inflammation); is diagnostic if torsion is <360 degrees, blood flow may allow testicle survival as long as surgery is performed within **4–6 hours** of onset.

Torsion of the appendix testis—Most common cause of testicular pain in boys age 2–10 years; gradual onset of pain and swelling with a small, tender mass on the upper pole of the testis; may be seen through the skin ("blue dot sign"); imaging shows increased blood flow; treatment is bed rest and nonsteroidal anti-inflammatory drugs (NSAIDs).

Epididymitis—Retrograde spread of a **urethral infection**; most common in **sexually active adolescents** (*Chlamydia, Mycoplasma, Neisseria gonorrhea*) and less commonly in prepubertal boys who have a UTI and an underlying anatomical abnormality (*E. coli* and other Gram-negatives); **scrotal edema, erythema, tenderness, and reactive hydrocele**; decreased pain with elevation of testis; obtain urinalyses (pyuria, bacteriuria) and Gram stain and culture of any urethral discharge; treatment is per the specific organism identified. If the diagnosis is not clear, imaging is required; surgical exploration may be necessary if torsion cannot be ruled out.

Orchitis—Gradual increase in tenderness and swelling of testes, most commonly with systemic signs and symptoms of viral infections, especially **mumps, varicella, or coxsackie**.

Testicular masses
- Painless hard mass with negative transillumination.
- **Prepubertal: more than one-third are malignant, most** of which are **yolk-sac tumors**, but also rhabdomyosarcoma and leukemia.
- In adolescents: almost all are malignant.
- **Best initial test:** ultrasound. Also draw blood for **alpha-fetoprotein (increased in yolk-sac tumors) and beta-human chorionic gonadotropin (increased in teratocarcinomas)**.
- Definitive diagnosis **surgical exploration** and biopsy; usually, radical orchiopexy is needed, except in a benign tumor in a prepubertal boy where removal of the mass alone may be accomplished.

Urethritis (boys and girls)—Presents with urinary **urgency, pyuria, and gross and microscopic hematuria**; urine cultures may be positive for bacteria (*Chlamydia*, or *Ureaplasma*), but **cultures are usually negative**; may occur after trauma; generally improves spontaneously, but for children >8 years of age, **doxycycline** for 10 days is the treatment of choice; if there is no resolution, cystoscopy should be performed to search for an underlying disorder.

Female Congenital Disorders

Imperforate hymen—Outflow tract obstruction presenting as **primary amenorrhea and pain** which begins with menarche; may be associated with defects of the vaginal canal; pelvic exam and **ultrasound** are usually needed to evaluate the obstruction; requires **surgical intervention**.

Labial adhesions—Labia minora with central adherence from just below the clitoris to the fourchette; mostly in girls <6 years of age; cause local inflammation and pooling of urine in the vagina → **recurrent vulvovaginitis and UTIs**; treatment of choice is application of **estrogen cream** for a week and then petrolatum or zinc oxide for 1–2 months after adhesions separate. Evaluate for underlying cause.

Female Acquired Disorders

Bartholin gland cysts—**Obstruction (mucus, infection, swelling) of Bartholin ducts**, allowing the normal fluid to build up and producing a cyst and; if infected, an **abscess** is produced; **cysts are small and painless (on either side of the vulva) and usually resolve; abscesses (very painful** and enlarging over 2–4 days) need to be drained if they do not drain spontaneously.

Ovarian torsion—Torsion of the **adnexum; intermittent sharp abdominal pain radiating down the ipsilateral leg;** usually associated with **ovarian cyst or tumor**; evaluate with **Doppler flow study and laparoscopy;** the procedure of choice is laparoscopic detorsion (recovery of ovarian function may occur).

Ovarian disorders—Present as **abdominal pain and mass**; ovarian follicular cysts present from birth to puberty and disappear spontaneously; functional ovarian cysts rarely present beyond the neonatal period; in adolescents, the most common ovarian mass is a **teratoma** (usually benign) followed by the **ovarian adenoma**. Ovarian malignancies are uncommon in children, (germ-cell tumors most common). Multicystic ovaries, chronic anovulation, hirsutism, acne, and obesity are characteristic of **polycystic ovarian syndrome** (increased androgens). Patients also have insulin resistance and compensatory hyperinsulinism, resulting in abnormal glucose metabolism, hypertriglyceridemia, and long-term cardiovascular complications; more common in first-degree relatives of women with the condition.

Uterine/vaginal bleeding—Most from: **foreign body** (most commonly toilet paper; foul-smelling discharge with vaginal bleeding suggests foreign body; plain radiography or ultrasound is helpful); blunt and penetrating **vaginal trauma** (possibility of **sexual abuse**); urethral prolapse (mucosa prolapses through meatus and bleeds easily), vascular malformations, anatomic abnormalities, **vulvovaginitis, ovarian cysts**, hemorrhagic cystitis, premature menarche (rare), **estrogen exposure**, thyroid disease, and tumors (benign and malignant); ectopic pregnancy, abortion (spontaneous, incomplete, or threatened), anovulatory cycles, and contraceptives

Vulvovaginitis—Vaginal discharge, erythema, tenderness, pruritus, dysuria, and bleeding; recurrent **nonspecific vaginitis** (coliform bacteria from fecal contamination; then streptococci and coagulase-positive staphylococci manually transmitted from the nasopharynx; also from irritants and tight clothing) **stops at puberty with estrogen increase and decrease in vaginal acidity**; treatment is with education regarding proper hygiene, wearing loose clothing, sitz baths with mild soap; if recurrent, treat with amoxicillin or a first-generation cephalosporin or topical polymyxin or estrogen cream. The most common causes of specific vulvovaginitis are *Gardnerella vaginalis* and *Candida* (and others less commonly). Treatment is per the specific organism cultured.

INFECTIOUS DISEASES

PREVENTION OF INFECTIOUS DISEASES

Table 15.1: Prevention of Infectious Disease in Select Settings

Setting/Situation	Prevention Issues
Child-care centers	• Increased risk in younger children, adult caregivers; is greater with **poor hygiene**; also more **antibiotic resistance** • Mostly respiratory (viruses, *S. pneumoniae*), diarrhea (viruses, parasites, bacteria) and skin infections (impetigo, scabies, pediculosis, tinea); **nasopharyngeal carriage** of *S. pneumoniae, N. meningitidis* • **CMV** transmission in saliva or urine contact (asymptomatic shedding) • Preventive methods: complete immunizations, exclude sick children and caregivers, adult vaccines for caregivers, **good hand-washing** (most important), appropriate hygiene for diaper changes, appropriate food handling, and frequent facility cleaning
Hospitals and offices	• Most common transmission **by hands** (all organisms); some airborne; also food and water contamination → outbreaks • **Office: separate well and sick children areas** (good triage); proper cleaning, disinfectant, and sterilization methods; hand-washing before and after each patient encounter • **Hospital:** surveillance by infection control committee, **hand-washing** (most important; preferred: waterless hand hygiene products) before and after each patient; **standard (universal) precautions** (gloves, gowns, masks, goggles, appropriate handling of sharps and materials contaminated with body fluids) • **Strict aseptic technique** for all invasive procedures and for catheter care • **Isolation:** contact (gowns, gloves with preferred single-room isolation), droplet (masks for close contact and preferred single-room isolation), and airborne (masks and single room with negative pressure ventilation)

(continued on next page)

Table 15.1: Prevention of Infectious Disease in Select Settings *(cont.)*

Setting/Situation	Prevention Issues
Vector-borne disease	• Restrict high-risk activities (especially in endemic areas) and keep indoors (in screened and protected areas) from dusk until dawn; **wear clothing to cover extremities.** • Spray clothing with **permethrin** and use permethrin-impregnated bed nets. • Spray with **DEET** (AAP: safe in children > 2 months of age and up to 30% concentration) every 6–8 hours, covering all body areas. • Assure community functioning of retention drainage basins and channels. • **Decrease ponding of water** (stagnation). • **Mosquito collection** and testing with mapping for disease surveillance and control • Good maintenance of home swimming pools, otherwise drain • Do not attract wild animals to property by offering food, leaving garbage uncovered, or leaving dropped fruit (from trees) in yard.
Recreational water use	• From swallowing water; or contact with contaminated water from pools, spas, or natural bodies of water • Mostly **diarrhea** from *Cryptosporidium* and *Giardia*, then *Shigella*, *Escherichia coli* 0157:H7, and noroviruses • Follow **CDC's Health Swimming Program** (emphasis on appropriate disinfecting of pools): water testing and response; maintain pool water to existing public-health requirements. • Provide **appropriate education to swimmers and parents** regarding unhealthy behaviors: swallowing water, no swimming with diarrhea, frequent bathroom breaks, change diapers in bathroom, wash child with soap and water before swimming, hand-washing after bathroom use.

Abbreviations: American Academy of Pediatrics, AAP; Centers for Disease Control, CDC; cytomegalovirus, CMV

INFECTIONS IN IMMUNOCOMPROMISED HOSTS

See also: Chapter 9; and later discussion of HIV in this chapter.

Table 15.2: Infections in the Immunocompromised Host

Condition	Major Issues
Malnutrition	• Especially with **protein energy malnutrition** → increased susceptibility to infection (especially opportunistic); secondary immune deficiencies • Prolonged diarrhea, anemia, nutrient deficiencies, and decreased growth • **Respiratory infections** (*S. pneumoniae*, *Haemophilus influenzae*, active TB), **chronic diarrhea**, measles, malaria, helminthic infections (all are protracted and prolonged)

(continued)

Condition	Major Issues
Asplenia	• Bacteremia and meningitis from *S. pneumoniae, H. influenza* type b, and *Neisseria meningitidis* • Increased risk **especially < 2 years of age** (poor antibody production), **sickle-cell anemia, other hemoglobinopathies, congenital or surgical asplenia** • > 5 years: better production of anticapsular antibodies and decreased risk of serious infection
Malignancy	• Major problem is **neutropenia (ANC < 500/mm³)** → increased risk of bacterial infection • Fever may be the only finding of infection with severe neutropenia; peripheral blood culture, culture of each catheter port, other cultures as needed, radiographic studies • **Most organisms:** Gram-positives (*S. aureus, S. pneumoniae,* coagulase-negative staphylococci, viridans streptococci) > Gram-negatives (*Pseudomonas aeruginosa, Escherichia coli, Klebsiella, Enterobacter, Acinetobacter*); also *Candida* and *Aspergillus*
Indwelling catheters	• Localized and systemic infections; usually from **bacteria of skin**; most from **central venous catheters** (greater risk in the very young, premature, and on TPN) • Most are Gram-positive cocci (over half are **coagulase-negative staphylococci**) > Gram-negatives > fungi • Erythema, tenderness, purulent discharge, or fever without a focus (sepsis) • Perform culture of the exit drainage and **quantitative blood cultures from the catheter and peripheral blood** (significantly greater number of catheter organisms compared to peripheral blood is consistent with catheter infection). • **For infection of a peripheral IV or central venous catheter:** remove and treat with antibiotics (unless with a normal host and uncomplicated infection with coagulase-negative staphylococci, then catheter removal is sufficient). **For long-term catheters (Broviac, Hickman):** parenteral antibiotics for 10–14 days without catheter removal (vancomycin plus third-generation cephalosporin); if blood culture still positive after 72 hours, then remove catheter and start antifungal therapy.
Burns	• Life-threatening infections with organisms from the burn wound • Usual **Gram-positive organisms, plus enteric organisms, including *P. aeruginosa*** • All third-degree and second-degree burns of >10% body surface area need to be **excised and grafted as soon as possible to prevent deep wound sepsis.** • Topical treatment with **silver nitrate, silver sulfadiazine, or mafenide acetate** • Consider short course of oral or IV penicillin for all acute burns.

Abbreviations: absolute neutrophil count, ANC; tuberculosis, TB; total parenteral nutrition, TPN

ANTIMICROBIALS

Table 15.3: Most Commonly Used Antibiotics*

Antibiotic Class	Specific Drugs	Activity Against	Comments
Beta-lactams	• A) **Amino-penicillins** (crystalline penicillin, ampicillin, amoxicillin) • B) **Semisynthetic penicillins** (nafcillin, oxacillin, cloxacillin [oral], dicloxacillin [oral]) • C) **Carboxypenicillins** and ureidopenicillin (carbenicillin, ticarcillin, piperacillin, mezlocillin, and azlocillin) • D) **Beta-lactamase inhibitor** (ampicillin-sulbactam, amoxicillin-clavulanate, piperacillin-tazobactam) • E) **Cephalosporins: first-generation** (cephalexin, cephradine, cefadroxil, cefazolin); **second-generation** (cefaclor, cefoxitin, cefuroxime, cefotetan, cefprozil); **third-generation** (cefixime, cefoperazone, cefpodoxime, ceftazidime, ceftriaxone, cefotaxime); **fourth-generation** (cefepime); **expanded-coverage, semi-synthetic** (cefdinir) • F) **Carbapenems** (imipenem, meropenem, ertapenem)	• A) Drug of choice for GBS, GABHS, *Treponema pallidum, L. monocytogenes,* and *Neisseria meningitidis* • B) Penicillinase-resistant; *S. aureus* and other Gram-positive organisms but not *S. epidermidis* and *Enterococcus* • C) Extended spectrum: *P. aeruginosa,* other Gram-negative enterics, *Enterobacter, Bacteroides* • D) Enhances activity against penicillinase-producing organisms, especially *S. aureus, Streptococcus, Haemophilus influenzae,* and *Moraxella catarrhalis* • E) **First-generation:** *S. aureus, Streptococcus, Escherichia coli, Klebsiella, Proteus;* **second-generation:** expanded coverage including *H. influenzae* and *M. catarrhalis;* better Gram-negative coverage; **third-generation:** Gram-positive and improved Gram-negative coverage; ceftazidime covers *Pseudomonas;* **fourth-generation:** Gram-positive and Gram-negative organisms, plus many with drug resistance; *P. aeruginosa* • F) Broadest Gram-positive and Gram-negative spectrum of any antibiotic; includes anaerobes and *Pseudomonas*	• Gram-negative coverage (including *H. influenzae*) limited due to increasing resistance • Limited by increasing methicillin-resistant *S. aureus* (MRSA) • Major uses of cephalosporins: **first-generation:** skin and soft-tissue infections; **second-generation**: UTI, sinopulmonary infections, soft-tissue infections; **third-generation:** more serious infections (sepsis, meningitis), CF patients (ceftazidime), febrile patients, neutropenic patients; **fourth-generation:** parenteral: meningitis, including *Pseudomonas;* **semi-synthetic** (cefdinir, Omnicef®): oral, extended spectrum; second-line drug for otitis media • Many types of allergic and other reactions; crossover between drug categories; diarrhea, enterocolitis; ampicillin rash (idiopathic), elevated liver enzymes, interstitial nephritis (methicillin); hematological abnormalities

(continued)

Antibiotic Class	Specific Drugs	Activity Against	Comments
Aminoglycosides	Gentamicin, tobramycin, amikacin, kanamycin, streptomycin, netilmicin	• Gram-negatives, *S. aureus*; synergy with beta-lactams against GBS, *Listeria monocytogenes, Pseudomonas, S. epidermidis,* viridans streptococci and *Enterococcus;* Streptomycin: atypical *Mycobacteria, Mycobacterium tuberculosis,* and *Francisella tularensis*	• Neonatal sepsis, Gram-negative sepsis, certain intraabdominal infections, UTIs, in CF patients, and in cancer patients with fever and neutropenia • Major adverse effects: ototoxicity and nephrotoxicity; follow peak and trough levels; adjust dose for decreased renal function
Lincosamide	Clindamycin	Some Gram-positive and some Gram-negative anaerobes and not for *Enterococcus*	• Important in treatment of MRSA (except for poor CNS penetration) • Also with a beta-lactam for invasive GABHS and anaerobic infections • Oral, parenteral, topical (acne), and vaginal cream • Major adverse effect: *Clostridium difficile* colitis
Macrolides	Erythromycin, azithromycin, clarithromycin	Gram-positives, *H. influenzae, Chlamydia trachomatis, Mycoplasma, Chlamydophila pneumoniae, Legionella*	• Increasing Gram-positive resistance • Drugs of choice for type I penicillin allergy • Azithromycin: very long half-life, so once-daily dosing, with shorter treatment; little GI side effects and no metabolic drug interactions; alternate drug for otitis media • Clarithromycin: decreased GI side effects but drug interactions like erythromycin • Erythromycin: has IV formulations; significant GI effects (may be used as a prokinetic agent); antagonizes hepatic CYP450 activity → increased levels of statins and theophylline; itraconazole may increase levels, and rifampin, phenytoin and carbamazepine may decrease levels

(continued on next page)

Table 15.3: Most Commonly Used Antibiotics* *(cont.)*

Antibiotic Class	Specific Drugs	Activity Against	Comments
Inhibitor of bacterial RNA polymerase	Rifampin	*M. tuberculosis, M. leprae*	• Most important in treatment of tuberculosis • Synergistic for *S. aureus* • Elimination of nasopharyngeal carriage of *N. meningitidis and H. influenzae* (close contacts of patient with meningitis)
Fluoroquinolones	Ciprofloxacin, levofloxacin, moxifloxacin, gemifloxacin	Broad-spectrum against Gram-positives and Gram-negatives (including *Enterobacter* and *Pseudomonas*), penicillin-resistant *S. pneumoniae*, MRSA (some), *Mycoplasma, Legionella*	• Oral, parenteral, topical ophthalmic and otic preparations • Not FDA-approved (joint destruction in juvenile animals not seen in humans) for oral or parenteral use in children, but safe when used for specific infections (selective GU infections, critically ill with Gram-negative infections and when no other oral medication is feasible) • Topically for eye infections, external ear infections; and ofloxacin (no toxicity in middle ear) for perforated tympanic membrane or tube otorrhea
Tetracyclines	Tetracycline hydrochloride, doxycycline, minocycline	Bacteriostatic; broad-spectrum against Gram-positives (not *Enterococcus*) and Gram-negatives, rickettsial diseases, Lyme disease, some parasites, *Mycoplasma, Chlamydia*	• If possible, use alternative agent for children < 8 years due to enamel hypoplasia and teeth-staining • Acne: in place of topical antibiotic • **Doxycycline: drug of choice for all ages for Rocky Mountain spotted fever; drug of choice for children > 8 years for Lyme disease** • Adverse effects: photosensitivity, teeth-staining may be permanent; pseudotumor cerebri, SLE-like syndrome (minocycline)

(continued)

Antibiotic Class	Specific Drugs	Activity Against	Comments
Sulfonamides	TMP/SMX, sulfisoxazole, sulfadiazine	Bacteriostatic; *E. coli, Proteus mirabilis, Klebsiella, Pneumocystis carinii* (TMP/SMX); *Toxoplasma gondii* (sulfadiazine)	• Lower urinary tract infections • Toxoplasmosis (sulfadiazine) • *P. carinii* pneumonia treatment and prophylaxis • Alternate prophylaxis for acute rheumatic fever (sulfadiazine)
Glycopeptide	Vancomycin	Limited to Gram-positives including *S. aureus* (and MRSA), coagulase-negative staphylococci, *S. pneumoniae* (and with resistant), *Enterococcus, Corynebacterium, C. difficile* and *Bacillus*	• Infections with coagulase-negative staphylococci, MRSA and resistant *S. pneumoniae* • Initial empiric treatment (with a third-generation cephalosporin) for bacterial meningitis in a child > 2 months • With other antibiotics in oncology patients with fever and neutropenia • Orally for pseudomembranous colitis (*C. difficile*) • Oto- and nephrotoxicity; flushing (red-man syndrome) with fast infusion; use slow infusion and follow peak and trough levels; adjust dose for decreased renal function

*See specific parasitic and viral illnesses for parasitic and viral drugs, respectively.

Abbreviations: cystic fibrosis, CF; central nervous system, CNS; group A beta-hemolytic streptococcus, GABHS; group B streptococci, GBS; gastrointestinal, GI; genitourinary, GU; methicillin-resistant S. aureus, MRSA; systemic lupus erythematosus, SLE; trimethoprim-sulfamethoxazole, TMP/SMX; urinary tract infection, UTI

SPECIFIC VIRAL PATHOGENS AND MAJOR CLINICAL PRESENTATIONS

Enteroviruses (polio and non-polio infections)

- Poliovirus
  - Only in humans; fecal-oral and respiratory spread; no U.S.-acquired case for 30 years (all were vaccine-associated with the old oral polio vaccine)
  - Majority are **asymptomatic** or minor nonspecific illness
  - In small number, **acute asymmetric flaccid paralysis and areflexia** (most of these with paralytic poliomyelitis); can have cranial nerve and respiratory muscle paralysis

- **Diagnostic test of choice:** viral culture of stool and throat as early as possible; any isolate is sent to the Centers for Disease Control (CDC).
- Treatment supportive.

• Non-polio enteroviruses (**coxsackievirus A and B, echoviruses, numbered enteroviruses**)
  - **Nonspecific febrile illness** most common: respiratory, gastrointestinal (GI), central nervous system (CNS), skin and cardiac findings; neonates at high risk for significant illness/mortality
  - Fecal-oral, respiratory, and perinatal vertical spread; fomite transmission; most common in summer and early autumn
  - Viral isolation from throat, stool, and rectal swabs, or any other site of infection (cerebrospinal fluid [CSF]); best evaluation is with **polymerase chain reaction (PCR) for viral nucleic acid**
  - Treatment supportive; contact precautions for hospitalized patients.
  - **Hand-foot-mouth syndrome**
    ◦ **Coxsackie A16** and enterovirus 71
    ◦ Fever, **oral vesicles which ulcerate** (present anywhere in the oral cavity), inflammation and **painful vesicles on hands (especially), feet**, groin, and buttocks; generally lasts 7–10 days
    ◦ Major issue is **hydration** (IV may be necessary) if child will not take oral fluids due to pain.

  - **Herpangina**
    ◦ Most are **coxsackie A**.
    ◦ Acute onset of fever and pharyngitis with ulcerating **posterior pharyngeal vesicles;** rest of the exam is normal; usually mild, lasting less than a week.

  - **Encephalitis (enterovirus 71) and meningitis (echovirus 9)**
    ◦ **Most common cause of viral meningitis (young infants) if immunized against mumps**
    ◦ Fever, nonspecific signs and symptoms (GI, respiratory), CNS findings (meningismus, irritability, vomiting, confusion, lethargy); resolves within 1 week

Adenoviral Infections

51 serotypes with 6 species; certain serotypes associated with specific clinical syndromes; most—acute upper airway infections, e.g., common cold, pharyngitis, and otitis media; **also certain serotypes (40, 41, and 31) with gastroenteritis.** Transmitted by respiratory tract secretions and fecal-oral route.

• **Pharyngoconjunctival fever** (fever plus pharyngitis plus conjunctivitis): community outbreaks from **contaminated swimming pools and fomites**
• **Nosocomial transmission:** infected equipment (**epidemic keratoconjunctivitis [conjunctivitis plus corneal involvement] from office ophthalmological equipment) and health-care workers
• Less common: **lower respiratory tract infection; hemorrhagic cystitis**

- More severe infection in young infants and immunocompromised (**pneumonia, meningitis, encephalitis**)
- Diagnosis: PCR of pharyngeal secretions, eye secretions, or in stool
- Treatment supportive.

Influenza Virus Infections

- Three antigenic types: **A, B, and C**; epidemic disease from A and B; influenza A classified by two surface antigens (influenza B not divided into subtypes): hemagglutinin (HA) and neuraminidase (NA). **Antigenic shift:** major changes leading to a new HA or NA (global pandemics); **antigenic drift** (only with influenza A at regular intervals → seasonal epidemics in winter): minor variation within the same subtype
- Droplet spread from person to person or by fomites; highest rates in schoolchildren with secondary spread; highest infectivity with peak of symptoms (viral shedding stops within 7 days of onset); higher morbidity rates (complications, hospitalization) in neonates and children with underlying conditions

Clinical presentation—Acute onset of fever and systemic findings (chills, rigors, headache, malaise, myalgia) and a nonproductive cough with respiratory symptoms increasing thereafter

Diagnosis—Serology is the best way to confirm the diagnosis: positive IgM (but not until day 10 of illness) or increase in IgG (but may take 4 weeks); early diagnosis with PCR of nasopharyngeal aspirates, serum, or stool, but repeated samples may be needed.

New guidelines for antiviral therapy and prophylaxis—Neuraminidase inhibitors oseltamivir and zanamivir are now the preferred drugs due to widespread resistance to the amantadine (amantadine [>1 year of age] and rimantadine [>13 years of age]; for influenza A only).

- Oseltamivir not approved for children <1 year of age (possible CNS toxicity) but been used during epidemics; it is given as a tablet or liquid (orally for 5 days).
- Zanamivir given by aerosol twice daily for 5 days (for children at least 7 years of age).
- Prophylaxis used for high-risk unimmunized children, unimmunized family members or health-care workers who are in contact with high-risk unimmunized children or those <6 months of age, and for control of outbreaks (to workers and children who are institutionalized). The greatest effect seen if therapy is started within 12 hours of symptom onset and should be started no later than 48 hours after symptom onset.

Treatment—mostly supportive

Measles, Mumps, Rubella, Varicella Zoster, Roseola, Fifth Disease

Table 15.4: Childhood Viral Exanthematous Diseases

Viral Illness	Spread and Contagion	Disease Confirmation	Prodrome	Exanthem	Complications
Measles	Infectious droplets or airborne spread; contagious from 1–2 days before onset of symptoms to 4 days after appearance of the rash	Single serum sample for IgM at initial visit; report to local or state Health Department	Fever plus cough, coryza, conjunctivitis (3 C's), then Koplik spots (pathognomonic) 1–4 days prior to rash (red lesions with blue-white central spots; begins on buccal surface at the premolars and spreads anteriorly)	Erythematous maculopapular rash; starts around hairline; spreads to forehead and downward over 7 days, then disappears in same direction by 10 days	Most common is otitis media; pneumonia (most common cause of death), diarrhea and vomiting, encephalitis (especially with the very young, people over age 20, with malnutrition, vitamin A deficiency, and underlying problems); SSPE: rare; occurs after 7–10 years (neurodegeneration and death)
Mumps	Infected respiratory secretions; maximal contagion 1–2 days prior to onset of parotitis to 5 days after onset with viral shedding up to 9 days	PCR, cell culture, or antigen detection from respiratory secretions, CSF, or urine; positive IgG or rise in acute to convalescent titers	1–2 days of nonspecific symptoms	Parotid enlargement and tenderness (some with submandibular) asymmetrical or symmetrical which peaks in 3 days and resolves over the next week	Most common is meningoencephalitis (5 days after parotitis, resolving in 7–10 days); adolescent/adult males: orchitis (after present with parotitis); oophoritis in females less common; sterility very uncommon; mumps pancreatitis (with or without salivary gland involvement)

(continued)

Viral Illness	Spread and Contagion	Disease Confirmation	Prodrome	Exanthem	Complications
Rubella	Direct or droplet contact or respiratory secretions; maximal contagion from 3 days before to 7 days after rash onset	Enzyme assay for IgG against rubella	Fever and other nonspecific findings plus lymphadeno-pathy (mostly posterior auricular, occipital, and posterior cervical). May have enanthem (Forchheimer spots; rose-colored/pete-chial lesions on soft palate); adolescents (more in females) and adults may have polyarthralgia and polyarthritis (mostly small hand joints)	Erythematous macules (looks similar to measles) begin on face and spread downward with disappearance of the rash proximally; lasts 3 days	Postinfectious thrombocytopenia (2 weeks after rash onset; mild, self-limited bleeding and petechiae); encephalitis (within 7 days of rash onset); rare progressive rubella panencephalitis (like SSPE); congenital rubella syndrome (see Chapter 1)
Varicella zoster	Airborne spread (rarely from zoster); also transplacental infection (see Chapter 1); highest contagion from 1–2 days before to shortly after onset of rash and persists until all lesions have crusted	Tissue culture from vesicular fluid or direct fluorescent antibody test of vesicle scraping or PCR of bodily fluid; also acute and convalescent sera	Fever and nonspecific findings 24–48 hours before rash onset	Chickenpox: Lesions first appear on trunk, face, and scalp and proceed outward; very pruritic erythematous macules → papules → vesicles → umbilication → crusting; lesions occur in crops over 7–10 days (longer with immuno-compromise)	Most common: secondary bacterial infections (skin scratching); encephalitis, acute cerebellar ataxia, pneumonitis, hepatitis, and progressive severe varicella (all more common with immunodeficiencies); zoster (reactivation of latent virus in dorsal root ganglia): vesicular lesions along a dermatome with pain and post-herpetic neuralgia; congenital varicella syndrome (see Chapter 1); higher risk of Reye syndrome with use of salicylates

(continued on next page)

Table 15.4: Childhood Viral Exanthematous Diseases *(cont.)*

Viral Illness	Spread and Contagion	Disease Confirmation	Prodrome	Exanthem	Complications
Roseola (exanthem subitum; HHV type 6)	Transmission usually to a young infant from asymptomatic shedding of secretions from close contacts; most infections between age 6–24 months (most seropositive by age 4 years)	Acute and convalescent sera with a rise in IgG titer or culture of virus in blood mononuclear cells	High fever (rises rapidly and persists for 3–7 days, then resolves acutely); nonspecific respiratory or GI symptoms prior to or with fever	As fever decreases, or within a few days of temperature normalization, rash begins on trunk (rose-colored maculopapular) and spreads outward over 1–3 days	Febrile seizure with acute rise of temperature to often >103° F (39.4°C); rare cause of meningo-encephalitis
Fifth disease (erythema infectiosum; parvovirus B19)	Replicates only in human RBC precursors; transmission by contact with respiratory secretions, exposure to contaminated blood, or perinatally; highest contagion just prior to rash onset (and not contagious with the development of rash)	Preferred method is parvovirus B19-IgM in the healthy person and PCR for the virus in immuno-suppressed	Fever plus nonspecific systemic symptoms	Macular erythema on cheeks (slapped-cheek appearance); then diffuse macular erythema on upper trunk and proximal arms, with rapid central clearing to a lacy-appearing (reticular) rash which may come and go for 3 weeks (no illness, no contagion)	Most important is chronic anemia in the immuno-suppressed, transient aplastic crisis (with hemolytic anemias, especially sickle-cell) and fetal aplastic anemia → hydrops fetalis (maternal infection in first 20 weeks of gestation)

Abbreviations: cerebrospinal fluid, CSF; gastrointestinal, GI; human herpesvirus, HHV; polymerase chain reaction, PCR; red blood cell, RBC; subacute sclerosing panencephalitis, SSPE

Notes on Table 15.4

- **Use of vitamin A for measles:** some children with measles have low levels of vitamin A (inversely correlated to illness severity); **AAP: vitamin A therapy** for children 6 months to 2 years of age who are hospitalized because of complications, and for those >6 months of age with immunodeficiency, clinical vitamin A deficiency, malabsorption, moderate to severe malnutrition, and/or recent immigration from areas with high measles mortality.

- Postexposure prophylaxis of measles: **vaccine to susceptible immunocompetent persons** within 72 hours of exposure (may prevent or modify) and for outbreaks: **monovalent measles vaccine** to children as young as 6 months; if given before first birthday, need re-immunization with measles-mumps-rubella vaccine (MMR) at 12–15 months as usual; **immune globulin** up to 6 days after exposure to **susceptible household contacts who are immunocompromised, pregnant, or <1 year of age** (not for those who have already received one dose of MMR)
- Neither mumps vaccine nor immune serum globulin is effective for postexposure prophylaxis; **most effective means of dealing with school outbreaks** is to exclude susceptible children from school until immunization.
- **Rubella: postexposure immunoglobulin for exposed susceptible women if pregnancy termination is not an option** (does not guarantee lack of fetal effects); need **rubella antibody testing** as soon as possible after exposure; positive IgG = immunity; if negative, perform second test in 2 weeks and if that is negative, again in 6 weeks (both re-tests negative = no infection; second and third tests positive = seroconversion); rubella vaccine after exposure to immunocompetent, non-pregnant people does not prevent illness
- **Breakthrough varicella:** in those vaccinated **at least 42 days** prior to rash onset caused by **wild-type virus**; usually milder with less contagion (but still keep out of school until all lesions have crusted); lesions beginning **<42 days** since the vaccine are caused by **vaccine strains.** Children with ≥**50 lesions** are as contagious as wild-type disease.
- **Varicella postexposure prophylaxis:** vaccine to susceptible children within 3–5 days of exposure; **varicella-zoster immune globulin (VZIG)** within 96 hours of appearance of rash in index case to susceptible household contacts, close-contact playmates, immunocompromised or pregnant, **newborns whose mothers develop the rash anywhere from 5 days before to 48 hours after delivery,** hospital exposure for preterm infants (≥28 weeks' gestation) if mother has no reliable history of varicella or positive serology and for preterm infants (<28 weeks or <1,000 g birth weight) regardless of maternal history or serology
- **Treatment of varicella:** consider **oral acyclovir** for people at risk for moderate to severe varicella (>12 years old, with chronic lung or skin disorders, on long-term salicylates, or receiving short or intermittent courses of corticosteroids [including inhaled]; also consider for secondary household cases [usually more severe illness than the index case]). **IV acyclovir** is recommended for pregnant women with severe complications, and for immunocompromised patients with either chickenpox or zoster (VZIG is not effective once the disease is established).
- Treatment of **severe herpesvirus 6 infections** in immunocompromised patients: ganciclovir or cidofovir
- Treatment of **parvovirus B19 infections** is supportive, unless transfusion is needed for anemia or aplastic crises; intrauterine transfusion has been used for fetal infection; consider IVIG for the immunocompromised patient.

Epstein-Barr Virus (EBV) Infections

- B-lymphotropic herpesvirus; most common cause of **infectious mononucleosis**; humans are the only source; transmission from **close personal contact from saliva or sexual intercourse** (viral excretion for months); lifelong intermittent excretion; period of contagion not determined
- **Clinical presentation:** most in young children are asymptomatic; older children have a nonspecific prodrome for 1–2 weeks with increasing **fever, pharyngitis (looks like streptococcal pharyngitis), lethargy, generalized lymphadenopathy (especially anterior and posterior cervical nodes), and splenomegaly. Maculopapular rash** may occur in a small number, but is very **common if treated with ampicillin or amoxicillin** (immune-mediated vasculitic rash). Most symptoms last 2–4 weeks with gradual recovery; some with fatigue for up to 6 months and occasionally for a few years; no evidence for chronic fatigue syndrome.
- **Complications: airway obstruction** (tonsillar and oropharyngeal lymphoid swelling), meningoencephalitis, **Guillain-Barré syndrome, splenic rupture** (rare), thrombocytopenia, hemolytic anemia, myocarditis
- Other EBV disorders: **Burkitt lymphoma** (primarily in Central Africa), nasopharyngeal carcinoma (primarily in Southeast Asia), CNS undifferentiated B-cell lymphomas, X-linked lymphoproliferative syndrome, and post-transplantation lymphoproliferative disorder.
- **Diagnosis: heterophil antibody** (IgM) appears in the first 2 weeks and gradually disappears over 6 months (slide agglutination test = **Monospot**) + **atypical lymphocytosis**; if negative, then the **single best test is the IgM to the viral capsid antigen (VCA)**, which is positive in the first 4 weeks to a few months. Past infection is indicated by a positive IgG-VCA, negative IgM-VCA, negative early antigen (EA) and positive EBNA (EBV nuclear antigen).
- **Management:** supportive (bed rest only for debilitating fatigue); **avoid contact sports** while splenomegaly is present; possible **short-course prednisone** if incipient airway obstruction, thrombocytopenia with bleeding, hemolytic anemia, seizures, or meningitis

Cytomegalovirus (CMV)

Herpesvirus member; only human strains produce human disease; transmitted by direct contact with secretions (saliva, urine, and sexual transmission), by vertical transmission (transplacental, intrapartum, or after birth; see Chapter 1), and by transfusions (eliminated with CMV-negative donors, with filtration to remove white blood cells [WBCs], or by freezing in glycerol or buffy coat removal). Persists in a latent form (WBCs and tissues; seropositive) with reactivation many years later (especially in immunocompromised); high rates of excretion in young children in day-care centers. Severe disease usually in a seronegative person or premature infant.

Clinical presentation—Asymptomatic or subclinical infections: most common in immunocompetent children; older children and adolescents: infectious mononucleosis–like syndrome (heterophil-negative) and/or hepatomegaly/hepatitis. In immunocompromised patients (especially with bone marrow transplantations and HIV): most as pneumonitis, then less so as hepatitis, retinitis, CNS disease, or GI disease

Diagnosis—Isolation of virus in cell culture from urine and other body fluids and tissues, or monoclonal antibodies or PCR; primary infection: seroconversion or simultaneous positive IgM and IgG (persist for life); recurrent infection: seropositive person with reappearance of viral excretion

Treatment—Recommended for immunocompromised: ganciclovir plus immune globulin; prophylaxis with ganciclovir or acyclovir reduces morbidity in transplant patients; ganciclovir for congenital disease prevents hearing deterioration; lifelong prophylaxis to AIDS patients who have a history of CMV disease to prevent recurrence

Herpes Simplex Infections

Herpes simplex virus (HSV)-1 and HSV-2 are transmitted from asymptomatic and symptomatic carriers; HSV-1: usually face and skin above the waist; direct contact with infected oral secretions or lesions (also genital infections from autoinoculation); HSV-2: more common in the skin below the waist and genitalia (sexually active); direct contact with infected genital lesions or secretions

- Neonatal infections more often **intrapartum** (see Chapter 1), and most are HSV-2.
- Patients with **primary infection** (greatest concentration of virus) shed virus for 1 to several weeks (recurrent infection for 3–4 days)
- Intermittent asymptomatic recurrent infections persist for life.

Clinical manifestations (after neonatal period)—Most primary infections are **asymptomatic or gingivostomatitis** (fever, painful ulcerative lesions of mouth and gingiva with or without vesicular lesions around the mouth). **Genital** (most common in adolescents and adults): vesicular/ulcerative lesions of the genitals and perineum.

Other clinical presentations—Cutaneous lesions (skin abrasion and contact with infected secretions during contact sports; **herpes gladiatorum), herpes whitlow** (infection of the paronychia; thumb-sucking with oral lesions or adolescents with exposure to infected genital secretions), **eczema herpeticum** (herpetic lesions concentrated in areas of eczematous involvement), **keratoconjunctivitis, encephalitis** (HSV-1; frontal, temporal cortex, and limbic system; coma and death in most if untreated), **aseptic meningitis** (most common cause of recurrent aseptic meningitis); severe, life-threatening infection in the immunocompromised

Diagnosis—Isolation of virus, antigen or by **PCR** (vesicular fluid, eye or mouth swabs, CSF)

Management—Only **acyclovir** has an **IV** formulation; **acyclovir, valacyclovir, and famciclovir are available orally** (the latter two having much greater oral bioavailability than acyclovir); for **gingivostomatitis**: oral acyclovir within 72 hours (decreased severity and duration); for **recurrence**: any of the three oral drugs shortens the duration; oral acyclovir for eczema herpeticum; any of the three drugs should be used to treat the **first episode of genital herpes** (reduces severity and duration but has no effect on subsequent infections); intermittent therapy or chronic suppressive therapy may be used for **recurrences; CNS infection, neonatal infection, and severe infection in the immunocompromised** should be treated promptly with IV acyclovir; **eye infections** should be referred to an ophthalmologist (topical trifluridine, iododeoxyuridine, and possible parenteral therapy).

Human Papillomavirus (HPV)

Small DNA viruses; species-specific; transmission by close contact; can produce epithelial warts and mucous membrane warts (anogenital, oral/nasal, conjunctival, and respiratory tract); nongenital warts acquired by minor skin trauma (especially hands and feet; common in children and adolescents); most prevalent sexually transmitted viral infection in the United States (anogenital infection). **Low-risk HPV** types 6 and 11 most common in genital warts (rarely progress to malignancy); high-risk (70% of cervical cancer) = types 16 and 18.

Clinical presentation—Most common venereal presentation is latent infection; external genital warts less common; most common clinically detected lesion in adolescent girls is the low-grade squamous intraepithelial lesion (LGSIL): most regress spontaneously, but small number can induce high-grade squamous intraepithelial lesions (HGSIL; less likely to regress; precancerous), which rarely progress to invasive cancer.

Diagnosis—Detection of viral DNA, RNA, or capsid protein; screen (within the first 3 years of intercourse) for cervical cancer with a **Papanicolaou (Pap) smear**, but is not confirmatory; women with atypical squamous cells should have the smear repeated in 4–6 months and if positive → **colposcopy**.

Treatment—Remove symptomatic **common warts** (most resolve spontaneously): cryotherapy, electrotherapy, salicylic acid preparations; **genital lesions** regress over extended period; if parents request, should be treated: electrosurgery, surgical excision, laser surgery, cryotherapy. Recommended patient-applied treatments: topical podofilox or imiquimod.

Rabies Virus

Worldwide infection of large variety of animals (only one known genotype in the United States); dog transmission: **majority of cases.** In the United States, raccoons are the most commonly infected, **then** skunks, bats, foxes, and coyotes (**no transmission from small mammals**); transmission through a bite with infected saliva (**higher chance of infection with bites on the face and hands**); virus replication in muscle → peripheral nerve along the axon → CNS → **brain and spinal cord** → anterograde through the peripheral nerve → innervated organs.

Clinical presentation—**Incubation period can be days to months;** the encephalitic form **begins with fever** and paresthesias/pruritus **at the site of the bite and along the extremity;** then intermittent periods of encephalopathy; **then** coma; hydrophobia and aerophobia develop **(brain-stem involvement)** → **choking and aspiration secondary to** spasms; death in 2–3 weeks. The other form is paralytic rabies: less frequent; ascending motor weakness **affecting the extremities and cranial nerves, plus some degree of encephalopathy.**

Diagnosis—Virus (saliva, brain biopsy) as well as antiviral antibody and viral RNA can be detected in serum or CSF.

Management—Nothing alters the course of the illness after symptoms are present, and death will occur. For household pets (dogs, cats, ferrets): **observe for 10 days and use prophylaxis only if animal develops signs of rabies;** if rabid or suspected of being rabid (bats, raccoons, skunks, coyotes, and foxes), **immediate immunization and rabies immune globulin.** After thorough cleansing of the wound (use antibiotics and tetanus prophylaxis as needed for a bite wound), use rabies immune globulin infused maximally around the wound and the rest injected into an arm or leg distant from the one that will be used for the vaccine; and inactivated vaccine (IM) on the same day and then on day 3, 7, 14 and 28.

Arboviruses

Group of viruses transmitted by mosquitoes (from birds and other vertebrate hosts) during warmer weather over most of the United States; most causes are due to West Nile encephalitis, St. Louis encephalitis, and the California encephalitis group; **less frequent causes are** western equine encephalitis, eastern equine encephalitis, and Colorado tick fever (transmitted by the wood tick). Prevalence rates vary geographically; symptoms and severity vary widely from asymptomatic or subclinical to severe meningoencephalitis (some with neurological sequelae) and death. Diagnosis is by testing acute-phase serum at least 5 days after onset of illness for virus-specific IgM; also, fourfold increase in acute and convalescent IgG titers; virus or RNA by PCR can be isolated in brain tissue. Treatment is intensive supportive care.

Human Immunodeficiency Virus (HIV, AIDS)

Almost all infections from HIV-1 (HIV-2 causes infection in monkey species and is a rare cause in children) and majority are **secondary to vertical transmission; smaller number are acquired between 13–19 years.** Transmission is by sexual contact, by contact with infected blood **(rare now)**, intrauterine, intrapartum **(60–70% of all)**, and **from breastfeeding (small number in industrialized countries)**. Increased risk with birth <34 weeks or birth weight <2,500 g, >4 hours of rupture of membranes.

Clinical presentation

- **Most infants are normal at birth, and then may develop** lymphadenopathy, hepatosplenomegaly, **chronic diarrhea, failure-to-thrive, oral candidiasis, or interstitial pneumonitis.**
- **Systemic and pulmonary findings** are more common presenting findings in children in the United States; higher incidence of **recurrent bacterial infections, lymphocytic interstitial pneumonitis (LIP),** early progressive neurological deterioration, and chronic parotid enlargement.

Infections/complications

- Most are **recurrent infections (mostly pneumonia and sepsis,** then others less commonly) with encapsulated bacteria and then other Gram-positive and Gram-negative organisms.
- **Opportunistic infections** with **severe decrease in CD4**; usually—**fulminant, primary infection** (most **common is *Pneumocystis carinii*); infections with atypical mycobacteria** (*Mycobacterium* *avian-intracellular* complex) now rare in children (good combination-drug regimens and prophylaxis to those with severe immunosuppression)
- **Most common fungal illness** is oral **candidiasis,** (may progress to esophageal disease); disseminated histoplasmosis, coccidioidomycosis, and cryptococcus are rare in children
- **Most common parasitic infections**—intestinal *Cryptosporidiosis* and *Giardia,* often presenting as severe **chronic diarrhea with malnutrition** and chronic liver inflammation with or without cholestasis (chronic hepatitis, portal hypertension, and liver failure).
- **Most prominent viral illnesses—herpes simplex** (chronic, recurrent), **varicella zoster** (severe, prolonged; chronic, recurrent), **CMV** (disseminated); also respiratory infections with **RSV and adenovirus;** there are also **chronic, recurrent HPV genital infections.**
- **LIP is the most common lower respiratory tract abnormality** (chronic, diffuse reticulonodular pattern; mild to moderate hypoxemia); *S. pneumoniae* is the most common bacterial pathogen; *Pseudomonas aeruginosa* more commonly with low CD4 counts and often leads to respiratory failure and death; increased incidence of **pulmonary and extrapulmonary tuberculosis (TB).**
- Malignancies in children occur less frequently; most are **non-Hodgkin lymphomas** and leiomyosarcoma (EBV-associated).

Diagnosis

- May test positive for transplacental HIV antibody up to **18 months** of age, so for all <18 months, need to test for HIV nucleic acid (**preferred test: HIV DNA PCR**); perform within **the first 48 hours of life**; if negative, need to re-test at ages 1–2 months and 4–6 months.
- For those ≥18 months of age, use a **screening enzyme immunoassay (EIA) and if positive, confirm with Western blot**.

Prevention of perinatal HIV transmission

- **Universal HIV testing** to all pregnant women, with repeat testing in the third trimester (<36 weeks) for those with higher risks; rapid tests are available (better than the standard EIA).
- **For HIV-positive mothers,** see Chapter 1.

Treatment—based on **viral load** (predicts rate of disease progression), **CD4 count** (risk of complications and opportunistic infections), and **clinical condition**. Use **combination of at least three drugs** (highly active antiretroviral therapy, **HAART**; nucleotide reverse transcriptase inhibitors, non-nucleotide reverse transcriptase inhibitors, protease inhibitors, and fusion inhibitors) to **suppress viral replication to undetectable levels**; should begin in a **child <1 year** of age as soon as the diagnosis is made (better with start of treatment at <3 months of age) and in an **older child who is symptomatic or who has any immune dysfunction**. Drug combinations are changed when the therapy becomes **ineffective** or when **toxicity or tolerance** develops (high mutation rate). All should receive **PCP prophylaxis** (trimethoprim-sulfamethoxazole, TMP/SMX) per current recommendations (age 6 weeks–1 year and >1 year based on CD4 count).

SPECIFIC BACTERIAL PATHOGENS AND MAJOR CLINICAL PRESENTATIONS

Infections covered in other chapters will not be discussed here.

Staphylococcus

Coagulase-negative staphylococci (CONS; *S. epidermidis, S. haemolyticus, S. saprophyticus*)

- Most from **contamination** (inhabitant of skin and mucous membranes) or **nosocomial infection**: intravascular catheter infections, prosthetic devices, CSF shunts, chemotherapy, and bone marrow transplantation; most common cause of late-onset sepsis in premature infants
- Draw two separate cultures to differentiate bacteremia from contamination (should grow within 24 hours, both cultures positive).
- Most strains are **methicillin-resistant**, so start empiric therapy with **vancomycin**.

Staphylococcus aureus

- Colonizes skin and mucous membranes of healthy people (anterior nares, skin)
- Most **nosocomial surgical site infections** (along with *P. aeruginosa*), most common causes of **nosocomial pneumonia**. Increasing amount of in-hospital and community infection with **methicillin-resistant *S. aureus*** (MRSA; carriage can persist for years)
- **Localized infections:** impetigo, furuncles, carbuncles, cellulitis, lymphadenitis, styes, wound infections, foreign-body infections; bacteremia → infection in any organ and abscess formation
- Many strains release **exotoxins**—produce localized disease (**bullous impetigo**) or generalized (**staphylococcal scalded-skin syndrome** [SSSS]): generalized erythema and exfoliation in young children (particularly neonates and infants). Older children tend to get bullous impetigo or a scarlet fever–type of eruption.
- **Food poisoning:** symptoms elicited by **enterotoxins**; usually from food handlers' hands and inadequate cooking or heating/refrigeration (bacteria multiply and produce heat-stable toxin). Short time from ingestion to acute, severe onset of nausea, cramps, vomiting, and usually diarrhea (usually lack of fever) for 1–2 days.
- **Toxic shock syndrome:** caused by toxin-producing *S. aureus* (**toxic shock-producing toxin-1**): fever, rapid onset of hypotension, vomiting, watery diarrhea, myalgia, conjunctival hyperemia, strawberry tongue, and an erythematous rash (with hand and foot desquamation), and multisystem organ disease; most occur in **young menstruating women using tampons** or other vaginal devices (now less than half of all cases); nonmenstrual disease in children and males: associated with infections (wound, skin, surgical, mucous membrane, trauma) and nasal packing.

Streptococcus

- **Group A streptococcus** (GAS; *S. pyogenes*): mostly upper respiratory tract and skin (impetigo) infections; increasing incidence of **severe invasive GAS infections** (bacteremia, streptococcal toxic shock, necrotizing fasciitis); more common with varicella infection, chronic illness, immunosuppression, and diabetes, and in the very young and the very old. Other infections: erysipelas, cellulitis, perianal dermatitis, prepubertal vaginitis, osteomyelitis, septic arthritis, endocarditis, and pneumonia
  - **Pediatric autoimmune neuropsychiatric disorder associated with *S. pyogenes* (PANDAS):** obsessive-compulsive disorder, tic disorders, and Tourette syndrome with relationship to GAS infection (proposed that these patients produce autoimmune antibodies that cross react with brain tissue, similar to Sydenham chorea); currently no recommendations for prophylaxis or immune therapy
- **Non-GAS or group B streptococci: viridans** streptococci (alpha-hemolytic) and beta-hemolytic groups; common colonizers of intact body surfaces; most common infections are with C and G (most have an **underlying medical disorder**; often animal contact with group C); most viridans streptococcal infections associated with **endocarditis and bacteremia in neutropenic patients**. Penicillin is antibiotic of choice.
- **Enterococcus** (*E. faecalis*): Gram-positive, catalase-negative anaerobes; normal GI inhabitants, colonizers of oral secretions, upper respiratory tract, skin, and vagina;

common **hospital-acquired infection** (mostly in newborns; early- or late-onset infection); often resistant to antibiotics; in older children: **urinary tract infections** (**UTIs**; primary infection or nosocomial) or **intra-abdominal abscesses** following intestinal perforation.

Corynebacterium diphtheriae

Gram-positive bacillus producing an **extracellular toxin**; transmission by close contact (inhabitant of mucous membranes and skin) with discharge from nose, throat, eye, and skin lesions; most common initial site of infection is the **tonsils and pharynx**, starting with pharyngitis (with or without fever) and tonsillar **pseudomembrane** formation which can progress posteriorly and may lead to **airway obstruction** (may need removal of the pseudomembrane and intubation); edema and enlarged lymph nodes cause a **"bull neck"** appearance; the major complications are **toxic cardiomyopathy** (heart failure, dysrhythmias) and **neuropathy** (cranial nerve, polyneuropathy, diaphragm paralysis). Specific **antitoxin** is the primary therapy with **erythromycin or penicillin** to eliminate and prevent transmission of the organism.

Bordetella pertussis

Gram-negative, pleomorphic bacillus; humans are only known source, with transmission from respiratory droplets; **adolescents and adults may have mild disease and spread to infants and others within a household**; most contagious during catarrhal phase and for 2 weeks after onset of cough; classic clinical presentation with first 2 weeks of upper respiratory symptoms (**catarrhal phase**) with a cough, then 2 weeks of a **severe paroxysmal cough with an inspiratory whoop and post-tussive emesis**, then **gradual improvement** over weeks to months; complications: pneumonia, **respiratory failure**, seizures, encephalopathy, and death (most severe in the first 6 months, in preterm infants, and in non-immunized). Direct immunofluorescence test for nasopharyngeal secretions, but it is of low specificity and variable sensitivity; the **most rapid and sensitive method is PCR of nasopharyngeal secretions** (culture requires special transport and special media, and is slow-growing); the drug of choice is a **macrolide** for 14 days, with full **treatment of all household members**. Infants under 3 months of age and anybody with respiratory distress should be admitted to the hospital.

Chlamydia trachomatis

Trachoma: most important preventable cause of blindness in the world (endemic areas); disease spread from **eye to eye**; flies are common vector; begins as follicular conjunctivitis in early childhood with healing → conjunctival scarring and an entropion (eyelid turns inward and the **lashes abrade the cornea**) → **ulceration** → **scarring and blindness**; the recommended treatment is a **single dose of azithromycin**.

Listeria monocytogenes

Aerobic, Gram-positive bacillus found widely in the environment; outbreaks from **food-borne transmission** (unpasteurized milk, soft cheeses, prepared meats, undercooked poultry, unwashed raw vegetables); **asymptomatic fecal and vaginal carriage in pregnant women** (see Chapter 1 for neonatal infection); in childhood: most have **meningitis or outbreaks from contaminated food presenting as fever and diarrhea**; treat severe infections with **IV ampicillin and an aminoglycoside**, and then ampicillin alone after clinical response (or for milder disease).

Kingella kingae

Gram-negative coccobacilli previously classified as *Moraxella*; inhabitant of the oropharynx (more in children) and **transmitted in child-care centers without causing disease**; most common infections are **osteomyelitis** (femur is the most common site) and **septic arthritis** (monoarticular; knee > hip > ankle; see Chapter 17) in children <5 years of age; is also associated with meningitis, pneumonia, and endocarditis. **Penicillin** is the drug of choice for beta-lactamase negative strains.

Bartonella henselae

Gram-negative bacillus → cat-scratch disease; cat fleas transmit the organisms between cats; human transmission occurs after a scratch from a cat or kitten; **may start with nonspecific findings, including fever; hallmark** is papules at the site of the scratch (linear) and then **1–2 weeks later**, adenopathy **in the nodes draining the site of infection**; the **nodes spontaneously suppurate** in less than one-third; **systemic findings** are much less common (hepatitis, encephalitis, pneumonia, hematologic, and others). **Parinaud oculoglandular syndrome:** inoculation of the conjunctiva with ipsilateral preauricular and submandibular adenopathy. **Nodes that do not drain spontaneously (2–4 months) and are symptomatic** should be drained by needle aspiration; **antibiotics** are recommended only with systemic findings (there is no difference in outcome with respect to node drainage in those treated and not treated with antibiotics) or in immunosuppressed persons (e.g., oral azithromycin and IV gentamicin).

Borrelia burgdorferi

Spirochete that is the cause of **Lyme disease**; most cases in the United States are in the **Northeast**, then **upper Midwest**, and then on the West Coast. The vector is the infected **tick** of the genus *Ixodes*. U.S. incidence is highest in children age 5–9 years and from April through October.

- **Early localized disease:** fever and nonspecific constitutional signs plus **erythema migrans** (red macule or papule that expands over days to weeks to form an annular erythematous macular lesion, if untreated)
- **Early disseminated disease:** nonspecific constitutional symptoms plus **multiple erythema migrans** (secondary lesions usually smaller than the primary) and represents

hematogenous and cutaneous dissemination; also high incidence of **cranial nerve palsies** (especially **VII**) and **eye problems** including conjunctivitis and **anterior uveitis**
- **Late disease: recurrent pauciarticular arthritis** (large joints, especially the knees); CNS manifestations are uncommon in children
- The most commonly used test for antibody detection is the **enzyme immunoassay with a Western blot** as confirmatory.
- The treatment of choice for early localized disease is **doxycycline for children >8 years old and amoxicillin for those <8**. Treatment almost always prevents progression of the disease.
- Early disseminated disease and late disease are treated with the same antibiotics but for a longer period; recurrent arthritis and CNS disease are treated with parenteral ceftriaxone or penicillin.

Rickettsial Disease

Rickettsia rickettsii is the most common (**Rocky Mountain spotted fever** [RMSF]) in the United States, and is the second most common vector-borne illness; **ticks** are the reservoirs and vectors, and transmit the agent to mammals during feeding. Most cases occur in the **southeastern U.S.** (dog tick) and less in the northern Rocky Mountain states (wood tick). Severe vascular obstruction (vasculitis) → gangrene and involvement of other organs (CNS, heart, lungs, GI tract, and kidneys), **disseminated intravascular coagulation (DIC)**, and **death** (or significant long-term sequelae)

- The major initial symptoms are **fever, headache, myalgia**, nausea, and vomiting (often with abdominal pain and diarrhea); **rash develops before the 6th day of illness** first on the **wrists and ankles** (macular, maculopapular, and then often **petechial, hemorrhagic** with **palpable purpura**) and spreads to the **palms and soles** and proximally to the rest of the body.
- The most widely used test is the **indirect immunofluorescence antibody assay**: titer-increase between acute and convalescent sera.
- **Doxycycline** is the drug of choice for children of any age, with treatment based on clinical likelihood of illness (best outcome if begun <5 days of illness).

Ehrlichiosis: infective agent from genus *Ehrlichia* and *Anaplasma*; Gram-negative cocci that cause human **monocytic ehrlichiosis (HME)** or **granulocytic ehrlichiosis (HGE)**; most cases of HME in southeastern and south central U.S., and HGE in north central and northeastern U.S.; transmitted by **tick bite**, (peak May through July); **similar clinical presentation to RMSF** but with **leukopenia (HME and HGE), neutropenia (HGA), anemia, thrombocytopenia**, hepatitis (hepatosplenomegaly), **hyponatremia** (in almost all), and rash; uncommon complications include severe pulmonary, CNS, cardiac, or renal involvement; the disease usually lasts 4–12 days. Diagnosis is demonstrated by seroconversion; PCR is fairly sensitive early in the disease; the drug of choice for all patients is **doxycycline**.

Brucellosis

Brucella species are small, Gram-negative coccobacilli; **humans are accidental hosts** (direct contact with wild or infected animals or unpasteurized dairy products); **increased risk with animal-based occupations** from inoculation through skin, inhalation, contact with conjunctival mucosa, or oral ingestion; children have a mild, self-limited disease compared to the more chronic disease in adults; nonspecific findings (fever, malaise, night sweats, weight loss, arthralgia, and myalgia with hepatosplenomegaly, lymphadenopathy, and arthritis). The organism may be recovered in the blood, bone marrow, or other tissues; also diagnosed with serum agglutination test or increase in acute to convalescent antibody titers. Relapses are common if undertreated—best regimen is doxycycline + rifampin for 4–6 weeks plus streptomycin IM or gentamicin IM **or** IV for 1–2 weeks; **for children <8 years of age:** use TMP/SMX plus rifampin for 4–6 weeks.

Pasteurella multocida

The most common human *Pasteurella* pathogen; **anaerobic**, Gram-negative coccobacilli or rods found primarily as pathogens in animals (**oral flora of almost all cats and up to half of dogs** and many other animals), with transmission occurring most commonly from the **bite of a cat or dog** (also respiratory-tract spread from animals to humans); most common manifestation is **cellulitis within 24 hours at the site of inoculation**, including a serosanguineous or purulent discharge plus fever, chills, and regional lymphadenopathy (may also have local infective complications, e.g., septic arthritis); drug of choice is an **aminopenicillin**.

Meningococcal Infections

Neisseria meningitidis: Gram-negative diplococcus; most common disease-producing strains are **A** (epidemics elsewhere in the world), **B, C, Y** (each accounting for about 30%), and **W-135** (**vaccine contains A, C, Y, and W-135**); **asymptomatic colonization of the upper respiratory tract with transmission through respiratory droplets (close contacts at increased risk)**; increased severity and recurrence in those with **terminal complement deficiencies, deficiency of C3 and properdin, and functional and anatomic asplenia**; patients are no longer contagious after 24 hours of appropriate antibiotic therapy.

Meningococcemia: abrupt onset of fever and nonspecific findings, with evidence of **poor perfusion** then the development of a **rash** (in only a small number of patients), which begins as **maculopapular or petechial and may develop into purpura fulminans** (purpuric rash, shock, heart and renal failure, adrenal hemorrhage, and death). The drug of choice is **high-dose penicillin G**.

Salmonella

Gram-negative bacilli with over 2,000 known serotypes; reservoirs for **nontyphoidal** *Salmonella* are animals (ingestion of **contaminated poultry, beef, fish, and dairy products**, also other contaminated foods, water, and pet reptiles).

- **S. typhi** is found only in humans; direct contact or contaminated fomite; most U.S. cases are acquired from **international travel**; prolonged fecal excretion (may be **prolonged with antibiotic therapy**); **typhoid fever:** high fever and constitutional symptoms, then **abdominal pain and tenderness, hepatosplenomegaly**, changes in mental status, and **rose spots** (maculopapular erythematous lesions appearing in crops over 2–3 days, mostly on lower chest and abdomen from days 7–10 of illness); course is usually 2–4 weeks without complications; rates of chronic carriage are low in children (increases with age and gallbladder disease).
- **Nontyphoidal organisms** (*S. typhimurium, S. enteritidis*, and others) cause asymptomatic carriage, **gastroenteritis**, bacteremia, and focal infections.
- No antimicrobial therapy for healthy children >3 months of age with noninvasive gastroenteritis; antibiotic treatment for typhoid depends on severity and resistance (amoxicillin, ampicillin, azithromycin, ceftriaxone, cefixime, or a fluoroquinolone) plus supportive therapy.

Shigella

Gram-negative bacilli with four species (*S. dysenteriae* is rare in the United States; **S. sonnei and then S. flexneri** are most common causes of dysentery); humans are the natural host, with fecal-oral transmission (also ingestion of contaminated food and water, fomite transmission, and intercourse); **more common in older children**; no chronic carrier state; **watery diarrhea to bloody diarrhea with systemic symptoms**; some organisms make toxin (**Shiga toxin**—*S. dysenteriae,* Shiga toxin-producing *E. coli*); the most common complication is **dehydration**; **neurological** abnormalities are the most common extraintestinal manifestations (meningismus, **seizures**, encephalopathy). Antibiotics are used to decrease the length and severity of illness, shedding, and infection of others: **ceftriaxone** may be used for empiric therapy (best initial treatment); alternative drugs include nalidixic acid or azithromycin.

Campylobacter

Gram-negative bacilli; **intestinal disease** usually associated with *C. jejuni* and *C. coli*; **extraintestinal disease** with *C. fetus* (neonates and debilitated hosts; bacteremia, meningitis, endocarditis); reservoir is the GI tract of domestic and wild birds and animals, with transmission from contaminated food, untreated water, or unpasteurized dairy products, or directly by the fecal-oral route; peak infection in early childhood and young adults; other immunoreactive complications can occur during the convalescent phase, including reactive arthritis (see Chapter 10), Reiter syndrome (arthritis, urethritis, conjunctivitis), erythema nodosum, and IgA nephropathy. **Antibiotics** (erythromycin or azithromycin) are indicated with dysentery, with any severe disease, and with any underlying problem or systemic presentation (parenteral aminoglycoside or carbapenem).

Yersinia enterocolitica

Gram-negative coccobacilli; principal source is **feral animals** (especially swine) **and pets** with transmission through contact with infected animals or contaminated food, water, or blood products; not as common in United States; fever, abdominal pain, and diarrhea that may **mimic appendicitis** (mesenteric adenitis); especially <7 years of age; systemic and focal complications are not common; also **postinfectious reactive complications** (as with *Campylobacter*); enterocolitis in healthy children is self-limited and should not be treated; systemic infection, infection in the very young, or in those with underlying conditions should be treated: most strains are sensitive to TMP/SMX for milder cases and parenteral third-generation cephalosporin with or without aminoglycoside for more severe.

Anaerobes

Clostridium botulinum: Gram-positive, spore-forming, obligate anaerobe occurring worldwide in soil, dust, and marine sediments; botulism is produced by the **neurotoxin** (heat labile): blocks neuromuscular transmission; death secondary to **airway and respiratory muscle paralysis**. All forms begin as **asymmetric, descending, flaccid paralysis beginning with muscles supplied by the cranial nerves (multiple bulbar palsies) and no fever**.

- **Infant botulism** (increased risk of spore ingestion from **honey**); almost all cases between ages 3 weeks–6 months; initial finding: **constipation**, lethargy, weak cry, decreased movement, and feeding difficulty; then **drooling, diminished gag and suck, oculomotor palsies, poor head control,** and **respiratory arrest**
- **Foodborne botulism:** outbreaks from many sources of canned (most common source—**home-canned foods**) and un-canned foods in all areas of the United States. **Wound botulism:** contamination of traumatized tissue (crush injuries, gross trauma) or injection of contaminated heroin
- Treatment of infant botulism is with human **botulism immune globulin (BIG, IV) and supportive care**; older patients with suspected botulism are treated with **1 vial of equine botulinum antitoxin**; antibiotics are only used for secondary infections and wound botulism.

Clostridium perfringens: widespread in nature and in raw meat and poultry; spores germinate during **slow cooling and storage** (common is with preparation of large quantities of food that are being kept warm); **enterotoxin** produced by the organism in the lower intestine produces symptoms; **sudden onset of watery diarrhea with severe, crampy midepigastric pain without fever resolving within 24 hours**; usually no treatment is required (supportive).

Clostridium tetani: normal inhabitant of soil and animal and human intestines; causes illness through effects of: **tetanus toxin** (binds to myoneural junction of skeletal muscle and in the spinal cord, then blocks inhibition to motor neurons); occurs worldwide and is **endemic in many developing countries**; greatest risk of infection with **contaminated wounds with devitalized tissue and deep puncture wounds**

- **Neonatal tetanus** (3–12 days of age; decreased ability to suck and swallow, constant crying, decreased movement, spasms, and rigidity) is very common in **Africa** (women not immunized and **nonsterile umbilical cord practices**).
- **Generalized tetanus: trismus** (lockjaw) and **severe muscle spasm**; intractable spasms of facial muscles: **sardonic smile** (risus sardonicus); progressively more severe over a week and generalized (extreme hyperextension: **opisthotonos**); **laryngeal and airway spasm** can lead to obstruction and death; **tetanic seizures: sudden, severe tonic contractions with high fever** while the patient is conscious and in extreme pain (no impairment of sensory or cortical function); in survivors, the symptoms decrease gradually over 2–4 weeks.
- The organism is not always visible on Gram stain and is hard to isolate, so the **diagnosis is a clinical one**.
- A single dose of **human tetanus immune globulin (TIG)** is the treatment as soon as possible (cannot be neutralized after axonal ascent) plus either **penicillin G or metronidazole** and muscle relaxants (diazepam).

Other anaerobic infections (*Bacteroides*, *Fusobacterium*, *Peptostreptococcus*, *Veillonella*, and others): **myonecrosis** (gas gangrene; *C. perfringens*), **skin and soft-tissue infections**, tissue ulceration caused by **pressure necrosis** and lack of adequate blood supply, **bites, and foreign bodies**; **genital tract infections** (pelvic inflammatory disease, vaginitis, tubo-ovarian abscesses); **intestinal rupture** (especially the colon; abscess, peritonitis); **respiratory system disease**: upper (chronic sinusitis, chronic otitis, peritonsillar abscess, deep pharyngeal node abscess, and periodontal disease) and lower (foreign-body obstruction, aspiration); and **brain abscesses and subdural empyema**

Treponema pallidum (acquired syphilis; see Chapter 1 for congenital)

- Mobile spirochete requiring **darkfield microscopy or direct immunofluorescent staining**; acquired by **sexual contact, perinatally, or by exposure to infected blood or tissues**
- **Primary syphilis:** syphilitic genital **chancre** (painless papule → clean, painless ulcer; very contagious) **and regional adenitis** 2–6 weeks after initial infection and heals in 4–6 weeks
- If not treated, develops **secondary syphilis** (spirochetes in the blood) 2–10 weeks after the chancre heals; **maculopapular rash that can cover the entire body, including the palms and soles; condyloma lata** (wartlike plaques around the anus and vagina); low-grade fever and constitutional symptoms with **generalized lymphadenitis**; other focal sites of infection including CNS, renal, hepatic, and ocular
- Without treatment, becomes **latent** within 1–2 months after the onset of the rash with **relapses over a year (early latent period**; no further relapses after 1 year).
- Without treatment, **late syphilis** develops: either asymptomatic (**late latent**) or symptomatic, which is **tertiary syphilis with cardiovascular, CNS, and gummatous lesions** (granulomas of the skin and musculoskeletal system).

- **Diagnosis: Best method**—organisms on darkfield microscopy or direct immuno-fluorescent staining, (not widely available); **screen with a nontreponemal test**—either the **VDRL** (Venereal Disease Research Laboratory) or the **RPR** (rapid plasma regain); gives **quantitative results that correlate with disease activity and decreases with adequate treatment**. Confirm positive results with an **antibody-specific treponemal test**: *T. pallidum* hemagglutination assay (TPHA), *T. pallidum* particle agglutination (TPPA), or fluorescent treponemal antibody absorption test (FTA-ABS). Not quantitative and become **positive after the initial infection and remain positive for life** (so are good for diagnosis of first episode and for a false-positive nontreponemal test). For neurosyphilis: CSF pleocytosis with increased protein and a **positive CSF VDRL** and neurological symptoms.
- **Treatment:** Primary, secondary, and early latent: **benzathine penicillin G** 50,000 U/kg IM (max. 2.4 million U, the adult dose); latent syphilis or of more than 1 year's duration, except neurosyphilis: same dosing of benzathine penicillin G given as **three weekly injections** (max. each dose 2.4 million U); neurosyphilis: **aqueous crystalline penicillin G** 200,000–300,000 U/kg/day divided every 4–6 hours for 10–14 days (max. 24 million U per day). For allergic patients other than with neurosyphilis or for children >8 years of age, use **doxycycline or tetracycline**; for others, **oral penicillin desensitization** (administered over 4 hours in the hospital).

Mycobacterium tuberculosis

- Non–spore-forming tubercle bacilli; acid-fast, weakly Gram-positive obligate aerobic rods
- Majority of U.S. cases are foreign-born (mostly children <5 years of age and young adults). **Person-to-person by airborne droplets from a person with cavitary pulmonary TB.** Highest risk in **urban, low-income areas in nonwhite persons** (highest in first-generation immigrants from high-prevalence areas); increased **drug resistance** throughout the world
- **Latent TB infections:** positive TB skin test with no physical or radiographic evidence of active disease; **TB disease** is infection where there are signs, symptoms, and/or radiographic findings of active disease and/or of extrapulmonary disease.

Diagnosis

- Isolation of the organism: attempt **sputum culture**, even though most younger children (and many adolescents) will not voluntarily produce sputum (induce with a nebulizer, chest percussion, and suctioning); **best method is an early-morning gastric aspirate** (before getting out of bed or eating) on three consecutive mornings using fluorescent staining methods and culture or PCR.
- **TB skin testing** (Mantoux): 5 tuberculin units of **purified protein derivative (PPD)** given intradermal; bacilli Calmette-Guérin (BCG) vaccine is not a contraindication (any person with a positive result then needs a chest x-ray). The test is read (diameter of induration in mm) 48–72 hours after placement by a trained person. **A negative test**

does not exclude latent disease or infection (various factors can lead to an initial non-reactive test). **Induration ≥15 mm** is a positive test for all children who are ≥4 years of age without risk factors; **induration ≥10 mm** is considered positive for those at risk of disseminated disease (children <4 and those with certain underlying medical conditions) and with increased exposure; **induration of ≥5 mm** is positive for those children in close contact with known or suspected TB cases, children already suspected of having the disease, or those on immunosuppressive therapy.

- Assess risk of exposure to TB during routine health-care visits; those with **increased risk of contact with contagious people or children with suspected disease should receive a PPD**; household evaluation is indicated if another member of the household converts from negative to positive. Initial PPD should be performed before the start of any immunosuppressive therapy.

Clinical presentation

Most childhood infections are **asymptomatic**.

- With disease, most common symptoms (1–6 months after infection): low-grade fever and nonspecific constitutional symptoms; infants are more likely to have symptoms (nonproductive cough, mild dyspnea, and failure-to-thrive) or evidence of bronchial obstruction (tachypnea, localized wheezing, decreased breath sounds).
- Primary TB complex (Ghon complex): **local infection at the site of entry with regional adenopathy (almost all are lung)**; most prominent finding is **large hilar adenitis** (which may cause bronchial compression and distal atelectasis); **pleural effusions** are common and generally asymptomatic; organism is carried to tissues via blood and lymphatics over the next 2 weeks to 3 months; **disseminated TB** always occurs and is usually asymptomatic (unless large number of organisms and a poor host response) and is more common in young children (high fever, productive cough, weight loss, night sweats; high incidence of meningitis and peritonitis); healing of the primary lesion occurs with **fibrosis, calcification** (takes 6–12 months), or **caseous necrosis** (liquefaction of the parenchyma; which could rupture into a bronchus and blood, leaving a **cavitary lesion**) → **military dissemination**
- **Reactivation** is rare in younger children (more common in adolescents) **extensive pulmonary infiltrates or cavities in the upper lobes**; symptoms: **fever**, malaise, anorexia, weight loss, **cough, hemoptysis, night sweats, chest pain** (with little or no physical findings)
- Relatively small numbers present with **extrapulmonary TB**. Most common form is **scrofula (superficial lymph nodes)**; presents as a gradual increase in nodes (firm, non-tender, and usually unilateral; often leads to caseating necrosis). Other extrapulmonary manifestations are **meningitis**, bone and joint (mostly **vertebral**) disease, skin, middle-ear and mastoid disease, and renal disease.

Treatment

- **Latent TB:** isoniazid (INH) for 9 months (if INH-susceptible); rifampin for 6 months (if INH-resistant)
- **Pulmonary and extrapulmonary disease** (non-meningitis): 2 months of INH plus rifampin plus pyrazinamide, then 4 months of INH plus rifampin
- **Meningitis:** 2 months of INH plus rifampin plus pyrazinamide plus either an aminoglycoside (streptomycin preferred) or ethionamide (until sensitivities are known) and prednisone for 6–8 weeks, followed by 7–10 months of INH plus rifampin
- Most common **adverse effects:**
  - **INH: hepatitis, liver enzyme elevation, peripheral neuritis**; pyridoxine (INH inhibition of pyridoxine metabolism) needed only for children on meat- or milk-deficient diets
  - **Rifampin:** vomiting, flulike illness, **hepatitis, thrombocytopenia, orange discoloration of secretions**
  - **Ethambutol: optic neuritis**, decreased red-green discrimination, GI-tract disturbances
  - **Pyrazinamide:** hepatotoxicity, hyperuricemia
  - **Streptomycin:** rash, **nephrotoxicity, auditory and vestibular toxic effects**
  - **Ethionamide:** GI disturbances, **hepatotoxicity**

Preventive methods

- **BCG vaccine:** live vaccine used in many countries around the world but not routinely in the United States; does not prevent infection with *M. tuberculosis* (has had little effect on control of TB throughout the world); has protective effect against miliary TB and meningitis in children. CDC recommends BCG use in infants and children with a negative PPD who are not infected with HIV for: a child who is continuously exposed to a person with contagious TB resistant to INH and rifampin, or who is continuously exposed to a person with untreated or ineffectively treated contagious pulmonary TB and the child cannot be removed from the exposure or given anti-TB therapy.
- **Control measures:** people exposed in the past 3 months to a contagious person should have a PPD and chest x-ray; all exposed household contacts under age 4 years and all those with any immunodeficiency should start INH (as long as active infection is excluded). Children with disease can return to child care and school after starting on appropriate therapy and showing significant improvement.
- **TB during pregnancy:** INH (and pyridoxine) plus rifampin plus ethambutol (all safe for the fetus) recommended for at least 9 months if mother has TB during pregnancy; and INH (after the first trimester) with latent TB
- **Congenital TB:** rare, but can occur with material bacteremia; if suspected, perform cultures (including placental), lumbar puncture, PPD (usually negative), and chest x-ray and the infant started on isoniazid plus rifampin plus pyrazinamide plus streptomycin until infection and sensitivities are confirmed. Corticosteroids are added if the newborn has meningitis.

Managing the newborn whose mother is at risk or has TB

- If the mother has **a positive PPD but is asymptomatic with a normal chest x-ray**, no separation from the newborn and no evaluation or therapy in the newborn. Evaluate all household members.
- If the mother has a **positive PPD and abnormal chest x-ray**, separate from newborn until she has been evaluated, including sputum cultures; if the x-ray, exam, and sputum are not consistent with active disease, no further separation; treat mother appropriately. Evaluate all household members.
- If x-ray or sputum shows **evidence of active TB**, institute treatment of the mother and start the newborn on INH; further separation only for evidence of drug resistance, noncompliance to treatment, or severe illness requiring hospitalization (until mother is considered to be noninfectious). Continue INH in the infant until mother's sputum cultures are negative for 3 consecutive months, then place a PPD on the infant. If positive, continue INH for another 9 months; if negative, discontinue the INH.
- **TB and breastfeeding:** INH is secreted in breast milk but there are no adverse effects; breast-fed infants do not need pyridoxine unless they are receiving INH.

Nontuberculous (Atypical) Mycobacteria

Most commonly seen in infected children: *Mycobacterium avium complex* (MAC; seen mostly with HIV and CF), *M. kansasii* (tap water), *M. marinum* (water in an aquarium), *M. fortuitum*, and *M. abscessus;* found in soil, food, water, and animals; usually as a result of skin abrasions, surgical incisions, or entry from the mouth, throat, or respiratory or GI tracts; most infections are localized at entry site with regional adenopathy; dissemination in immunocompromised persons (MAC); no person-to-person transmission.

Most common clinical presentation in children is cervical lymphadenitis (MAC), otitis media (*M. abscessus;* contaminated tympanostomy tubes), central catheter infections (*M. fortuitum*), skin infection (*M. abscessus, M. fortuitum,* and *M. marinum*), osteomyelitis (MAC, *M. kansasii, and M. fortuitum*), and lung disease (MAC, *M. kansasii, M. abscessus*). **Definitive diagnosis** is by isolation of the organism; **may have a positive PPD** (usually <10 mm). **Therapy** of adenitis is by complete surgical excision (no advantage to anti-TB drugs); otherwise, therapy is specific to the organism.

FUNGAL PATHOGENS
Candida Species

Most infections from *Candida albicans;* other species cause infections in compromised hosts, premature infants, and those with central venous catheters. *C. albicans* is present on the skin and in the mouth, intestinal tract, and vagina; infants are colonized in the GI, respiratory tract, and skin in the first 2 weeks of life. The **organism grows** on blood agar.

Infections in immunocompetent children

- **Diaper dermatitis:** confluent erythema (papular) with erythematous **satellite lesions** in the perineum; often with **antibiotic use**; treatment with frequent diaper changes, aeration, and the use of **a topical antifungal** (nystatin, clotrimazole, miconazole) and possibly a **topical corticosteroid** for 1–2 days.
- **Oral thrush:** white plaques on lips, tongue, buccal mucosa, and palate; attempt at removal leads to **punctate bleeding**; uncommon after first year; **use of antibiotics** may lead to recurrent/persistent infection (if no underlying cause, may be first sign of **immunodeficiency or endocrine disorder**). Treatment is with **oral nystatin** (to each side of the mouth four times per day).
- **Vulvovaginitis:** common in **pubertal and adolescent girls** (oral antibiotic use, poor hygiene, oral contraceptives, pregnancy); in prepubertal girls, is usually from prolonged antibiotic use or diabetes; presents with pain or itching, vulvar/vaginal erythema, and a **white, cheesy vaginal discharge**. Treatment is with vaginal creams or troches of nystatin, clotrimazole, or miconazole, **or a single oral dose of fluconazole** (also for persistent infection).

Infections in immunocompromised children

- **Catheter infections:** increased risk if **neutropenia, broad-spectrum antibiotic** use, and **prolonged TPN** (especially with intralipids); risk for disseminated disease; treatment is **removal of the catheter and IV amphotericin B** for 2–3 weeks.
- **Cancer and transplant patients: neutropenia** from chemotherapy (significant increased risk after 5 days); if **fever and neutropenia** present for **at least 5 days, amphotericin B** is started as empiric therapy (or voriconazole or caspofungin, which are newer and safer drugs); significantly increased in **bone-marrow transplant patients** due to prolonged neutropenia (most infection in lung, kidney, liver, and spleen); **fluconazole** usually used prophylactically (also in solid-organ transplant patients).
- **HIV:** most common are oral thrush and diaper dermatitis; also severe, persist **mucocutaneous candidiasis** (progressing to esophagitis), dermatitis; treatment is usually with systemic **itraconazole or fluconazole. Chronic mucocutaneous candidiasis** is associated with immunodeficiency (primary defect of T-lymphocyte responsiveness to *Candida*), endocrine disorders (diabetes, Addison disease), and may involve the esophagus and larynx.

Infections in neonates

Increased with **very low birth weight, prolonged central venous catheter use** (especially with TPN), prolonged mechanical ventilation, abdominal surgery, and use of broad-spectrum antibiotics; sepsis, renal fungal balls, CNS abscess, endocarditis

- **Parenteral amphotericin** for systemic candidiasis (nephrotoxic; use **lipid-complex formulations** if impaired renal function); add **flucytosine** for CNS and kidney infections; **fluconazole, voriconazole, or itraconazole** is very useful for renal infections; **caspofungin** may be used with resistant organisms or failure of other therapies.

Aspergillus

Mold on decaying vegetation and in soil; **most common cause of infection** is *Aspergillus fumigatus;* **route of transmission** is inhalation of conidia (asexual fungal spores) → respiratory tract colonization; is no person-to-person spread. Immunocompromised (especially with respect to neutrophil function) are at risk for dissemination and invasive disease; skin infection can follow direct contact with traumatized skin.

Noninvasive disease

Otomycosis: mycelia in the ear canal that leads to chronic ear infections (tropical and subtropical regions); skin infection: nosocomial; mostly in premature neonates and immunocompromised persons; sinusitis: chronic infection of one sinus; aspergilloma: fungal balls in bronchi and seen with TB, bronchiectasis, pulmonary cysts, and congenital heart disease; the **major risk** is hemoptysis.

Invasive disease

Seen with **immunocompromised** patients with **prolonged neutropenia or impaired phagocytic function**; most: sinusitis, pneumonia, skin infection (ecthyma gangrenosum), and eye infection (endophthalmitis); less common: CNS, bone, and heart. **Drug of choice** is parenteral voriconazole.

Hypersensitivity

Most common is **allergic bronchopulmonary aspergillosis**: can complicate chronic pulmonary disease (steroid-dependent asthma and cystic fibrosis); **definitive diagnosis**: reversible airway obstruction, elevated serum IgE, peripheral blood eosinophilia, a positive *A. fumigatus* scratch test, *A. fumigatus*—IgG antibodies, pulmonary infiltrates, and bronchiectasis (diagnostic without this finding). **Acute exacerbations** are treated with oral prednisone, usually for 6 weeks; antifungal therapies are not yet recommended in children; end result is **pulmonary fibrosis**.

Histoplasma

Histoplasma capsulatum is endemic in the eastern and central U.S., especially **the Ohio, Missouri, and Mississippi river valleys** (grows in **moist soil, facilitated by bird and bat droppings**); spores are spread with wind or disturbances of soil; infection occurs when **inhaled. No person-to-person transmission**. Can be grown on standard fungal media; rapid identification is with detection of the polysaccharide antigen in serum, urine, or bronchoalveolar lavage by radioimmunoassay.

Causes symptoms in very few, most with acute pulmonary disease (**flulike with chest pain, hilar adenopathy, and mild pulmonary infiltrates for up to 2 weeks**). Inhalation of large numbers of spores can produce more severe respiratory symptoms, prolonged fever, and weight loss, with **erythema nodosum** in adolescents. Children <2 years can develop **progressive disseminated histoplasmosis** (rare). Children with severe or prolonged disease should be treated with **amphotericin B**. Itraconazole is effective for the treatment of mild disseminated disease in HIV patients.

Coccidioides

Coccidioides immitis is **found in soil of dry, arid areas** of California (San Joaquin Valley; Valley fever), Arizona, New Mexico, northern Utah, and Texas; **infection** is through inhalation of dust-borne arthroconidia (dust storms, earthquakes, digging); **no person-to-person transmission**.

Primary infection (respiratory) is asymptomatic or mild **in the majority of children; symptomatic disease**: dry cough, chest pain, and frequently a rash (diffuse erythematous maculopapular, erythema multiforme, and tibial erythema nodosum); **chest x-ray** shows consolidation and hilar or mediastinal lymphadenopathy. Rarely infection disseminates and looks similar to progressive primary TB. There may be residual lesions (cavities, granulomas, or fibrocavitary pulmonary disease). An **IgM** is positive in the first few weeks after the appearance of symptoms; a **DNA probe** can identify the organism in cultures.

Therapy for those at high risk for disseminated disease: **amphotericin B** initially for severe, disseminated disease (non-CNS), and **fluconazole** for CNS infections; **fluconazole, ketoconazole, itraconazole, or voriconazole** for less severe infections.

PARASITIC PATHOGENS

Helminths

Table 15.5: Most Common Helminthic Infections in the United States

	Enterobius vermicularis	*Ascaris lumbricoides*	*Necator americanus*	*Taeniae*	*Cysticercosis*
Infection	Pinworm infection (roundworm; nematode)	Ascariasis (nematode)	Hookworm (nematode)	*Taenia solium* (pork tapeworm) and *T. saginata* (beef tapeworm) (cestodes)	Infection with the intermediate stage of *T. solium*
Epidemiology	Most common helminthic infection in United States; more common in temperate regions	Most common helminthic infection in the world; more common in tropical regions; in United States, highest prevalence in preschool children	*N. americanus* is most common cause in United States; larvae in warm, moist soil, especially rural areas where human feces used for fertilization and with poor sanitation	Worldwide animal inhabitant; only adult stages in human intestine	Most common worldwide parasitic infection of the CNS (neurocysticercosis); poor sanitation and fecal fertilization near cattle and swine; eggs found only in human feces (humans are the only definitive host)

(continued)

	Enterobius vermicularis	*Ascaris lumbricoides*	*Necator americanus*	*Taeniae*	*Cysticercosis*
Acquisition and spread	Fecal-oral spread (contaminated fingers, nails, clothing, bedding); within families and institutional settings	Hand-mouth or from contaminated raw fruits and vegetables	Penetrates skin, or by ingestion	Raw or undercooked infected meat	Ingestion of undercooked contaminated pork
Pathogenesis	Inhabit ileocecal region; females migrate to perianal area at night to deposit eggs	Ova hatch in small intestine → larvae → penetrate intestinal wall → migration to lungs via veins (pulmonary ascariasis) → swallowed with coughing → intestine → adult worms	After skin penetration → venous circulation → lungs → swallowed → intestine (or after ingestion) → male and female worms attach to intestinal wall → deposit eggs. Cause bleeding (rupture of capillaries in lamina propria); can remain up to 5 years.	Ingestion → anterior segment (scolex) anchors to bowel wall and adds flattened segments (proglottids) distally over 2–3 months; the last segment contains many eggs → passed into stool	Ingestion → intestinal infection with adult worms; eggs produced liberate oncospheres, which cross the intestinal wall and spread hematogenously to any organ (especially muscle and brain) → produce fluid-filled cyst with a single protoscolex
Clinical presentation	Nocturnal perianal pruritus	Most without symptoms; most common are pulmonary (cough, dyspnea, pulmonary infiltrates plus blood eosinophilia) and intestinal or biliary obstruction (cholecystitis, pancreatitis)	Most common is Fe-deficiency anemia, hypoalbuminemia and edema (from blood loss proportional to number of worms); if prolonged: decreased growth and development; may have abdominal pain, diarrhea, and anorexia, and cough during pulmonary phase	Nonspecific abdominal findings positive for anal pruritus; proglottids can be seen during stool passage	Almost all present with seizures; any neurological (including spinal cord) finding or change in behavior or cognition; also eye disease, myositis, carditis

(continued)

Table 15.5: Most Common Helminthic Infections in the United States *(cont.)*

	Enterobius vermicularis	*Ascaris lumbricoides*	*Necator americanus*	*Taeniae*	**Cysticercosis**
Diagnosis	Place cellophane tape to perianal area in A.M.; preserve in ethyl alcohol for microscopic exam; also wet mount of stool from rectal exam	Characteristic eggs in fecal smears	Eosinophilia and characteristic eggs on fecal smear	Proglottids in stool samples; the scolex is species-diagnostic	Proglottids may be seen in feces only in some; serum antibody testing is sensitive; CSF shows eosinophilia; need MRI: most common finding is single cyst (and may see the protoscolex within) with significant calcification
Treatment	Single PO dose mebendazole or albendazole, repeat in 2 weeks	No good Rx for pulmonary phase; intestinal: albendazole, mebendazole, or pyrantel pamoate	Albendazole, mebendazole, or pyrantel pamoate (may need combination and multiple doses); rare need for Fe supplementation or blood transfusion	Praziquantel or niclosamide	Natural history is to resolve spontaneously; treat seizures; may need VP shunt if there is ventricular obstruction; albendazole (with corticosteroids initially) is the drug of choice: enhances resolution of lesions and decreases recurrent seizures; not indicated for only degenerating or calcified lesions; does not lead to change in acute symptoms

Abbreviations: central nervous system, CNS; cerebrospinal fluid, CSF; ventriculoperitoneal, VP

Entamoeba histolytica

Pathogenic species of *Entamoeba* causing **amebiasis**; most cases in the United States are in **travelers to endemic areas or immigrants**; **transmission** by the fecal-oral route or contaminated food or water; ingestion of cysts → exocysts in small intestine form trophozoites → colonize lumen of the colon and may invade mucosa

Clinical presentation

- Ranges from asymptomatic cyst passage to colitis (amebic dysentery; colicky abdominal pain, diarrhea with tenesmus, blood, mucus, but few leukocytes and little constitutional symptoms) or extraintestinal disease (mainly hepatic abscess from disseminated infection even months to years later).
- **Presents** as fever; abdominal pain with a tender, enlarged liver; increased hepatic enzymes; increased erythrocyte sedimentation rate (ESR) and anemia; **more severe disease** (rapidly progressing) in very young or malnourished patient.

Diagnosis—Antigen in stool by enzyme immunoassay, **microscopic exam of fresh stool; serum antibody tests.**

Treatment—**For moderate to severe intestinal symptoms or extraintestinal disease:** metronidazole or tinidazole, followed by paromomycin or iodoquinol; **for asymptomatic cyst excreters**: treat with paromomycin or iodoquinol. Image-guided aspiration of cysts.

Toxoplasma gondii

- **Obligate intracellular protozoa (only known species of *Toxoplasma*)** that is present in animals throughout the world
- **Transmission** mostly orally, transplacentally (**primary maternal infection during gestation**; see Chapter 1) or in a transplanted organ or blood transfusion (seropositive donor with latent infection)
- **Latent encysted eggs** persist for life (tissue cysts mostly in skeletal muscle, CNS and cardiac muscle)
- Usually newly infected cats (**definitive hosts**; from other infected cats or by ingestion of contaminated meat) excrete oocytes (then must sporulate before infective)
- **Human infection** from cat or by ingestion of raw or undercooked contaminated meat (sheep, pigs, cattle are intermediate hosts)

Acquired toxoplasmosis

- Most cases are **asymptomatic**. Symptoms are **nonspecific** if present (fever, rash, malaise, arthralgia, myalgia)
- **Most common sign** is cervical adenopathy (tender and nonsuppurative; resolves without treatment); also hepatosplenomegaly, hepatitis, meningitis, encephalitis, brain abscess, pneumonitis, pericarditis, and myocarditis, but these are all uncommon
- **Ocular disease** (chorioretinitis; can become reactivated years later) occurs in a small number (most from congenital infection)
- **Disseminated disease** (especially CNS) occurs primarily in those with **HIV**, with malignancies, and on immunosuppressive therapies.

Diagnosis—**Specific IgM antibodies** and **increase in acute to convalescent IgG titers**; also, **PCR** may be performed on urine, blood, CSF, and amniotic fluid

Treatment—Treat the following with **pyrimethamine plus sulfadiazine (plus folinic acid)**: severe, persistent acquired infections; those with organ damage or ocular disease; those who are immunosuppressed. Once disease has occurred in a patient with HIV, the patient requires lifelong suppressive therapy.

Pneumocystis carinii (jiroveci)

- **Extracellular parasite (now classified as a fungus,** based on DNA analysis) found in the lungs of mammals around the world (especially **rodents**); **organisms** (cysts containing sporozoites) **are not transmitted from one species to another**; suggested that those infecting humans be called *P. jiroveci*; **mode of transmission is unknown**; most people have asymptomatic infection (seroconversion) in the first 4 years of life.

- In the U.S., most commonly seen as an interstitial plasma-cell pneumonitis in immunocompromised (*Pneumocystis* pneumonia, PCP; see Chapters 7 and 9, and previously in this chapter). **Severe, life-threatening disease with HIV** (most commonly at 3–6 months of life), **congenital defects** in cell-mediated immunity or in persons on immunosuppressive therapy (including during induction of remission for leukemia and lymphoma).

Diagnosis—**Demonstration of organism in lung tissue** (best way is with open-lung biopsy in younger children and transbronchial biopsy in older ones) **or respiratory tract specimens** (bronchoalveolar lavage, tracheal aspirate); chest x-ray shows **bilateral, diffuse granular alveolar disease** beginning in the **perihilar area** and spreading peripherally and lastly to the apices.

Treatment—Drug of choice is **IV TMP-SMX** (oral for mild disease); if patient cannot tolerate (adverse reactions) or is unresponsive, then **IV pentamidine** (high incidence of adverse effects). Most include a **corticosteroid** early in the disease for moderate to severe illness.

Plasmodium (malaria)

- Intracellular protozoa transmitted to humans by blood-feeding of **the female *Anopheles* mosquito** (and much less commonly by blood transfusion, contaminated needles, and perinatally); four human species: ***P. falciparum, P. malariae, P. vivax, P. ovale***; highest areas of transmission in the world are **Africa, Asia, and South America** (endemic in over 100 countries); most cases in U.S. are from travelers or immigrants.
- In humans, cause fever, anemia (hemolysis, RBC splenic sequestration, and bone marrow suppression), immunologic dysfunction, and tissue hypoxia (vascular damage and obstruction leading to cerebral, cardiac, pulmonary, intestinal, and liver failure).

Clinical presentation

May have nonspecific prodromal symptoms; then paroxysms of high fever with rigors, pallor, jaundice, sweats, headache, myalgia, abdominal pain, vomiting, and diarrhea alternating with fatigue; some with severe signs and symptoms including decreased consciousness, hepatosplenomegaly, severe anemia, thrombocytopenia, hypotension, hypoglycemia, hyperkalemia, and/or respiratory obstruction. May have recurrences after primary attack from survival of erythrocytic forms in blood, or more long-term from release of merozoites from the liver. Sickle hemoglobin and hemoglobin F are protective.

Diagnosis—Consider in a **child with a fever** who has **traveled to an endemic area in the past year**. Perform thick (scan large numbers of RBCs) and thin (identify species and percentage of infected RBCs) RBC smears; obtain multiple samples per day for 3 consecutive days; also available is a monoclonal antibody test in a test strip for fingerprick sample for *P. falciparum*.

Table 15.6: Characteristics and Treatment of Malarial Species

	P. falciparum	*P. malariae*	*P. vivax*	*P. ovale*
Severity	Most severe; considered a medical emergency; huge parasitemia infecting both immature and mature cells	Mildest form; most chronic form	Less severe than *P. falciparum*	Least common; similar to *P. vivax*; often concurrent infection with *P. falciparum*
Timing and chronicity of symptoms	Symptoms often within a month of return from an endemic area; periodicity of symptoms less common than with others	Periodicity of symptoms every 3–4 days; long-term asymptomatic parasitemia because of persistence in RBCs	Periodicity of symptoms every other day; long-term relapses because of continued release of merozoites from hepatocytes	Periodicity of symptoms every other day; long-term relapses because of continued release of merozoites from hepatocytes
Complications	Serious complications: cerebral malaria, pulmonary edema, renal failure, respiratory failure, severe anemia, and vascular collapse; more common cause of congenital malaria	Nephrotic syndrome (immune complex deposition)	Hypersplenism: can cause splenic rupture (most with trauma) and death; more common cause of congenital malaria	Hypersplenism: can cause splenic rupture (most with trauma) and death
Treatment	**Uncomplicated:** 1) Chloroquine-sensitive: oral chloroquine phosphate 2) Chloroquine-resistant: quinine sulfate plus either doxycycline, tetracycline, or clindamycin OR Atovaquone-proguanil OR Mefloquine **Severe:** quinidine gluconate IV plus doxycycline, tetracycline, or clindamycin (doxycycline and clindamycin may be given IV)	**Uncomplicated:** chloroquine phosphate **Severe:** quinidine gluconate IV plus doxycycline, tetracycline, or clindamycin (doxycycline and clindamycin may be given IV)	**Uncomplicated:** 1) Chloroquine-sensitive: chloroquine phosphate plus primaquine phosphate 2) Chloroquine-resistant: quinine sulfate plus either doxycycline, tetracycline, or primaquine phosphate OR Mefloquine plus primaquine phosphate **Severe:** quinidine gluconate IV plus doxycycline, tetracycline, or clindamycin (doxycycline and clindamycin may be given IV)	**Uncomplicated:** chloroquine phosphate plus primaquine phosphate **Severe:** quinidine gluconate IV plus doxycycline, tetracycline, or clindamycin (doxycycline and clindamycin may be given IV)

Abbreviations: red blood cells, RBCs

Prevention

As in Table 15.1 + **chemoprophylaxis** (per the CDC):

- When traveling to areas **without chloroquine-resistant** *P. falciparum*: **chloroquine phosphate or hydroxychloroquine sulfate** (may be better tolerated; GI disturbances, headache, dizziness, blurred vision) once per week starting 2 weeks before travel through 4 weeks after leaving endemic area; if unable to take either, then **atovaquone-proguanil** (must weigh at least 5 kg [11 lb]; not for use in pregnancy or severe renal failure), **doxycycline** (not for children <8 years or pregnant women; GI side effects, photosensitivity, esophagitis), or **mefloquine** (not with cardiac conduction abnormalities or major psychiatric disorders).
- When traveling to areas with **resistant** *P. falciparum*: **mefloquine** weekly (2 weeks before to 4 weeks after), **atovaquone-proguanil** daily (2 days before travel through 7 days after leaving the area), or **doxycycline** daily (2 days before travel through 4 weeks after leaving area). Mefloquine is the only drug that is safe during pregnancy.
- When traveling to areas with **multidrug resistance: doxycycline or atovaquone-proguanil** as above. **Anti-relapse therapy for** *P. vivax and P. ovale*: **primaquine** (must rule out glucose-6-phosphate dehydrogenase [G6PD] deficiency first; if present, can cause fatal hemolysis) only for persons who have had prolonged exposure (decreases risk of relapses).

ENDOCRINE DISORDERS 16

EVALUATION OF STATURE (HEIGHT)

Short Stature

Definition—Height **less than 2 standard deviations (S.D.) less than the mean for age and sex**

- **Growth velocity** (GV) refers to the pattern of growth seen on the child's growth curve
- Normal growth pattern follows 1–2 major percentiles upward, which occurs with an appropriate increment in growth between measured points; **normal growth velocity represent overall health**
- **Abnormal growth velocity** represents a deviation from this normal upward pattern/ (may occur from birth or be acquired after a previous period of normal growth)

Evaluation

- Document where the child is on the growth curve and identify the growth velocity as normal or abnormal.
- **Measure the parents** and ask about **heights of other family members**; this is important for **familial short stature**, and the best estimate of **ultimate height potential** in the child (position on the growth curve at 2 years of age is most consistent with **mid-parental height**).
- Perform a thorough history and physical, including neurological evaluation, developmental assessment, nutritional history and assessment, review of systems, and family history (hereditary diseases, endocrine disorders, genetic syndromes). Assess for any previous or current medical (chronic illness, endocrine disorder) or nutritional problems which may play a role in the child's growth.
- Generally, **nutritional problems and chronic illnesses are seen with an initial decrease in weight prior to change in growth velocity and so there is a decreased weight/height ratio**; whereas other causes for short stature are seen with an **age-appropriate weight/height or increased ratio** (i.e., a decrease in growth velocity is the primary problem).
- Physical exam is most important determinant of possible genetic disorder, which may be associated with short stature (pattern of dysmorphic features).

- Do not initially perform a wide variety of laboratory tests; for the most part unhelpful.
- **Best initial test:** radiograph of nondominant hand and wrist, which is called a **bone age** (BA; looking for **skeletal maturation** compared to norms in the atlas of Greulich and Pyle)
- With normal growth, BA matures in close approximation to chronological age (CA), but in conditions of aberrant growth → delayed or even advanced.
- BA is closely related to **stage of sexual maturity** than is CA.
- The more delayed the BA, the greater is the **potential for continued (catch-up) growth**; advanced BA, premature epiphyseal closure → ultimate height < genetic potential (**stunted adult height**).
- Specific laboratory tests should be performed when a differential (or specific) diagnosis may be suggested by the history and physical.
- **Constitutional delay:** weight and height normal at birth, then slowing over the first year with **short stature (but normal growth velocity)** during childhood and a **delayed pubertal growth spurt and sexual development**; one or both parents will usually have a **history of the same pattern** with **normal adult height**. Because of the delay in BA, there is the potential for adult height based on genetic potential (midparental height estimate)

Bone Age Delayed (BA < CA)

- **Growth velocity normal:** constitutional delay*
- **Growth velocity abnormal:** chronic illness, nutritional disorder, endocrine disorder
  - **Decreased weight/height:** malnutrition, chronic illness, psychosocial deprivation
  - **Increased weight/height:** endocrine disorders

Bone Age Normal (BA = CA)

- **Growth velocity normal:** familial short stature
- **Growth velocity abnormal:** genetic syndromes, TORCH infections, teratogenic effects, skeletal dysplasias (increased weight/height)

Figure 16.1: Differential Diagnosis of Short Stature

Tall Stature

- **Defined as height >2 S.D. above the mean (>97.5%).**
- Most are due to **familial tall stature**—the parents (and perhaps other siblings) are tall, and the child has been tall throughout childhood with a **normal growth velocity** and has no positive medical history or physical findings. No evaluation is needed.
- Children with **exogenous obesity** commonly have rapid growth and in the absence of other findings, no evaluation needs to be done.
- If the history and/or physical exam is suggestive of an abnormal reason for tall stature (e.g., syndromic) or if there is accelerated growth velocity, then a diagnostic workup should be performed.

- Most important first step is to obtain a **BA** (will be close to the chronological age in cases with normal GV, or **advanced to various degrees** with pathological acceleration of growth).

Examples of other etiologies of tall stature
- Genetic: Klinefelter syndrome, XXY, Marfan syndrome
- Inborn errors of metabolism: homocystinuria
- Endocrine: hyperthyroidism, androgen or estrogen deficiencies or resistance (persistent open epiphyses and continued growth), McCune-Albright syndrome, excess growth hormone production, causes of precocious puberty
- Fetal overgrowth syndromes, e.g., Beckwith-Wiedemann syndrome

Management—Sex hormones (testosterone for boys, estrogen for girls) aids in epiphyseal closure; used for continued growth with estimated adult height (based on BA) of **more than 3 S.D. above the mean** in a child with psychosocial problems due to his height. Sex hormone use needs to be started no later than at the beginning of puberty.

PITUITARY DISORDERS

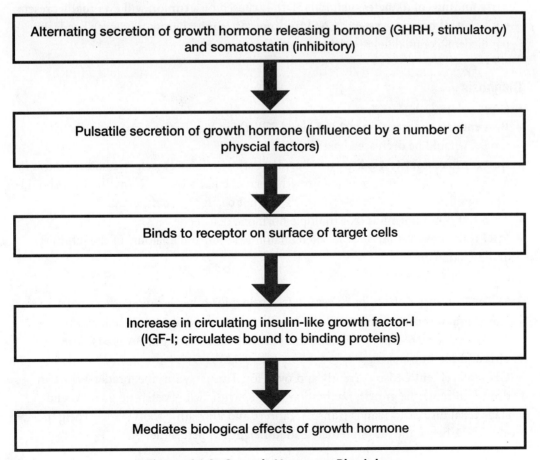

Figure 16.2: Growth Hormone Physiology

Hypopituitarism

Etiology

- May present as **isolated growth hormone deficiency or multiple hormonal deficiencies**.
- **Congenital causes:** gene mutations (often with positive family history), and anatomic abnormalities (hypoplasia, aplasia).
- **Congenital isolated growth hormone deficiency**—from deletions in the growth hormone gene (autosomal recessive, dominant, and X-linked inheritance), receptor mutations, or from an abnormality in the insulin-like growth factor (IGF)-1 gene (or binding protein or receptor).
- **Acquired causes:** any lesion (tumor, infection, trauma, vascular, hypoxic) that damages the hypothalamus or pituitary; usually presents with multiple hormone abnormalities; the most common cause is a **craniopharyngioma**.

Clinical presentation

- **Congenital:** normal birth weight and height, then **decreased growth** over first year; thyroid and adrenal deficiencies: severe **hypoglycemia**, other signs and symptoms of **hypothyroidism** (see below), seizures, **mineralocorticoid deficiency**; with **hypogonadism**: boys have a **microphallus** and various dysmorphic features.
- **Acquired: severe growth failure** then **thyroid (hypothyroid) and adrenal (hypoadrenalism) atrophy; lack of sexual maturation or regression with amenorrhea in girls; early findings of diabetes insipidus** (DI). If caused by a **tumor**, will eventually present with **central nervous system (CNS) findings** (after initial growth failure): headache, papilledema, cranial nerve palsies, visual disturbances.

Diagnosis

- **BA is delayed.**
- **Best endocrine screening test** is a blood IGF-1 and binding protein levels, matched to the BA (should be decreased based on BA).
- **Best confirmatory test** is a growth hormone stimulation test (safe method is to give IV arginine and then perform blood growth hormone [GH] level). Normally there should be a significant rise in GH levels, which will not occur with deficiency.
- Then **test other hormones** for multiple hormone deficiency
- **MRI is the best test** for an associated anatomic lesion and anatomy of the pituitary and hypothalamus.

Treatment—Growth hormone therapy (see below for other hormone therapies)

- Start **human recombinant GH (r-hGH)** as soon as the diagnosis is made (subcutaneously 6–7 days per week until growth is slowing and BA is >14 years in girls and >16 in boys).
- **GH replacement** is also currently approved for: Turner syndrome, Prader-Willi syndrome, intrauterine growth retardation (IUGR) with lack of catch-up growth, end-stage renal disease (if plan is transplantation), and idiopathic short stature (height <2.25 S.D. below the mean predicted adult height 5th percentile.

- **Potential complications with r-hGH:** leukemia (usually with other risk factors), increased risk of type 2 diabetes mellitus (DM), development of hypothyroidism or adrenal insufficiency, gynecomastia, pseudotumor cerebri, and joint abnormalities (worsening scoliosis)

Central Diabetes Insipidus (DI)

ADH and accompanying protein (neurophysin-II) synthesized in hypothalamus and stored in posterior pituitary

Released from increase in serum osmolality (main regulator of osmolality-osmoreceptors in hypothalamus) and secondarily from decreased blood volume (carotid sinus baroreceptors)*

Acts on vasopressin-2 receptors in the kidney to increase permeability of the renal collecting system to water; then thrist mechanisms occur

Figure 16.3: Antidiuretic hormone (ADH) and water homeostasis

*Volume is regulated primarily by the renin-angiotensin system with antidiuretic hormone (ADH) and natriuretic peptides (endothelial cells of vascular smooth muscle → stimulation of sodium excretion and inhibition of ADH release).

Etiology—**Gene mutations** (autosomal dominant), **malformations**, or acquired lesions (**post-surgical, trauma, infection, malignancy** [especially germinoma, pinealoma, large craniopharyngioma or optic glioma, leukemic or histiocytic infiltrates]), **drugs** (alpha-adrenergics, opiate antagonists, phenytoin)

Clinical presentation—**Severe polyuria and polydipsia** in infancy + intermittent fever, **hypernatremia, dehydration, and concentrated urine**; nocturia, enuresis, and weight loss in older children (acquired)

Diagnosis
- Clinical presentation (**pathological polyuria and polydipsia**) with:
  - **Serum osmolality >290 mOsm/kg and urine osmolality <290 mOsm/kg**
  - If serum osmolality is <300 mOsm/kg but >270 mOsm/kg, need a **water deprivation test** for confirmation and to distinguish between central and nephrogenic DI (see Chapter 14).

Treatment—For neonates and young infants: **increased free water** alone; for older children: use **long-lasting analog DDAVP (desmopressin)**, the **intranasal form** for better dosing. For acute-onset DI (e.g., postsurgical), use **IV aqueous vasopressin** (pitressin) with limitation of fluid intake (to avoid hyponatremia).

Hyperpituitarism

Primary is rare—most from **pituitary adenomas: prolactinoma** (most common pituitary tumor of adolescence), **corticotropinoma** (most common prepubertal adenoma; ACTH-producing), and **somatotropinoma**. The more common reason for increased secretion of any pituitary hormone is **secondary** (primary problem in the target gland with negative feedback).

Prolactinoma

- Much more common in **girls**
- Clinical findings: **headache, visual deficits (with large tumors), amenorrhea in girls, galactorrhea (principal finding)**; some develop findings of **hypopituitarism** (growth hormone) or **hyperpituitarism** with increases in growth hormone and/or TSH
- Diagnosis: **increased serum prolactin level**; then **MRI of brain** for lesion
- Treatment: most respond well to **bromocriptine** (dopamine agonist) or the long-acting cabergoline

Increased growth hormone production (from somatotropinoma, or due to other causes)
- Continued open epiphyses lead to **gigantism** (and acromegaly with closed epiphyses in adults)
- Clinical findings: significant **acceleration of growth velocity**, possible behavioral and visual changes and other **findings of a CNS lesion**; most occur (adenoma) around the **start of puberty**; many due to **McCune-Albright syndrome** (autonomous hyperfunctioning of many glands due to activation of cyclic AMP [cAMP] receptors: tall stature, precocious puberty, abnormal skin pigmentation, and skeletal fibrous dysplasia).
- Diagnosis: **best initial screen:** serum IGF-1 and binding protein (age-adjusted value will be increased); **confirmation:** oral glucose suppression test—administration of glucose then blood GH level; **MRI of brain** for causative lesion
- Treatment: tumors removed by **transsphenoidal surgery**, but may not lead to a complete cure; if GH levels are not normalized, then **radiation therapy** with added **somatostatin analog (octreotide)**; bromocriptine may be used additionally for those that also secrete prolactin.

PUBERTAL DISORDERS

Increased adrenocortical androgens at 6–8 years of age (adrenarche); low levels of luteinizing hormone (LH) and pulsatile discharge of gonadatropin releasing hormone (GnRH) from the hypothalamus prior to puberty

Increasing LH pulses (and synergy with follicle stimulating hormone ([FSH]) with progression of puberty → increased gonadal size

Increasing production of sex hormones (estradiol and testosterone) with daytime LH pulses → secondary sexual characteristics, bone growth and skeletal maturation (estrogens responsible)

Figure 16.4: Sex Hormone Physiology

Testicular Hypofunction

Etiology and evaluation

- **Primary hypogonadotropism (testicular = hypergonadotropic hypogonadism):** congenital absence of testes (genetic, familial), rudimentary testes (autosomal recessive or X-linked), multiple malformation syndromes (Klinefelter, Noonan, and others; see Chapter 2), chemotherapy, radiation, and testicular injury. May be evident at birth or at the time of puberty **without development of secondary sex characteristics and prepubertal appearance.**
  - Diagnosis: **low levels of testosterone with increased levels of LH and FSH.** A karyotype (and genetic evaluation) should be performed for the diagnosis of Klinefelter or other chromosomal anomalies (primarily Klinefelter variants) or non-chromosomal syndromes.

- **Secondary hypogonadism (central = hypogonadotropic hypogonadism):** testes are normal but remain prepubertal due to lack of stimulation of gonadotropin (decreased gonadotropin-releasing hormone [GnRH]). The most common etiologies are: Prader-Willi syndrome, Kallmann syndrome (X-linked; isolated gonadotropin deficiency with anosmia, mid-face defects, and renal agenesis), other syndromes, CNS malformations, or acquired lesions causing hypopituitarism (tumor, infection, trauma, chronic illness, malnutrition and anorexia nervosa).
  - Diagnosis: **prepubertal blood levels of LH and FSH and low levels of testosterone.** A **GnRH-stimulation test will not increase levels of LH** (will remain nondetectable, prepubertal). Prior to the onset of puberty must **differentiate from constitutional**

delay. (BA and family history may be helpful.) Other pituitary hormones should also be measured. If puberty has not occurred by age 15 years, a **course of testosterone** should be given; with constitutional delay, this should lead to the beginning of pubertal development and an increase in growth velocity. **Genetic evaluation** should be performed for any findings suggestive of specific syndromes. An **MRI is the best test for anatomic evaluation** of acquired lesions.

Management—Replacement therapy with a **long-acting testosterone** beginning at age 11–12 years and **human chorionic gonadotropin (hCG)** for testicular growth and spermatogenesis

Gynecomastia

- Defined as **breast tissue in a male**; common finding

- Pseudogynecomastia (adipose tissue) in overweight boys vs. true gynecomastia (glandular breast tissue) = of **estrogen:androgen imbalance**

- May be present in newborns (maternal estrogen stimulation) or early puberty (**physiological pubertal gynecomastia**) as asymmetric or symmetric, often tender enlargement of the breasts, lasting up to 2 years. Only finding is a **decreased ratio of testosterone to estradiol**. For severe, persistent cases, consider **danazol** (anti-estrogen) or, rarely, surgery.

- Other causes: familial (X-linked or autosomal dominant), hyperthyroidism, adrenal steroid biosynthetic defects, or an exogenous source of estrogen

Ovarian Hypofunction

- **Primary hypogonadism (ovarian = hypergonadotropic hypogonadism):** no prepubertal clinical findings except for Turner syndrome. Also, **pure ovarian dysgenesis** (without the features of Turner syndrome) and müllerian dysgenesis (both present as primary amenorrhea with increased blood levels of gonadotropins and ultrasound showing streak ovaries); mixed gonadal dysgenesis: mosaics presenting as **ambiguous genitalia** at birth (or female with short stature or male phenotype). **Both gonads should be removed** (germ cell tumors). Less commonly, other abnormal karyotypes (may be associated with mental retardation), other genetic syndromes, drugs, radiation, or autoimmune dysfunction (with or without other autoimmune disorders).

- **Secondary hypogonadism (central = hypogonadotropic hypogonadism):** problem with the hypothalamus or anterior pituitary leading to **low levels of LH and FSH;** most commonly the result of **hypopituitarism.** May be isolated deficiency (Kallmann syndrome) or other genetic syndromes (girls with Prader-Willi syndrome). The same diagnostic tests are done as with males, except **estradiol** is the sex hormone measured instead of testosterone.

  - **Polycystic ovary syndrome** (PCOS; Stein-Leventhal syndrome): most common cause of **anovulatory infertility; secondary amenorrhea, obesity, hirsutism, and bilaterally enlarged polycystic ovaries** (felt on exam at the onset of puberty; seen on ultrasound); also associated with **insulin resistance and the metabolic syndrome** (see below). Findings; **increase in LH and LH:FSH ratio with a decrease in sex hormone binding globulin → increase in dehydroepiandrosterone sulfate (DHEAS) and free testosterone**. Treatment is with **weight control** (and possibly an **oral hypoglycemic agent** with glucose intolerance), ovarian suppression with **oral contraceptives containing nonandrogenic progestins** (desogestrel and testolactone), and **spironolactone for hirsutism**.

Management—Early use of r-hGH for Turner syndrome; **replacement therapy with estrogen** at age 12–13 years to induce puberty, then monthly cycling of estrogen and progesterone (withdrawal bleeding on no-medication days)

Precocious Puberty

Defined as onset of puberty at **<8 years of age in a female or <9 years of age in a male**

Etiology

- Incomplete (partial):
  - **Premature adrenarche:** early onset of **sexual hair** (due to early maturation of **adrenal androgen production**) with **no other changes in sexual maturation**; somewhat **advanced height and skeletal maturation**; no treatment is needed.
  - **Premature thelarche: early breast development in girls**; most common presentation is in the **neonatal period with regression** over the first years of life—often **familial or sporadic**; no other signs of sexual maturation, and normal (undetectable) levels of LH and FSH. Later onset (after 3 years) is more consistent with **true isosexual precocity**, exogenous estrogens, or functioning follicular cysts.
  - **Premature menarche:** rare; may be idiopathic with few episodes and normal pubertal development and menstrual cycles; most prepubertal vaginal bleeding is due to other causes (trauma, foreign body, sexual abuse).

- True sexual precocity:
  - **Central precocious puberty:** usually sporadic or familial, and **idiopathic in girls** (much higher incidence); boys commonly have a **CNS lesion**. Girls more commonly have **initial anovulatory cycles; advanced height, weight, and skeletal maturity, → early epiphyseal closure and stunted adult height** without treatment. **Acquired lesions:** the most frequent is a **hypothalamic hamartoma** (GnRH-secreting neurons); also, other hypothalamic lesions or damage (irradiation); besides precocious puberty, may present with findings of a **CNS tumor** (including seizures) and **DI**.
    - **Diagnosis:** significant increase in LH and FSH with increased levels of serum testosterone in boys; in girls, estradiol is low during early puberty and then increases (i.e., the normal physiology). A **GnRH stimulation test → significant increase in LH** in boys; LH may remain low in girls, so the **best test is to stimulate with the GnRH analog leuprolide and obtain a serum estradiol** (which will then be elevated). **MRI** should be performed for the possibility of an acquired lesion.

- ° **Treatment: GnRH agonists (drug of choice = leuprolide acetate)** desensitize the cells to the effects of endogenous GnRH and stops pubertal progression and height and skeletal advancement (with increase in adult height); sexual features regress and hormones return to prepubertal levels.
- - **Peripheral precocious puberty (precocious pseudopuberty):** some sexual characteristics appear but there is no activation of gonadotropin secretion; may be isosexual or heterosexual (develop features of the opposite sex). **LH and FSH levels are low (prepubertal) with increased androgens (testosterone, DHEAS) or estrogen (estradiol).**
  - ° Causes—male: **gonadotropin-secreting tumors** (hCG-secreting hepatoblastoma; stimulates LH receptors in Leydig cells of testes → increased testosterone with low LH and FSH levels), **other tumors** (teratomas; teratocarcinomas; choriocarcinomas of the CNS, liver, and mediastinum; associated with **increased hCG and alpha-fetoprotein**), Leydig cell tumors, adrenal tumors, **CAH**, or exogenous androgens. **Abdominal-pelvic imaging** may be necessary.
  - ° Causes—female: **McCune-Albright syndrome** (see above), **ovarian tumors and functional cysts**, adrenal tumors (may be virilizing; increased testosterone, DHEAS), **CAH** (may be virilizing), exogenous estrogen. **Abdominal-pelvic imaging** may be necessary to find the cause.

DISORDERS OF SEXUAL DIFFERENTIATION

Presence of Y chromosome with SRY (testes-determining factor) on short arm

↓

Undifferentiated gonad (6 weeks): germ cells develop into Leydig cells and supporting cells into Sertolii cells

↓

Sertoli cell differentiation produces anti-müllerian hormone (AMH), causing involution of precursors to cervix, uterus, and fallopian tubes

↓

8–12 weeks gestation: placental chrionic gonadotropin peaks and stimulates Leydig cells to produce testosterone-development of wolffian duct in to seminal vesicles, vas deferens, and epididymis

↓

Testosterone then decreased to low levels maintained by LH from the fetal pituitary; required for penile growth

↓

In cells, some testosterone converts to dihydrotestosterone (DHT) by α-reductase and very small amount to estradiol by aromatase; functional androgen receptor needed for testosterone and DHT to develop external genitalia

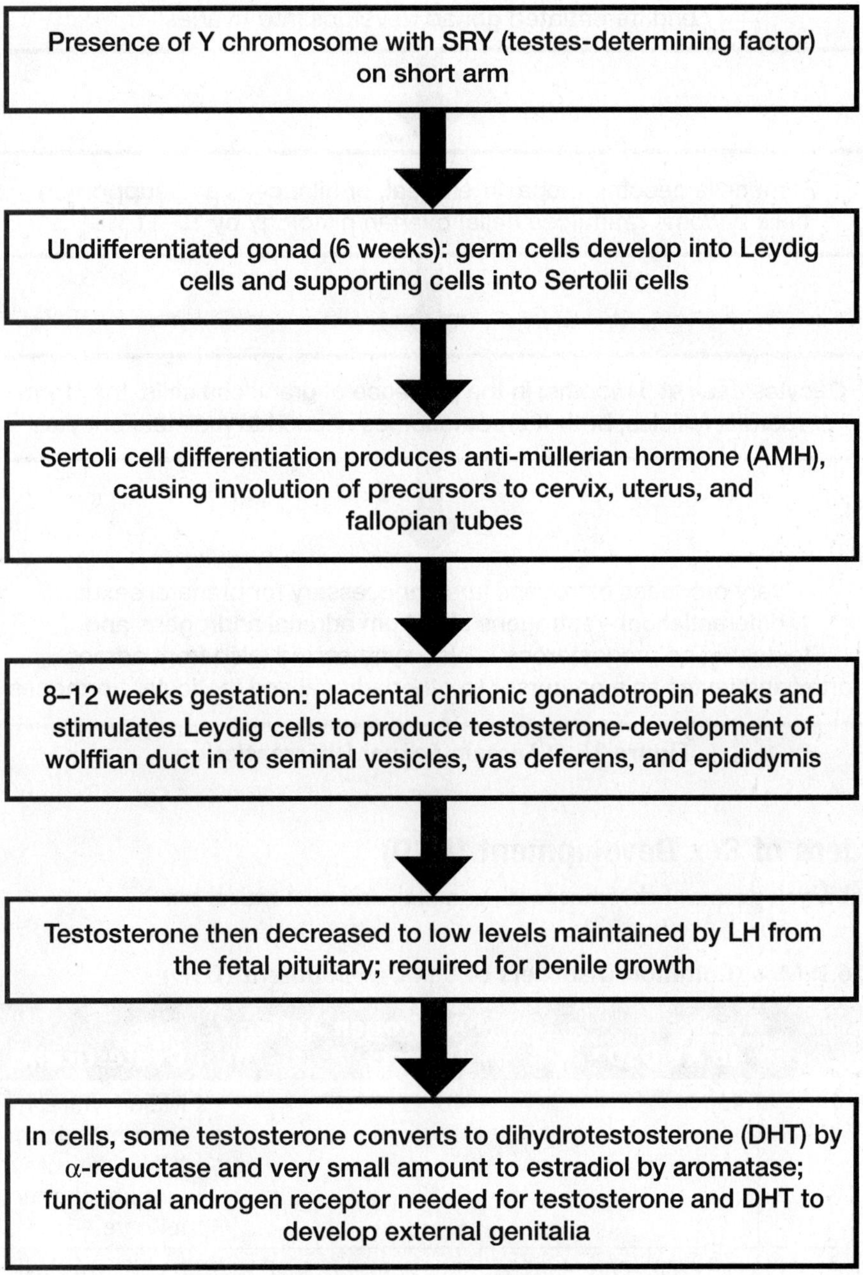

Figure 16.5: Male Sexual Differentiation

Without a Y chromosome and the SRY site (and AMH and testosterone) and with normal 46 XX chromosome, undifferentiated gonad develops into ovaries

Germ cells become theca, interstitial, or hilar cells and supporting cells become granulosa cells; ovarian histology by 10–11 weeks

Oocytes peak at 5 months; in the presence of granulosa cells, they form primordial follicles; both X chromosomes needed to maintain oocytes

Ovary produces estrogens (are unnecessary for prenatal sexual differentiation)—estrogens also from adrenal androgens and testosterone progesterone is also synthesized (also from adrenal cortex and testes as a precursor to other adrenal and testicular hormones)

Figure 16.6: Female Sexual Differentiation

Disorders of Sex Development (DSD)

Atypical development of chromosomal, gonadal, and anatomical sex

Table 16.1: Most Common Disorders of Sex Development (DSD)

	46,XX DSD	46,XY DSD	Androgen Action Defects	Ovotesticular DSD
Genotype	46,XX	46,XY	46,XY	Majority are 46,XX; then mosaicism (46, XX/46,XY, of which half are chimeras); few are 46,XY
Gonads	Ovaries (no AMH present)	Difficult to find but almost always testes (rudimentary to normal)	Testes in inguinal canals, labial/scrotal folds, or abdominal cavity	Ovary and testicular tissue present in the same or opposite gonads; most common are ovotestes unilaterally or bilaterally

(continued)

	46,XX DSD	46,XY DSD	Androgen Action Defects	Ovotesticular DSD
External genitals	Virilized (clitoral hypertrophy, labial/scrotal fusion)	Incomplete virilization, ambiguous features to phenotypic female; no pubertal sex changes in most	From normal male to undervirilized male to severe ambiguity to female phenotype; some forms may have pubertal secondary sex changes; sex rearing depends on phenotype	Ambiguous (atypical); may be highly virilized with no uterus and good testosterone function (raised as males); if no uterus with little virilization and minimal testosterone function, raised as females
Internal organs	Normal tubes and uterus	Testes, epididymis, vas deferens, or müllerian structures	No müllerian structures; wolffian duct structures present	May or may not have a uterus
Most common etiologies	-Most common is CAH (see CAH section in this chapter). -Aromatase deficiency (decreased estrogen, increased androgens → some degree of virilization and hypergonadotropic hypogonadism seen at puberty) -Androgenic progestins given during pregnancy (for threatened abortion) -Maternal ovarian or adrenal androgen-producing tumors	-Deletion or mutations of the short arm of the Y chromosome and/or the SRY region (various genetic syndromes) → müllerian structures (no AMH) -Enzymatic defects in the synthesis of testosterone by the fetal testes -Defect in Leydig cell differentiation (lack of LH receptors) → hypoplasia or aplasia -Lipoid CAH -Persistent müllerian ducts (defects in AMH gene → low levels of AMH; cryptorchidism + fallopian tubes and uterus)	-5 α-reductase deficiency (autosomal recessive) → decreased DHT (increased testosterone-to-DHT ratio) -Most common are the androgen-insensitivity syndromes (X-linked).	Most causes unknown; sporadic

Note: Most important initial diagnostic steps are to determine the genetic sex (karyotype) and to determine if a uterus and ovaries are present (ultrasound); if a uterus is present and there are no palpable gonads, the diagnosis is usually a virilized XX; if there is no uterus and no palpable gonads, the diagnosis is usually an undervirilized XY.

Abbreviations: anti-müllerian hormone, AMH; congenital adrenal hyperplasia, CAH; dihydrotestosterone, DHT

THYROID DISORDERS

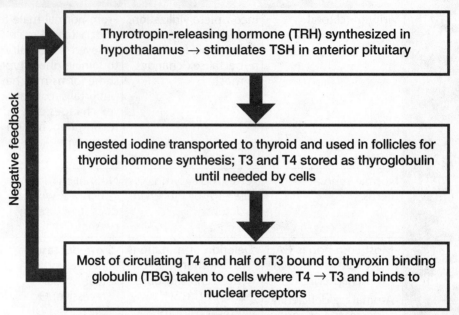

Figure 16.7: Thyroid Hormone Physiology

Thyroid hormones: T3 (the physiologically active hormone): 4 times more potent than T4 but only one-fifth is secreted; the rest is from deiodination of T4 in other tissues; only small amounts of T3 and T4 circulate as unbound hormones (T4 bound to TBG and other carriers and T3 to albumin); reverse T3 is metabolically inert. TBG can be increased or decreased in various conditions and with different drugs, but variations in levels are not associated with clinical findings.

Thyroid Goiters

Goiters

- **Congenital:** usually due to a synthetic defect in thyroxine synthesis or maternal antithyroid drugs that cross the placenta; also congenital transient hyperthyroidism from maternal Graves disease; may be sporadic with no identifiable cause

- **Acquired:** most are due to lymphocytic thyroiditis (see below) or are sporadic; may present as hypothyroid or euthyroid; other causes: certain drugs (lithium, amiodarone), treatment with iodide preparations for long periods

  - Colloid (simple) goiter: occurs most commonly in females around puberty; remains euthyroid; cause unknown; decreases in size over time

  - Multinodular: contains single or multiple palpable nodules; may be due to mild thyroid stimulation over time; usually euthyroid (uncommonly hyperthyroid); associated with McCune-Albright syndrome

Thyroid Nodules and Cancer

- Solitary nodules are common and are **usually benign** (benign adenoma, cyst, developmental abnormalities, associated with lymphocytic thyroiditis).

- Most are **nonfunctioning** and the patient is **euthyroid**; initial **ultrasound** to determine nodule size and appearance; if thyroid tests show a decrease in TSH, a **radionuclide scan** can then be used to determine if it is a **hot (i.e., functioning) nodule**. The most accurate diagnosis (pathology) is **fine-needle aspiration**.

- Increased **risk of thyroid cancer** if nodule is large, fixed, or hard, or is associated with cervical adenopathy or vocal cord paralysis

- Thyroid cancer is rare in children; seen mostly as an autosomal dominant condition, as a result of **radiation, or with chronic lymphocytic thyroiditis.**

- Most cancers are **papillary**, follicular > medullary

- Presentation is usually with a painless nodule or goiter; nodules in medullary cancer may be calcified.

- Medullary carcinoma may be sporadic or familial (autosomal dominant), or may occur as part of MEN type IIA or IIB.

- Treatment is **subtotal to total thyroidectomy** (with ablative radiotherapy and then thyroid hormone).

Hypothyroidism

Congenital hypothyroidism

- Most common cause is **thyroid dysgenesis** (hypoplasia, aplasia, or ectopic gland)
- Usually sporadic (familial less commonly)
- **Biochemical defects in thyroid hormone synthesis** with or without a **goiter**
- **Transplacental passage of thyroid autoantibodies from maternal autoimmune disease and presenting as transient congenital hypothyroidism** (3–6 months)
- Radioiodine administration during pregnancy (by mistake), maternal iodine exposure
- **Central hypothyroidism** due to thyrotropin-releasing hormone (TRH) or TSH deficiency

Clinical presentation—Usually **asymptomatic at birth (transplacental passage of moderate amounts of T4,** but still significantly decreased for neonatal screening diagnosis) with signs and symptoms over the first months of life; initial findings: **prolonged physiological jaundice** (due to delayed maturation of glucuronyl transferase), **widely patent fontanels (posterior fontanel) and cranial sutures**, and an increase in head circumference (due to brain myxedema). Other findings of hypothyroidism develop slowly: lethargy with increased sleep, poor feeding, decreased appetite, constipation, and decreased crying. Suggestive physical findings: **large, protruding tongue; hypotonia; umbilical hernia; cold, mottled skin; edema; coarse, brittle, and scant hair; decreased temperature and heart rate**. Longstanding, untreated hypothyroidism (by 3–6 months) may result in **growth failure, developmental retardation (including mental retardation)**, delayed tooth eruption, anemia, and heart failure.

Diagnosis—**Neonatal screen measures T4** and TSH; low T4 will identify primary hypothyroidism. Thyroid hormones will show a **decrease in T4 and free T4 (fT4) with an increase in TSH for primary hypothyroidism and a decrease in TSH, T4, and fT4 in central hypothyroidism**. A **radionuclide scan** determines thyroid dysgenesis or a synthetic defect (normal-size gland in the correct location with an increase in uptake). Genetic studies can be performed to detect the specific defect.

Treatment—**Oral levothyroxine** returns the thyroid hormones to normal and **suppresses the TSH to a normal range**. Growth will catch up, and **normal growth indicates adequate therapy**. Early diagnosis and treatment for normal growth and intelligence and prevention of irreversible brain damage.

Acquired hypothyroidism

—Most commonly due to **chronic lymphocytic thyroiditis (Hashimoto, autoimmune)** and may be associated with type I or II polyglandular syndromes; **increased incidence with Down, Turner. and Klinefelter syndromes**; other causes (not common): medications containing iodides, radiation, surgery, infiltrative (histiocytosis), or cystinosis.

Chronic lymphocytic thyroiditis: autoimmune disease with antithyroglobulin, antiperoxidase, and thyrotropin receptor–blocking antibodies → gland hyperplasia (infiltration with lymphocytes and plasma cells) and follicular atrophy. May present as a goiter (euthyroid or hypothyroid; diffuse, firm, nontender increase in thyroid) or as atrophic hypothyroidism. Twice as common in females, most commonly presenting in early adolescence (but can appear at almost any age); there may be familial cases (autosomal dominant with decreased penetration in males).

Clinical presentation—First sign is **decreased growth velocity** (and delayed BA) with or without a goiter; then the common signs and symptoms of hypothyroidism (**lethargy, increased sleep, constipation, cold intolerance, increased weight, skin myxedema, muscle weakness**); with severe long-standing disease, can have neurological findings, ileus, adrenal insufficiency, heart failure, respiratory failure, hyponatremia, bradycardia, and a hyperplastic increase in the pituitary and sella (leading to headaches, visual disturbances, and other endocrine findings).

Diagnosis—**T4 and fT4 may be normal or decreased, but there will be an increase in TSH and presence of serum antithyroid antibodies.**

Treatment—**Levothyroxine if hypothyroid**; must follow labs, as the disease may be self-limiting; goiter size deceases but persists, to some degree, for years; also, antibodies vary and also persist for years.

Hyperthyroidism

Almost all cases are due to **Graves disease (autoimmune production of thyroid-stimulating antibodies, leading to a diffuse toxic goiter)**; transplacental antibodies from mothers with Graves disease may affect neonates transiently (remits in 6 weeks to 4 months), but may be severe. Other causes are uncommon (functioning thyroid nodule, McCune-Albright syndrome, TSH-secreting pituitary tumors).

Graves disease: production of thyrotropin receptor–stimulating antibodies (TRS-Ab) and also thyrotropin receptor–blocking antibodies (TRB-Ab), with findings from net effect of the two → **diffuse goiter, generalized hyperplasia of the lymphatic tissue and of the retro-orbital tissues (exophthalmos)**. Girls affected boys, most often with a positive family history (and associated with HLA-B8 and -DR3) for some form of autoimmune thyroid disease (and/or other HLA-D3–associated disorders such as Addison disease, celiac disease, myasthenia gravis); most common presentation is early to middle adolescence.

Clinical presentation—**Gradual** symptoms: **emotional lability and motor hyperactivity** (tremors, restlessness), then **decreased sleep, increased appetite and eating but with weight loss, and decreased school performance**. Thyroid size is variable (as are the other findings); skin flushed, with increased sweating, and there may be cardiovascular effects e.g. tachycardia, palpitations, arrhythmias (atrial fibrillation), and heart failure. There may be an acute outpouring of thyroid hormones leading to a **thyroid crisis** (storm): increased temperature, severe tachycardia and heart failure, and seizures which, if untreated, may lead to coma and death.

Diagnosis—**Increased T4, T3, fT4, fT3, and decreased TSH with positive autoantibodies (TRS-Ab in most)**

Treatment—Primary treatment is still **antithyroid drugs** (with radioiodine ablation in some children over 10 years of age)—either **methimazole** (may be associated with less adverse effects; more potent with longer half-life → once per day dosing) or **propylthiouracil** (PTU; three-times-per-day dosing, but is less protein-bound so less crosses the placenta and into breast milk). Radiotherapy or subtotal to total thyroidectomy is indicated for suboptimal response. For severe initial symptoms (including thyroid crisis), a **beta-blocker (propranolol)** is needed for sympathetic blockade (and IV fluids, glucocorticoids, and digitalis may be needed for severe disease).

PARATHYROID DISORDERS AND DISORDERS OF CALCIUM-PHOSPHORUS HOMEOSTASIS

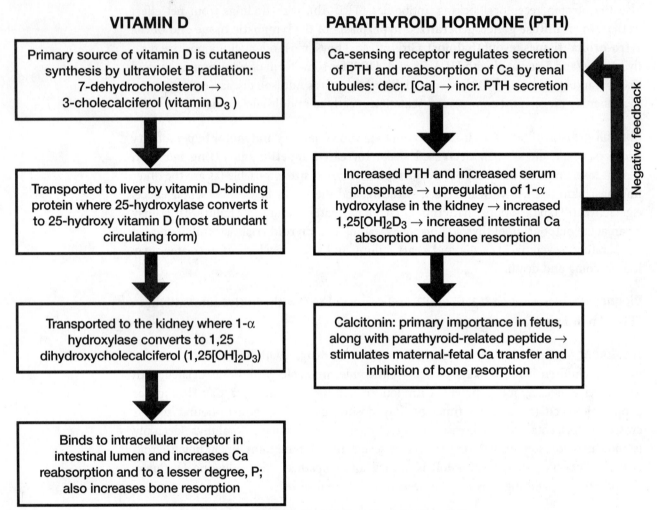

Figure 16.8: Vitamin D and Parathyroid Physiology

Hypoparathyroidism

Neonatal: functional immaturity of parathyroid gland in first days of life, especially in preterm infants, sick infants, and infants of diabetic mothers (transient, mild, asymptomatic hypocalcemia in healthy infants to symptomatic hypocalcemia in very small or sick infants); suppression of neonatal parathyroid hormone (PTH) by **maternal hyperparathyroidism** (transient hypocalcemia but may be symptomatic).

Infants and older children: parathyroid aplasia/hypoplasia (**DiGeorge and other 22q11-deletion syndromes**), other inherited hypoparathyroidism (X-linked recessive, autosomal recessive, autosomal dominant; may have dysmorphic features), mitochondrial DNA mutations, as a complication of surgery (thyroid), **autoimmune** (parathyroid antibodies associated with other autoimmune disease), infiltrative (hemosiderosis, copper in

Wilson disease), or idiopathic. **Other causes of hypocalcemia** include nutritional deficiency (rickets), magnesium deficiency (impairs release of PTH and leads to hormone resistance), increased inorganic phosphate (laxatives, enemas, inorganic phosphate poisoning, early in the treatment of acute lymphoblastic leukemia), and vitamin D deficiency (see below).

Clinical presentation—**Muscle pains, cramps, paresthesias, carpopedal spasm, Chvostek sign, Trousseau sign, and seizures**; long-standing: cataracts, tooth abnormalities (including delayed eruption), mental deterioration

Diagnosis—**Low serum Ca (and ionized), increased serum P, low to normal alkaline phosphatase, low 1,25-[OH]$_2$D$_3$, normal Mg, low PTH**

Treatment—Emergency: (neonatal tetany) **IV 10% Ca gluconate** while monitoring heart rhythm plus **1,25-D$_2$ (calcitriol) orally**; then **oral calcitriol plus supplemental calcium and adequate dietary Ca intake**

Pseudohypoparathyroidism

Albright hereditary osteodystrophy: genetic defect in hormone receptor adenylate cyclase system; parathyroid gland is normal or hyperplastic with **increased levels of PTH due to PTH resistance** (with or without abnormalities of other G-protein–coupled receptors, e.g., TSH, glucagon, gonadotropins); presents with **skeletal abnormalities and tetany**; diagnosis with **decreased serum Ca, increased serum P and alkaline phosphatase, and increased PTH.**

Hyperparathyroidism

Most from **secondary hyperparathyroidism** due to vitamin D deficiencies, malabsorption, chronic renal disease, or pseudohypoparathyroidism; **primary disease:** diffuse hyperplasia (familial; severe hypocalcemia in the neonate), transient neonatal hyperparathyroidism (mothers with hypoparathyroidism or pseudohypoparathyroidism → chronic intrauterine exposure to hypocalcemia), benign adenoma (familial, or part of MEN I or II). Other causes of **hypercalcemia:** familial benign hypercalcemia (autosomal dominant; Ca-sensing receptor gene mutation; asymptomatic with normal PTH), granulomatous disease (sarcoid, tuberculosis [TB]), malignancy (solid tumors, leukemia, lymphoma), hypervitaminosis D, hypophosphatasia (inactive alkaline phosphatase), Williams syndrome.

Clinical presentation—**Muscle weakness, fatigue, anorexia, nausea, vomiting, constipation, headache, abdominal pain** (may be with acute pancreatitis), **fever, polydipsia, and polyuria.** Long-standing: nephrocalcinosis, renal calculi, bone changes, decreased height (vertebral compression), seizures, mental retardation.

Diagnosis—Increased serum Ca (and ionized), decreased P, decreased Mg, normal to increased alkaline phosphatase, increased PTH (in relation to serum Ca), resorption of periosteal bone on x-rays (along margins of fingers) with or without radiographic signs of rickets

Treatment—All cases of primary hyperparathyroidism require **surgical exploration** with removal of adenomas and parathyroidectomy with severe disease.

Vitamin D Disorders, Rickets

Clinical findings in rickets: abnormalities of the extremities (valgus or varus deformities, tibial and femoral bowing, wrist and ankle enlargement); **rachitic rosary, craniotabes** and frontal bossing, craniosynostosis, delayed fontanel closure, delayed dentition, kyphoscoliosis, **fractures**, and symptoms of hypocalcemia.

Radiographic findings: thickening of growth plates (widening of the distal metaphases; wrists and ankles), metaphyseal fraying (loss of distinct border), metaphyseal cupping (becomes flat or concave; best at distal ends of radius, ulna, and fibula), rachitic rosary

Table 16.2: Other Causes of Rickets (see also Chapter 3)

	Vitamin D Deficiency	Vitamin D–Dependent Rickets Types I and II	Hypophosphatemic Rickets	Rickets of Prematurity
Epidemiology	Most common cause	—	X-linked hypophosphatemic rickets is the most common cause of rickets due to hypophosphatemia; autosomal dominant is much less common.	Most common in infants <1,000 g, ill, on TPN and with diuretic and cortico-steroid use; also if fed unsupplemented breast milk or standard (non-preterm) infant formulas (low in Ca and P)
Cause	Poor intake, inadequate cutaneous synthesis (see Chapter 3)	Type I: autosomal recessive; mutation for 1 α-hydroxylase Type II: autosomal recessive; mutation for vitamin D receptor → no response to 1,25-D_2	X-linked: increased renal phosphate excretion and decreased production of 1,25-D_2 Autosomal dominant: decreased resorption of proximal tubular phosphate and decreased production of 1,25-D_2	Premature birth interrupts Ca and P transfer from the mother to the fetus; insufficient Ca and P postnatally with Ca and P losses

(continued)

	Vitamin D Deficiency	Vitamin D–Dependent Rickets Types I and II	Hypophosphatemic Rickets	Rickets of Prematurity
Features	Clinical features of rickets (see text)	Type I: presents in first 2 years with any feature of rickets Type II: presents from infancy to adulthood, depending on severity; most-severe forms with alopecia	X-linked: rickets with abnormalities of the lower extremities, decreased growth velocity, and delayed dentition Autosomal dominant: incomplete penetrance and variable age of onset; variable features of rickets	1–4 months after birth: decreased growth, fractures, and classic findings of rickets
Laboratory values	Increased PTH → normal to low Ca and decreased serum P (renal losses and decreased intestinal absorption); increased alkaline phosphatase, decreased 1,25-D_2 with severe deficiency (1 α-hydroxylase is upregulated)	Type I: Normal 25-D but low 1,25-D_2; serum Ca normal to low with decreased serum P and increased PTH and alkaline phosphatase Type II: greatly increased levels of 1,25-D_2, otherwise all other values the same as type I	Increased renal P excretion → decreased serum P; increased alkaline phosphatase; normal Ca and PTH and inappropriately low 1,25-D_2	Decreased P → increased 1,25-D_2 → bone resorption; serum Ca may be low, normal, or even high; increased alkaline phosphatase
Treatment	Initial replacement vitamin D and calcium, then maintenance and adequate dietary Ca and P	Type I: calcitriol Type II: very high doses of 1,25-D_2 and oral Ca (for partially functioning receptor); if no response, long-term IV calcium	Oral phosphorus and calcitriol	Careful weekly screening with provision of sufficient Ca, P, and vitamin D in TPN and oral feedings (increased provisions for rickets)

Abbreviations: parathyroid hormone, PTH; total parenteral nutrition, TPN

Secondary vitamin D deficiencies: Decreased absorption of fat-soluble vitamins with cholestatic liver disease, bile acid metabolism defects, pancreatic insufficiency, general malabsorption diseases, protein-losing enteropathies, surgical resection; also increased degradation (phenobarbital, phenytoin, isoniazid [INH], rifampin).

ADRENAL DISORDERS

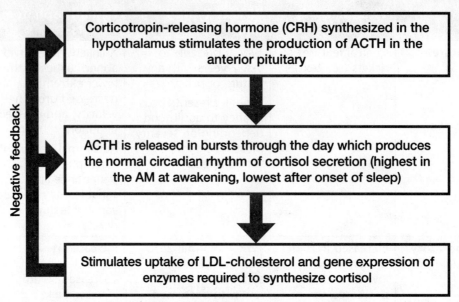

Figure 16.9: Adrenal Hormone Physiology

Aldosterone is regulated mainly through the renin-angiotensin system and serum potassium; ACTH has only a short-term effect: decreased intravascular volume → increased renin production in the kidney → cleaves angiotensinogen produced by the liver → angiotensin I (inactive) → angiotensin-converting enzyme (ACE) in the lungs and other tissues cleaves to the active angiotensin II, which is cleaved to angiotensin III; II and III are the stimulators of aldosterone.

Primary Adrenal Insufficiency

Inherited: most common is **CAH** (see below); other less uncommon etiologies: adrenoleukodystrophy (impaired oxidation of very long-chain fatty acids in peroxisomes with CNS demyelination → degenerative disease), adrenal hypoplasia (hypogonadotropic hypogonadism, and cryptorchidism in boys), isolated familial glucocorticoid deficiency, disorders of cholesterol synthesis and metabolism.

Acquired: Addison disease: autoimmune (antiadrenal cytoplasmic antibodies) → lymphocytic infiltration of cortex with preservation of the medulla; may occur as part of type I or II polyendocrine syndrome; others uncommon: infection (TB, meningococcemia), hemorrhage, certain drugs (anticonvulsants, ketoconazole and others)

Clinical presentation—Deficiency of cortisol with or without aldosterone deficiency. **Effects of cortisol deficiency: hypoglycemia with ketosis** (utilization of fatty acids for energy), anorexia, nausea and vomiting, decreased cardiac output, and vascular tone → **orthostatic hypotension** and shock. Effects of **aldosterone deficiency:** decreased reabsorption of Na → **hyponatremia, hypovolemia** → decreased glomerular filtration rate (GFR) → decreased excretion of free water → increased ADH→ decreased plasma osmolality and hyponatremia; decreased K excretion → **hyperkalemia**. Increased ACTH: **increased pigmentation** (melanocyte-stimulating hormone). Young infants mostly have inborn errors, infection, adrenal hypoplasia, and adrenal hemorrhage, and present with anorexia, nausea, and vomiting with a rapid onset of electrolyte and volume abnormalities leading rapidly to shock and death. Older children typically have Addison syndrome with a more gradual onset, starting with muscle weakness, malaise, anorexia, vomiting, weight loss, and orthostatic hypotension, and then hypoglycemia, ketosis, hyponatremia, and (late-onset) hyperkalemia.

Diagnosis—Hypoglycemia, ketosis, hyponatremia, hyperkalemia, acidosis, dehydration with increased BUN; **serum cortisol and aldosterone are decreased and ACTH and plasma renin activity are increased. Most definitive test** = testing serum cortisol levels before and after IV administration of ACTH (cortisol levels fail to increase after ACTH). Can test for **antiadrenal antibodies** for Addison disease, specific cortisol precursor enzymes for biosynthetic defects, very long-chain fatty acids for adrenoleukodystrophy, and imaging for adrenal anatomy (hypoplasia, hyperplasia, masses).

Treatment—Emergency treatment: **IV glucose, normal saline (NS), and fluid replacement, treat hyperkalemia, high-dose IV hydrocortisone**; chronic replacement with **oral hydrocortisone and fludrocortisone** (mineralocorticoid)

Secondary Adrenal Insufficiency

Most common is **abrupt cessation or too-fast tapering of administered corticosteroids**; less common: ACTH deficiency as part of pituitary or hypothalamic dysfunction (usually with other pituitary hormones; from destructive lesions, surgery, radiation; see discussion above), congenital pituitary lesions alone or with other midline structures (septo-optic dysplasia)

Clinical presentation—There is **no problem with aldosterone synthesis**, as the adrenal gland is intact and the renin-angiotensin system is not involved, so the problem is cortisol deficiency: **hypoglycemia, ketosis, weakness, orthostatic hypotension**, and any other involved hormones and/or effects of an expanding CNS lesion.

Diagnosis—**Hypoglycemia, ketosis, acidosis, decreased cortisol and ACTH with normal aldosterone and plasma renin activity**

Treatment—Glucocorticoids

Congenital Adrenal Hyperplasia (CAH) (Simplified)

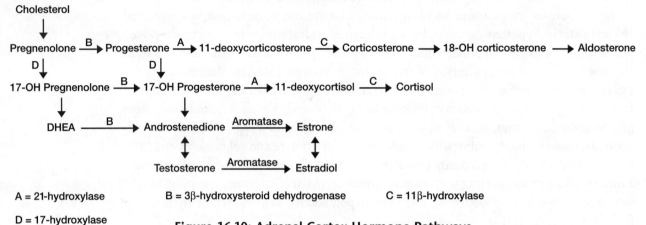

Cholesterol

Pregnenolone —B→ Progesterone —A→ 11-deoxycorticosterone —C→ Corticosterone —→ 18-OH corticosterone —→ Aldosterone

17-OH Pregnenolone —B→ 17-OH Progesterone —A→ 11-deoxycortisol —C→ Cortisol

DHEA —B→ Androstenedione —Aromatase→ Estrone

Testosterone —Aromatase→ Estradiol

A = 21-hydroxylase   B = 3β-hydroxysteroid dehydrogenase   C = 11β-hydroxylase

D = 17-hydroxylase

Figure 16.10: Adrenal Cortex Hormone Pathways

Biochemistry

- 21-Hydroxylase is required for the synthesis of **cortisol and aldosterone**
- Most common presentation and most severe form is **salt-losing form (hypoaldosteronism)**; the rest can synthesize aldosterone and are not salt-losing
- Salt-losing + non-salt-losing forms = **classic 21-hydroxylase deficiency**
- Nonclassical form (small number) → mild increase in levels of androgen
- Precursor **17-hydroxyprogesterone** accumulates (just prior to the block) and causes **shunting into androgen pathway** → **increased androstenedione and testosterone** (from 8–10 weeks' gestation) → **virilization** to various degrees in the female (clitoral enlargement, partial to complete labial fusion, and urogenital sinus)
- Females have ovaries and normal internal organs

Clinical presentation

- **Salt-losing form presents as primary adrenal insufficiency** over the first few weeks of life (as described above).
- **Males in either form appear normal at birth so are more likely to be sick and die with the salt-losing form.**
- **Females are virilized** to varying degrees.
- If not treated (the non-salt-wasting form), there are **progressive androgen effects after birth**: increased growth velocity and skeletal maturation, precocious puberty in males (testes remain prepubertal), and further masculinization in females (with no breast development or menarche unless treatment is begun).

The Other Most Important CAH Syndromes

- **11-β-hydroxylase deficiency:** 11-deoxycortisol is not converted to cortisol, so there is increased secretion of ACTH → increased precursor synthesis → androgen shunting but no decrease in aldosterone synthesis; hypertensive secondary to increased deoxycorticosterone; signs of androgen excess as in 21-hydroxylase deficiency.

- **3-β-hydroxysteroid dehydrogenase deficiency:** decreased synthesis of cortisol, aldosterone, and androstenedione but increased secretion of dehydroepiandrosterone (DHEA); salt-wasting crisis; boys are incompletely virilized, girls are mildly virilized; postnatal precocious adrenarche (DHEA); girls have hirsutism, irregular menses, and polycystic ovarian syndrome (PCOS); boys have hypogonadism.

- **17-hydroxylase deficiency:** cannot synthesize cortisol, but corticosterone is normal so there is no adrenal insufficiency; excess deoxycorticosterone → hypertension, hypokalemia, and suppression of the renin-angiotensin system; cannot synthesize sex hormones, so males present with ambiguity or as phenotypic females, and females have failure of sexual development at puberty.

Diagnosis—Hypoglycemia, hyponatremia, hyperkalemia, and acidosis; **increased 17-hydroxyprogesterone,** decreased cortisol, increased plasma renin activity and decreased aldosterone, increased androstenedione and testosterone. The **best test** is to measure 17-hydroxyprogesterone before and after an IV bolus of ACTH (large increase). **Prenatal diagnosis** chorionic villus sampling (CVS) at 10–11 weeks for those who have already had a child with CAH. The **newborn screen** (done in some states) measures 17-hydroxyprogesterone but there are a number of false positives. Positive values need to be retested at 2 weeks.

Treatment—Daily **hydrocortisone** (and increased amounts with any stress) and **fludrocortisone** (with aldosterone deficiency) plus sodium supplementation if needed.

Cushing Syndrome

Hypersecretion of ACTH by the pituitary **(Cushing disease),** or of glucocorticoids by the adrenal or exogenously; **endogenous Cushing syndrome:** most in infants from a **functioning adrenocortical tumor** (most are **malignant** carcinomas; fewer are benign adenomas) → **increased cortisol, aldosterone, androgens, and estrogens. Cushing disease** is caused most commonly by a **pituitary adenoma** (may be a microadenoma and difficult to find) in children >7 years of age → **bilateral adrenal hyperplasia;** less commonly from **ectopic production of ACTH** from a **neuroblastoma**, **Wilms tumor**, ganglioblastoma, and others. It may also be part of MEN I syndrome.

Clinical findings—Moon facies, generalized obesity, abdominal striae, decreased growth velocity, delayed pubertal changes, amenorrhea, hypertension, androgen effects (hirsutism, acne, deepened voice, phallic enlargement), hyperglycemia, increased incidence of infection, osteoporosis (pathological fractures), headache, weakness

Diagnosis—Loss of cortisol circadian rhythm. The **best screening test** is a single-dose dexamethasone suppression test (if given at 11 P.M. there will be no decrease in the 8 A.M. cortisol measurement). To determine the etiology: give an IV bolus of corticotropin-releasing hormone (CRH); with **ACTH-dependent Cushing disease** there will be large increase in ACTH and cortisol, but with **adrenal tumors** there will be no increase. A **CT scan is the best study of the adrenals** for a tumor, and an **MRI with contrast of the brain for a pituitary lesion.**

Treatment—Transsphenoidal pituitary microsurgery is the treatment of choice for a pituitary adenoma. With an ACTH-secreting metastatic tumor, the adrenal(s) should be removed. For a unilateral benign cortical adenoma, remove the adrenal; if bilateral, then bilateral subtotal adrenalectomy.

Primary Hyperaldosteronism

Increased secretion of aldosterone independent of the renin-angiotensin system; females have unilateral **aldosterone-secreting adenomas** and males have **bilateral micronodular hyperplasia.**

Clinical presentation—Most with **moderate to severe hypertension** (headache, dizziness, visual changes) and **chronic hypokalemia** (polyuria, polydipsia, muscle weakness, intestinal paralysis), fatigue, and decreased growth.

Diagnosis—**Decreased serum K with metabolic alkalosis and hypernatremia;** plasma aldosterone is increased with low plasma renin activity (better is increased ratio of plasma aldosterone to renin activity).

Treatment—**Surgical removal** of tumor; if bilateral hyperplasia, need **aldosterone antagonist** (spironolactone, eplerenone)

Pheochromocytoma

Catecholamine-secreting tumor from chromaffin cells; almost all arise from the **adrenal medulla** but may occur anywhere along the **sympathetic chain.**

Clinical presentation

- Most common between ages of 6–14 years and on the right side (20% are bilateral)
- May be autosomal dominant inheritance or part of **neurofibromatosis,** von Hippel-Lindau disease, or MEN IIA or IIB
- Secretion of large amounts of **epinephrine and norepinephrine significant hypertension** (up to 260/210 mm Hg) that is more often **sustained**
- **Hypertensive signs and symptoms** are present (headache, dizziness, palpitations) with sweating and abdominal pain. Growth failure, precordial pain, pulmonary edema, and heart and liver failure. There may be **hypertensive encephalopathy** (seizures). Retinal exam—papilledema, hemorrhages, exudates, and arterial constriction.

Diagnosis—Increased blood or urinary catecholamines; children predominantly excrete norepinephrine and its metabolites, **vanillylmandelic acid (VMA) and metanephrine**. With neuroblastoma, hypertension is uncommon and dopamine and homovanillic acid (HVA) are excreted. Most can be imaged with **ultrasound, CT, or MRI; use ^{131}I-metaiodobenzylguanidine scan** (taken up by chromaffin cells) for possible extra-adrenal tumors.

Treatment—**Preoperative alpha- and beta-blockade and fluid-loading**; then thorough transabdominal exploration with tumor removal; 10% are malignant.

DIABETES MELLITUS (DM)

Type 1
Autoimmune destruction of pancreatic beta cells → low to absent levels of endogenous insulin

- **Genetic susceptibility** (primarily increased risk with HLA-DR3 and -DR4) association with other autoimmune disease
- Onset mostly during childhood with a **peak in adolescence**
- Onset felt to be linked to **environmental triggers** (dietary, infectious, chemical), including psychosocial stress.

Pathophysiology—Catabolic state with low insulin levels → decreased glucose utilization by muscle and fat and initial **postprandial hyperglycemia**; with further autoimmune destruction and decreasing insulin levels → increased hepatic glycogen breakdown and gluconeogenesis → **fasting hyperglycemia**. When serum (glucose) **renal threshold** for glucose reabsorption (>180 mg/dL) → **osmotic diuresis → dehydration, electrolyte abnormalities, and loss of calories**. Counterregulatory hormones are secreted (glucagon, GH, cortisol, and epinephrine) → more glucose production and impairment of insulin secretion, accelerated lipolysis, and less lipid synthesis; fatty acids are used for fuel and are metabolized to **ketone bodies**. These accumulate to produce a **metabolic acidosis** and are excreted in the urine (**diabetic ketoacidosis, DKA**).

Clinical presentation—Initially **intermittent polyuria and nocturia**; then **more persistent polyuria with polydipsia**; loss of calories in the urine leads to **polyphagia, loss of weight and body fat**. With very low insulin levels and continuation of the pathophysiology, **DKA** ensues: nausea, vomiting, abdominal pain, weakness, dehydration, orthostatic hypotension, Kussmaul breathing, a fruity breath (from acetone).

Diagnosis—**Classic symptoms plus nonfasting blood glucose of >200 mg/dL with or without ketonuria** is diagnostic; DKA: electrolyte abnormalities, **increased anion gap metabolic acidosis, hyperosmolality, and ketonuria**.

Management

Table 16.3: Management of DKA

Metabolic Abnormality	Physiology	Initial Therapy	Effect	Subsequent Therapy
Hyperglycemia	Giving insulin from the start of treatment moves glucose intracellularly, decreases hepatic glucose production, and stops the movement of free fatty acids to the liver.	Insulin infusion (without bolus) at 0.1 U/kg/hr	Continued decrease in hyperglycemia	Add 5% dextrose to the infusion when serum glucose is <250 mg/dL; if serum glucose is <180 mg/dL and no further acidosis, discontinue infusion and switch to SQ insulin with oral feeds; if continued acidosis, continue IV rehydration but decrease insulin infusion until acidosis is corrected.
Dehydration	Osmotic diuresis leads to dehydration and hyperosmolality; need to re-expand the intravascular volume and replace losses	Initial bolus with NS or Ringer's lactate (20 mL/kg; can be repeated), then volume correction over 24–36 hours with 0.5 NS + K-phosphate + K-acetate	Initial fast volume expansion, then gradual rehydration; along with insulin infusion, decreases hyperglycemia and leads to increased renal perfusion and excretion; once the serum glucose is <180 mg/dL, osmotic diuresis stops and rehydration improves	Gradual rehydration from 24–36 hours, depending on severity; too fast of a decrease in osmolality may lead to increased risk of cerebral edema; as above, add 5% dextrose to IV when serum glucose <250 mg/dL; may change to PO fluids and feeding with SQ insulin when no further dehydration, electrolyte shifts, and correction of acidosis
Metabolic acidosis	Low insulin infusion rates stop the release of fatty acids and the production of ketoacids.	Insulin infusion and IV rehydration	Gradual decrease in ketoacids, ketonuria and increase in plasma pH; ketogenesis continues until all fatty acid substrates in the liver are used	Discontinue insulin infusion and IV rehydration based on improvement in plasma pH and not ketonuria (may persist).

(continued)

Metabolic Abnormality	Physiology	Initial Therapy	Effect	Subsequent Therapy
Na loss	There is total body loss of Na, but a moderate hypernatremic dehydration (free-water loss plus effect of increased aldosterone) and initial serum Na is low to normal (dilution due to hyperglycemia and increased Na-free lipid fraction; see Chapter 3); Na increases by 1.6 mmol for every 100 mg/dL decrease in serum glucose.	Initial bolus of isotonic saline with hypernatremic dehydration keeps most of the fluid in the intravascular space; then hypotonic (but not less than 0.45% NaCl) saline to replace free-water deficit	Serum Na gradually increases and then stabilizes in the normal range with rehydration.	Continued IV NaCl replacement until rehydrated, with a normal serum Na (135–145 mEq/L) and minimal acidosis (pH >7.30)
K loss	Dehydration leads to activation of the renin-angiotensin-aldosterone system with increased potassium excretion → total-body loss of K (also due to osmotic diuresis and ketonuria); but initial serum K is normal to increased due to movement of intracellular K to the serum (catabolism and acidosis).	Add potassium supplement as a combination of K-phosphate and K-acetate (added buffer); may need 40–80 mEq/L of K (must monitor frequently); monitor ECG.	May see dramatic drop in serum K, then gradual stabilization of serum K to the normal range but continued losses until catabolic process is reversed and diuresis is controlled; takes days for restoration of intracellular K	As above, continued IV therapy until full rehydration, no further electrolyte shifts, and correction of acidosis
Phosphate loss	Total-body loss of phosphate; but with catabolism and acidosis, phosphate is also moved from the intracellular space to the serum, and initial serum level will be normal to increased	Add K supplement as a combination of K-phosphate and K-acetate (added buffer); may need 40–80 mEq/L of K (must monitor frequently)	May see a dramatic drop in serum phosphate, then gradual stabilization of serum phosphate to the normal range but continued losses until catabolic process is reversed and diuresis is controlled; takes days for restoration of intracellular phosphate	As above, continued IV therapy until full rehydration, no further electrolyte shifts, and correction of acidosis

Abbreviations: normal saline, NS; subcutaneous, SQ

Insulin therapy

- Replacement insulin dose based on pubertal status (0.7 U/kg/day prepubertal, 1.0 U/kg/day mid-pubertal, and 1.2 U/kg/day late pubertal); initial dose should be about 70% of these values; most have residual beta-cell function at first (**"honeymoon period"**) with a gradual increase in requirements over the next few months; insulin changes per self-monitoring.
- **Rapid-acting bolus insulin analogs** (lispro and aspart)—absorbed much faster and do not need to dissociate first → distinct periods of action + little longer-term decreased effect and little overlap the next dose.
- **Better control of increased postprandial glucose and between-meal or nighttime hypoglycemia.**
- The **long-acting analogs** (glargine and detemir) have a much more physiological 24-hour response (Lente and Ultralente insulins no longer available); usually given as a single daily dose in older children and may be given twice daily in younger. Given as 25–30% of total daily dose in infants and toddlers and 40–50% of total daily dose in older children and adolescents. Remaining total daily dose given as bolus for three meals. Also pre-mixed combinations (Humalog Mix, NovoLog Mix).
- Dosing schedule initially based on blood glucose level and then, more **accurate dosing with carbohydrate content of meals and the blood glucose**.
- Subcutaneous infusion pump may allow for normal insulin levels and increased flexibility in management and lifestyle; may be better metabolic control and decreased risk of severe hypoglycemia.
- Intensive (tight glucose) control shown to **decrease microvascular complications** (retinopathy and nephropathy) and **neuropathy**, but there is an increased **risk of hypoglycemia**.

Monitoring

- **Self-monitoring** of blood glucose: **≥4 times/day** prior to meals and at bedtime; when starting on insulin and with any adjustments, need values at 12 A.M. and 3 A.M. to test for nocturnal hypoglycemia.
- Ideal values are **80 mg/dL fasting glucose to 140 mg/dL after meals (60–220 mg/dL is acceptable; based on age)**; if the A.M. fasting glucose is high: adjustment is made with the long-acting P.M. dose, or a bedtime snack bolus may be added. For other postprandial values that are high, the previous-meal dose would be adjusted.
- Continuous glucose monitoring systems are also available for closer monitoring.
  - **HbA₁c: glycosylated Hb:** fraction of hemoglobin (Hb) to which glucose has been non-enzymatically bound; increased values are correlated to higher serum glucose for longer periods of time; represents **average glucose concentration for the preceding 2–3 months. Good levels: 6–7.9%; fair levels: 8–9.9%; poor levels: ≥10%.**

Nutrition

Total daily calories based on surface area from standard tables; ideal distribution is **55% carbohydrate, 30% fat, 15% protein**; 70% of carbohydrates should be **complex, with limitation of sucrose and simple sugars**; a diet high in **fiber** and the **low ratio of polyunsaturated to saturated fatty acids.**

Carbohydrate counting used to adjust insulin dosage, and meal plans based on **groups of food exchanges**; calories should be: **20% breakfast, 20% lunch, 30% supper, with 10% each from three daily snacks.**

Exercise—Any type of exercise allowed, but limited at any time by **hypoglycemia**; regular exercise provides **better glucose regulation**; need an **additional carbohydrate exchange** prior to exercise and **available glucose** during and after any exercise; if episodes of hypoglycemia, insulin dose on the day of exercise should be decreased.

Short-term complications

- **Major complication is hypoglycemia**; most children have mild episodes weekly and more significant episodes few times per year; more likely in young infants and toddlers, so should use less intense control.
- **Symptoms:** pallor, sweating, hunger, tremors, tachycardia (all due to catecholamine surge); with further decline (decreased cerebral glucose): drowsiness, confusion, personality changes, and impaired judgment, which could lead to seizures and coma. Need a source of **emergency glucose at all times** (5–10 g) with glucose check 15–20 minutes later. If oral administration not possible, need **glucagon injection kit**; if still no better, transport to Emergency Room for **IV glucose**.
- **Dawn phenomenon:** seen mostly when NPH is used as basal insulin at supper and in the evening; overnight growth hormone secretion and increased insulin clearance leads to a mild elevation of A.M. glucose; this is a normal physiology in nondiabetic children who can compensate with increased insulin.
- **Somogyi effect:** rare finding; high A.M. glucose due to rebound from a late-night or early-morning hypoglycemic episode with an exaggerated counterregulatory response (but most children who become hypoglycemic overnight remain so).

Type 2

Etiology—**Insulin resistance** at skeletal muscle, increased hepatic glucose production, decreased insulin secretion, and worsening of hyperglycemia over time (decreased insulin gene expression). Has a stronger genetic component than type 1. **No autoimmune pancreatic destruction** (but autoimmune markers may be present); aggravated by environmental factors, **especially low physical activity and a high-calorie, fatty diet.**

Epidemiology—Is now **epidemic in U.S. children**; more frequently seen in **non-white Americans** (Hispanic Americans, African Americans, Asian Americans, Native Americans, Pacific Islanders). Average age at onset: 13–14 years (**range 10–19 years**).

Clinical presentation—More **commonly insidious onset (abrupt with type 1), obesity is present (not common in type 1)**, mild or absent polyuria and polydipsia (typical of type 1), plus findings of **metabolic syndrome** (syndrome X; not typically present in type 1):

- Glucose intolerance with insulin resistance
- Hyperinsulinemia
- Hypertension
- Obesity
- Dyslipidemia
- Acanthosis nigricans

Most present with **moderate hyperglycemia and no weight loss** (may have recent weight gain), may **have mild DKA (ketoacidosis in up to one-quarter and ketonuria in up to one-third) at onset** with the stress of another illness (more common in African Americans). PCOS may also be present in pubertal girls (see above).

Diagnosis

- **Impaired glucose tolerance:** fasting blood glucose of 110–125 mg/dL *or* 2-hour oral glucose tolerance test glucose ≥140 but <200 mg/dL
- **Diabetes:** symptoms of DM plus a random plasma glucose =200 mg/dL *or* fasting blood glucose ≥126 mg/dL *or* 2-hour oral glucose tolerance test glucose ≥200 mg/dL

Screening—Current American Academy of Pediatricians (AAP) recommendations: **overweight child** (body mass index [BMI] >85% for age and sex) **at 10 years of age or onset of puberty** (whichever is first) **plus** any two of the following:

- Family history of type 2 DM in first- or second-degree relative
- High-risk race/ethnicity (non-white Americans: Hispanic Americans, African Americans, Asian Americans, Native Americans, Pacific Islanders)
- Signs of, or conditions associated with, insulin resistance (metabolic syndrome findings)
- Screen **every 2 years with a fasting blood glucose** (preferred method).

Treatment

- First and **most important**: nutritional education and improved exercise level (increased physical activity and weight loss are often unsuccessful)
- **Insulin** required at diagnosis with dehydration, high glucose levels, and ketoacidosis/ketonuria, usually for a few weeks

- **Only oral hypoglycemic agents that are FDA-approved are metformin (biguanide preferred) and glimepiride (sulfonylurea).** With diagnosis (or after initial insulin therapy), start with **metformin** (decreases hepatic glucose production; contraindicated with significant hepatic or renal disease; often results in weight loss).
- If control is not achieved, add **glimepiride** (may cause weight gain).
- If still lack of control, refer to endocrinologist (preferred use of **insulin** at this point; monotherapy not sufficient in most over time

Maturity-Onset Diabetes of Youth (MODY)

- Genetic abnormality with early-onset (**9–25 years**) type 2 DM, **autosomal dominant** inheritance, and a defect in insulin secretion (six types, based on mutated gene) from mild glucose intolerance to severe diabetes.
- **Criteria for diagnosis:** DM for at least three generations, evidence of autosomal dominant transmission, diagnosis prior to age 25 years
- Need molecular analysis of currently known gene mutations (most specific test) to facilitate diagnosis and management (severity, prognosis).

ORTHOPEDIC DISORDERS AND SPORTS MEDICINE

CONGENITAL SYSTEMIC AND ANATOMIC ABNORMALITIES/DISORDERS

Osteogenesis Imperfecta

Defects in type I collagen → abnormal bone development; most common genetic cause (autosomal dominant) of **osteoporosis**.

Clinical presentation—**Easily fractured bone plus blue sclera plus early deafness.** Main morbidities and causes of death are from cor pulmonale, decreased pulmonary function with recurrent infections, and central nervous system (CNS) complications.

- **Type I: mild**; recurrent fractures from mild to moderate trauma (decreased incidence after puberty); blue sclera and early hearing loss
- **Type II: perinatally lethal**; stillborn or death within first year of life; intrauterine growth retardation (IUGR) plus many intrauterine fractures and bowing of extremities; rib fractures and small thorax → **respiratory insufficiency**
- **Type III: progressively deteriorating**; also may have intrauterine fractures; postnatal fractures with mild trauma → deformities; extreme short stature, vertebral compression, and scoliosis.
- **Type IV: moderately severe**; fractures from birth or after starting to walk; moderate bowing of extremities and short stature; decreased incidence of fractures after puberty

Diagnosis—Biochemical studies or DNA testing from **skin fibroblast culture or leukocytes**; prenatal diagnosis (chorionic villus sampling [CVS]) for families with previously affected child; ultrasound detection of abnormalities in early second trimester

Management—**Supportive treatment**: genetic counseling, physical therapy, management of fractures, correction of deformities; currently no cure

Skeletal Dysplasias (Chondroplasias)

Genetic group of disorders of skeletal development and growth; gene mutations → skeletal abnormalities (with secondary complications) and non-skeletal problems; some types **may be lethal** in-utero. Abnormalities seen on **fetal ultrasound** or in the neonatal period.

Abnormalities in different proteins → many different recognized clinical presentations, from **mild to severely affected** individuals with **predominant short limb, short trunk, or both**.

Diagnosis—Primarily through **clinical recognition** based on findings, family history, in-utero findings, and **radiographs of the entire skeleton**. Molecular genetic testing with **prenatal diagnosis**. It is important to make the distinction between lethal and non-lethal varieties in order to plan for course of therapy.

Examples

- **Achondroplasia syndromes:** short limbs due to **proximal limb shortening (rhizo-melic, i.e., femur)**. **Thanatophoric dysplasia** is similar with very short stature, **small thorax with severe respiratory distress**; diagnosed **antenatally or at birth**; **most common lethal chondroplasia**, often stillborn or early death.
- **Spondyloepiphyseal dysplasias:** autosomal dominant; **short trunk** and limbs (to lesser degree); **may be lethal** or present in a milder form; x-rays show **abnormal development of vertebral bodies and of epiphyses**; severity of the radiographic changes is proportional to the clinical severity
- **Diastrophic dysplasias:** autosomal recessive; defective sulfation of **cartilage proteins**; **very short extremities**, short hands, **proximal thumb displacement**, severe scoliosis, clubfoot, and restricted joint movements; **severe and progressive**, but usually with a **normal life span**
- **Camptomelic dysplasia:** seen in **newborns** with **short bones, bowing of the lower legs, cervical spine abnormalities, respiratory distress, defects of other organs**; death usually due to **respiratory distress** in the neonatal period
- **Asphyxiating thoracic dystrophy (Jeune syndrome):** autosomal recessive; seen in the **newborn** with **long, narrow thorax, very short ribs, and respiratory distress secondary to pulmonary hypoplasia**; slightly short limbs and postaxial polydactyly. Most commonly **die in neonatal period or early infancy**; if infant survives, the rib cage grows and respiratory function improves.

Arthrogryposis Multiplex Congenita

Newborn with multiple rigid joint deformities, contractions, and dislocations (especially the hip, then the knee); antenatally with **decreased fetal movement** (fetal immobility; see Chapter 2) and polyhydramnios. There may be **limb involvement** with defective or absent muscles, with a systemic neurological or myopathic disorder or in association with other major anomalies and specific syndromes.

Diagnosis

- The **clinical exam and x-rays** are best for diagnosis.
- Use **CT or MRI for brain and spine anatomy, muscle biopsy** for suspected primary myopathy, or **blood molecular DNA testing** for a specific suspected genetic disorder.

- Most common etiologies: **intrauterine constraint**, maternal and/or intrauterine factors leading to **decreased fetal movements**, primary skeletal disorders (bones, joints, and associated tissue), primary myopathies, specific syndromes associated with arthrogryposis and CNS or spinal disorders.

Management—Treatment of deformities with all nonsurgical and surgical means

Torticollis

Lateral bending of the head and neck to one side and rotation of the head and neck to the opposite side (see Chapter 2).

Diagnosis—Thorough antenatal history, neurological evaluation, **plain films of the cervical spine**; follow up as needed with **MRI of the brain and spine**

Management—For congenital muscular torticollis, **stretching exercises begun early** are successful in almost all; for negative results or for other causes, surgery is usually needed.

Klippel-Feil syndrome: congenital fusion of one or more cervical vertebrae with anomalies of the cervical spine; short neck, restricted neck movement with torticollis; association with genitourinary (GU) abnormalities most commonly, then with auditory, neurologic, cardiovascular, and other musculoskeletal abnormalities

Polydactyly and Syndactyly

- Polydactyly: most common deformation of the fingers and toes; presence of one or more extra digits or parts of digits (hands or feet). **Preaxial:** next to the thumb in the hand, next to the great toe in foot. **Postaxial:** next to the 5th finger or toe; may also be **centrally placed**. May occur bilaterally and associated with other anomalies or genetic syndromes (e.g., Trisomy 13, Ellis-van Creveld Syndrome). Depending on extent of digit formation, simple ligation or surgery is needed for removal.
- **Syndactyly:** incomplete or complete (skin, tendon, and bone) webbing between digits; often with a family history; may be isolated or as part of a syndrome; surgical treatment only for those with functional impairment or when associated with polydactyly

Scoliosis

Congenital or developmental lateral curvature of the spine of greater than 10 degrees; most are **idiopathic** (genetic role); the **infantile type** (birth to 3 years of age), is rare, and resolves spontaneously; **juvenile** (uncommon; from age 3–10 years), and **adolescent (most common;** from 11 years of age); during adolescence, girls are at greater risk for more significant degrees of curvature (equal sex distribution in younger ages). **Other causes:** congenital (embryonic abnormality often with vertebral anomalies and organ anomalies; genetic predisposition), connective tissue disorders and syndromes, neuromuscular disorders, certain metabolic disorders, post-traumatic, and tumors.

Clinical presentation—Presents at birth or later in childhood or adolescence with mild to severe spinal curvature; idiopathic generally seen during **school screening program** and may present with **back pain**.

Diagnosis

- Initial inspection (anterior and lateral) looking for **asymmetries**, and then **forward bending at the hips (Adams test)** showing **asymmetry of the posterior chest wall** (elevation of one shoulder) and lateral shift of the trunk
- May be an apparent **leg-length discrepancy**
- View trunk from the side to evaluate the degree of **kyphosis and lordosis**
- Careful neurological exam needed for any possible underlying causes
- Next step is radiographic evaluation: **standing posterior-anterior and lateral views of the entire spine** to measure degree and pattern of curvature and underlying spinal anomalies
- **MRI** should be obtained if there is a suspicion of an underlying cause (CNS or spinal)

Management

- Observation—the **majority of curves do not progress**; exercise or any kind of manipulation is not effective; **bracing** may be effective in idiopathic scoliosis to prevent further progression, but does not decrease the curve.
- **Idiopathic:** risk of curve progression correlates to the amount of growth remaining (skeletal maturity) and the degree of curvature; curves <30 degrees rarely progress after skeletal maturity; whereas those >45 degrees may slowly progress. Curves 25 to 45 degrees may be treated with bracing; surgery (implant rods) is performed in skeletally immature children with thoracic curves >45 degrees and lumbar curves of 35–40 degrees; in skeletally mature individuals, surgery is performed for curves >50–55 degrees.

Kyphosis

Greater forward angulation in the thoracic spine compared to physiological (normal is about 40 degrees); **curves >50 degrees** are generally a cosmetic issue, but also may be related to back pain; may be **flexible or rigid**; **flexible kyphosis (postural)** is common in adolescents—they can correct their posture voluntarily, and supine hyperextended x-rays show complete correction and **no vertebral pathology**; this is **non-progressive** and **no therapy** is required; **congenital kyphosis** is due to abnormality in formation of the vertebral body; may be associated with an **underlying primary disorder**. Major complication is paralysis due to cord compression. Most common form of **structural kyphosis** is **Scheuermann type**, caused by wedging of at least three vertebrae (more common in adolescent males). Treatment is individualized.

Coxa Vara and Valgus

Coxa vara: congenital or acquired decrease in angle of shaft and head/neck of femur; presents with a painless limp after the onset of walking, with later development of increasing pain that may be referred to the knee. Exam shows leg held in external rotation, and with decreased abduction and internal rotation, and muscle atrophy with or without shortening of the extremity; bilateral involvement—waddling gait and lumbar lordosis. It may be acquired (as **coxa valgus**) secondary to bone or joint infections, neuromuscular disease, trauma, avascular necrosis, slipped capital-femoral epiphysis, or metabolic bone disease.

Leg-Length Discrepancy

- Defined as leg discrepancy >2 cm. Produces gait **asymmetry** with small compensatory lumbar curvature.
- **Congenital:** isolated defects in growth of the femur, tibia, or fibula; skeletal dysplasias, neurofibromatosis, and syndromes associated with vascular anomalies.
- **Acquired:** from untreated developmental hip dysplasia, trauma, neurologic disease, tumor, inflammatory and infectious bone and joint diseases, acquired coxa vara, and severe scoliosis.
- **Assessment:** Assess for underlying cause **radiographic procedures and views of hips and legs** are needed.
- **Treatment:** Goal is to **decrease leg-length difference to <2.5 cm at skeletal maturity.** Some cases only need observation; others are treated with orthoses or limb-shortening or -lengthening procedures.

Developmental Dysplasia of the Hip (DDH)

Newborn hips that are **subluxated** (partial contact between femoral head and acetabulum), are **dislocated**, and/or have **malformed acetabula**; **teratogenic** if occurs early in-utero (12th–18th week) and is often associated with **neuromuscular disorders or dysmorphic syndromes**; normal infant with either **prenatal** (increased occurrence in final 4 weeks of pregnancy); **intrauterine constraint and with breech presentation and oligohydramnios** or **early postnatal** (infant positioning with **ligamentous laxity**, e.g., swaddling); genetic factors involved; **greater incidence in females** (susceptible to maternal hormonal relaxin leading to ligamentous laxity); **highest risk are girls with positive family history (especially if breech position).**

Diagnosis

Many false positives and negatives regardless of diagnostic test—no signs are pathognomonic. In newborns, observe for **signs of asymmetry:** difference in limb length, decreased movement in abduction, asymmetric thigh-gluteal folds in prone; **Barlow maneuver:** sensation of unstable hip (dislocation with "clunk") with gentle adduction and posterior pressure. **Ortolani maneuver:** reduction of already dislocated hip—lift abducted hip anteriorly to hear/feel **"clunk."** By 8–12 weeks of life, these tests no longer possible due to increased muscle tightness. At 3–6 months, the most reliable exam is showing limitation of abduction with asymmetry of thigh folds, and positive **Galeazzi sign** (relative shortness of femur with hips and knees flexed).

Imaging: Adjunct to clinical exam; **x-rays are more reliable at age 4–6 months** (ossification centers develop in the femoral head). **Real-time ultrasonography is most accurate in first month of life** (and until age 4 months). Minor degrees of instability in first month almost all resolve without treatment.

Management (current recommendations by American Academy of Pediatrics [AAP])

- All newborns need to be screened by **physical exam**.
- If **positive Barlow or Ortolani** (not any soft sign), **refer immediately to orthopedic surgeon**; majority of abnormal findings will resolve within 2 weeks. Do not order ultrasound or x-ray, i.e., treatment decisions based on results of exam. **Triple diapering is not recommended** (lack of efficacy data).
- If exam results **equivocal,** perform **follow-up exam in 2 weeks**. If exam is positive, **refer immediately to orthopedic surgeon**. If Barlow and Ortolani tests are negative but diagnosis still suspected (and/or with risk factors: girls, positive family history, breech) perform **ultrasound or refer to orthopedic surgeon at 3–4 weeks of age**. If test results negative and patient is low-risk, then follow with normal well-child care. **Hips must be examined at every visit.** Any time there is exam evidence of possible dislocation, **must be confirmed radiographically**.
- **Pavlik harness is used for all degrees of hip dysplasia (up to 6 months)**, full-time for 6 weeks—almost all resolve; failure rate after 6 months is more than half because of difficulty keeping child in the harness; for infants **age 6 months–2 years, closed reduction under general anesthesia is initial therapy**—hip is moved to the reduced position with good range of motion (ROM) and is casted; if fails, open reduction (**usually needed in a child older than age 2 years**).

Internal Tibial Torsion

Tibia is **turned medially** (internally rotated) and result is **intoeing** in the ambulatory child; usually presents in the second year of life. Management is **observation and reassurance—spontaneous resolution and normal growth and development** with continuation of walking (usually complete correction occurs over early childhood).

Metatarsus Adductus

Adduction of the forefoot relative to the hindfoot at the tarsal-metatarsal joints; midfoot and hindfoot are normal; most common cause is **abnormal intrauterine positioning**; leads to **intoeing with abnormal shoe wear** in a walking child; treatment based on rigidity and amount of deformity, mostly nonoperative. For flexible: stretching exercises with or without splinting; if no improvement in 4–6 weeks, then **serial casting** and orthoses; if residual or no response: surgery at age 4–6 years.

Talipes Equinovarus (Clubfoot)

Misalignment of calcaneo-talar-navicular joints → **hindfoot deformity (hindfoot varus and equines and forefoot plantarflexion and adductus)**; all associated with calf atrophy; most are flexible deformations due to **abnormal intrauterine positioning** with a genetic influence; secondary causes (neuromuscular disorders) are more rigid and more difficult to treat. **X-rays are recommended** to demonstrate malalignment among tarsal bones. Treatment is first with **manipulation and serial casting**; most require some type of **surgery**, and then **orthoses**.

Pes Planovalgus (Flexible Flatfeet)

- Normal longitudinal arch when examined in non-weight-bearing, but have a **midfoot sag and hindfoot valgus during standing**; flexible (normal ROM) to rigid; common in young infants and children (physiologic ligamentous laxity), which improves during mid-childhood with normal development of longitudinal arch; familial ligamentous laxity generally persists into adolescence.
- No x-rays for asymptomatic cases; if symptoms present, x-rays to assess deformity.
- Small number with symptoms or abnormal shoe wear treated with **medial arch supports** for symptom relief (does not change foot shape); severe cases associated with connective tissue disorders, hereditary sensory-motor neuropathies, and Down syndrome, and generally require custom orthoses; tight Achilles tendon and persistent symptoms generally require surgery.

ACQUIRED DISORDERS

Nursemaid Elbow

Subluxation of the annular ligament (attaches radial head to the proximal ulna); if **longitudinal distal traction** is applied suddenly to the radius in a young child (where the radial head is not as bulbous; typically, holding a child's outstretched arm as he falls), then **ligament may slip proximally off the head**. Uncommon after age 5 years. There is **immediate pain and limitation of supination**. Diagnosis is clinical; no x-rays needed. **Treatment:** put pressure over radial head with one hand, and extend and rotate forearm into supination (may feel a click) → immediate relief of pain.

Back Pain

Many possible causes: most common is **trauma from acute injury or overuse** (repetitive physical activities); also diskitis, osteomyelitis, abscess, rheumatic disease, primary tumors, metastases from other primary malignancies, kyphoscoliosis, intraabdominal or pelvic diseases (referred pain), spondylolysis, and spondylolisthesis. Thorough history, physical **(including abdominal and possible pelvic exams)** and **neurological and musculoskeletal evaluation** with **initial plain x-rays** further evaluation with bone scan, CT, MRI, or brain/spinal cord.

- **Spondylolysis:** unilateral or bilateral defects in the connection of the superior and inferior articular facets (most common at L5); acquired secondary to **repetitive hyperextension → stress fracture →** pseudoarthrosis (false joint); more common with wrestlers, weight lifters, gymnasts, and football players
- **Spondylolisthesis:** forward slip of the involved vertebra (of spondylolysis) on the one below it; **common cause of adolescent back pain**

Clinical presentation—Spondylolysis: presents with **low back pain that radiates to buttocks with hamstring spasm, exacerbated by hyperextension of spine**; spondylolisthesis: **lumbar back pain plus radiculopathy and bowel/bladder dysfunction** (nerve root compression) plus loss of spinal mobility and gait disturbance. Pain related to infection, inflammation, or neoplasm is more likely to be constant (even with rest) and causes awakening from sleep.

Diagnosis—**Plain films** with various views first; if normal, obtain **bone scan with single-photon emission CT scan (SPECT)** and **MRI** for nerve root involvement.

Management—If **asymptomatic with spondylolysis**, no treatment; with pain: modification of activity, physical therapy, oral analgesics, and lumbosacral orthoses for several months; heals in most; if inadequate response, then surgery. With **spondylolisthesis:** individualize therapy; higher degrees of slippage in skeletally immature children generally require surgery.

Femoral Anteversion

Most common deformity, presenting as intoeing; more common in young toddlers and early school-age girls; acquired most commonly secondary to **abnormal sitting habits ("w" position)**; there is some degree of generalized ligamental laxity. **Entire leg is inwardly rotated with restriction of external rotation;** clinical diagnosis, x-rays not necessary; treatment is mostly observation with **correction of abnormal sitting pattern;** usually corrects with growth by age 8–10 years; surgery with large degree of rotation and functional impairment.

Apophysitis

Inflammation at the insertion of a muscle group from **repetitive motions** during periods of rapid growth **→ microfractures at the cartilage insertion site with inflammation**

- **Calcaneal apophysitis:** most common cause of heel pain in children (Sever disease). Manage conservatively with nonsteroidal anti-inflammatory drugs (NSAIDs), decreased activity, stretching, and orthoses.
- **Little League elbow:** apophysitis of the medial epicondyle from throwing, repetitive wrist flexion and extension, or weight-bearing on hands (gymnastics); medial elbow

pain; treat with no throwing for 4–6 weeks, then stretching and strengthening exercises and 1–2 weeks of progressive functional throwing

- **Osgood-Schlatter disease:** traction apophysitis of **tibial tubercle** and patellar tendon; **pain and swelling over tibial tubercle** in a growing child (typically, late childhood; adolescence in an athlete) **aggravated by repetitive activities**; resolves with skeletal maturity; x-ray demonstrates apophysitis. Management—**rest, restriction of activities**, with or without knee immobilization and isometric exercises; symptoms usually heal within 12–24 months.

Avascular Necrosis (Legg-Calve-Perthes disease)

- Unknown etiology; **temporary disruption of blood flow to the capital-femoral epiphysis** → impaired epiphyseal growth and **femoral head deformity**
- Males (very active; often with delayed skeletal maturity) affected to a greater degree than females
- Peak incidence in early to mid-childhood.

Clinical presentation—Usually **insidious onset of limp with or without pain** (may be **referred to anteromedial thigh or groin**); onset often preceded by trauma. Exam: decreased internal rotation and abduction with or without mild hip-flexion contracture.

Diagnosis

- **AP and lateral frog-leg plain films** show widening of the joint space, **lateralization and flattening of the femoral head**, with a ragged-appearing growth plate; with healing → re-ossification → new bone formation → return to normal of bone density → **joint remodeling until skeletal maturity**.
- Presentation from mild to severe, depending on amount of femoral head involved. Later presentation (>9 years of age, with less time until skeletal maturity) does worse; joint symptoms typically later in life.

Management—Primarily **conservative**: decreased activity, physical therapy to maintain hip ROM; with increasing severity: bed rest with or without traction; surgery for severe, nonresponsive cases

Slipped Capital-Femoral Epiphysis (SCFE)

Femoral head remains in acetabulum as neck of femur rotates anteriorly → **displacement of the metaphysis at the physeal plate**; involvement of mechanical and anatomical factors: more common in an **obese (most closely associated factor) adolescent male during the adolescent growth spurt**; may have associated endocrine abnormality

Clinical presentation—Most frequent is **chronic development of a limp with subtle hip pain** (weeks to months); may then have an **acute severe exacerbation of pain** in hip area with **inability to bear weight,** or may present acutely at the start; pain may be in the thigh or groin or **referred to the knee**; may be bilateral; hip held in external rotation with or without apparent leg-shortening.

Diagnosis—AP and lateral **frog-leg plain films**—**widening and irregularity of the physis (pre-slip)** to anterior displacement of femoral neck overlying femoral head (slip); if not diagnostic, CT scan is accurate.

Management—**Spica cast or surgical pinning**; unless significant slippage, then **surgical realignment procedures** with pinning. Order thyroid function tests to rule out hypothyroidism. **Complications**—osteonecrosis and chondrolysis.

Infections

Table 17.1: Transient Toxic Synovitis, Osteomyelitis, and Septic Arthritis

	Transient Toxic Synovitis	Osteomyelitis	Septic Arthritis
Anatomic location	Hip joint (mono-articular)	More at the end of bones (tibia, femur, humerus, and fibula most common); in young infants, contiguous joint and multiple sites may also be involved	Majority with LE joints (knee, hip, fibula, ankle) and smaller number with UE (shoulder, wrist)
Etiology	Probably viral or hyper-sensitivity; may involve minor trauma	*Staph. aureus* is the most common cause in all age groups, including neonates (then GBS and Gram-negatives); *K. kingae* may be next most common; then, in older children, *Streptococcus* spp., *Pseudomonas. aeruginosa* (almost all with deep foot punctures); in sickle-cell: *Salmonella* spp., *Staph. aureus, Strep. pneumoniae.* Most with hematogenous spread; others from closed trauma, penetrating injury, open fracture, foreign body, bites, nosocomial, and with immunocompromise.	Most from *Staph. aureus* in all ages; then GABHS, *Strep. pneumoniae,* and *K. kingae*; gonococcus in sexually active adolescents; majority from hematogenous spread and then direct inoculation from a contiguous focus (injuries, nosocomial infection, foreign bodies, intra-articular injection)
Epidemiology	Toddler to mid-childhood	More common in infants and toddlers; half by age 5 years; males greater (more trauma)	More in infants and toddlers; half by age 2, most by age 5 years

(continued)

	Transient Toxic Synovitis	Osteomyelitis	Septic Arthritis
Clinical presentation	Prior nonspecific viral syndrome, then acute onset of pain (groin, anterior thigh, knee), limp, and mild decreased ROM; afebrile or low-grade fever	Acute onset of fever, pain, decreased movement, limp, refusal to bear weight, localized signs of inflammation (soft-tissue response)	Early subtle signs in neonates, may be associated with adjacent osteomyelitis; older: acute-onset fever, pain, swelling, erythema, warmth, limb, refusal to walk, decreased ROM
Diagnosis	AP and lateral hip x-rays normal; ultrasound may show small effusion; CBC and ESR normal; if concern regarding septic arthritis, aspirate joint; MRI or bone scan may be needed for any concern about contiguous osteomyelitis	-Blood culture for all; elevated WBC, ESR, CRP -Initial plain films to exclude other causes; may see soft-tissue changes after 3 days and bone changes after a week or two -MRI is the best test for anatomic detail and to aid in bone aspiration; bone scan useful for possible multiple sites -Definitive diagnosis with bone aspiration for Gram stain, culture/sensitivity, and possible PCR (*K. kingae* is difficult to culture)	-Blood culture in all; elevated WBC, ESR, CRP; if GC is suspected, cervical, anal, and throat cultures -Plain films are normal in over half; may show widening of joint capsule, soft-tissue edema, or obliteration of normal radiographic findings -Ultrasound-guided (especially for hip) joint aspiration for Gram stain, culture/sensitivity; need repeat daily joint aspiration for another 1–2 days for effusion to resolve -Bone scan useful for sacroiliac joint; if suspect adjacent osteomyelitis, need MRI

(continued on next page)

Table 17.1: Transient Toxic Synovitis, Osteomyelitis, and Septic Arthritis *(cont.)*

	Transient Toxic Synovitis	**Osteomyelitis**	**Septic Arthritis**
Management	Symptomatic: decreased activity + NSAIDS for pain; usually recover in 3 weeks	-Initial empirical antibiotics for most likely organism; **neonates:** nafcillin or oxacillin plus third-generation cephalosporin (*Staph. aureus*, GBS, and Gram-negatives); **older children:** nafcillin or oxacillin and cefotaxime (*Staph. aureus*, streptococci, and *K. kingae*; if Hib is suspected, use third-generation cephalosporin; if MRSA or anaerobes are suspected, substitute the nafcillin/oxacillin with vancomycin or clindamycin); **sickle-cell:** nafcillin or oxacillin plus third-generation cephalosporin -Adjust antibiotics to the best sensitivities, when available; if no organism recovered and patient is not better, re-aspirate. -Duration of therapy depends on organism, clinical improvement, and normalization of ESR. -May usually switch from IV to PO meds (depending on sensitivities to meds that can be delivered orally; need serum bactericidal titer ≥1:8) if clinically improved with decreasing ESR -Surgery if frank pus obtained (needs to be drained), lack of improvement, penetrating injury, or retained foreign body, and chronic osteomyelitis (sinus tracts)	Initial empirical antibiotics as for osteomyelitis, then adjust meds per sensitivities; usual duration 10–14 days for streptococci and *K. kingae*; longer for staphylococci and Gram-negatives plus need clinical improvement and ESR normalization. Surgery for all hips (emergency) or lack of improvement.

Abbreviations: C-reactive protein, CRP; erythrocyte sedimentation rate, ESR; group A beta-hemolytic streptococcus, GABHS; group B streptococci, GBS; gonococcus, GC; Haemophilus influenzae type b, Hib; Kingella kingae, K. kingae; lower extremity, LE; methicillin-resistant Staph. aureus, MRSA; nonsteroidal anti-inflammatory drugs, NSAIDs; polymerase chain reaction, PCR; range of motion, ROM; upper extremity, UE; white blood cell, WBC

Bone Neoplasms

Table 17.2: Benign and Malignant Bone Tumors and Bone Cysts

Osteosarcoma	• Most common malignant (highly) bone tumor in children; most during adolescent growth spurt • Genetic and acquired predispositions (hereditary retinoblastoma, familial cancer syndrome, irradiation, others) • Metaphyses of long bones • Deep bone pain with limp and swelling with night awakening; palpation of a tender mass with decreased ROM • X-ray: mixed lytic and blastic changes with new bone formation = sunburst pattern; need MRI of bone with biopsy and metastatic workup (CT of chest and bone scan; metastases to lungs and bones) • Preoperative chemotherapy and complete surgical excision with postoperative chemotherapy and rehabilitation (up to 70% 5-year survival if no metastases; up to 20% with metastases); also removal of metastatic lung nodules
Ewing sarcoma	• Next most common malignant bone tumor; most with specific chromosomal translocation • Undifferentiated sarcoma of **neural crest origin** • Equally located between extremities and central skeleton • Presents similarly to osteosarcoma; also respiratory distress with chest involvement; cord compression with vertebral involvement; often with systemic symptoms (fever, weight loss) • X-ray: lytic lesion with periosteal reaction (**onionskin appearance**); **MRI** entire bone for anatomy; evaluate for metastases: **CT chest, bone scan, and bone marrow aspiration and biopsy**; treatment with **multiagent chemotherapy** preoperatively → shrinkage of tumor and decrease in pain; local **radiation and/or surgery**; similar prognosis as with osteosarcoma
Osteoid osteoma	• Small tumor, mostly on proximal femur or tibia • Presents at 5–20 years of age • Continuous and gradual increase in pain, **often worse at night, relieved by ASA**; may have limp, muscle weakness, and atrophy • X-ray: **round-oval lucency** of metaphysis or diaphysis surrounded by **sclerotic bone**; some may not be seen and **CT** should then be performed • Management is **surgical removal.**
Osteochondroma	• One of most common benign bone tumors; rare malignant degeneration to a chondrosarcoma • Most common at 5–15 years of age • **Metaphysis** of long bone, especially distal femur, proximal humerus, or proximal tibia • May be asymptomatic; increases in size until skeletal maturation; bony, **non-painful mass** • X-ray: mass on a **stalk or with a broad base extending from bone surface with a cartilage cap** covering the lesion • **No routine removal** unless large and symptomatic

(continued on next page)

Table 17.2: Benign and Malignant Bone Tumors and Bone Cysts *(cont.)*

Osteoblastoma	• Most commonly involve the vertebrae, but may affect any bone • Progressive growth with local bone destruction • **Insidious**-onset dull ache with or without neurological symptoms (if vertebral) • X-ray: **variable** changes that may look malignant, so **biopsy** is generally needed • Treatment: **surgery**
Fibromas	• **Common fibrous bone lesions** in children >2 years of age • **Usually asymptomatic** but may present with **pathological fracture**; exam is generally normal • X-ray: eccentric **lucency with sharp margins** in **metaphyseal cortex** with **long axis parallel to the bone**; may be multiple or bilateral • No biopsy (characteristic x-ray) or treatment (regress with skeletal maturity) unless very large (possible pathological fracture)
Unicameral bone cyst	• Can occur at any age, but rare under 3 years and after skeletal maturity (most then resolve spontaneously) • Majority are **asymptomatic**, may present with pathological fracture with minor trauma • X-ray: solitary central lucency with a sharp margin within the medulla; most in **proximal humerus or femur** • Allow fracture to heal, then **aspirate cyst** and inject corticosteroid.
Aneurysmal bone cyst	• Large, deep space with blood and solid pieces of tissue; most on femur, tibia, spine • Occurs <20 years of age • **Progressively growing**; presents with pain and swelling; if vertebral involvement: compression and neurological findings • X-ray: eccentric destruction and expansion of metaphysis with sclerotic rim of bone • Surgical treatment—may recur

Abbreviations: acetylsalicylic acid, ASA; range of motion, ROM

Childhood Fractures

- **Buckle (torus) fracture:** compression fracture at junction of metaphysis and diaphysis; most common at **distal radius**; heals in 3–4 weeks with **immobilization**
- **Plastic deformation:** seen only in children; force produces **microscopic failure on the convex side** but not to the concave side of the bone, **no visible fracture line**; small angulations correct with growth
- **Greenstick fracture:** bone is bent; failure on the convex side of the bone but the **fracture line does not go completely through to the concave** (this side has plastic deformation); treatment: breaking the bone on the concave side, or it will recoil back.
- **Complete fracture:** fracture line completely through the bone
  - **Spiral fracture:** produced by a rotational force; reduced easily
  - **Oblique fracture:** diaphysis is at 30 degrees to the bone axis; very unstable
  - **Transverse fracture:** reduced using the intact periosteum from the concave side

- **Epiphyseal fractures:** around the growth plate; potential for deformity; most frequently at the distal radius; **five Salter-Harris types** (predicts outcome and guides therapy), as follows:
  - **I and II:** separation through physis (I); or fracture through portion of the physis, extending to the metaphysis (II); treat with closed reduction
  - **III and IV:** through portion of the physis, extending through the epiphysis and into the joint (III) or across the metaphysis, physis, and epiphysis (IV); requires **anatomic alignment**
  - **V:** not diagnosed initially; presents in the future as growth disturbance; **crush injury** to the physis

SPORTS MEDICINE

Injury prevention

- **Decrease playing time** in **hot weather** with **frequent water breaks** and **headgear removed** to decrease heat-related illness; **modify activity based on environmental temperature.**
- **Adequate hydration prior to exercise**
- Teach ways to **decrease likelihood of specific mechanisms of injuries** and penalize those who do not follow rules.
- Remove environmental hazards.
- Use appropriate and **proper-fitting protective equipment**
- Appropriate **safe training practices** with emphasis on flexibility; warm-up and warm-down sessions
- **Avoid overtraining and overuse injuries** (repetitive microtrauma, see Acute Sprains section below).
- Appropriate **rehabilitation of old injuries** before returning to play

Evaluation for Sports Participation

- Directed history and physical (past medical history, surgical history, medications, allergies, immunizations, nutritional, review of systems, and physical exam, including neurological) and **screening musculoskeletal exam:** identify possible problems, with possible exclusion **or delay from play**, or certain types of activities (increased risk of injury or death in those with certain medical conditions); different state requirements, but the minimum is an **annual exam 3–6 weeks prior to onset of training in healthy athletes**
- If no symptoms or problems that require further investigation, then no screening labs needed; **standardized questionnaires** available and almost all problems identified by history. Most common identified problems are **previous non-rehabilitated injuries**. Any suspected cardiac disease—12-lead ECG, echocardiogram, and then possibility of Holter monitor and stress test. Recommendation for participation with respect to specific cardiac diagnosis done with consultation from cardiologist. Sudden death due to unsuspected cardiac problems.

- Examples of problems that need to be addressed and may cause increased risk with certain activities: hypertension, arrhythmias, obesity, visual disturbances, bronchospasm, inguinal hernia, scoliosis, contagious disease, acute and chronic injuries
- **Disqualification and limitations** are set by a qualified physician with the help of subspecialty consultants and expert guidelines.

Acute Sprains, Strains, and Contusions

Types

- **Sprain:** injury to ligament or joint capsule; graded from 1–3 (torn fibers with no laxity of ligament, to all fibers torn with complete joint laxity)
- **Strain:** injury to muscle or tendon; graded from 1–3 (mild pain with little weakness, to complete rupture of muscle or tendon with marked weakness)
- **Contusion:** crush injury to any soft tissue
- **More severe injuries** suggestive of structural changes: **acute signs and symptoms with immediate swelling, deformity, or bone or joint instability**
- **Overuse injuries: repetitive microtrauma** greater than rate of repair in muscle, tendon, bone, cartilage; more common in **sports with the same repetitive motion**. Most frequent factor is **training error**: increasing intensity and duration too quickly; scarring and abnormal tissue develops which lead to **tendinopathies**; goal is to eliminate causative factors in order to prevent reinjury.

Initial evaluation

- First, check peripheral pulses and capillary refill, gross motor and sensory function (**assess neurovascular injury**) → maintain vascular and skeletal stability. Immediate orthopedic consultation: vascular compromise, nerve compromise, or open fracture; deep laceration over a joint; uneducable dislocation; displaced fracture; complete tendon tear.
- Apply pressure to any site of bleeding.
- Cover wound with sterile saline-soaked gauze, pad, and splint.

Return to Play

Rehabilitation program starts on the day of the injury, and proceeds slowly and gradually.

- **Limit further injury, control swelling and pain, and minimize losses of strength and flexibility:** ice (plastic ice bag to skin 20 minutes continuously three or four times per day until swelling resolves), slings, crutches, analgesia (NSAIDs), elastic wrap compression (limits further bleeding and swelling), elevation (promotes venous return and limits further swelling); initiate isometric strengthening and ROM exercises as soon as possible.

- **Improve strength and flexibility while allowing healing of internal structures**: remove protective devices when no further pain with daily activities; see physical therapist or athletic trainer to develop program of stretching.
- Attain **near-normal strength and flexibility and further improve/maintain cardiovascular fitness**: controlled conditioning with weights or elastic bands
- **Return to exercise without restriction with near-normal strength, flexibility, endurance, and proprioception:** start sport-specific exercises and progress in a stepwise manner; any activities, as long as there is no pain within 24 hours of the activity
- Each injury related to a specific sport has very specific conditions and steps in returning to play.

Heat Illness

- **Greater risk of heat illness in children** due to increased ratio of surface area to body mass and greater heat per kg of body weight produced; decreased perspiration and blunted thirst response
- **Heat stress (mild)**
  - **Heat cramps:** most common; mild dehydration and salt depletion; mostly involving calf and hamstring—late in activity (muscle fatigue); **treatment:** oral hydration with electrolyte drinks and gentle stretching. Return to play if no problem with performance.
  - **Heat syncope:** fainting after prolonged exercise secondary to depleted intravascular volume
  - **Heat edema:** mild edema of hands and feet with initial heat exposure; resolves with time
  - **Heat tetany:** carpopedal spasm/tingling due to hyperventilation; **treatment:** move to a cooler area and decrease rate of breathing

- **Heat exhaustion:** rectal temperature 100–103°F (37.7–39.4°C) with or without mild CNS dysfunction (headache, dizziness, syncope) and nausea, vomiting, and weakness; **treatment:** move to cool area, cool with fans, remove excess clothing, ice over groin and axilla, oral hydration (IV if cannot take PO), monitor rectal temperature; if no rapid response, transfer to Emergency Room (ER)
- **Heat stroke:** rectal temperature >104°F (40°C) with CNS dysfunction and potential tissue damage; usually intense exertion and profuse sweating; medical emergency (increased mortality); **treatment:** immediate whole-body cold-water immersion with constant monitoring; discontinue when rectal temperature 101–102°F (38.3–38.8°C); IV fluids (normal saline or Ringer's lactate); immediate transport to ER; needs to be cleared by physician before any return to play

Concussion

Any decrease in neurological or cognitive function after a traumatic event with or without loss of consciousness: remove from activity, examine medically, and monitor regularly over hours (**Sport Concussion Assessment Tool; SCAT**); return to play is gradual with accomplishment of stepwise series of tasks before full play.

- **Simple concussion:** no signs or symptoms; resolves over 7–10 days; gradual return to play after being asymptomatic
- **Complex concussion:** persistent symptoms or cognitive impairment (focal neurological findings, any cognitive impairment, symptoms from multiple concussions); needs **formal neuropsychological testing**. If focal findings or worsening of symptoms then **neuroimaging**. Increased risk with persistent vomiting, prolonged headache, persistent short-term memory loss, seizure, Glasgow Coma Scale <15, or signs of a basal or depressed skull fracture.

Neck Injuries

- Most common injury is **soft tissue**; **assume fracture** if midline cervical pain, pain on ROM, focal neurological defects, or loss of consciousness.
- **Brachial plexus injury** (C5-T1): usually upper trunk (C5–C6); presents with unilateral burning, paresthesias, and arm weakness; usually resolves quickly. With bilateral involvement or persistent signs and symptoms, discontinue play and obtain **MRI**.

Management

- **Immobilize with C-spine brace.**
- Obtain AP, lateral, oblique, and open-mouth x-rays before immobilizer is removed.
- If active extension and flexion is not possible, **CT** is needed (undiagnosed fracture on plain films).
- **MRI** for possible ligamentous or spinal cord injuries
- If no positive findings: immobilize neck with soft collar with rest and use anti-inflammatory medications.
- Start ROM exercises as soon as possible and return to play with full-strength ROM and sports-specific neck function.

Shoulder Injuries

- **Clavicle fracture:** direct blow to the clavicle, or from fall on lateral shoulder or outstretched hand; almost all are mid third, which requires **arm sling**; for displaced medial or lateral third fracture: obtain immediate orthopedic consult
- **Acromioclavicular (AC) separation:** acromion is hit directly with the humerus adducted → acromion is forced inferiorly and medially; tenderness at AC joint with **palpation of step-off between clavicle and acromion**; most treated with sling and analgesics, then ROM exercises and strengthening of rotator cuff; worse types with ligament tear and fascial detachment require surgery

- **Anterior dislocation:** falling with **hand outstretched and arm straight**, or making forceful contact with another player; feels like **shoulder popped out, then severe pain**; anterior displacement of humeral head → **bulge in anterior shoulder** with or without neurological findings. **Treatment:** reduce shoulder; when x-ray is normal, immobilize for a week with early ROM and strengthening exercises; after at least three dislocations → surgery
- **Rotator cuff tendinopathy:** most injury to the supraspinatus; **shoulder pain at top of arc of motion** and at rest and with activity; weakness and pain with strength testing. **Treatment:** ice, rest, stretching, strengthening exercises, analgesics, physical therapy

Elbow Injuries

- Most are **posterior dislocations:** falling back on an **outstretched arm with elbow extended**; possible compromise of **brachial artery** (intact if positive radial and ulnar pulses) and **radial, ulnar, and median nerves**; olecranon process is displaced behind the distal humerus; **reduce** with gentle longitudinal traction to forearm with gentle upward pressure of distal humerus; if not possible, pad and place in sling and send to ER.
- **Chronic injuries from overuse syndromes:** if **onset of acute pain,** need x-rays to assess for **avulsion of the medial epicondyle**; adolescents with fused apophysis are likely to have an **ulnar collateral ligament tear** (ultrasound or MRI to assess; surgery if complete tear). **Tennis elbow** (more common in adults) = **lateral epicondylitis**. Best prevention of these is to stop performing the task with the onset of elbow pain.

Wrist Injuries

Fractures are most common injury; almost **half of all fractures in children**; most from fall on **outstretched hands**, the vast majority of the **distal radius and ulna**; most are **torus (buckle) or greenstick fractures.**

Knee Injuries

Types

- **Acute inability of weight-bearing within a few minutes of the injury** likely to be a **serious injury** (fracture, patellar dislocation, anterior cruciate ligament [ACL] tear, or meniscal tear). Also, **if swelling occurs within a few hours: likely to be a hemarthrosis due to a serious injury**—likely an **ACL tear** (direct blow, hyperextension) and orthopedic consultation and surgery are required immediately.
- **Posterior cruciate ligament tears** are rare; usually due to a direct blow to an area of the proximal tibia; usually nonsurgical treatment
- **Medial collateral ligament (MCL):** blow to outside of the knee; **lateral collateral ligament:** from varus knee stress; uncommon; both are outside the joint, so not much effusion or disability; nonsurgical treatment

- **Meniscal tears:** same as ACL: hemarthrosis, joint pain; requires **immediate orthopedic consult**
- **Patellar dislocation:** non-contact injury; lateral dislocation with bleeding into the joint; nonsurgical treatment
- **Patellofemoral stress syndrome:** most common cause of **anterior knee pain**; diagnosis of exclusion; diffuse pain, may be bilateral; no swelling; history of change in activity; if medial patellar tenderness or pain with compression of joint without effusion or other positive findings, then no imaging is required. Treatment is nonsurgical and gradual return to play.

Initial therapy—Hinged brace immobilization, crutches, compression, and elevation; plain films required if isolated patellar tenderness, fibular head tenderness, inability to flex 90 degrees, inability to bear weight for four paces immediately and in the ER

Lower Leg and Ankle Injuries

- **Shin splints: medial tibial stress syndrome**
  - Most common overuse injury of the lower leg
  - Diffuse tenderness over lower tibia
  - If **tibial stress fracture**, tenderness is **more focal and severe**
  - Both caused by traction of soleus on tibia
  - X-ray: initially normal in shin splints and stress fracture for first few weeks; later, periosteal reaction with a stress fracture; bone scan is the most sensitive: (normal in shin splints); MRI best test of stress fracture
  - **Treatment:** ice, rest, NSAIDs, correcting training errors, non-weight-bearing activities

- **Ankle injuries** are **most common acute athletic injury**; almost all **are sprains**
  - **Examine neurovascular status** (do not move ankle); then check for other findings (edema, ecchymoses, anatomic abnormalities) and ROM.

- **Ankle plain films** if malleolar pain, unable to bear weight, or bone tenderness over posterior distal tibia or fibula; **foot plain films** if pain in area of midfoot or bone tenderness over navicular or 5th metatarsal
- **Initial treatment:** rest, ice, compression, and elevation for 48–72 hours; rehabilitation on day of injury with isometric exercises, and gradual return to play with full ROM and near-normal strength, otherwise recurrent injuries are likely

DERMATOLOGICAL DISORDERS

LESIONS AND DISORDERS SEEN IN NEWBORNS AND INFANTS

Erythema Toxicum

- **Description:** Transient eruption in full-term infants (less common in preterms), in first days of life. Small, yellow-white papulo-pustules on an erythematous base. Any area except palms and soles; clumps of lesions in different areas or more diffuse.
- **Causes:** Unknown; not infectious
- **Diagnosis:** Clinical characteristics; staining contents of lesion shows eosinophils (not necessary to do)
- **Treatment:** None

Transient Neonatal Pustular Melanosis

- **Description:** Transient, benign eruption of newborns at birth; more common in black infants; early appearance of pustules which rupture → ring of fine scale → hyperpigmented macules (may persist for a few months); may have all stages of lesions present anywhere, but especially forehead, neck, and lower back.
- **Causes:** Unknown; not infectious
- **Diagnosis:** Characteristic presentation + pustules filled with polymorphonuclear cells (PMNs), debris and few eosinophils
- **Treatment:** None

Infantile Acropustulosis

- **Description:** Common, transient eruption in young infants (2 months—first year) more common in black males. Small to medium-size erythematous papules → vesiculo-pustular lesions → open and crust before healing; recurrences and remissions over first 2 years mostly on hands and feet (especially palms and soles), ankles and wrists.
- **Causes:** Unknown; not infectious

- **Diagnosis:** Characteristic presentation; lesions contain neutrophils and occasional eosinophils
- **Associated findings:** Intense pruritus
- **Treatment:** Oral first-generation antihistamines (for nighttime sedation) and topical corticosteroids for pruritus

Salmon Patch

- **Description:** Localized vascular ectasia in newborns. Light pink (salmon-flesh color) macule with irregular border. Posterior neck, glabella, eyelids, and forehead; symmetric (both sides of midline or both eyelids); lesions on posterior neck and central forehead may persist, others fade.
- **Causes:** Unknown reason for occurrence
- **Diagnosis:** Characteristic location and appearance
- **Treatment:** None

Mongolian Spots

- **Description:** Common, pigmented macules that fade over first few years of life; mostly in dark-skinned newborns. Blue-black to gray with irregular borders. Mostly presacral, back, posterior thighs and legs; multiple lesions widely distributed and in less common locations (e.g., shoulder)
- **Causes:** Melanin-containing melanocytes in the dermis that have had arrested migration
- **Diagnosis:** Characteristic appearance, and onset at birth
- **Treatment:** None

Port-Wine Stain (see also Chapter 22)

- **Description:** Vascular malformation present at birth; dilated capillaries in the dermis. Pink-purple (color of port wine) macular discoloration of skin, with sharp edges. Most on unilateral head and neck. Complications dependent upon association with a specific syndrome. If in trigeminal distribution, may be part of Sturge-Weber syndrome (see Chapter 22); also part of Klippel-Trenaunay syndrome and, other conditions.
- **Diagnosis:** Characteristic area and distribution; permanent lesion (does not fade)
- **Treatment:** Best Rx is pulsed-dye laser begun early in infancy; leads to normal skin without scarring

Hemangiomas

- **Description:** Vascular tumor; (most common tumor in children) proliferation of vascular endothelium. **Superficial:** bright red, protrudes above skin, sharp borders (verrucous-like). **Deep:** more diffuse, smoother, less defined, and may have a bluish color at base. Most **mixed**, with elements of superficial and deep. Occurs anywhere; but most on face, scalp, chest, and back.

- **Diagnosis:** Characteristic appearance; begins first 2 months of life and expands rapidly (over first year), then becomes stable and involutes by 5–9 years.
- **Associated findings:** With various syndromes: **Kasabach-Merritt syndrome:** life-threatening hemorrhage and severe anemia from large hemangiomas (that do not regress) with thrombocytopenia, hemolytic anemia (microangiopathic), and coagulopathy
- **Complications:** Infection, ulceration, bleeding; large lesions may interfere with vital functions (eye, nose, mouth, perianal); can extend internally (tracheal) and may cause specific problems, depending on location (e.g., respiratory distress)
- **Treatment:** Most just observed (will eventually involute); treat large lesions with functional impairment with pulsed-dye laser and corticosteroids; hemangiomas of Kasabach-Merritt syndrome may need surgery, irradiation, embolization, and chemotherapy.

Nevus Sebaceous (of Jadassohn)

- **Description:** All skin elements but mostly sebaceous glands, formed from primary epithelial germ cells. Small, oval or linear, slightly elevated, yellow-orange plaque with sharp borders, most common on the scalp in an area of alopecia, less so on neck and trunk.
- **Diagnosis:** Characteristic appearance and histopathology on biopsy
- **Associated findings:** May be associated with eye, central nervous system (CNS), and skeletal defects
- **Complications:** Can dedifferentiate into epithelial tumors (basal-cell carcinoma)
- **Treatment:** Total excision before adolescence

Ectodermal Dysplasias

- **Description:** Disorders (about 30 genotypes) causing defects (need at least two for diagnosis) of the skin, nails, hair, teeth, and glands. Most common is **anhydrotic ecto-dermal dysplasia** (X-linked recessive, autosomal recessive, and dominant forms): partial or complete absence of sweat glands, abnormal dental development, and decreased hair; newborns present with peeling, dry, wrinkled, hypopigmented skin; scalp hair, eyebrows, and lashes are fine and sparse; infants present with episodes of high fevers (no sweating; decreased saliva and tears); characteristic dysmorphic facial features. Can occur over entire body.
- **Diagnosis:** Scalp biopsy is the best test.
- **Associated findings:** High incidence of atopy, ear and eye abnormalities, and gastro-esophageal reflux; may occur with immune defects
- **Complications:** High body temperatures, fluid and electrolyte loss, corneal damage, failure-to-thrive
- **Treatment:** Protection from high temperatures, use of artificial tears, early dental therapy

Harlequin Fetus

- **Description:** Autosomal recessive ichthyosis; disorder of cornification with hyperkeratosis and scaling. Thick, hard, cracked skin at birth, with horny plates → facial disfigurement, constriction of fingers and toes, flattened nose and ears, severe ectropion (eversion of eyelid margins with skin maceration, conjunctival inflammation, and keratitis), everted lips; may have absent nails and hair. Can occur over entire body.
- **Diagnosis:** Clinical presentation; prenatal diagnosis possible with fetoscopy and microscopy of amniotic fluid cells
- **Associated findings:** Decreased joint mobility, immobile hands and feet, increased incidence of infections, respiratory distress
- **Complications:** Most die in initial days to weeks of life; survival leads to chronic ichthyosis and neurological defects.
- **Treatment:** Humidified, heated incubator; high IV fluids; and careful monitoring of electrolytes, emollients, and oral retinoids

Collodion Baby

- **Description:** Presentation of congenital ichthyosis. Usually autosomal recessive due to various mutations. At birth, covered with thick, tight membrane (looks like oiled parchment [collodion]), which is shed (desquamates in large sheets) eventually; otherwise, similar features to harlequin fetus; new membrane may form in localized areas after several weeks. Can occur over entire body.
- **Diagnosis:** Clinical appearance; molecular genetic diagnosis
- **Associated findings:** May evolve into other forms of ichthyosis.
- **Complications:** Hypothermia, dehydration, infection, aspiration pneumonia
- **Treatment:** High humidity, IV fluids, emollients

Inherited Ichthyosis

- **Description:** Most common forms of ichthyosis to present as collodion babies. Autosomal recessive lamellar ichthyosis and congenital ichthyosiform erythroderma; different gene mutations.
- **Lamellar ichthyosis**—collodion baby, then after shedding the membrane → large, dark scales with little erythema. In **congenital ichthyosiform erythroderma**—persistent erythroderma and white-appearing scales. Can occur over entire body.
- **Diagnosis:** Clinical appearance following collodion shedding; skin biopsy, molecular genetic testing
- **Associated findings:** Severe pruritus; ectropion; nail abnormalities; alopecia; small, flattened ears
- **Complications:** Bacterial colonization with secondary infection; eye problems (ectropion); severe cosmetic issues
- **Treatment:** High humidity, IV fluids, emollients, keratolytic agents (lactic acid), and oral retinoids

HYPERPIGMENTED AND HYPOPIGMENTED LESIONS

Lentigines

- **Description:** Permanent deposits of melanin with increased number of melanocytes in epidermis. Cause is unknown; not related to sun exposure. Small, round, dark-brown macules can occur anywhere on the body.
- **Diagnosis:** Characteristic features and histology
- **Associated findings: LEOPARD syndrome** (multiple lentigines syndrome): generalized, symmetric distribution of **l**entigines, **E**CG abnormalities, **o**cular hypertelorism, **p**ulmonic stenosis, **a**bnormal genitals, growth **r**etardation, and sensorineural **d**eafness; also **Peutz-Jeghers syndrome:** melanin-producing macules of lips and mucous membranes with gastrointestinal (GI) polyposis (see Chapter 13)
- **Complications:** If associated with syndromes
- **Treatment:** If numerous, laser therapy.

Café-au-Lait Spots

- **Description:** Hyperpigmented, light brown to tan macules with sharp smooth borders of various sizes; at birth or later in life; presence of 1–3 is normal. Can occur anywhere on body.
- **Diagnosis:** Typical appearance; part of diagnosis of neurofibromatosis type I
- **Associated findings:** Increased numbers of large café-au-lait spots with McCune-Albright syndrome (see Chapter 16) and neurofibromatosis type I (see Chapter 22)
- **Complications:** If associated with above syndromes
- **Treatment:** None; management of associated condition

Incontinentia Pigmenti

- **Description:** Rare inherited ectodermal disorder with skin, eye, and dental abnormalities. Mosaic condition due to random X-inactivation of an X-linked dominant gene (lethal in males). Erythematous linear streaks in first weeks of life, and plaques of vesicles, → verrucous plaques, → various patterns of hyperpigmented (key feature) patches; phases may overlap. Initial lesions more common on limbs and trunk (circumferentially); hyperpigmentation more on the trunk.
- **Diagnosis:** Unique linear configuration of vesicles, filled with eosinophils and high blood eosinophilia; axilla and groin always involved with hyperpigmented phase; characteristic histopathology
- **Associated findings:** Alopecia, dental defects, CNS and eye abnormalities
- **Complications:** Severe dental problems; gross motor problems; mental retardation; seizures; paralysis; severe eye problems, including optic-nerve atrophy
- **Treatment:** Skin lesions are benign; other associations and complications are treated individually.

Albinism (Congenital Oculocutaneous Albinism; OCA)

- **Description:** Partial or complete failure of melanin formation, but normal melanocytes. Different gene defects and inheritance patterns; OCA-1 due to decreased tyrosinase activity. Complete lack of visible pigment (most severe form): white hair and skin, and blue or pink iris; near-normal to near–OCA-1 appearance with **OCA 2** (most common worldwide): little or no melanin at birth → accumulation of red-yellow pigment in childhood → light-brown skin color in white children and yellow-brown skin in black children. Occurs on skin, hair, and eyes.
- **Diagnosis:** Clinical pattern; molecular diagnosis
- **Associated findings:** Photophobia, nystagmus, decreased visual activity
- **Complications:** Visual problems; OCA-2 may improve with aging; skin malignancies
- **Treatment:** Protective clothing and broad-spectrum sunscreen; careful evaluation for possible skin malignancies

Vitiligo

- **Description:** Generalized or localized areas of hypopigmentation; possible immunological abnormality. Most have generalized form: symmetric pattern of white macular patches with hypopigmentation of the entire skin; with localized disease may be dermatomal distribution, or may occur on benign moles. Can occur over any body part.
- **Diagnosis:** Characteristic appearance and histopathology
- **Associated findings:** Autoimmune associated diseases
- **Complications:** May occur with syndromes with eye, ear, and CNS abnormalities
- **Treatment:** Potent topical steroids, tacrolimus or pimecrolimus for localized areas; more extensive: narrow-band ultraviolet B (UVB) light; minimize sun exposure; cover-up cosmetics

VESICULOBULLOUS DISORDERS

Erythema Multiforme

- **Description:** Abrupt eruption from blister cleavage line in sub-epidermis; cell-mediated immune response → damage to keratinocytes and release of cytokines. Papular lesion with an erythematous outer border, an inner pale ring, and a dark-purple to necrotic center (target lesion); may have lesions of the lips and buccal surface only (i.e., the only involved mucosal surface); resolves in about 2 weeks. Occurs most commonly on extensor surfaces of the arms; less so elsewhere.
- **Diagnosis:** Characteristic appearance and histopathology
- **Associated findings:** Most common association with herpes simplex (especially with certain HLA types) and may have recurrent lesions with recurrent herpes simplex virus (HSV) infections; other causes often not found
- **Complications: Does not** progress to Stevens-Johnson syndrome.

- **Treatment:** Symptomatic relief from emollients, antihistamines, and nonsteroidal anti-inflammatory drugs (NSAIDs)

Stevens-Johnson Syndrome

- **Description:** Widespread cutaneous and mucosal vesicles and bullae; significant mucous membrane morbidity; may be a hypersensitivity reaction. Initial erythematous macules → central necrosis to form vesicles, bullae, and denuded areas → ulcerations and crusting (with bleeding); skin tenderness minimal, but mucosal pain severe; crops of new lesions over 4–6 weeks. Widespread lesions on face, trunk, and extremities with involvement of at least two mucosal surfaces (eyes, oral, airway, GI, anogenital).
- **Diagnosis:** Characteristic findings (skin lesions and two mucosal surfaces) and histopathology
- **Associated findings:** Most common infectious cause is *Mycoplasma pneumoniae*; also certain drugs: anticonvulsants, antibiotics, and NSAIDs; most severe form is **toxic epidermal necrolysis** (triggered by drugs) with extensive skin and mucous membrane involvement, and toxicity.
- **Complications:** Corneal ulceration, anterior uveitis, pneumonitis, hepatitis, enterocolitis, acute tubular necrosis (ATN), fluid loss with dehydration and electrolyte imbalance, infections
- **Treatment:** Supportive: skin cleansing and compresses, IV fluids, analgesics, topical anesthetics, management of mucosal lesions, and ophthalmology consult with daily eye exams and topical ocular corticosteroids

EPIDERMAL DISORDERS

Psoriasis

- **Description:** Proliferation and abnormal differentiation of keratinocytes with inflammation of epidermis and dermis; most likely secondary to an immune defect. Erythematous papules → plaques with sharp, irregular borders → thick, silver-like scale; may begin in first 20 years of life; rare in neonate (may present as diaper dermatitis). Most common areas are scalp, extensor surfaces of extremities, genitals, gluteal fold, and umbilicus; new lesions in sites of trauma (Koebner response).
- **Diagnosis:** Clinical pattern and histopathology
- **Associated findings:** Nail involvement; **guttate psoriasis** occurs mostly in children: acute, large appearance of many small, round lesions (look like the typical larger plaques); mostly on trunk, face, and proximal limbs; often with onset after a streptococcal infection
- **Complications:** Lifelong remissions and exacerbations; psoriatic arthritis
- **Treatment:** Topical corticosteroids, vitamin D analogs or retinoids for skin lesions, and phenol/saline solutions and tar shampoo to remove scalp scales; children with extensive disease who have failed topical therapy should receive narrow-band UVB phototherapy; more severe disease treated with immunomodulators and oral retinoids.

Pityriasis Rosea

- **Description:** Benign skin eruption in children and young adults with unknown cause (viral suspected). Starts with the solitary Herald patch (may occur anywhere): large, round, erythematous lesion with raised border and fine scales; then 5–10 days later, widespread symmetric eruption of small, pink to brown, oval to round lesions with a raised border, covered by a fine scale; lasts 2–12 weeks with postinflammatory hypo- or hyperpigmentation; generalized eruption mostly over trunk and proximal limbs.
- **Diagnosis:** Herald patch preceding generalized eruption; long axis of generalized lesions is aligned with the cutaneous cleavage lines, forming a "Christmas tree pattern" on the back
- **Associated findings:** May be mildly pruritic
- **Treatment:** Emollient for significant scaling; and lubricating lotion and oral antihistamine for pruritus, or low-potency topical corticosteroid

KERATINIZATION DISORDER

Ichthyosis Vulgaris

- **Description:** Most common disorder of abnormal keratinization; autosomal dominant or polygenic, with onset usually in first year. Mutation leading to abnormal cornification. Most have only a slight roughening of the skin surface; others have scaling; more often in winter (may go away in warmer months), and improves with age. Mostly on extensor surfaces, primarily legs; flexural areas are spared.
- **Diagnosis:** Histopathology to differentiate from other forms of ichthyosis
- **Complications:** None; there are other forms of ichthyosis that are more severe and may be part of genetic syndromes.
- **Treatment:** Decrease scaling with daily emollient or lubricant.

ECZEMATOUS DISORDERS (SEE ALSO CHAPTER 8 FOR ATOPIC DERMATITIS)

Contact Dermatitis

- **Description:** Nonspecific skin injury from prolonged repetitive contact with an irritant (irritant contact dermatitis: saliva, abrasive materials, soaps, detergents, bubble bath, medications) or a delayed hypersensitivity reaction (allergic contact dermatitis: T cell–mediated reaction from an antigen in contact with the skin, followed by sensitization.) **Irritant dermatitis** dependent on underlying irritant and location. **Allergic dermatitis** acute, erythematous, and eczematous, e.g., rhus dermatitis (poison ivy, oak, sumac): linear streaks of vesicles with slightly raised patches of extremely pruritic erythema; to prevent new areas of involvement, must use soap and water to remove antigen that is retained on the skin and under the nails (also remove and wash clothing). Occurs anywhere in contact with the irritant or sensitizing agent (e.g., exposed areas of skin for rhus dermatitis, earlobes for nickel dermatitis, feet from shoe dermatitis).

- **Diagnosis:** Recognition of appearance of lesions with respect to exposure to an irritant or a contact allergen; if confusion: patch testing
- **Associated findings:** Specific to the irritant/allergen and area of reaction
- **Complications:** Massive bullous reactions with significant swelling; secondary infection
- **Treatment:** Elimination of the agent, cool compresses, topical steroids, and oral antihistamines; more severe cases treated with oral corticosteroids

Seborrheic Dermatitis

- **Description:** Chronic inflammatory disease activity of sebaceous glands in infancy and adolescence. Cause unknown. Infantile form (not related to development in adolescence) begins in first month of life and worsens over first year; often starts as diffuse or focal scaling and crusting of the scalp (cradle cap); formation of greasy, scaly, erythematous, papular areas of skin. Patchy, focal with spread to any area; predilection for face, neck, behind ears, axillae, and diaper area; in adolescence, usually more localized: mostly scalp and intertriginous areas, eyelids, external ear canal
- **Diagnosis:** Clinical appearance, timing, and pattern, but may be hard to distinguish from psoriasis and atopic dermatitis
- **Associated findings:** Atopic dermatitis; mild to marked pruritus; hair loss
- **Complications:** With immune dysfunction: dermatitis with chronic diarrhea and failure-to-thrive
- **Treatment:** Antiseborrheic shampoo (selenium sulfur, tar) used daily; topical corticosteroids, tacrolimus or pimecrolimus, wet compresses

HAIR LOSS

Traction Alopecia

- **Description:** Tightening of the skin on the scalp (applied scalp traction) → trauma to the hair follicle from tight braids, etc. Broken hairs and inflammatory papules in patches. Mostly at the scalp margin
- **Diagnosis:** History and pattern of hair loss with broken hairs
- **Associated findings:** Regional adenopathy
- **Complications:** Scarring of hair follicles, if chronic
- **Treatment:** Discontinue use of traction methods of hair-styling.

Trichotillomania

- **Description:** Compulsive, chronic pulling and twisting of hair; more common in females. Most related to obsessive-compulsive disorder; also related to emotional stress. Irregular areas of incomplete hair loss with broken hairs; scalp is usually normal, but may be chronic folliculitis and mild bleeding. Mostly occurs on crown, and occipital and parietal areas.

- **Diagnosis:** History in association with psychiatric problem
- **Associated findings:** Other body hair may also be traumatized
- **Complications:** Trichobezoars; atrophy and fibrosis → irreversible hair loss
- **Treatment:** Behavioral therapy and psychiatric medications

Alopecia Areata

- **Description:** Rapid loss of hair; small number with family history; may have autoantibodies to other tissues. Cause is unknown. Rapid loss of hair in round to oval patches on scalp and other areas of body; most with onset under 20 years of age; skin appears normal, with mild perifollicular inflammation.
- **Diagnosis:** Clinical presentation
- **Associated findings:** Atopic disease, autoimmune disease, nail changes
- **Complications:** If there are other associations, as above
- **Treatment:** Any therapy is not completely effective and may be associated with problems or complications: topical, intradermal, or systemic corticosteroids, topical minoxidil; spontaneous remission usually occurs.

Telogen Effluvium

- **Description:** Sudden loss of large amounts of hair with brushing, washing, combing; also accounts for normal loss of hair in infants in first months of life. Premature conversion of growing hairs (anagen) to resting hairs (telogen) from a number of precipitating causes (fever, surgery, sudden weight loss, stress, other causes) with hair loss later. Remaining hairs are intact, with telogen bulbs present and no inflammation.
- **Diagnosis:** History and clinical presentation
- **Treatment:** Usually, hair loss is not severe and hair re-grows in about 6 months.

Tinea Capitis

- **Description:** Dermatophyte infection of the scalp, more common in black school-age children. Most from *Trichophyton tonsurans* (contact with infected hairs and epithelial cells on other persons or from being shed into common environments); less from *Microsporum canis* (cats and dogs), and few from other microsporum and trichophyton species. Various forms: **black-dot ringworm**: small, circular patches of alopecia, with the hair broken off close to the follicle; **diffuse, scaly, with minimal hair loss** that looks more like seborrhea; **chronic diffuse alopecia with adenopathy**; **kerion**: inflammatory, granulomatous mass with pustules; may present with fever, pain, and adenopathy; results in permanent hair loss with scarring
- **Diagnosis:** KOH preparation of broken hair showing spores; planted broken hairs on Sabouraud medium for fungal growth. Fluorescence of infected hair with Wood's lamp. (Trichophytum will not fluoresce.)
- **Complications:** Possible hair loss with scarring; pruritus

- **Treatment:** Oral griseofulvin for 8–12 weeks; discontinue only after negative culture; treat patient and family with sporicidal shampoo (selenium sulfide or ketoconazole shampoo).

INFECTIONS

Impetigo

- **Description:** Superficial bacterial infection. Most from nonbullous impetigo by *Staph. aureus* (spread from the nose to the skin, and then infects; any age), then group A beta-hemolytic streptococci (GABHS; skin is first colonized, then infection, then colonization of the nasopharynx; usually in preschool children); next common is bullous impetigo: *Staph. aureus* phage group 2, mostly in infants and young children. **Nonbullous:** initial vesicle or pustule → honey-colored plaque → crusts; may be spread to other parts of body by fingers, towels, clothing; **bullous:** flaccid, clear bullae which rupture, leaving a rim of scale and a central erythematous moist area; is localized staphylococcal scalded skin syndrome (SSSS).
- **Diagnosis:** Gram stain and culture of the lesion or fluid from an intact blister; for bullous impetigo, blood cultures are rarely positive with local lesions in healthy children
- **Associated findings:** Nonbullous: mild pruritus, regional adenopathy and spread; SSSS with more generalized infection with *Staph. aureus* phage group 2
- **Complications:** More common with bullous: septicemia, pneumonia, osteomyelitis, septic arthritis; acute poststreptococcal glomerulonephritis with nephritogenic strains of GABHS
- **Treatment:** Topical mupirocin ointment (bactericidal) is the drug of choice. With bullous lesions, widespread nonbullous lesions, lesions that are spreading, or those near the mouth: use an oral beta-lactamase drug (best cure rates with erythromycin) unless there is known widespread resistance.

Staphylococcal Scalded Skin Syndrome (SSSS)

- **Description:** Generalized cutaneous involvement with systemic illness in children under 5. Phage group 2 *Staph. aureus* with foci of infection in the nasopharynx and, less commonly, the umbilicus, urinary tract, conjunctivae, and blood. Hematogenous spread of staphylococcal exfoliative toxins A or B. Fever and nonspecific findings plus skin tenderness prior to onset of rash, then diffuse bright erythema and possible development of sterile, flaccid bullae; conjunctivae are inflamed and purulent; radial fissuring and crusting around the eyes, nose, and mouth, and a positive **Nikolsky sign** (gentle tangential force produces separation of areas of epidermis) and large sheets of epidermis peel away to leave moist, denuded skin (desquamation phase after 2–5 days); heals without scarring in 10–14 days. Occurs over entire body.
- **Diagnosis:** Classic presentation, Nikolsky sign (also present in toxic epidermal necrolysis but only at sites of erythema and with a drug ingestion and without radial crusting); intact bullae are sterile (different from bullous impetigo): obtain cultures from

any localized site of infection and blood; subcorneal-granular layer split on skin biopsy (usually not necessary)

- **Complications:** Secondary infection, septicemia, dehydration and fluid abnormalities, hypothermia
- **Treatment:** Parenteral beta-lactamase drug plus clindamycin to inhibit bacterial toxin synthesis; IV fluids and close attention to electrolyte balance; careful cleansing of skin with application of emollients

Cellulitis

- **Description:** Subcutaneous bacterial infection of loose connective tissue with some involvement of the dermis (but not epidermis); usually secondary to a break in the skin. *Strep. pyogenes* and *Staph. aureus*, then other streptococcal species and other organisms with immunocompromise or diabetes. Area of erythematous inflammation and tenderness with indistinct lateral margins (is deep) with systemic findings (fever) and regional adenopathy. Occurs anywhere there has been skin trauma from any cause.
- **Diagnosis:** Aspirate from the point of maximal inflammation, but positive in only up to one-third; blood culture may be positive in up to one-fourth of cases; is basically a clinical diagnosis
- **Associated findings:** Constitutional signs and symptoms, regional adenitis, lymphangitis
- **Complications:** Abscess formation, septicemia, osteomyelitis, septic arthritis, necrotizing fasciitis, glomerulonephritis from *Strep. pyogenes*
- **Treatment:** Empiric treatment with a beta-lactamase if patient is non–toxic appearing; if systemic signs are present or if patient does not improve on oral therapy within 24–48 hours, use IV oxacillin or nafcillin (may add vancomycin or clindamycin with severe toxicity and concern for resistance); neonate receive a sepsis evaluation and IV oxacillin or nafcillin plus an aminoglycoside.

Tinea Versicolor

- **Description:** Benign, cutaneous fungal infection, localized to the stratum corneum; hypo- or hyperpigmented macules/patches on the chest and back; may chronically recur. Caused by the yeast *Malassezia furfur* (indigenous flora rich in sebum); especially in warm, humid environments and with increased sweating, occlusive clothing, malnutrition, and immunodeficiency. Varies per skin type: reddish-brown (in white person) to hypo- or hyperpigmented areas in darker-skinned person; macules covered with fine scales which enlarge to form confluent patterns (little to no pruritis). Mostly on the neck, upper chest, back, and upper arms
- **Diagnosis:** Characteristic appearance plus KOH preparation showing spores and hyphae; Woods lamp gives a yellow-gold fluorescence
- **Complications:** Involved areas do not tan after sun exposure
- **Treatment:** Not eradicated permanently from skin; recurs; topical selenium sulfide, an imidazole, or terbinafine cream; or orally with an imidazole

Tinea Corporis, Pedis, Cruris, and Unguium

- **Description:** Dermatophyte infection on the skin, feet, groin, and nail plate, acquired from direct contact with infected persons or pets or from infected hairs and scales. **Tinea corporis**: mostly from *Trichophyton rubrum*, *T. mentagrophytes*, and *M. canis*. **Tinea cruris**: *T. rubrum* and *Epidermophyton floccosum*. **Tinea pedis**: *T. rubrum*, *T. mentagrophytes*, and *E. floccosum*. **Tinea unguium**: *T. rubrum* and *T. mentagrophytes*.
  - **Tinea corporis**: dry, erythematous, elevated scaly papules that spread outward and clear centrally (ringworm; central clearing does not always occur).
  - **Tinea cruris**: mostly in adolescent males; more in obese persons with increased sweating and tight clothing; small, red, raised, scaly erythematous patch on inner aspect of thigh that spreads peripherally and becomes vesicular (bilateral irregular areas with sharp borders and hyperpigmented scaly center).
  - **Tinea pedis**: more in preadolescent and adolescent males; in toe webs and on soles—fissuring, maceration, and peeling, with papules, vesicles, and pustules; usually malodorous, tender, and pruritic; may be transmitted in swimming pools and shower facilities.
  - **Tinea unguium**: most occur with tinea pedis; superficial white patches or more invasive subungual infection, which may cause the nail to break off.
- **Diagnosis:** Clinical appearance plus KOH preparation and culture
- **Treatment: Tinea corporis**: a topical imidazole, terbinafine, or oral itraconazole. **Tinea cruris**: loose cotton underwear and a topical imidazole. **Tinea pedis**: no occlusive footwear, dry between toes, absorbent antifungal powder; topical imidazole. **Tinea unguium**: an oral imidazole or terbinafine

Scabies

- **Description:** Skin infestation caused by burrowing and release of toxic antigenic substance by the female mite *Sarcoptes scabiei*. Mite burrows into the stratum corneum, deposits eggs and fecal material (scybala). Begins as small red papules that become excoriated, crusted, or scaly and form threadlike burrows; infants may not present with burrows and may have papules, vesicles, pustules, and bullae with an eczematous dermatitis (intense pruritis). In infants: primarily on the palms, soles, face, and scalp, but can involve the entire body. In older children and adolescents: interdigital areas, wrist flexors, ankles, axillae, buttocks, areola, groin.
- **Diagnosis:** Place a drop of mineral oil on a fresh papule, scrape with a #15 scalpel blade, and examine microscopically for mites, eggs, and scybala.
- **Complications:** Eczematous dermatitis, secondary infection, lymphangitis
- **Treatment:** Permethrin 5% or 1% lindane (not in young infants; neurotoxic) to entire body (not face) for 8–12 hours and reapply in 1 week; treat entire household and wash clothing, towels, and bed linens in hot water; there is no further transmission 24 hours after initial treatment.

Molluscum Contagiosum

- **Description:** Cutaneous viral infection causing wartlike lesions; most common in schoolchildren, the immunocompromised, and persons with atopy. Caused by poxvirus; direct contact with infected persons or fomites or autoinoculation. Skin-colored, smooth, domed papules with a central umbilication containing a cheesy plug. Especially on face, eyelids, neck, axillae, thighs, groin, and genitals (sexually active adolescents).
- **Diagnosis:** Central plug containing cells with virus can be expressed out and examined microscopically with KOH, Wright stain, or Giemsa stain showing a rounded, lobulated, cup-shaped mass of cells.
- **Complications:** Can spread rapidly to large areas
- **Treatment:** Curettage in children who can tolerate mild pain; in younger children, use cantharidin (not on face) and cover with bandage (aids in formation of blister that can then be removed); imiquimod to the face

Warts

- **Description:** Cutaneous viral infections causing discrete lesions. Caused by human papillomavirus of various types from direct contact, autoinoculation, or fomites.
- **Common warts** (verruca vulgaris), mostly from human papillomavirus (HPV)-2 and -4: distinct papules with rough hyperkeratotic surface containing thrombosed dermal capillary loops. **Common warts** occur mostly on fingers, hands, face, knees, and elbows; **plantar warts**, mostly from HPV-1: flush with surface due to constant pressure, with hyperkeratosis and pain. **Flat warts** from HPV-3 and -10: small, pink to brown, slightly elevated papules with minimal keratosis; many may appear on the face, arms, back of hands, and knees, particularly after trauma. **Genital warts,** mostly types 6 and 11 in sexually active adolescents; condyloma acuminatum are mucous membrane warts: fleshy, moist papillomas in the perianal area, labia, vagina, penis; also in oral mucosa; may form large masses; children may acquire genital warts from birth, inoculation by common warts, or from sexual abuse.
- **Diagnosis:** Clinical appearance
- **Complications:** Certain types of **genital warts** (16, 18) are major risk for development of cervical cancer; less commonly, **other non-genital warts** may cause squamous cell carcinoma of the skin, mucous membranes, and larynx.
- **Treatment: Common warts**: half disappear spontaneously within 2 years; pare away excess keratin with scalpel until thrombosed capillaries can be seen; then treat with liquid nitrogen, cryotherapy, pulsed-dye laser, or topically with salicylates in collodion (slow). Treat **plantar warts** with 40% salicylate plasters and then remove keratin debris with prolonged soaking and an emery board. **Condyloma** may be treated with 25% podophyllin or imiquimod cream.

Pediculosis

- **Description:** Infestation of human host by one of three obligate parasites (lice): **body lice** (*Pediculus humanus corporis*); **head lice** (*P. humanus capitis*), and **pubic lice** (*Phthirus pubis*); only the body louse is a vector of human disease (typhus, relapsing fever, trench fever). **Body lice:** females deposit eggs (nits) in seams of clothing and are tightly attached but not to human hairs; nymphs and adults feed on blood, inject saliva into the host, and deposit fecal matter on skin; sensitization occurs and then symptoms; poor hygiene → lice in clothing and bedding; red macules/papules with small hemorrhagic center that becomes excoriated. **Head lice:** small eggs laid in proximal hair shafts and become adherent; intense pruritus → scratching and secondary pyoderma with regional adenopathy; from head-to-head contact and fomites (towels, brushes, combs). **Pubic lice:** transmitted from skin-to-skin or sexual contact, usually in adolescents; oval nits attached to hair shafts plus moderate to severe pruritus and excoriation; small, gray spots on pubic area, abdomen, and thighs (maculae cerulea).
- **Diagnosis: Body lice:** history and clinical appearance. **Head lice:** nits are detectible with hand lens or microscope. **Pubic lice:** nits may be seen on hair shafts.
- **Associated findings:** Extreme pruritus; eczematous dermatitis, secondary infections; regional adenopathy
- **Complications:** Secondary disease from the body louse
- **Treatment: Body lice:** improve hygiene; launder all clothes, towels, and bedding in hot water; lindane or permethrin to eradicate eggs and lice. **Head lice:** regular brushing and combing to remove nits; permethrin cream rinse, lindane shampoo, or malathion in isopropyl alcohol (not for young infants); throw away brushes and combs. **Pubic lice:** permethrin or lindane shampoo; wash all clothing, bed linens, and towels in hot water.

ACNE

Background/etiology: increased **adrenal androgens** at puberty leads to **abnormal keratinization** of follicular epithelium with **impaction** of keratinized cells within the follicular lumen plus increased activity of **sebaceous production of sebum** and proliferation of *Propionibacterium acnes* → increased formation of **free fatty acids** by hydrolyzation of sebum triglycerides → **inflammatory reaction**

Types of Lesions

- **Comedones:** noninflammatory lesions from dilated, epithelial-lined follicular sac filled with keratinous material, lipid, and bacteria; **open comedone** (blackhead) has a pilosebaceous opening where the plug may be seen; **closed comedone** (whitehead) has a very tiny opening and becomes inflammatory much more easily
- **Inflammatory papule/nodule:** developed from a comedone that has ruptured its contents into dermis → inflammatory response; if inflammation is close to the surface, it results in a **papule or pustule**; if deeper, a **nodule** develops
- **Nodulocystic lesions:** liquefied masses of inflammatory debris which form from suppuration and giant-cell reaction to keratin and hair

Severity, Clinical Presentation, and Treatment of Acne

Table 18.1: Acne: Severity, Clinical Presentation, and Treatment

Severity	Clinical Presentation	Treatment Options	Notes on Medication
Mild	Mostly open and closed comedones with a few small papules and pustules; mostly on central face	**Topical retinoid:** primary treatment; apply once nightly; comes in various strengths, gradual increase as tolerated (may start every other day and then increase) *or* **Azelaic acid** once or twice a day	**Retinoids:** tretinoin, adapalene, or tazarotene; anti-comedonal, anti-inflammatory, and keratolytic; main side effects are irritation and dryness **Azelaic acid:** mild antimicrobial and keratolytic
Moderate	Increased numbers of comedones, papules, and pustules; lesions may involve upper chest, deltoid, and upper back (more common in males)	**Topical retinoid plus Benzoyl peroxide** once or twice daily; may use benzoyl peroxide in the A.M. and topical retinoid at night *or* **Topical antibiotic** (clindamycin or erythromycin) applied once or twice per day; more effective in a combined product with benzoyl peroxide *or* **Oral antibiotic** if no response to topical therapy alone, or if topical therapy not tolerated, or with moderate to severe inflammatory disease; once or twice daily for at least 6–8 weeks, followed by decrease to minimal effective dose	**Benzoyl peroxide:** mainly an antimicrobial; does not cause increased microbial resistance; gel formulations are preferred; main side effects: irritation and drying **Topical antibiotics:** clindamycin or erythromycin for inflammatory acne; not as effective as benzoyl peroxide or oral antibiotics; do not use alone (not anti-comedonal, and may lead to resistance) **Oral antibiotic:** tetracycline or derivative (doxycycline, minocycline) or erythromycin; decrease growth and activity of *P. acnes* and are anti-inflammatory; never use in combination with topical antibiotics; possible resistance and side effects

(continued)

Severity	Clinical Presentation	Treatment Options	Notes on Medication
Moderately severe	Many comedones, papules, and pustules with few deeper inflamed nodules; more extensive involvement of the trunk and shoulders	**Topical retinoid plus benzoyl peroxide plus oral antibiotic** *or* **Isotretinoin** (Accutane®) if no response to conventional therapy	Increase dosages as tolerated to achieve control. **Isotretinoin** (13-cis-retinoic acid): standard oral course of 16–20 weeks (may need additional courses); keratolytic, anti-inflammatory, reduces *P. acnes*, anti-comedonal, and decreases sebum; teratogenic: must adhere to a pregnancy prevention program (signed statement, birth control, and pregnancy monitoring); also must rule out liver disease and hyperlipidemia prior to treatment, and re-check labs in 4 weeks (increases serum triglycerides and cholesterol)
Severe	Nodulocystic acne: many small papules, pustules, and comedones; plus larger number of deep, painful nodules and cysts on face and upper trunk; more widespread involvement of trunk and shoulders	**Topical retinoid plus benzoyl peroxide plus oral antibiotic** *or* **Isotretinoin** (Accutane®) if no response to conventional therapy	In addition to isotretinoin, intralesional corticosteroid injection for painful nodulocystic lesions Consider hormonal agents (estrogen-containing oral contraceptives) or spironolactone for women who are unresponsive to antibiotics and not candidates for isotretinoin.

ADOLESCENT MEDICINE 19

ADOLESCENT DEVELOPMENT

Development During Early Adolescence (11–14 Years)

Physical Growth and Development
- Onset of puberty; sexual maturity rating (SMR) stage 1–2
- Female growth spurt 6–12 months before menarche; boys later with an increased peak growth 2–3 years after girls and continued growth for 2–3 years after girls have stopped; voice changes
- Changes in mean body fat and lean body mass

Sexual Development
- Increasing anxiety/interest in sexuality
- Beginning of consolidation of sexual orientation
- Individual and mutual sexual exploration, experimentation, and questioning
- Most common form of sexual behavior is masturbation.

Psychosocial Development
- Primary interest is with peers (same sex) over family; increasing desire for autonomy, independence, and privacy; express developing sense of personal identity.
- Development of adult relationships other than parents as role models
- Adjustment to middle school—more challenging social environment; development of a sense of achievement and self-esteem
- Mood swings and attempts at independence may lead to arguments with parents.

Cognitive Development
- Rapid cognition development; transition from concrete operational thinking to logical, abstract, and idealistic thinking
- Self awareness increases; mostly with respect to external characteristics
- Onset of puberty; sexual maturity rating (SMR) stage 1–2

- Female growth spurt 6–12 months before menarche; boys later with an increased peak growth velocity 2–3 years after girls and continued growth for 2–3 years after girls have stopped; voice changes
- Gender-specific changes in mean body fat and lean body mass

Sexual Maturity Rating (SMR)

Table 19.1: Sexual Maturity Rating (*from Tanner:* Growth at Adolescence, *2nd ed., Blackwell Scientific Publications, Oxford, England, 1962*)

SMR Stage	Boys	Girls
1	No pubic hair, with preadolescent testes and penis	Preadolescent pubic hair, and breast appearance
2	Little pubic hair, long with some pigment; some penile enlargement; enlarged scrotum with slight texture, still pink	Small amount; straight pubic hair on medial labia with slight pigmentation; small breast/papilla mound with increased areolar diameter
3	Small amount of pubic hair, curling, darker; penis longer, testes larger	Increased amount of darker hair with start of curling; enlarged breast and areola without contour separation
4	Coarse, curly pubic hair, similar to adult but less in quantity; glans and breadth of penis increased in size; larger testes, scrotum darkening	Less than adult but coarser, curly; secondary mound of areola and papilla
5	Pubic hair spread to medial thighs; adult distribution; adult-size penis and testes/scrotum	Adult appearance with spread to medial thighs; areola part of breast contour with nipple projection; mature-appearing

Abbreviations: sexual maturity rating, SMR

Development During Middle Adolescence (15–17 Years)

Physical Growth and Development

- Growth accelerates, stopping at 16 years for girls and 18 years in boys; weight parallels height; muscle mass and strength increase; lean body mass increases in boys and decreases in girls with the accumulation of subcutaneous body fat.
- SMR 3–4
- Menarche is reached between SMR 3–4 in almost all girls.
- Increase then stabilization of vital capacity, blood pressure, and hematocrit

Cognitive Development

- Formal operations—further development of logical and abstract thought; complex reasoning, inductive and deductive reasoning, inferential thinking
- Ability to see understand actions in a moral and ethical sense; development of personal code of ethics
- Extensive questioning and analysis

Psychosocial Development

- Peers are the key reference group for developing important behaviors.
- Further separation from family; possible strained relationships; driving force is increased freedom and unsupervised time (onset of driving)
- Central focus is school and related activities.
- Appearance remains important but become more accepting of their body image
- Increased experimentation with risky behaviors
- More introspection, idealism, and concern for the future and available opportunities
- Highest risk of mental health problems (mood disorders, conduct disorders, learning disorders)

Sexual Development

- Sorting out of sexual identity; experimentation (does not necessarily reflect ultimate sexual orientation)
- Dating and superficial relationships (not with respect to intimacy)
- Sexual knowledge and risks do not always control behavior.
- Sexual activity is highly variable.

Development During Late Adolescence (18–21)

Physical Growth and Development

- SMR 5
- Growth of facial and chest hair; may have onset of male-pattern baldness
- Physical development complete
- Ending of linear growth in males

Cognitive Development

- Cognitive skills continue to develop (perhaps through 3rd decade).
- Full, independent analysis of situations, events, mores, ethics
- Sense of self identity with refinement of value system
- Thinking about perspectives for the future (school, work, career, military, marriage)

Psychosocial Development

- Increasing thoughts about others
- Decreased adult supervision with increasing autonomy and eventually emancipation
- Emotional and physical separation from family
- Increasing stress and responsibilities may lead to experimentation with drugs and alcohol.
- Peer group and values become less important.
- Emotions are steadier and more constant.

Sexual Development

- Empathy develops (needed for meaningful relationships).
- Need/capacity to commit to some form of relationship
- More serious relationships involving love and commitment
- Consolidation of sexual identity

PREVENTIVE HEALTH CARE

General Concepts for Adolescent Health-Care Visits

- Address the **concerns of the adolescent and parents**, and offer guidance.
- Beginning in early adolescence, should start to spend **part of each visit with the adolescent alone** to discuss any sensitive issues; make clear that the parent will be immediately notified if there is **concern regarding a life-threatening situation**.
- Increase the amount of time **communicating with the adolescents themselves** (as opposed to the parent) to create a supportive environment; increases the chances of **effective prevention and risk-reduction counseling**.
- Comprehensive adolescent developmental and behavioral assessment tools are helpful (**HEADSS**—**h**ome, **e**ducation/**e**mployment, peer group **a**ctivities, **d**rugs, **s**exuality, **s**uicide) with more in-depth questioning for potential problems; or use of **questionnaires developed for screening** (adolescent and parent input; questionnaires completed prior to visit).
- Physicians must be aware of **state laws regarding confidential health services for adolescents**, confidential policies, and limits (abuse, suicidal/homicidal intent, injuries from violence; see below).
- The physician's role is to help the adolescent choose **responsible and health-promoting behaviors;** physician should recognize various **risk levels** based on developmental tracking.

Adolescent Visits (yearly)

Per AAP's Recommendations for Preventive Pediatric Healthcare, each annual visit should include:

- Interval history and changes in health status: problems and concerns since the last visit addressed to **both the parent and the adolescent**
- Observation of **parent–youth interaction** (depending on age, if a parent accompanies), both verbal and nonverbal interactions
- **Developmental surveillance:** determine whether the adolescent is developing in an appropriate fashion (cognitive, emotional, moral, social, and physical) with respect to family relationships, relationships with others, stress, self-confidence and well-being, responsible decision-making, healthy lifestyle, and engagement in the community.
- **Physical exam:** complete physical exam with emphasis on measuring and plotting **height, weight, body mass index (BMI), and blood pressure**; careful inspection of the **skin** for common (acne) and less common (acanthosis nigricans) findings, and for self-inflicted injury, possible drug use, and any body art or accessories (tattoos and piercings); examine **back** for curvature abnormalities; **breast exam** in females, evaluate for gynecomastia in males; **male genital exam**: visual inspection for sexual maturity rating (SMR) and evidence of sexually transmitted illnesses (STIs), and examine testicles for abnormalities; **female**: visual inspection for SMR and evidence of STI, and pelvic exam if warranted (sexual activity or specific problems)
- **Screening: Snellen test**, once in early adolescence and at any other ages where risk screening suggests a problem; evaluate **hearing** if risk screening indicates a possible

problem; **tuberculosis (TB) testing**, depending on exposure and risk status (see Chapter 15); **dyslipidemia screening** with risk factors; screen for **chlamydia and gonorrhea if sexually active**, and additional screening for syphilis and possibly HIV depending on results of risk screening; obtain a **urine human chorionic gonadotropin (hCG)** if patient is sexually active without contraception, has missed menses, or has amenorrhea; **Pap smear** if sexually active or within 3 years of onset of sexual activity; **alcohol and drug screening** if positive on initial risk screening assessment

- **Anticipatory guidance:** oral hygiene, nutrition, physical exercise, body image, limiting screen time (i.e., on computer, watching TV); relationships to family, peers, and community; school performance, non-academic activities, coping and mood regulation; sexuality issues, STIs, pregnancy, tobacco, alcohol, drugs, violence and injury prevention, nonviolent conflict resolution

ADOLESCENT GYNECOLOGY

Pelvic and Breast Exams

- **Indications for first pelvic exam** (American College of Obstetrics and Gynecology): age 21 if not sexually active and without specific problems, otherwise within 3 years of becoming sexually active or with: abnormal vaginal discharge, unexplained dysuria or abdominal pain, severe dysmenorrhea, or acute phase of menstrual irregularities. If none are present, the **first gynecological encounter should be at 13–15 years of age** (no routine pelvic exam) for educational discussion regarding issues related to sexuality.

- History may initially be taken with a parent, depending on adolescent's age; otherwise, issues are **confidential**; most important factor is to develop rapport.

- Method for pelvic exam:
  - Exam in **absence of parent but with a female chaperone,** and **communicate** throughout exam
  - Dorsal lithotomy position with appropriate size speculum
  - **Inspect** vulva, **palpate** Bartholin glands; inspect, measure clitoris (should be <10 mm in width); inspect hymen; perform **speculum exam;** perform **bimanual exam** with single digit in virginal girl.

- Most common adolescent breast problem is either a **benign breast cyst or fibroadenoma**; repeat in 2 weeks if a mass is found (cysts vary during the menstrual cycle); if there is a **persistent mass on three cycles,** refer to a surgeon. Cancerous lesion is very rare in an adolescent (more commonly associated with a serous, serosanguineous, or bloody discharge); **mammography should not be used** because the breast tissue is too dense and the lesion is usually not seen; **ultrasound** is appropriate for a cyst vs. a solid mass, and **color Doppler study** for a fibroadenoma vs. a breast abscess.
  - **Mastalgia** is common: cyclical swelling and tenderness, most prominent during the premenstrual period; **benign breast changes** may be nodular, have poorly localized tenderness or pain radiating to the axilla and arm. Treatment: heat, firm support, analgesia, hormonal therapy, and evening primrose oil.
  - Breast discharge is uncommon; **normal/benign** is white; infection is purulent and malignancy is as indicated above.

Sexually Transmitted Illnesses

Increased risk in adolescence with: early age at onset of sexual activity, lack of consistent condom use, anal sex, drug and alcohol use, trauma, abuse and violence, poverty, limited access to adolescent health care, and/or an uncircumcised penis

Clinical presentations

- **Male urethritis:** urethral discharge and/or dysuria; most asymptomatic or minimal symptoms; most common pathogens are *Chlamydia trachomatis* **and** *Neisseria gonorrhea*; diagnosis with Gram stain, culture (and polymerase chain reaction [PCR]) of the urethra, and any discharge; if gonorrhea or chlamydia cannot be found with culture and PCR, then probably due to *Ureaplasma urealyticum* **or** *Mycoplasma genitalium* (no diagnostic tests are easily available, so this is labeled as nongonococcal, non-chlamydial urethritis).
- **Vaginitis:** superficial infection of the vaginal mucosa; vaginal discharge with or without vulvar inflammation, pruritus, and odor; colonization without infection but with discharge is **bacterial vaginosis** (not an STI but increased incidence with sexual activity); main infections are **candidiasis and trichomoniasis.**
- **Cervicitis:** deeper infections in the cervix; may present with irregular or increased bleeding, mucopurulent discharge, or erythematous cervix that bleeds easily; most are from *C. trachomatis* **and** *N. gonorrhea*, less commonly from herpes.
- **Pelvic inflammatory disease:** upper genital tract infection: **endometritis, salpingitis, tubo-ovarian abscess, and pelvic peritonitis;** *N. gonorrhea* and *C. trachomatis* are the most common etiologies in younger adolescents; with aging and recurrence, increased incidence of *Mycoplasma hominis*, **group B streptococci (GBS)**, other streptococci, anaerobes, *Escherichia coli*, and *Gardnerella vaginalis*. **Minimal criteria** for diagnosis are: lower abdominal tenderness, adnexal tenderness, or cervical motion tenderness in a sexually active female with no other cause for illness; other associations: increase in dysmenorrhea, vaginal discharge, abnormal vaginal bleeding, urinary symptoms, and fever. **Empiric treatment** is initiated if any of the primary signs are present; further workup includes culture for *N. gonorrhea*, PCR for *C. trachomatis*, microscopy of vaginal secretions, urinalysis and culture, pregnancy test, CBC, erythrocyte sedimentation rate (ESR), and rapid plasma reagin (RPR); pelvic ultrasound is indicated for certain specific findings.
- **Genital ulcers:** ulcerative lesion exposed to sexual contact, most on the penis and vulva; also can be oral or rectal; most causes are **herpes**, and much less commonly **syphilis and chancroid** (*Haemophilus ducreyi*).

Diagnosis of vaginal discharge

- *Candida:* white, floccular discharge with pH <4.5 and no amine odor; wet preparation shows mycelia
- *Trichomonas:* gray-yellow discharge with pH >4.5 and positive amine odor; WBCs and trichomonads present; best test is culture; treatment is with metronidazole or tinidazole

- **Bacterial vaginosis:** gray-yellow discharge with pH >4.5 and positive amine odor; clue cells present, with few WBCs and no lactobacilli seen
- **Cervicitis:** gray-yellow discharge with pH >4.5 and positive amine odor; no trichomonads or clue cells seen; WBCs seen but no lactobacilli

Dysmenorrhea

- **Painful menstrual cramps** (lower abdominal and low back with radiation to upper thighs); present to some degree in the **majority of adolescent girls**
  - **Primary:** no pelvic pathology; begins at time of menstrual cycle and lasts up to 3 days; accompanied by headache, nausea, vomiting; assessed with **rectoabdominal exam** (pelvic exam if sexually active); treated with **nonsteroidal anti-inflammatory drugs (NSAIDs;** prostaglandin synthetase inhibitors) or **oral contraceptive**
  - **Secondary:** due to a **structural abnormality** (pain beginning with menarche and with bleeding), **endometriosis** (increasing severity of pain and chronic pelvic pain worse with bleeding), or **foreign body**; diagnose with pelvic exam, ultrasonography, and possibly laparoscopy; congenital lesions with obstruction are treated surgically; endometriosis treated hormonally and/or surgically
  - **Premenstrual syndrome (PMS):** breast tenderness, headache, fatigue, bloating, and behavioral signs and symptoms (irritability, mood swings, depression, lack of concentration); occurs during the second half of the menstrual cycle and ends with onset of menstruation; not common in adolescents and not related to dysmenorrhea; some effectiveness with NSAIDs (mefenamic acid), diuretics, and other medications

Amenorrhea

- Absence of menses
  - **Primary:** no menses by age 14 with no secondary sex characteristics, or by age 16 with secondary sex characteristics
    ◦ Exclude pregnancy first (less likely with primary compared to secondary amenorrhea).
    ◦ With normal puberty, perform pelvic exam and ultrasound; most likely diagnosis is a müllerian duct system abnormality resulting in obstruction (most: **imperforate hymen**).
    ◦ With delay of pubertal changes, obtain follicle-stimulating hormone (FSH) and leuteinizing hormone (LH); low levels are consistent with **constitutional delay, chronic illness, malnutrition**, anorexia nervosa, and hypopituitarism (isolated gonadotropin-releasing hormone [GnRH] or with other hormones); high levels are consistent with **hypergonadotropic hypogonadism** (see Chapter 14), and genetic analysis and pelvic ultrasound are needed.
  - **Secondary:** absence of vaginal bleeding for at least 3 months after menarche
    ◦ Exclude pregnancy first (most common cause of secondary amenorrhea).
    ◦ With no hirsutism or virilization: measure FSH, LH, thyroid-stimulating hormone (TSH), and prolactin; presence of high FSH and LH is diagnostic of **ovarian failure**; abnormality of TSH is indicative of **primary or central hypothyroidism;**

high prolactin is consistent with a **prolactinoma; if LH and FSH are low, check endometrial status with a progesterone challenge test** (if no withdrawal bleeding, there is not enough estrogen priming, or there is an abnormal uterus or an obstruction).

○ With hirsutism and/or virilization: obtain serum testosterone, dehydroepiandrosterone sulfate (DHEAS), and LH/FSH ratio; there are moderate elevations of all in **polycystic ovarian syndrome** (PCOS; see Chapter 14); elevated DHEAS suggests congenital adrenal hyperplasia, and 17-OH-progesterone should be measured; an extremely high level of DHEAS and/or testosterone suggests an androgen-producing tumor.

- Establishing the underlying cause may permit a specific correction; if not, hormone therapy based on the presence of a low-estrogen state is indicated.

Abnormal Uterine Bleeding

- **Dysfunctional uterine bleeding:** anovulatory cycles (usually in **first year of cycles**); presents as **menorrhagia** (excessive amount and duration of uterine bleeding occurring regularly) and **metrorrhagia** (irregular bleeding between regular periods); **no pathological cause found,** no extrauterine bleeding; represents most cases
- **Organic causes:** small percentage of cases; most common causes: **ectopic pregnancy, threatened abortion, hormonal contraceptives,** endometriosis, and coagulopathy; other, less common causes: infection, foreign body, neoplasia, and trauma.
- Establish severity of bleeding with a **hemoglobin (Hgb) and hematocrit (Hct)** to determine need for hospitalization and initial therapy (iron supplementation, cycling with oral contraceptives, curettage).

Contraception

- **Counseling of adolescents:** physicians should make adolescents aware of the various types of contraception, how to use them, and the advantages and disadvantages of each, including possible side effects; **failure rates** need to be reviewed for each, and an understanding and plan for failure need to be stated by the adolescent; a pelvic exam is required first; there should be close follow-up.
- Types of contraception:
  - **Condoms and spermicidals** (nonoxynol-9, foams, jellies, creams, suppositories): when used together, there is a lower failure rate with no significant side effects (possible contact vaginitis and mucosal damage from spermicides) compared to either alone; they are inexpensive, can be purchased without a prescription, require no advanced planning, and **protect against STIs,** spermicidals must be placed before each intercourse.
  - **Diaphragms and cervical caps:** used less by adolescents because of the need for insertion and use with a jelly; there are no significant side effects.
  - **Intrauterine devices (IUDs):** plastic devices of varying sizes and shapes that need to be placed (by the physician) into the cervical os; may or may not contain copper or progesterone; make implantation less likely and are very effective; major side effect is

increased **risk of infection**; should be considered the **last resort for adolescent contraception**.

- **Hormonal therapy:** contains either an **estrogen** (ethinyl estradiol; prevents LH surge and inhibits ovulation) **plus a progestin** or a **progestin alone** (affects fallopian tube transport to decrease the likelihood of fertilization and implantation); **compliance** is a major issue with respect to failure rate (significant if three doses are missed).

  ◦ **Combination pills:** short-term negative effects: transient nausea and weight gain; short-term positive effects: shorter menses, increased high-density lipoprotein (HDL) with estrogen, decrease of dysmenorrhea, improvement of acne with nonandrogenic progestins; rare risks in adolescents: thrombophlebitis, hepatic adenomas, myocardial infarction, glucose intolerance; **contraindications:** liver disease, breast disease, anything in which a **hypercoagulable state** would be a problem (increases level of factor VIII and decreases antithrombin III), migraines, known or suspected pregnancy; also available as a transdermal patch and as a vaginal contraceptive ring

  ◦ **Progestin only:** used if there are potential problems with the use of estrogen; **less reliable**; higher incidence of both amenorrhea and increased bleeding; may be used as an IM depot drug (medroxyprogesterone, Depo-Provera) in patients where compliance may be an issue; major side effect is **bone mineral density loss** (and risk of osteoporosis later in life); should not be used for more than 2 years

  ◦ **Emergency contraception:** intervention window of **up to 120 hours if unprotected sex** (greatest risk of pregnancy in mid-cycle); combined pills (in United States) with ethinyl estradiol and either norgestrel or levonorgestrel disrupts the luteal phase → decreases the risk of pregnancy by 75%; also an FDA-approved prepared kit containing 2 tablets of levonorgestrel only; most common side effect is nausea and vomiting; must check for pregnancy prior to dispensing and 2 weeks after; pills are self-administered, after obtaining by physician prescription.

Adolescent Pregnancy

Epidemiology

- **United States has highest teen birth rate among all industrialized nations**; highest rates in women **18–19** years old
- **Birth rates have decreased regularly since the 1990s**, especially for **African Americans and 15-17-year-olds**; also **decreased pregnancy rates** (births, miscarriages, abortions, stillbirths) primarily due to delay in onset of sexual activity and increased use of contraceptives
- Increased teen pregnancy rates seen with: lower socioeconomic groups, poor school performance, families with low education, single-parent families, families where one or both parents were teen parents
- **Teenage fathers** tend to have decreased educational levels and to be involved with illegal substances and illegal activities.
- Adolescent women have the highest rates of experiencing **violence during pregnancy** (proportional to poor outcome); adolescent mothers tend to have **increased depression**

after birth; tend to quit school and **remain behind in education** (thus limiting income); **substance use** increases again after pregnancy (most quit during); many become **pregnant again within 2 years** (half result in births with even later entry into prenatal care).

- **Pregnancy complications:** higher risk of complications (but most pregnancies do not have serious complications; highest rates of poor outcome with the youngest): STIs, anemia, pregnancy-induced hypertension, eclampsia, poor weight gain, **decreased birth weight, extreme prematurity and very low birth weight (VLBW) babies; increased perinatal morbidity and mortality, neonatal deaths and postneonatal mortality, and sudden infant death syndrome (SIDS)**

- Children of adolescent mothers have increased incidence of behavioral problems, higher school drop-out rate, and higher rate of incarceration in males, and tend to become adolescent parents; improved outcomes with consistent, positive involvement from the father and community programs.

- Initial diagnosis with typical findings suggesting pregnancy and **enlarged uterus with cervical cyanosis and softening**; need to obtain a **qualitative urine or blood β-hCG,** which is positive 7 days after implantation; a quantitative β-hCG (positive 7 days after fertilization) is more sensitive and specific but much more costly and may be used under certain circumstances (suspicion of ectopic pregnancy, molar pregnancy, retained placenta after abortion). **Home urine tests** have decreased sensitivity and specificity and should always be followed with an in-office β-hCG.

- **Physician counseling:** assessment of **psychosocial/emotional** aspects of pregnancy; **discuss options;** discuss involvement of adolescent mother's **parents and** the baby's **biological father;** discuss plans for the mother to continue her **education;** discuss discontinuation of **substance use;** provide nutritional information; test for STIs; assess for and discontinue possible **teratogens;** start folic acid, calcium, and iron supplementation; **refer to obstetrician as soon as possible**.

SUBSTANCE ABUSE

General Concepts

- **Epidemiology:** most commonly used drugs by adolescents in the United States are **alcohol (the vast majority by age 21 years) and tobacco; marijuana** is the most common illicit drug; next are inhalants (more common in younger adolescents), then anabolic steroids; rise in the use of prescription drugs (Vicodin®, oxycodone, Percocet®), "club drugs," and "date rape drugs" (methylenedioxymethamphetamine [MDMA; "Ecstasy, X"], ketamine ["special K"], ephedrine ["herbal ecstasy, herbal X"], nitrites ["poppers"], and others)

- **Contributing factors:** biological, genetic, negative behavioral traits, social and peer groups, familial dynamics and support, school issues, and psychological issues (risk vs. coping factors)

- **Clinical presentation:** most adolescents present with **no obvious physical findings;** most are found during evaluation of **motor vehicle accidents and intentional injuries** (in the Emergency Room); may present with an overdose suggestive of the drug's class of action; changes in growth and development, changes in sleep, personality, and mood; decreased school performance; menstrual abnormalities; seizures, onset of specific psychiatric illness, or physical evidence of drug use (IV tracks, needle marks, nasal mucosal injury)

- **Laboratory evaluation: blood and urine drug screens** (alcohol, amphetamines, barbiturates, benzodiazepines, cannabinoids, cocaine, methaqualone, opiates, and phencyclidine); other than in an emergency setting, urine screens are performed **with informed choice to confidentiality**; there should be **no involuntary screening in older, competent adolescents** unless there are strong medical indications. **Indications for screening**: psychiatric symptoms, significant changes in school performance or daily behavior, evaluation of serious motor vehicle accidents (or recurrent accidents), or other injuries; for monitoring of recovery.

- Diagnosis (*Diagnostic and Statistical Manual of Mental Disorders*, 4th ed. [DSM-IV])
  - **Substance abuse:** a maladaptive pattern of drug use with significant impairments: failure to fulfill major obligations at school, home, and work; drug use with respect to circumstances that are physically hazardous; drug use resulting in legal problems; continued use of drugs despite persistent social or interpersonal problems caused or worsened by the effects of the substance
  - **Substance dependency:** chronic and progressive disease process; loss of control over use; compulsion for drug-taking and the establishment of an altered state where one requires continued administration of the substance in order to feel good
  - Requires a comprehensive diagnostic approach with history, physical exam, mental status exam, self-reporting assessment tools, standardized tests, and laboratory screening

- **Role of the physician:** yearly screening questions and anticipatory guidance regarding drug use, recognition of adolescents at risk with more in-depth interviewing and evaluation (questionnaires; histories from parents, other relatives, teachers, friends); evaluation and preparation for referral (rating systems based on drug type, circumstances, timing, frequency, mental status and functional status); determining stage of abuse (from potential use, to experimenting, to regular use, to regular use with preoccupation of getting high); referral for treatment, coordination of care, office support and counseling
  - **Prevention:** probable drug experimentation to some degree in the developmentally normal adolescent; delay experimentation/use as long as possible, make the use as limited as possible and prevent use entirely while driving. (Center for Substance Abuse Prevention, National Registry of Effective Prevention Programs)

- Chronic treatment programs
  - Brief interventions and strategic family interventions, multidisciplinary family treatment, motivational enhancement therapy, cognitive-behavioral therapy, individual and group counseling, 12-step programs, pharmacologic
  - Outcomes are primarily correlated to amount of use and consistency of attendance at post-treatment groups; also correlated to peer drug use, presence of learning problems, and other psychobehavioral issues.

Specific Drugs

Table 19.2: Summary of Specific Drugs

ALCOHOL	
Epidemiology	More deaths in young people than all illicit drugs combined; up to half of all adolescent trauma admissions are alcohol-related; earlier use is correlated to later alcohol-related problems
Pharmacology	Rapidly absorbed in stomach, then to liver for metabolism: most by alcohol dehydrogenase → acetaldehyde by removal of 2 H^+ (contributes to excess production of triglycerides and fatty liver); at higher levels, through the hepatic microsomal enzyme system (decreased metabolism of drugs → accumulation, increased effect and toxicity)
Acute effects, toxicity, and adverse effects	CNS depressant; vasodilatation and hypothermia; grogginess, euphoria, decreased short-term memory, diuresis (inhibition of ADH); very high levels lead to respiratory depression, erosive gastritis, and alcoholic pancreatitis
Diagnosis	Suspect in any disoriented, lethargic, or comatose adolescent; need a blood level or breath test (good correlation); legal intoxication at 80–100 mg/dL (0.08–0.10%); elevation in liver enzymes; increased risk of death >200 mg/dL (median lethal dose: 500 mg/dL)
Treatment	If respiratory depression, need mechanical ventilation until liver metabolizes the alcohol; consider dialysis for levels >400 mg/dL
Long-term complications	Fatty liver → necrosis → inflammation (alcoholic hepatitis) → fibrosis (cirrhosis)

TOBACCO	
Epidemiology	More U.S. deaths than combined from all substances and firearms; most smokers start by age 12; almost all become adult smokers; also increased exposure from secondhand smoke and smokeless tobacco (decreasing use)
Pharmacology	Absorbed by many areas of the body; affects nicotine acetylcholine receptors in the brain
Acute effects, toxicity, and adverse effects	Increased chronic cough, wheezing, and sputum production; decreased hepatic metabolism of certain drugs (theophylline); increased risk of myocardial infarction with concurrent estrogen use; decreased birth weight if tobacco use during pregnancy
Treatment	Counseling from health-care professionals effective in stopping; nicotine-replacement treatment plus behavioral modification; formal cessation program
Long-term complications	Cardiovascular morbidity and mortality; malignancies

(continued on next page)

Table 19.2: Summary of Specific Drugs *(cont.)*

MARIJUANA	
Epidemiology	More than 40% in United States at age 15–16 years
Pharmacology	From *Cannabis sativa*; tetrahydrocannabinol (THC) fraction of the resin contains the hallucinogenic properties (can be synthesized); rapidly absorbed from inhalation (peak onset: 10 minutes) or orally (peak onset: 60 minutes); certain drugs interact with THC to potentiate sedation (e.g., alcohol) stimulation (cocaine), or antagonism (phenytoin)
Acute effects, toxicity, and adverse effects	Elation, euphoria, decreased short-term memory, poor performance on tasks requiring concentration, loss of judgment, increased appetite; hypothermia, tachycardia, hypertension, antiemetic effect; hallucinations are rare
Diagnosis	Urine drug screen
Long-term complications	Withdrawal symptoms in 24–48 hours after discontinuing; airway and pulmonary dysfunction with long-term use; related to adult-onset psychosis; memory and attention impairment

INHALANTS	
Epidemiology	Popular with younger adolescents; glue (toluene) and gasoline (by breathing deeply into a paper bag containing a soaked cloth), and volatile nitrites (amyl nitrite, butyl nitrite; more popular with older adolescents and young adults)
Pharmacology	Rapid action and short effect; toluene is excreted in the urine as hippuric acid, which can be tested for; abnormal blood studies with various complications; diagnosis more likely with complications or death
Acute effects, toxicity, and adverse effects	Psychoactive effects: euphoria, relaxation, pleasant hallucinations, excitement (effects vary between compounds); acute toxicities: cerebral edema, pulmonary edema, myocardial dysfunction, arrhythmias, hypotension, sudden death
Diagnosis	Difficult, except possibly for toluene (as above); acute intoxication: weakness, restlessness, nystagmus, dysarthria, disruptive behavior, hallucinations
Treatment	Respiratory and cardiovascular support
Long-term complications	Varies per drug used: widespread brain damage and cognitive abnormalities (mild to severe); gross and fine motor abnormalities; pulmonary dysfunction, liver and renal dysfunction, bone marrow suppression, impaired immunity, rhabdomyolysis, hearing and vision loss

(continued)

ANABOLIC STEROIDS

Epidemiology	Mostly used by competitive athletes of both sexes, predominantly males
Pharmacology	Anabolic-androgenic steroids (nandrolone, stanozolol, methenolone, oxandrolone, tibolone, testosterone preparations) are class III drugs, possession/use is illegal and punishable as a felony; myotrophic action at androgen receptors; psychological effects; also other performance-enhancing drugs that are available OTC: androstenedione/DHEA, creatine, ephedra
Acute effects, toxicity, and adverse effects	Most immediate effect is acne, then hirsutism and striae; in males: gynecomastia and breast pain, testicular atrophy, and azoospermia; females: breast atrophy, clitoral enlargement, menstrual abnormalities (more are irreversible in females); in both sexes, serious psychological effects with high doses: rage, mania, depression
Diagnosis	Complete history with clinical signs; urine tests are typically performed only in high-level competitive sports programs
Treatment	Supportive
Long-term complications	Addiction and dependence; hepatomegaly, hepatitis, abnormal lipid profile, increased risk of hepatocellular carcinoma, hypertension, decreased tendon strength, growth retardation with accelerated skeletal maturation; problem behaviors (other substance abuse, violent behaviors)

OPIATES

Epidemiology	Overall, not commonly used in adolescence (increased use among suburban middle-class adolescents); very high addiction rate; associated increased rates of violence, criminal behavior, and incarceration; overdose is leading cause of death among drug users
Pharmacology	Heroin is a semisynthetic preparation (as is oxycodone and hydromorphone); morphine and codeine are naturally derived from opium; synthetic compounds are methadone, meperidine, propoxyphene, and pentazocine; heroin is hydrolyzed to morphine with hepatic conjugation before urinary excretion within 24 hours; can be injected SQ or IV (immediate onset of action), snorted, taken orally, or smoked; often mixed with fentanyl (up to 100 times more potent than morphine), which is responsible for many deaths
Acute effects, toxicity, and adverse effects	Euphoria, CNS depression, respiratory depression, vasodilatation, miosis, pulmonary edema, constipation, hypotension, bradycardia, decreased reflexes, seizures, stupor, coma, hypothermia; most adverse effects related to lack of sterile technique (needles): skin infection, thrombophlebitis, endocarditis, hepatitis, cerebral microabscesses, HIV
Diagnosis	Clinical presentation; heroin metabolite detected in urine for up to 48 hours; give IV naloxone → pupil dilation
Treatment	IV naloxone every 5 minutes plus supportive respiratory and cardiovascular care; detoxification with methadone or buprenorphine (greater rate of detox with less risk of addiction) plus drug treatment program
Long-term complications	Physiologic addiction and withdrawal (abstinence syndrome over 24–36 hours): yawning, lacrimation, mydriasis, insomnia, muscle cramps, diarrhea, tachycardia and systolic hypertension; complications with respect to adverse effects and acute problems described above

(continued on next page)

Table 19.2: Summary of Specific Drugs *(cont.)*

AMPHETAMINES	
Epidemiology	Second to marijuana as the most common illicit drug used by high-school seniors; methamphetamine is preferred because of potency, ease of absorption, and multiple modes of administration (oral, snorting, smoking)
Pharmacology	CNS effects through release of neurotransmitters and indirect catecholamine agonist effect; high doses are serotonergic; effects are dose-related
Acute effects, toxicity, and adverse effects	Sympathomimetic: tachycardia, hypertension, increased temperature, hyperreflexia, mydriasis, diaphoresis, seizures, arrhythmias (ventricular irritability and decreased conduction); psychosis may lead to violence
Diagnosis	Clinical presentation plus urine screen
Treatment	Haloperidol or droperidol for agitation and delusional behaviors; sedation with a benzodiazepine; supportive therapy
Long-term complications	Withdrawal: early agitation and depression with desire for further drug use, followed by decreased physical and mental energy and loss of interests, then drug craving returns; cerebrovascular damage and psychosis

COCAINE	
Epidemiology	Overall use has decreased, but increased use of crack cocaine among adolescents
Pharmacology	Alkaloid extracted from *Erythroxylum coca* (South America); supplied as the hydrochloride salt in crystalline form; crack cocaine: smoking of the cocaine alkaloid is highly addictive; rapidly absorbed from the nasal mucosa and is detoxified in the liver with the metabolite excreted in urine
Acute effects, toxicity, and adverse effects	Stimulant and sympathomimetic (and local anesthetic): euphoria, increased motor activity, diaphoresis, increased energy, mydriasis, tachycardia, hypertension, hyperthermia, paresthesias, seizures; can be lethal, especially if combined with other drugs; added diluents can alter the perceived effects
Diagnosis	Clinical presentation plus urine screen
Treatment	Intensive supportive care; outpatient care or residential treatment centers
Long-term complications	Depression and social withdrawal, poor school performance, increased risk-taking behaviors and illegal activities; suicidal ideation; hepatitis, HIV, death

HALLUCINOGENS	
Epidemiology	Most commonly used in adolescents are LSD and MDMA (Ecstasy, X), then phencyclidine (angel dust)
Pharmacology	LSD found in rye fungus; morning glory seeds contain derivatives; MDMA is synthetic similar to mescaline; PCP is also synthetic and easy to make in home labs; very small drug amounts alter serotonergic neurotransmitters; rapid absorption; PCP inhibits neuronal reuptake of catecholamines; supplied in various forms
Acute effects, toxicity, and adverse effects	**LSD:** dilated pupils, nausea, flushing; dizziness, elevated temperature, tachycardia, altered vision and hearing, delusions, body distortions, and paranoia. **MDMA:** euphoria, nausea, hyperthermia, blurred vision, increased sensations, increased emotional energy; anxiety, panic, psychosis; liver, kidney and cardiovascular failure. **PCP:** euphoria, hallucinations, emotional lability, psychosis; hypotension, arrhythmias, hyperreflexia, muscle rigidity, ataxia, nystagmus, seizures, coma. Death may occur with any of these drugs.

(continued)

Diagnosis	Clinical presentation plus urine screen
Treatment	Remove from any aggravating situation and try to re-establish reality; eliminate all stimulatory input (place in a dark, quiet room); supportive therapy, including possible gastric lavage for oral ingestion and IV diazepam for agitation
Long-term complications	Changes in brain function affecting cognition and memory; damage to serotonin-containing neurons (effects on mood, pain sensitivity, aggression, sleep, and sexual activity)

Abbreviations: antidiuretic hormone, ADH; central nervous system, CNS; dehydroepiandrosterone, DHEA; lysergic acid diethylamide, LSD; methylenedioxymethamphetamine, MDMA; over-the-counter, OTC; phencyclidine, PCP; subcutaneous, SQ; tetrahydrocannabinol, THC

EATING DISORDERS

Diagnostic Criteria

Table 19.3: Diagnostic Criteria for Eating Disorders (*from* Diagnostic and Statistical Manual of Mental Disorders, *4th ed. [DSM-IV]*)

Anorexia Nervosa	Bulimia Nervosa	Binge Eating
• Refusal to maintain body weight at a minimally normal value for age and height (with body weight less than 85% of expected; BMI <17.5 in those >17 years of age is suggestive) • Intense fear of gaining weight or becoming obese, which does not diminish as weight loss progresses • Disturbance in experiencing one's own body weight/shape on self-evaluation (looking "fat" in the face of emaciation) or denial of seriousness of low-weight situation • Absence of at least three consecutive menstrual cycles in postmenarchal females • Restrictor (severe limitation of intake of carbohydrates and fat) or bulimic subtypes (binge-eating with purging–induced vomiting or cathartics)	• Recurrent episodes of binge-eating: eating a large amount of food in a short period of time (<2 hours), and a sense of lack of control over eating during the episode • Inappropriate compensatory behavior to prevent weight gain: self-induced vomiting, laxatives, diuretics, enemas, excessive exercise • Occurrence of above at least twice/week for at least 3 months • Self-evaluation is significantly influenced by body shape and weight • Does not occur exclusively during episodes of anorexia nervosa • Divided into purging and non-purging types	• Recurrent episodes of binge-eating similar to bulimia nervosa • Episodes associated with: eating very rapidly, eating until very full, eating large amounts when not feeling hungry, eating alone due to embarrassment about quantity eaten, and/or feeling disgusted, depressed, or guilty after eating • Marked distress regarding binge-eating • Occurs at least 2 days/week for at least 6 months • Does not occur with compensatory behaviors and not exclusively with either anorexia nervosa or bulimia nervosa

Abbreviations: body mass index, BMI

Clinical presentation

Anorexia and bulimia: much overlap of findings: excessive weight loss and malnutrition, fatigue, irritability, lethargy, weakness, dizziness; sore throat, hoarseness, and dental caries in bulimia (induced vomiting), with many possible findings at presentation or over time:

- **Dehydration and electrolyte abnormalities** (often with rapid fluctuation): hypocalcemia, hypophosphatemia, hypokalemia, hypochloremic alkalosis, magnesium abnormalities (all can be due to laxative abuse, malabsorption, vomiting, diuretics, and water-loading)
- **Cardiorespiratory:** shortness of breath, chest pains, severe bradycardia, irregular pulse, postural hypotension, ECG abnormalities and arrhythmias, decreased cardiac output, congestive heart failure (late finding from rapid rehydration and refeeding)
- **Renal:** elevated BUN (dehydration and decreased glomerular filtration rate [GFR]), proteinuria, hematuria, pyuria with negative cultures
- **Bone:** low bone density → bone pain, stress fractures
- **Hematological:** bone marrow hypoplasia → anemia, leukopenia, and thrombocytopenia (uncommon)
- **Gastrointestinal:** delayed gastric emptying → abdominal pain, vomiting, constipation; elevated amylase (parotid swelling, pancreatitis)
- **Skin:** dry, lanugo hair, scarring on back of knuckles, enamel erosions/poor dentition (both signs of self-induced vomiting)
- **Endocrine:** amenorrhea, delayed sexual maturation, loss of diurnal variation in cortisol secretion, high growth-hormone secretion with low somatomedin C levels, low thyroxine, syndrome of inappropriate antidiuretic hormone secretion (SIADH), hypothermia
- **Psychological:** social isolation with poor peer relations, low self-esteem, anxiety, dependence and regression, depression (most common psychological disorder with bulimia), suicidal ideation, obsessions, perfectionism, substance abuse, bipolar disorder (less common), personality disorders

Binge-eating: Weight gain (does not have to be obese), gastric rupture (rare), negative self-esteem, impaired social functioning, higher degree of psychological problems (but lower than bulimia), major depressive disorder (major comorbid condition) and anxiety disorders; alcohol abuse

Diagnosis

- Thorough medical, developmental, psychosocial, sexual, family, and dietary/medication history.
- Complete physical, neurological exam, and psychosocial assessment
- Plot weight, height, BMI, and head circumference, and compare to previous points on growth curves.
- **Screening labs:** CBC, ESR (usually low), chemistry panel with liver enzymes/liver function tests, and urinalysis;
- Other tests to consider depending on presentation: lipid panel, amylase, ECG, echocardiogram, bone densitometry, LH and FSH, thyroid studies, and cortisol.

Treatment

- Assessment and treatment by a **multidisciplinary team**: psychological monitoring, individual and family psychotherapy, behavioral modification, interpersonal therapy (relationship stressors), nutritional rehabilitation, and pharmacology (comorbid depression, obsessive-compulsive disorder [OCD]).
- **Indications for hospitalization:** comorbid psychiatric conditions; suicidal ideation; very poor motivation to recover; severe bradycardia; hypotension; dehydration or electrolyte disturbances; hypothermia; cardiac, renal, or hepatic dysfunction or failure of outpatient management.
- Other types of treatment, depending on the patient's stability: **psychiatric residential treatment** (medically stable; requires structured supervision at meals and bathroom times), **day treatment** (medically stable; needs structure to help to gain weight), **intensive outpatient psychiatric treatment** (motivated, accepts support, self-sufficient in eating and lack of weight-losing behaviors).

LEGAL ISSUES (SEE ALSO CHAPTER 6)

- In the United States, **individual states** determine whether or not a minor can consent to treatment without parental knowledge (some have age limitations, usually 12–15 years).
  - **With suspicion of STI**, public health statutes allow physician to examine any sexually active adolescent with adolescent's consent.
  - Consent to treatment for **drug abuse or mental health treatment**
  - Most states allow contraception on adolescent's own consent; right to an abortion varies among states.
  - Parental consent not needed for: **emancipated minors, emergencies** (physician's judgment that delaying treatment for parental consent would jeopardize health or life), or with the **mature minor rule** (minors who are mature enough to understand their illness and the potential risks and benefits of treatment) as long as the therapy is clearly beneficial and within the standards of medical care.

- In general, **confidentiality issues** go along with self-consent except with issues of **mandatory reporting (abuse) or self-imposed dangers**; need to make that clear to the adolescent and try to obtain assent (see Chapter 6).

EMERGENCY MEDICINE

HEAD TRAUMA

Causes/Effects

- **Child abuse** (see Chapter 6), **contact, and inertial injuries**
- Contact injuries—the head strikes an object (or vice versa) → a **skull fracture, cerebral contusion, and/or intracranial hemorrhage**
- Inertial injuries—rapid acceleration-deceleration → movement of the brain → **diffuse axonal injury**
- Secondary injury occurs afterward → **cerebral edema**, release of inflammatory mediators and free radicals, hemorrhage, hypoxemia, **increased intracranial pressure**, hypotension, **loss of cerebral autoregulation**, and cell death.

Evaluation

- **Primary survey** for a neurological defect assessed quickly: **level of consciousness** (AVPU: alert, responsive to verbal commands, responsive to pain or unresponsive) and **pupil size and reactivity**
- **Secondary survey** after initial stabilization (of airway, breathing, circulation) is with the **Pediatric Glasgow Coma Scale** (PGCS; total score 15)
  - With any significant head injury: assess **eye opening** (from none to spontaneous; 0–4), **verbal response** (depending on age: older, none to oriented; young children and infants, appropriate words, smiling, fixing, and following; from 0–5), and **motor response** (none to obeys commands; 0–6)
  - Any child with a PGCS ≤8 with an abnormal CT → **admit to the pediatric intensive care unit (PICU) for intracranial pressure (ICP) management**. The radiographic procedure of choice is a **non-contrast head CT scan**.

Management

Prevent secondary injury:

- **Intubate** any child with PGCS <8; use **hyperventilation resulting in mild-moderate hypocarbia** for cerebral vasoconstriction and decrease in cerebral blood flow and ICP;

no vigorous, long-term hyperventilation (may lead to too great a degree in decrease of cerebral blood flow and cerebral oxygenation).

- **ICP monitoring** (intraventricular catheter to also drain cerebrospinal fluid [CSF] if ICP increases) for PGCS ≤8 with CT abnormality; **maintain cerebral perfusion pressure** (mean arterial pressure less ICP) **at 40 mm Hg**
- **IV mannitol** to decrease ICP (increases survival) with careful attention to **hypovolemia**
- Treat hypotension (cardiac pressors): needed for **control of cerebral perfusion pressure** and adequate systemic tissue perfusion and oxygenation
- Control **hyperthermia**.
- **Neurosurgery consult** for possible emergent surgery (evacuation of a focal hemorrhage)

POISONING

Risks

- Greatest risk—**children <5 years of age** and adolescents (toxic exposure: more likely intentional or occupational)
- Almost all in **home**, and **ingestion** is most common—most from **common household products** (<5 years), and pharmaceuticals/drugs (adolescents)
- Death secondary to unintentional poisoning is uncommon.

Prevention

- Product safety measures: **child-resistant packaging**
- **Poison prevention education** as part of early well-child care visits
- **Poison-proofing child's environment:** appropriate storage and labeling, products out of reach, locked cabinets and drawers, child-resistant caps
- **Early recognition** of signs of exposures and **plan of action** in case poisoning occurs
- Use of **online resources** and use of **poison control emergency telephone number**
- **Carbon monoxide detectors** with alarms in all homes and boats; proper installation and maintenance of all **fuel-burning appliances**; yearly inspection of furnaces, water heaters, gas pipes, and fireplace chimneys; do not use **fuel-burning space heaters** in unvented places and without monitoring
- Inspect **automobile exhaust systems** regularly; never leave car running in enclosed space.
- Do not use **charcoal grills, lanterns, hibachis, or camp stoves** indoors or in a tent or camper.

Evaluation of Unknown Substances

- Need accurate, problem-oriented history
  - **Description of toxin:** read **labels**; if not available, consult **poison control center** immediately.

- Pattern of **toxic syndromes** (toxidrome) with respect to ingredients on label
- Estimate the **amount of exposure** (needed for management): number of pills remaining in a bottle, amount of liquid remaining (assume difference to be taken dose); relate to child's age and weight; length of time in contact with skin or eyes
- **Time of exposure and time lapse** since exposure: may be a delay in effects or peak toxic concentrations
- **Progression of symptoms**
- Consider any **underlying disease/medications** for possible potentiation of effects or drug interactions.

Therapeutic Options

- Home monitoring with small doses in an asymptomatic patient; need phone follow-up within 30–60 minutes, then again in 1–3 hours; consider consultation with poison control center
- If possibility of a large dose, transport to the Emergency Department (ED); bring any emesis and containers from ingestion.
- **Prevent absorption**
  - **Wash skin** exposure with soap and water; **flush eyes** if exposed.
  - **Fresh air, oxygen** for inhaled toxins
  - **Activated charcoal** (slurry with water): decreases absorption and increases elimination of some drugs (see later sections for specifics); airway reflexes must be present or intubation is needed; a gastric tube may be needed, and repeat doses may improve removal
  - **Whole-bowel irrigation:** large volume of **nonabsorbable polyethylene glycol electrolyte solution** (GoLYTELY®) into the stomach for certain substances (see later sections for specifics); may lead to **fluid and electrolyte imbalance**
  - **Emesis with ipecac is no longer routinely recommended** (delay in onset of action and poor yield); also contraindicated with caustics and hydrocarbons.
  - **Gastric lavage:** aspirate stomach contents and then flush with normal saline; **no data on effectiveness in children** (small tubes needed; remove only a small amount of the contents); use only in older children and in select situations (see later sections)
  - **Dialysis:** primarily for severe toxicity with methanol, ethylene glycol, large symptomatic ingestions with salicylates, theophylline, and lithium
  - **Hemoperfusion:** blood is passed through a column of a resin; rarely used (perhaps for large ingestions of salicylates or theophylline); many risks

Specific Poisonings

Table 20.1: Acetaminophen (APAP)

Facts	✓ Single or combination product as liquid, tablets, capsules, suppositories ✓ Most common overdose ingestion (including death) in the United States and most common cause of **acute liver failure** ✓ Most do well; younger children have the best outcomes.
Pharmacology/ toxicity	✓ **Therapeutic levels:** 10–20 µg/mL; **serum overdose peak levels at 2–4 hours** after ingestion ✓ Maximum daily dose for children is 80 mg/kg (max. 2.6 g; **10–15 mg/kg every 4–6 hours**); **minimum toxic dose is 150 mg/kg**; hepatotoxicity at **250 mg/kg** ✓ Almost all drug metabolized in liver; toxicity via formation of **NAPQI**, which is not detoxified after a certain level, → **hepatic necrosis.**
Clinical presentation	✓ **Up to 24 hours after ingestion: asymptomatic or nonspecific signs and findings** (nausea, vomiting, dehydration, diaphoresis, pallor); beginning of **elevation of liver enzymes** ✓ **24–72 hours after ingestion:** initial symptoms decrease or resolve; **right upper quadrant pain with or without hepatomegaly**; tachycardia, hypotension (volume loss); further increase in liver enzymes with **liver function abnormalities** (elevated PT, bilirubin). ✓ **3–5 days after ingestion: initial symptoms may reappear**; liver failure, and if severe, encephalopathy (hyperammonemia) ± renal failure and cardiomyopathy; hepatic necrosis and acute tubular necrosis; possible death from **multiorgan failure or cerebral edema** ✓ **5–14 days after ingestion:** complete recovery or death; **no chronic hepatic dysfunction**
Management	✓ Assess airway, breathing, circulation, and fluid status: IV fluids and labs. ✓ Possible toxic/unknown dose, obtain **initial acetaminophen level and at 4 hours after ingestion** (if no significant level within 4 hours, there will be no hepatotoxicity); **plot 4-hour value of a single acute ingestion on the Rumack-Matthew nomogram** (predicts risk of hepatotoxicity at a single level in time; use through 24 hours); follow liver enzymes (hepatic injury at >1,000 IU/L), liver function tests, glucose, electrolytes, BUN, creatinine, and urinalysis. ✓ **Activated charcoal if presents within 4 hours** ✓ Treat with **oral NAC per protocol within 24 hours of toxic ingestion** (detoxifies NAPQI); **prevents hepatotoxicity if started within 8 hours; IV NAC for:** GI bleeding, caustic ingestion, altered mental status, pregnancy, or inability to tolerate oral ✓ **Liver transplant** if severe hepatotoxicity

Abbreviations: N-acetyl-p-aminophenol, APAP; gastrointestinal, GI; N-acetylcysteine, NAC; N-acetyl-benzoquinoneimine, NAPQI; prothrombin time, PT

Table 20.2: Salicylate

Facts	✓ Many oral and topical preparations ✓ Incidence of poisoning has decreased due to use of other analgesics/antipyretics.
Pharmacology/ toxicity	✓ Converted to **salicylic acid** after ingestion → metabolized in **liver** and then eliminated ✓ Inhibits Krebs cycle enzymes, uncouples oxidative phosphorylation → decreased ATP and increased lactate → **anion gap metabolic acidosis** ✓ **Respiratory center stimulant** → **respiratory alkalosis** → hypokalemia and hypocalcemia ✓ Increased cellular metabolism → depletion of intracellular glucose and hyperthermia ✓ Causes **vomiting and insensible fluid losses with dehydration** ✓ **Neurotoxicity** ✓ **Hepatotoxicity**: fatty infiltration, increased liver enzymes, hyperammonemia ✓ Hypoprothrombinemia and platelet dysfunction → **bleeding**
Clinical presentation	✓ **First 12 hours**: nausea, vomiting, **tinnitus** (clue), hyperthermia and CNS changes; with severe toxicity: tachycardia, hyperventilation (tachypnea and hyperpnea) from direct respiratory stimulation → **respiratory alkalosis and alkaluria with urinary excretion of sodium and potassium bicarbonate.** ✓ **Within hours to 12–24 hours** after ingestion: **paradoxic aciduria with continued respiratory alkalosis** (after significant urinary potassium loss) ✓ **From 4–6 to more than 24 hours** after ingestion: **dehydration, hypokalemia, worsening metabolic acidosis**
Management	✓ **Screen:** add few drops of **ferric chloride** to 1 mL urine; if salicylate present, urine turns to brown-purple → need quantitative salicylate level ✓ Obtain **ABG**: most common is **primary respiratory alkalosis and primary metabolic acidosis**; also follow electrolytes, BUN, creatinine, glucose, liver function tests, and urinalysis (pH, specific gravity). ✓ Obtain **initial and serial (every 2 hours until peak then every 4–6 hours until nontoxic) salicylate blood concentrations** (therapeutic level 15–30 mg/dL; symptoms >30 mg/dL and **possible death with 6-hour level >100 mg/dL**); peak overdose concentration at 4–6 hours. Done nomogram is no longer felt to be useful (only indicates severity of toxicity based on 6-hour level of non-enteric aspirin). ✓ **Activated charcoal** (may need additional doses if serum salicylate level plateaus) **with or without gastric lavage**; if enteric-coated aspirin ingested or levels do not decrease after activated charcoal → **whole-bowel irrigation.** ✓ **Alkalinization of blood and urine (IV sodium and potassium bicarbonate) to pH 7.5** prevents reabsorption of salicylate from urine and keeps salicylate in blood and out of tissue; continue at least until salicylate level is in the normal range. ✓ **Hemodialysis** if salicylate level >120 mg/dL acutely or >100 mg/dL at 6 hours post-ingestion, renal failure, refractory acidosis, seizures, coma, or noncardiogenic pulmonary edema

Abbreviations: arterial blood gas, ABG; adenosine triphosphate, ATP; central nervous system, CNS

Table 20.3: Ethylene Glycol

Facts	✓ Solvent in car radiator antifreeze ✓ Effects and management similar to methanol (windshield-washing fluid, industrial solvents)
Pharmacology/toxicity	✓ Metabolized first by alcohol dehydrogenase in the liver and then aldehyde dehydrogenase → **glyoxylic acid and oxalic acid** (both toxic); oxalic acid combines with calcium, → **hypocalcemia and calcium oxalate crystals.**
Clinical presentation	✓ **1–12 hours postingestion:** nausea, vomiting, inebriation, drowsiness, and metabolic acidosis ✓ **12–24 hours:** hypocalcemic effects: muscle pain, tetany, arrhythmia ✓ Then heart failure, renal failure, cerebral edema, and seizures
Management	✓ Screen: **Na fluorescein** (added to antifreeze) in the urine fluoresces with a Woods lamp ✓ Blood levels do not correlate with toxicity; can estimate serum levels from the osmolar gap. ✓ Follow electrolytes, BUN, creatinine, Ca, and ECG monitoring. ✓ Absorption is too rapid for activated charcoal use or gastric contamination. ✓ **Alkalinize with IV sodium bicarbonate** ✓ Current antidote (has replaced ethanol) is **fomepizole** (competitive inhibitor of alcohol dehydrogenase; no significant adverse effect). ✓ Moderate to severe cases require **hemofiltration or hemodialysis.**

Table 20.4: Carbon Monoxide

Facts	✓ Most frequent **toxic exposure** in the United States ✓ From incomplete combustion of organic matter (gas, oil, wood, charcoal) ✓ Most common exposures: **house fires, fuel-burning heaters** (especially in poorly ventilated rooms) ✓ More fatalities if **intentional exposure** ✓ Risks increased in **the very young**, very old, **fetuses** (fetal Hgb binds CO more than adult Hgb), and chronically ill ✓ People who live or work together may be affected; more in the winter months (may be a clue to diagnosis)
Pharmacology/toxicity	✓ Decreases oxygen-carrying capacity of hemoglobin (300 times greater binding than oxygen) and tissue oxygen uptake (**shifts oxy-Hgb curve to the left**); interrupts mitochondrial electron chain → produces **free radicals** → aids in the **inflammatory response, multiorgan failure, DIC, and neurological sequelae** ✓ **Vasodilatation, myocardial depression, and arrhythmias**

(continued)

Clinical presentation	✓ **Nonspecific, viral-like symptoms: headache** (most common), dizziness, nausea, loss of consciousness, shortness of breath, and loss of muscle control ✓ **Cherry-red skin is usually a postmortem finding; skin usually pale, mottled, cyanotic** (hypoxia and cardiac depression) ✓ **Pulse oximetry may be normal** (wavelengths from oxy-Hgb and carboxy-Hgb are read the same by the machine); but will be a **difference with oxy-Hgb saturation measured by spectrophotometer.** ✓ Seizures, memory loss, other neurological findings ✓ Most frequent long-term morbidities are **neurologic and neuropsychiatric problems.**
Management	✓ **ABGs** (cannot use calculated oxygen saturation; PaO_2 normal; assess acid-base status) and **carboxy-Hgb levels by direct spectrophotometry of venous sample;** asymptomatic patients with carboxy-Hgb levels <**10%** can be discharged; patients with mild symptoms treated with **100% oxygen for 4 hours** and complete improvement can be discharged home; follow-up at 24–48 hours and the following month (**delayed neurological findings up to 1 month)** ✓ CBC (Hgb concentration), complete metabolic panel, urinalysis, creatine kinase (rhabdomyolysis), cardiac enzymes (if chest pain, heart disease or risks), coagulation studies, chest x-ray with any pulmonary symptoms, ECG (arrhythmias, ischemia) ✓ Airway, breathing, circulation; **100% oxygen** (significant decrease in half-life of carboxy-Hgb) until asymptomatic and low carboxy-Hgb levels; **intubate if severely hypoxic, obtunded, or comatose;** cardiac monitoring ✓ Do not use bicarbonate: acidosis shifts the curve to the right and allows oxygen uploading to tissues (acidosis corrects gradually with oxygen). ✓ **Hyperbaric oxygen** with levels at least 15%, moderate to severe poisoning with neurologic symptoms, myocardial dysfunction, or in symptomatic pregnant patients

Abbreviations: arterial blood gas, ABG; carboxyhemoglobin, carboxy-Hgb; disseminated intravascular coagulation, DIC; hemoglobin, Hgb; oxygen-hemoglobin, oxy-Hgb

Table 20.5: Organophosphates

Facts	✓ Most widely used **insecticides** worldwide; similar findings with carbamates ✓ Most poisoning in children from **home exposure**—dermal, ingestion, inhalation ✓ Also used in chemical nerve agents ✓ Most morbidities and anoxic injury due to **respiratory failure** ✓ Deaths have decreased.
Pharmacology/ toxicity	✓ Results in reversible or irreversible (at about 18 hours after exposure) **cholinesterase inactivation → accumulation of Ach at synapses (nicotinic and muscarinic effects)** ✓ **Nicotinic effects:** skeletal muscle depolarization and fasciculations; **muscarinic:** smooth-muscle contractions (GI, bladder, secretory glands) and cardiac conduction delay ✓ Wide range of CNS effects ✓ Cholinergic effects also seen with **poisonous mushrooms,** but there will not be any nicotinic effects (weakness, muscle fasciculations).

(continued on next page)

Table 20.5: Organophosphates *(cont.)*

Clinical presentation	✓ Most common symptoms (**DUMBBELS**; less commonly seen in children): **d**iarrhea/defecation, **u**rination, **m**iosis, **b**ronchorrhea, **b**radycardia, **e**xcitation (muscle)/emesis, **l**acrimation, **s**alivation plus also GI cramps (or **SLUDGE**: **s**alivation, **l**acrimation, **u**rination, **d**efecation, **G**I distress, **e**mesis)
	✓ Other findings: wheezing, pulmonary edema, respiratory muscle weakness, paralysis, tachycardia, hypertension
	✓ CNS findings: **altered level of consciousness (most common in children)**, lethargy, restlessness, anxiety, confusion, dysarthria, headaches, ataxia, seizures, coma
Management	✓ **RBC cholinesterase level** to document exposure; does not correlate well with degree of exposure or symptoms
	✓ Follow CBC, electrolytes, BUN, creatinine, chest x-ray if pulmonary symptoms, ECG
	✓ Airway (intubation if needed), IV fluids, monitoring
	✓ **Decontamination by removal of all clothing and washing with soap and water**
	✓ **Atropine** (antagonizes **muscarinic effects**) for at least 24 hours or until atropine signs appear (dry, flushed skin; dilated pupils; increased heart rate)
	✓ **Pralidoxime** (primarily affects **nicotinic receptors**; breaks the bond with the enzyme); must be used early because will not work if irreversible effects are present; use with muscle weakness (including respiratory)
	✓ Treat unresponsive seizures with a benzodiazepine.

Abbreviations: acetylcholine, Ach; central nervous system, CNS; gastrointestinal, GI; red blood cell, RBC

Table 20.6: Hydrocarbons

Facts	✓ Many products from petroleum and wood including fuels, solvents, furniture polish, paints, glues, propellants, refrigerants, cleaning products, turpentine, pine oil
	✓ Unintentional and intentional ingestion, inhalation, dermal exposure and recreational drug use (see Chapter 19)
	✓ Worse cases in children **<5 years** (most of the unintentional exposures)
	✓ **Pulmonary toxicity** causes most morbidity and mortality.
Pharmacology/ toxicity	✓ Compounds with **higher volatility and low viscosity**—inhaled/aspirated into the respiratory system (most common complication).
	✓ Hypoxia, ARDS, GI irritation, arrhythmias, myocardial damage, coronary vasospasm, CNS effects (including encephalopathy), peripheral neuropathy, and death
	✓ Also hemolysis, bone marrow toxicity, hepatic and renal failure, renal tubular acidosis
	✓ Direct skin toxicity can result in severe burns.
Clinical presentation	✓ **Coughing, choking, vomiting, cyanosis** with pulmonary aspiration
	✓ Mucosal irritation, chemical burns
	✓ Hyperthermia, tachypnea, wheezing, rales, nausea, abdominal pain, arrhythmias, headache, lethargy, dizziness, ataxia, seizures, coma

(continued)

Management	✓ **Chest x-ray in all symptomatic children** (initially normal; positive findings of aspiration/inhalation may take hours); **obtain 6 hours after ingestion** if patient is to be discharged (asymptomatic); **any symptomatic patient should be admitted and observed for 12 hours:** follow pulse oximetry.
	✓ With poor oxygenation: **early intubation and ventilation (with PEEP) plus bronchodilators**
	✓ **Cutaneous decontamination** as soon as possible
	✓ **Induction of emesis is contraindicated,** and **gastric lavage** is indicated only with highly toxic substances (CHAMPS: **c**amphor, **h**alogenated hydrocarbons, **a**romatic hydrocarbons, heavy **m**etal-containing hydrocarbons and **p**esticide-containing hydrocarbons) and **only after intubation;** activated charcoal does not bind and is not useful.

Abbreviations: arterial blood gas, ABG; acute respiratory distress syndrome, ARDS; central nervous system, CNS; gastrointestinal, GI; positive end-expiratory pressure, PEEP

Table 20.7: Common Plants

Facts	✓ Most common reported plant exposures in the United States from **Caladium, Dieffenbachia, and Philodendron**
	✓ Commonly found in homes and offices
	✓ Most in children **<5 years old** from chewing and swallowing; also dermal and ocular exposure
Pharmacology/toxicity	✓ Presence of calcium oxalate crystals and proteolytic enzymes
Clinical presentation	✓ **Burning and irritation of oral mucosa;** swelling, drooling dysphagia and respiratory distress (all very uncommon)
Management	✓ No lab studies or imaging studies are indicated.
	✓ Upper airway endoscopy with severe swelling, respiratory findings
	✓ Ophthalmology exam for eye contamination
	✓ **Decontamination:** remove all plant pieces and rinse mouth with water; gastric decontamination is not needed.
	✓ **Analgesics** for pain (possibly corticosteroids for severe swelling)
	✓ Report all cases to poison control center for tracking.

Table 20.8: Iron

Facts	✓ Products are available in many homes (often look like candy)
	✓ Most from **children <6 years** who have ingested pediatric multivitamins
	✓ Worse cases in children **<3 years old**
Pharmacology/toxicity	✓ Severity proportional to amount of **elemental iron** ingested (number of tablets and percentage of elemental iron in each)
	✓ Signs of toxicity with **10–20 mg/kg** elemental iron; serious if **>60 mg/kg**
	✓ Mitochondrial toxin: disrupts oxidative phosphorylation → free radical formation and lipid peroxidation
	✓ **Corrosive to GI mucosa** (allows for unregulated absorption); systemic toxicity, hepatocellular injury (and fibrosis), increased pulmonary vascular resistance, and myocardial depression
	✓ **Anion gap metabolic acidosis** (conversion of free plasma iron to ferric chloride), lactic acidosis (interruption or cellular respiration), hypovolemia, hypoperfusion, and cardiogenic shock
	✓ **Coagulopathy**—inhibition of thrombin formation and reduced levels of clotting factors
Clinical presentation	✓ **First 6 hours: hemorrhagic vomiting, diarrhea, and abdominal pain**; may lead to **shock**
	✓ **6–12 hours** after exposure: if mild, may have **actual recovery**; but if moderate to severe, **recovery is temporary** (time for iron to distribute through body); lethargy, tachycardia, and tachypnea.
	✓ **12–24 hours: multiorgan damage: metabolic acidosis, coagulopathy,** shock, arrhythmias, CNS findings, seizures
	✓ **2–3 days** after ingestion: **hepatic injury**
	✓ **2–6 weeks** after ingestion: **scarring of the GI tract** (pyloric obstruction, cirrhosis; rare)
Management	✓ **Serum iron levels:** generally correlate with clinical severity (**mild = <300 μg/dL; moderate = 300–500 μg/dL; severe = >500 μg/dL**); obtain level at **2–6 hours after ingestion**; TIBC, WBC counts, serum glucose and deferoxamine challenge test are no longer considered useful.
	✓ **Abdominal x-ray:** may show radiopaque particles (not completely absorbed yet); obtain pre- and post-GI decontamination
	✓ IV fluid resuscitation and cardiovascular stabilization
	✓ **No gastric lavage** (iron particles are large and sticky in gastric contents)
	✓ **Whole-bowel irrigation** until repeat x-ray shows no more particles
	✓ **IV deferoxamine infusion** (binds absorbed iron) for estimated dose **>60 mg/kg or serum iron >500 μg/dL** or with any severe, persistent findings; use until clinical improvement, 6–24 hours.
	✓ Particles remaining in the GI tract after decontamination **need to be removed** endoscopically or surgically.

Abbreviations: central nervous system, CNS; gastrointestinal, GI; total iron-binding capacity, TIBC; white blood cell, WBC

Table 20.9: Cyclic Antidepressants

Facts	✓ Antidepressants: three-ring (tricyclic) or newer four-ring structure
	✓ Also used for migraine prophylaxis, chronic pain syndromes, nocturnal enuresis (imipramine), and other psychiatric diagnoses
	✓ Most: amitriptyline, desipramine, imipramine, nortriptyline, doxepin, clomipramine, amoxapine, and maprotiline
	✓ Incidence of overdose has increased, but most common antidepressant in toxic doses is now the **SSRIs**.
Pharmacology/ toxicity	✓ In overdose, pharmacokinetics are altered and elimination is prolonged → increased toxic effects
	✓ **Blocks neuronal uptake of norepinephrine, serotonin, and dopamine** in the CNS and peripheral nervous system; also **alpha-blocking** (vasodilatation with profound hypotension) and **anticholinergic effects** and **blocking of fast sodium channels in myocardial cells**
	✓ Toxicity at doses of **10–20 mg/kg/day** (therapeutic doses at 5–10 mg/kg/day) with significant effects at **>20 mg/kg/day**
	✓ Most serious effects are **CNS** (sedation, depressed mental status, seizures) and **cardiovascular** (heart block, ventricular arrhythmias, asystole).
Clinical presentation	✓ **Anticholinergic effects first:** dry skin, mydriasis, urinary retention, hypoactive/absent bowel sounds, hyperthermia, and myoclonic twitching
	✓ **CNS effects more frequently in children** (than cardiovascular effects): drowsiness, delirium, seizures, coma, respiratory depression (with respiratory arrest at any time)
	✓ **Cardiovascular:** sinus tachycardia most common; then vasodilatation with hypotension, shock, arrhythmias, heart block, and asystole
Management	✓ Follow CBC, electrolytes (**anion gap; hypokalemia**), BUN, creatinine, urinalysis, **ABGs (mixed acidosis)**; serum drug levels not readily available; screen with urine toxicology
	✓ Monitor **ECG (widening of QRS to >100 msec or a large R wave in a VR correlates with arrhythmias and seizures;** at least **6–8 hours** if asymptomatic and **24 hours** of normal findings for the symptomatic patient
	✓ Airway, breathing, circulation; IV fluids and pressors (**epinephrine** drug of choice) as needed
	✓ **Alkalinize with sodium bicarbonate to pH 7.45–7.55** (increases protein binding, stabilizes arrhythmias, increases blood pressure); monitor ECG, pH, and serum potassium closely.
	✓ **Administer activated charcoal.**
	✓ **Gastric lavage is helpful with significant ingestions if performed within 1 hour** after ingestion; **intubation should occur first** (and with any clinical deterioration).
	✓ Treat seizures with a **benzodiazepine.**
	✓ Treat arrhythmias: (**phenytoin**)

Abbreviations: arterial blood gas, ABG; central nervous system, CNS; selective serotonin reuptake inhibitor, SSRI

Table 20.10: Cough and Cold Preparations

Facts	✓ Toxicity from **antihistamines** (diphenhydramine, brompheniramine, chlorpheniramine), **decongestants** (pseudoephedrine and phenylephrine), and antitussives (**dextromethorphan**)
	✓ Most are asymptomatic or mildly symptomatic and are in children <6 years old (intentional more common in adolescents).
Pharmacology/toxicity	✓ Toxicity of **antihistamine** preparations from the **anticholinergic effects** (like atropine): competitive inhibition of **muscarinic receptors** to acetylcholine in the peripheral and CNS.
	✓ **Decongestants:** direct **catecholamine release**, blockage of reuptake and slowing of metabolism; direct effect on muscles and glands and respiratory/ CNS **stimulation**
	✓ **Dextromethorphan:** synthetic opioid acting at CNS opiate receptors; no analgesic or addictive properties; causes **serotonin syndrome** (agonist of serotonin transmission and inhibits reuptake); has become a recreational drug with large doses causing effects similar to PCP
Clinical presentation	✓ **Anticholinergic effects** (from antihistamines): agitation, fever, urinary retention; dry, hot, flushed skin and mydriasis; tachycardia, arrhythmias, nausea, vomiting, rhabdomyolysis, visual hallucinations, respiratory depression, ARDS, ECG abnormalities
	✓ **Catecholamine effects** (from decongestants): elevated blood pressure with reflex bradycardia → postural hypotension; hyperthermia, hyperexcitability, hallucinations, psychosis, seizures, intracranial bleeding
	✓ **Serotonergic** (from dextromethorphan or SSRIs, or many other drugs; see Chapter 19): mydriasis, nystagmus, agitation, tachycardia, autonomic instability (hypertension), increased bowel sounds (diarrhea), hyperreflexia, clonus, tremor
	✓ **Effects are often mixed** due to combined products in preparations; also, specific drugs may be associated with specific adverse effects.
Management	✓ Obtain electrolytes, CBC, plasma creatine kinase, screen for APAP, salicylates (often in formulations); emergency drug screens are not helpful in management; ECG
	✓ Airway, breathing circulation; IV fluids, glucose, oxygen, and naloxone (if decreased level of consciousness)
	✓ **Activated charcoal; most effective within 1 hour of ingestion**
	✓ Dystonic reactions *not* thought to be due to antihistamines: **diphenhydramine** IV frequently
	✓ Dystonic reactions to antihistamines: use **IV diazepam**; *do not* use **physostigmine** (anticholinergic) unless directed to do so by a poison control center because of severe, life-threatening complications.
	✓ Treat seizures with **lorazepam.**
	✓ Treat serotonin syndrome by managing each symptom separately; and use **cyproheptadine** (nonspecific serotonin antagonist) or newer, more specific antagonists.

Abbreviations: N-acetyl-p-aminophenol, APAP; acute respiratory distress syndrome, ARDS; central nervous system, CNS; phencyclidine, PCP; selective serotonin reuptake inhibitor, SSRI

DROWNING

Epidemiology

- Most common cause of accident-related death, next to motor vehicle accidents
- In United States: largest group is children age 1–14 years (higher in ethnic minorities)
- Most in **natural fresh water** (high rates in adolescents); then residential **swimming pools** (higher rates in young children); then bathtubs; and last, saltwater.
- Over half of infant drownings in the first year at domestic sites; over half in **bathtubs** during brief periods of lack of supervision (also in buckets, toilets, sinks, washing machines; falling in headfirst and unable to right the body to free the head)
- Large number of drownings in children >2 years of age in **hot tubs and spas** due to entrapment (from suction)
- Increased use of **alcohol-related drowning**, especially in ages 16–20 years; many involved with **watercraft**
- Significant increase in risk with chronic illness **(epilepsy)**
- Also from **child abuse/neglect and homicide**

Major Clinical Aspects Related to Pathophysiology

- Most drownings do not aspirate large amounts of water (early laryngospasm) small number who have vomited and aspirated gastric contents, but large amounts of water may be swallowed
- Progressive hypoxia → loss of consciousness → severe hypoxia, medullary depression → terminal apnea
  - **Saltwater drowning:** hypertonic pulmonary aspirate/swallowing → osmotic gradient → fluid drawn into the alveoli → **inactivation of surfactant** (acute respiratory distress syndrome; ARDS); with massive aspiration and ingestion (rare) → fluid shifts into the lungs and gastrointestinal (GI) tract → **hypernatremia and hemoconcentration** (exacerbated by cerebral DI)
  - **Freshwater drowning:** hypotonic fresh water → **washout of surfactant** (the effect is the same but due to a different reason) and with massive aspiration/ingestion, may be **hyponatremia and hemodilution** → hypo-osmolality, **intravascular hemolysis, hyperkalemia, hemoglobinuria, and renal tubular damage** (exacerbated by cerebral and pulmonary damage, causing syndrome of inappropriate antidiuretic hormone secretion SIADH).
  - Pulmonary hypoxic injury, direct injury from aspiration (dependent upon what is in the aspirate and degree of toxicity), and pneumonia
- Initially, **increase in heart rate and blood pressure** → **reflex bradycardia** (and arrhythmias in some) → decreased cardiac output and delivery of oxygen to tissues; up to 4 minutes of hypoxia → **myocardial hypoxia** and pulseless electrical activity.
- **Hypoxia-ischemia** → **progressive, irreversible injury** to most organs; **central nervous system (CNS) injury is the most common cause of mortality and long-term morbidities.**

- Other major injury and morbidities: acute tubular necrosis, renal failure, disseminated intravascular coagulation (DIC), thrombocytopenia, hypoxic GI damage, hepatic injury, pancreatic injury, and sepsis
- **Hypothermia:** significant due to **conductive and convective heat loss** and aspirating/swallowing cold water; as core temperature decreases **below 35°C (95°F)**, → decreased cognitive function, strength, coordination, → loss of consciousness with respiratory insufficiency → bradycardia, decreased cardiac output, and cardiac arrest

Major Therapeutic Issues

- **Immediate cardiopulmonary resuscitation (CPR) increases** the likelihood of a good outcome.
- With emergency personnel and equipment:
    - **100% oxygen with bag-and-mask ventilation as soon as possible**.
    - **Nasogastric (NG) tube** for gastric decompression and prevention of aspiration with vomiting
    - If suspicion of a foreign body—**chest compressions and back blows**, not abdominal thrusts.
    - **Cervical spine**—immobilized in case of a cervical injury; rare unless with a diving or boating accident.
    - **Passive re-warming**—drying the skin, removing wet clothing, and using blankets.
    - If no spontaneous respirations and decreased circulation, **intubate and use positive end-expiratory pressure (PEEP) with positive pressure ventilation (PaCO2 initially 35–40 mm Hg)**; monitor oxygen saturations (**keep >90%**) and ECG.
    - Establish **venous access** (or intraosseous if necessary): **bolus normal saline or Ringer's lactate**, and begin infusion.
    - Cardiac pressor of choice is **epinephrine** for maintenance of blood pressure and perfusion.
    - **Defibrillate** for ventricular fibrillation or pulseless ventricular tachycardia.

- All children with submersion should be hospitalized and monitored for at **least 6–12 hours**, even if asymptomatic; with minimal symptoms, may worsen **4–8 hours** after submersion (most will become symptomatic by 18 hours).
    - If still in arrest upon entry to the ER, continue to **treat aggressively** and try to stabilize (prognosis in the ER cannot initially be determined); no response after prolonged CPR is predictive of death or a persistent vegetative state (stop CPR **after 25–30 minutes** without response).
    - Measure **core body temperature** at the tympanic membrane (correlates most closely with brain temperature); need **continuous temperature-monitoring**; re-warming:
        - **Active re-warming methods** (warmed IV fluids, warmed oxygen, gastric or bladder lavage with warmed saline, and other methods) are used **with moderate to severe hypothermia** (<32°C [89.6°F]) to increase body temperature more rapidly
        - No active re-warming with temperature of **32–37.5°C (89.6–99.5°F)** and **continued unresponsiveness with adequate spontaneous circulation**.

- No human studies demonstrating that therapeutic hypothermia improves the outcome of drowning patients, but in resuscitated comatose patients, core temperature should be **prevented from going above 37.5°C (89.6°F)** in the first 24–48 hours (exacerbates hypoxic-ischemic encephalopathy)
  - Appropriate IV fluids to **maintain euglycemia** (no added glucose if hyperglycemic); IV glucose bolus and then infusion with added dextrose if hypoglycemic; correct electrolyte abnormalities

- Adequate **oxygen and PEEP** need to be utilized to **maintain oxygen saturations >90%**; if adequate spontaneous respirations, continuous positive airway pressure (CPAP) or biphasic positive airway pressure (BiPAP) may be used.
  - **Avoid permissive hypercapnia, but no excessive hyperventilation** (cerebral vasoconstriction and hypoperfusion): maintain **PCO$_2$ at 35–40 mm Hg**.
  - Use a **beta-2-agonist** for bronchoconstriction.
  - May need specialized therapies, such as high-frequency ventilation or inhaled nitric oxide

- **Continuous ECG monitoring, blood-pressure monitoring, and frequent arterial blood gases (ABGs) via an arterial catheter**; echocardiogram for cardiac function; central venous catheter to monitor preload and pulmonary arterial catheter
  - **Epinephrine** infusion is the drug of choice for continued hypotension and cardiac dysfunction after hypoxic-ischemic events.

- No routine head CT or MRI unless to evaluate for trauma
  - **Increased ICP** is usually a poor outcome.
  - No routine EEG monitoring except for evaluation of seizures or brain death.

- Other issues: aggressive control of fever, no prophylactic use of antibiotics but based on clinical findings/deterioration and cultures; renal failure is managed with fluid restriction, diuretics, and dialysis; GI ischemia: bowel rest, NG suction, and proton pump inhibitors

Prognostic Indicators

- Initial factors associated with **good outcome**: submersion <5 minutes; immediate CPR; resuscitation <10 minutes with return of spontaneous circulation, normal sinus rhythm, neurological responsiveness, reactive pupils; **possible** neuroprotective effects if drowning in icy water <5°C (<41°F)
- Initial factors associated with **bad outcome**: delay in CPR, submersion >10 minutes, resuscitation >25 minutes, arrhythmias, neurological unresponsiveness, nonreactive pupils
- The **best prognostic factor of long-term CNS outcome** is the neurological exam/progression in the first 24–72 hours; if consciousness is regained in 48–72 hours, unlikely to have serious neurological sequelae; without spontaneous purposeful movements and brain-stem function at 24 hours, outcome is poor.

BITES
Dog, Cat, Human

Table 20.11: Clinical Features and Management of Domestic Bites

	Dog	Cat	Human
Wound characteristics	Abrasions, punctures, lacerations, crush, tissue avulsion	Usually deep puncture wounds	Occlusion (upper and lower teeth come together) or clenched-fist injury (just contacts tooth)
Incidence of infection	Small if <8 hours to treatment	More than half with early onset	High risk
Increased risk of infection	Hands, feet, genitals, deep punctures, crush injury, tendon or bone injury, foreign material, delay of treatment >24 hours	Hands, feet, genitals, deep punctures, tendon or bone injury, foreign material, delay of treatment >24 hours	Hands, feet, genitals, foreign material, delay of treatment >24 hours
Most common organisms	*Staph. aureus and Pasteurella multocida*, *Staph. intermedius*, *Capnocytophaga canimorsus*; over half with mixed anaerobes	Predominantly *P. multocida*; also *Staph. aureus*; otherwise similar to dog	Nontypeable *Haemophilus influenzae*, alpha-streptococci, beta-lactamase–producing aerobes. *Eikenella corrodens* and **mixed anaerobes** (especially with clenched fist)
Management	• Aerobic and anaerobic cultures **if >8 hours**, with obvious infection, deep and extensive or immunocompromise • Anesthetize, clean, and irrigate with normal saline; débride devitalized tissue; consult surgery for severe wounds	• Aerobic and anaerobic cultures **in all**, unless very trivial • Otherwise, same care as for dog bite	• Aerobic and anaerobic cultures in all • Consider **hepatitis B** immunization (depending on immunization status) if instigator at high risk. • Otherwise same care as for dog bite

(continued)

	Dog	Cat	Human
Management (continued)	• **Do not suture infected wounds or those >24 hours**; delay closure of all **hand wounds**; primary closure of facial wounds if within **6 hours**. • Antibiotics except for most superficial wounds: **amoxicillin-clavulanate** orally or IV **ampicillin-sulbactam or ticarcillin-clavulanate** (for more severe wounds, obvious infection or signs of toxicity); if penicillin allergy, best coverage for both aerobes and anaerobes is azithromycin • Check **tetanus status** and administer tetanus toxoid if needed (see Chapter 4). • **Rabies**, depending on status of animal and known rabies in the community (see Chapter 15) • Follow-up in **24–48 hours**	(See previous page)	(See previous page)

Snake Bite

Background/toxicity—In the United States, majority of venomous bites are **pit vipers** (subfamily of true vipers; triangular heads, elliptical eyes, and a pit between the eye and nose) = **rattlesnakes, copperheads, and cottonmouths**; other venomous U.S. snake (mostly in Texas and the Southeast) is the **coral snake** (black and red bands separated by yellow bands). Pit vipers cause **tissue necrosis, vascular leak, and a coagulopathy** (possible hemorrhagic shock, renal failure, and ARDS); coral snakes release a **neurotoxin**.

Clinical presentation

- **Pit vipers:** rapid onset of pain and swelling (usually extremity); venom progression proximally; edema and ecchymoses; severe cases result in tissue necrosis; systemic features: nausea, vomiting, sweating, muscle fasciculations, and facial tingling. Worse cases associated with **severe clotting abnormalities**, generalized edema, arrhythmias, and shock.
- **Coral snake:** minimal pain due to no cytotoxicity, but **rapid progression of paralysis and death** secondary to respiratory failure (neurotoxin).

Management

- Determine if the snake is poisonous; the majority are not → **local wound care.**
- If venomous, **immobilize the extremity and transport directly to the ER**; do not use ice or tourniquet (evidence that there is increased risk of ischemia).
- Start **venous access** and draw labs (CBC, platelets, prothrombin time [PT], partial thromboplastin time [PTT], fibrinogen and fibrin degradation products, creatine kinase, BUN, creatinine and type and cross; these labs need to be followed periodically).
- On the skin, mark the area of the present location of edema and necrosis to compare with progression.
- **Clean and irrigate** wound; **tetanus** prophylaxis if necessary
- **Antivenin**, depending on the severity and progression
  - Animal-derived immunoglobulins that bind and neutralize the protein in venoms; four are FDA-approved for commercial use in the United States
  - May cause **immediate (anaphylaxis) and delayed hypersensitivity reactions (serum sickness**; 5–21 days later); consider pretreatment with IV diphenhydramine and methylprednisolone
  - In general, **rattlesnake bites require treatment** (only mild local swelling with no progression does not require treatment) and **copperhead bites do not.** CroTAb (ovine-derived; less immediate hypersensitivity and serum sickness compared to equine-derived *Crotalidae* polyvalent antivenin) is the antivenin of choice for pit vipers; best if given within **4 hours**; not effective after **12 hours**; cottonmouth bites are dependent on severity and progression; **coral snake antivenin** should be given **prophylactically** as soon as possible to prevent effect of **neurotoxin** (once symptoms have started, it is not effective).

Arachnid Bites

Black widow spider

Background/toxicity—Found in all of the United States (more in the South); shiny black spider with a **bright-red or orange abdomen** (classic hourglass appearance in only one species); found in protected places; releases a **neurotoxin** → presynaptic release of acetylcholine and norepinephrine → **excessive muscle depolarization and autonomic hyperactivity**

Clinical presentation—Initial bite → 2–3 mm, pale area with a red border; within 1 hour there is a **dull, crampy pain** which spreads to the entire body, including the **chest and abdomen (boardlike)** plus nausea, vomiting, sweating, **agitation, hypertension** (hypertension and agitation distinguish abdominal findings from a surgical abdomen). All symptoms resolve in 24–48 hours, but pain may be severe.

Management—**IV opiates** for pain and **benzodiazepine** for muscle relaxation; try conservative management first, but if severe (including autonomic instability) then **antivenin** is indicated (much less anaphylactic risk and serum sickness than snake antivenin; rapid resolution of symptoms)

Brown recluse spider

Background/toxicity—Lives in dark, undisturbed places; most potent species in river areas of the Midwest and the South (less potent ones in other areas of United States); small body with longer legs and **dark, violin-shaped mark on thorax**; venom contains **hyaluronidase and sphingomyelinase, which lyses cell walls and causes significant skin necrosis**

Clinical presentation—Initial pinprick bite, then within 2 hours—a painful, depressed blue lesion with rim of inflammation then **fever, chills, nausea, vomiting, and possible hemolysis** (directly from the toxin); a **hemorrhagic blister forms in 1–2 days, which sloughs and leaves a necrotic ulcer** (can enlarge and involve full skin thickness of skin)

Management—Most improve with **symptomatic care** (decreased pain in a few days); admit any significant bite for monitoring and pain control, **hydration, and maintenance of urine output** (if significant hemoglobinuria); local wound care for the skin lesion, which usually heals in weeks

Scorpion

Background/toxicity—The only significantly venomous species in United States is found in Southwest desert; stinger at the end of a six-segment tail releases venom that is **neurotoxic** → release of acetylcholine and **stimulation of sympathetic and parasympathetic nervous systems**.

Clinical presentation—Mild **local burning to severe pain**; severe cases with **autoimmune dysfunction** within 1 hour: agitation, irritability, salivation, blurred vision, muscle twitching, hypotension, tachycardia, tachypnea, and nystagmus; **small children** have an increased risk of autoimmune dysfunction, multiorgan failure, and death.

Management—Localized pain treated with **ice and analgesics** (decreases in 24 hours); severe reactions require hospitalization for **sedation and observation**; symptoms generally improve over 24–48 hours; if there is cardiopulmonary compromise, consider **antivenin** (not FDA-approved; obtain from Arizona Poison Control; rapid resolution of symptoms)

HEMATOLOGY/ONCOLOGY 21

RED BLOOD CELL DISORDERS

Nutritional Anemias

Table 21.1: Nutritional Anemias

	Iron Deficiency	Folate Deficiency	B12 Deficiency
Epidemiology	Highest incidence from **6 months to 2 years, and adolescence**	Uncommon; usually related to **undernutrition** and/or selective diets; breastfeeding mother with poor nutrition	Inadequate intake rare in children (poor maternal nutrition in a breast-fed infant or in a child); usually due to **pernicious anemia** or another primary problem
Physiology	Fe needed for the production of **heme proteins**; smaller amount stored as **ferritin** and **hemosiderin**; storage depletion leads to anemia	Absorbed in **proximal intestine**; circulates in plasma as THF, used primarily for **purine biosynthesis**; causes **arrest of nuclear maturation** (nuclear immaturity with respect to cytoplasm → **megaloblastic anemia**)	B12 binds to **intrinsic factor** in the stomach → transported to **terminal and is absorbed**; acts as a cofactor in enzymatic reactions and activation of folinic acid; DNA synthesis impaired due to **arrest of nuclear maturation from a decrease in folate derivatives**
Causes	Decreased intake (**cow's milk <1 year of age**; malabsorption), increased needs (chronic hemolysis) or blood loss	Decreased intake (**goat's milk**), decreased proximal intestinal absorption (**malabsorption, medications**), **antifolate medications** (methotrexate, azathioprine, sulfonamides), congenital THF deficiency, increased use (**chronic hemolysis, pregnancy**) or increased loss	Inadequate intake, inadequate absorption (**ileal disease** or **decreased/absent intrinsic factor**, pancreatic insufficiency, parasitic illnesses, intrinsic intestinal disease), impaired transport from intestine (congenital absence of transport molecules; familial)

(continued on next page)

Table 21.1: Nutritional Anemias (cont.)

	Iron Deficiency	Folate Deficiency	B12 Deficiency
Signs and symptoms	Lethargy, decreased appetite, irritability, **pica**, behavioral changes; pallor, **stomatitis**, tachycardia, systolic murmur, decreased blood pressure; heart failure if severe	Findings related to anemia; no neurological findings; **malnourishment**, possible abnormal stooling due to malabsorption	Anemia (and possibly pancytopenia), **glossitis, stomatitis, hyperpigmentation, decreased vibratory sensation (dorsal columns), psychiatric changes (dementia)**
Laboratory findings	-**Microcytic, hypochromic anemia** of underproduction: **decreased MCV and reticulocytes** -**Anisocytosis** (variable sized RBCs)—**normal to increased RDW** -Additional studies: increased FEP, decreased serum Fe and ferritin, decreased transferrin saturation, increased TIBC	-**Macrocytic anemia** with underproduction: **increased MCV and decreased to normal reticulocytes** -**RDW normal** -Smear: macrocytosis with **hypersegmented neutrophils** (at least 6 nuclear segments) -May also have decreased WBCs and platelets	-**Macrocytic anemia** with underproduction: **increased MCV and decreased to normal reticulocytes** -**RDW normal** -Smear: macrocytosis with **hypersegmented neutrophils** -May also have decreased WBCs and platelets
First step in management	If diagnosis is suggested, give a **trial of iron replacement for a month**: should see a **reticulocytosis within a week** (repeat reticulocytosis count in 5–7 days) and the **Hgb should increase by at least 1 g/dL in 1 month**; if not, consider other causes (thalassemia, lead, chronic disease); perform other Fe studies at this time.	Best test is RBC folate level, which includes THF	-May need bone marrow exam if more than one cell line affected; bone marrow shows **asynchrony of RBC precursors (nuclear/cytoplasmic)** -**Schilling test**: measure serum B12 before and after giving B12, then again using B12 plus intrinsic factor: ◦ **B12 increases after oral B12:** dietary cause ◦ **B12 increases only with oral B12 plus intrinsic factor:** pernicious anemia ◦ **No increase in B12 after intrinsic factor,** due to one of the other causes
Therapy	Continue iron (calculation based on **elemental iron**) for another 3 months.	**Folate supplementation;** change or eliminate causative drug, treat underlying intestinal problem	**Vitamin B12 with or without intrinsic factor**

Abbreviations: free erythrocyte protoporphyrin, FEP; hematocrit, Hct; hemoglobin, Hgb; mean corpuscular volume, MCV; red blood cell, RBC; red-cell distribution width, RDW; 5-methyl tetrahydrofolate, THF; total iron-binding capacity, TIBC

Table 21.2: Pure Red Cell Aplasia/Hypoplasia

	Blackfan-Diamond Anemia	Transient Erythroblastopenia of Childhood (TEC)
Etiology	Inherited (X-linked, autosomal recessive or dominant) defect of RBC progenitor cell → **decreased RBC production**	**Post-viral transient immune erythroid suppression with complete recovery**
Clinical presentation	-**From birth to early infancy** with anemia and heart failure (if severe) -**Short stature** (IUGR, LBW), facial dysmorphic features, **triphalangeal thumbs**, various renal anomalies	1–3-year-old previously well with **gradually increasing pallor and fatigue (over days) after a nonspecific viral illness**
Laboratory findings	-Decreased Hb and Hct -**Increased Hb F** -Macrocytosis (**increased MCV**) -Normal to moderate decreased WBCs with normal to increased platelets -Bone marrow aspirate—**markedly decreased numbers of erythroid precursors with normal myeloid precursors and megakaryocytes**	-**Normocytic, normochromic with very low reticulocytes** -Hb usually 5-7 g/dL -Smear: **normal RBC morphology** -May have very mild neutropenia -**RBC adenine deaminase is normal to low.** -Bone marrow (usually not needed)—**decreased to absent RBC precursors with other lines normal**
Management	Initial therapy with **prednisone** (most respond with long-term survival; leukemia rare complication); wean to alternate day and the smallest dose to keep [Hb] about 10 g/dL -For failures, use IV methylprednisolone, then **anabolic steroids**, then chronic blood transfusions with chelation; can also try hematopoietic growth factor (IL-3) -**Bone marrow transplant** if histocompatible sibling	-Packed RBC transfusion if hemodynamic instability (unusual)—follow CBC regularly—usually recovery in **1–2 months**

Pancytopenias

Table 21.3: Pancytopenias

	Fanconi Anemia	Aplastic Anemia
Etiology	Autosomal recessive pancytopenia; **characteristic chromosomal abnormalities;** higher prevalence in certain ethnic/geographic groups	**Inherited** (defect in stem cell) or **acquired** (transient, reversible or irreversible) cause of decreased hematopoietic cells resulting in **pancytopenia:** -**Inherited:** Shwachman-Diamond syndrome and others beside Fanconi -**Acquired:** infection (e.g., EBV, HIV, parvovirus B19), radiation, drugs (e.g., chloramphenicol, NSAIDs, chemotherapy), or immune (hypogammaglobulinemia)
Clinical features	-Age of diagnosis **birth to 50 years** (median 7); **characteristic birth defects: short stature, radial and thumb anomalies (hypoplastic or absent** and many others), abnormal skin pigmentation (including **café-au-lait spots**), GU abnormalities, and many others (eye, hearing, cardiovascular, GI, developmental) -**Petechiae, bruising, and bleeding** are generally the first signs, then worsening anemia, then repeated infections.	-Signs and symptoms of anemia, petechiae, bruising, bleeding, recurrent infections (depending on degree of neutropenia)
Laboratory findings	-Pancytopenia -**RBCs are macrocytic.** -**Increased Hgb F** -**Normal RBC adenine deaminase** -Bone marrow: **loss of erythroid, myeloid, and platelet precursors; hypocellular or aplasia with a fatty marrow** -Prenatal diagnosis: chromosome breaks in cells (CVS or amniocentesis), or known mutations in fetal cells	-**Pancytopenia with decreased reticulocytes** -Anemia is **macrocytic.** -**Increased Hgb F** -Bone marrow: **hypocellularity with decreased (to varying degrees) erythroid and myeloid precursors and megakaryocytes**
Complications	Median survival 30 years; death due to **bone marrow failure, then leukemia** (AML or myelomonocytic), then various solid tumors (older patients)	Bone marrow failure and death with severe suppression; some with moderate suppression recover

(continued)

	Fanconi Anemia	Aplastic Anemia
Management	-**Transfuse** for anemia associated with hemodynamic changes; **transfuse platelets and neutrophils for significant decreases; also G-CSF.** -Long-term treatment of choice—**stem cell transplant from an HLA-matched sibling** (prevents bone marrow failure and leukemia). -**Androgens** (oxymetholone) used if transplant not an option. -Various surgeries, depending on the associated abnormalities.	Treatment of choice is **allogenic bone marrow transplant** (cure); if no donor is available then antithymocyte globulin plus cyclosporine with IL-3 and G-CSF; high-dose corticosteroids and androgens if antithymocyte globulin is unavailable.

Abbreviations: acute myelogenous leukemia, AML; chorionic villus sampling, CVS; Epstein-Barr virus, EBV; granulocyte colony-stimulating factor, G-CSF; genitourinary, GU; hemoglobin, Hgb; interleukin, IL; red blood cell, RBC

Lead Poisoning

Background/etiology—Highest risk in **toddlers** (put things in their mouths); sources: **old paint** (still may have lead in old buildings), some **glass, batteries, cosmetics, jewelry, toys, pottery, lead soldering on water pipes, airborne** from factories that smelt lead; also through **inhalation and transdermal absorption**; defined as blood lead level **(BLL) >5 μg/ dL.** Higher risk in minorities and lower socioeconomic status (SES).

Physiology—Most lead is sequestered in bone (for several years), the rest to the blood and soft tissues; **interferes with heme synthesis** at three enzymatic steps → decreased hemoglobin (Hgb) and increased toxic products

Clinical presentation—**Decreased appetite, abdominal pain and constipation**, possible **pica**; pallor and fatigue (**anemia); neurobehavioral changes**: hyperactivity, inattention, personality changes, change in school performance; **encephalopathy** (at levels >70 μg/ dL): vomiting, papilledema, ataxia, seizures, decreased consciousness, hypertension and bradycardia, decreased respiratory effort, and coma

Laboratory findings—Hypochromic, microcytic anemia, basophilic stippling, decreased reticulocytes, normal red-cell distribution width (RDW), normal serum Fe, total iron-binding capacity (TIBC), and ferritin; **increased free erythrocyte protoporphyrin** (FEP); screening with fingerstick lead level → if positive, need **venous blood lead level**; long-bone x-rays: lead lines (distal metaphyses radiolucency; chronic lead exposure; growth-arrest line)

Treatment

- **BLL 10–14 μg/dL:** confirm with venous BLL in 1 month; if still elevated, educate family regarding lead exposure and repeat level in 3 months
- **BLL 15–19 μg/dL:** same as above; repeat level in 2 months

- **BLL 20–44 μg/dL:** confirm with BLL in 1 week; notify Health Department: need environmental inspection and determination of Pb exposure with cleanup and family education; follow BLL to confirm decrease back to normal
- **BLL 45–69 μg/dL:** venous BLL within 2 days; complete evaluation as above plus **remove from environment** (if not possible, hospitalize); **chelate with oral succimer or, if hospitalized, IV ethylenediaminetetraacetic acid (EDTA)**; monitor CBC, electrolytes, and liver function
- **BLL ≥70 μg/dL: immediate confirmation of BLL and hospitalization for IV chelation with dimercaprol (bronchoalveolar lavage [BAL]) and EDTA** (does not cross blood–brain barrier, so need additional chelators; increased risk of encephalopathy)

Hemolytic Anemias

Table 21.4: RBC Membrane Defects

	Hereditary Spherocytosis	Hereditary Elliptocytosis
Etiology	Autosomal dominant or recessive (most common in Northern Europeans); due to ankyrin defects (RBC cytoskeleton protein) → abnormally shaped RBC (**hyperchromic microspherocytes**) → trapped in and **removed by the spleen → hemolytic anemia**	Dysfunction of α- and β-spectrin; **autosomal dominant** results in **common mild disease; autosomal recessive: more severe** types; life-threatening hemolytic anemia in homozygotes; same pathophysiology as spherocytosis; highest frequency in malarial zones
Clinical features	-Any age, including **hemolytic disease in newborns**; severity and progression depend on rate of destruction vs. production of RBCs -**Mild to moderate anemia with slight increase in spleen size and mild to moderate jaundice** (small number require many transfusions and develop Fe-overload and poor growth) -**Episodes of acute exacerbated anemia** with **aplastic crisis** (parvovirus B19) or **folate deficiency** (with chronic hemolysis → megaloblastic changes) or with **hypersplenism**	**Mild asymptomatic** (or silent carrier state) to **severe transfusion-dependent disease** with **acute exacerbations** and life-threatening hemolysis, depending on the type of disease (and inheritance); may present as severe **hemolytic disease in the newborn**, requiring exchange transfusion

(continued)

	Hereditary Spherocytosis	Hereditary Elliptocytosis
Laboratory findings	-Anemia with **increased reticulocytes** -**Normal MCV, increased MCHC, increased RDW** -Smear: **spherocytes** present -Bone marrow: **erythroid hyperplasia** -**Osmotic fragility test:** tolerate less swelling when RBCs are suspended in a hypotonic salt solution	-Depending on type and severity, may have no or little anemia with no reticulocytosis to **severe anemia with reticulocytosis** -More severe disease: **low MCV, increased RDW, elliptocytes, poikilocytes, cell fragments, and osmotic fragility** -Specific protein abnormalities and genetic mutations may be determined.
Management	**Splenectomy** for moderate to severe disease (cures anemia and jaundice; only partially eliminates hemolysis; delay until age 3–5 years); **transfusions** (exchange transfusion in neonate) with decreased Hgb associated with hemodynamic compromise; **folate supplementation** with chronic hemolysis	Same as spherocytosis

Abbreviations: hemoglobin, Hgb; mean corpuscular Hgb concentration, MCHC; mean corpuscular volume , MCV; red blood cell, RBC; red-cell distribution width, RDW

Table 21.5: RBC Enzyme Defects

	Pyruvate Kinase Deficiency	G6PD Deficiency
Etiology	Products of glycolysis are depleted (lactate and **ATP**) → loss of K and water across the RBC membrane and cell contraction → **premature splenic destruction; autosomal recessive** with many mutations; increased in Northern European and Chinese descendants	Most common abnormality of the hexose monophosphate shunt; low production of **NADPH** → decreased glutathione peroxidase and reductase → **glutathione becomes oxidized** → **methemoglobin and sulfhemoglobin** → **denatured hemoglobin precipitates as intracellular inclusions** (Heinz bodies) → **removed in spleen** with intravascular hemolysis; higher in **Mediterranean, African American, Chinese,** and then Northern European heritage
Clinical features	Severity varies widely: **mild disease** presenting later in life (or not at all) to **severe hemolysis in the newborn**; anemia, jaundice, splenomegaly	-Minimal or no hemolysis except with **oxidative stress** (primaquine, pamaquine, sulfonamides and sulfones, nitrofurans, ASA, probenecid, dimercaprol, APAP, naphthalene, and fava beans) or **infection.** -**Acute-onset** pallor, jaundice, hepatosplenomegaly, abdominal pain, dark urine, tachycardia, and possibly shock -May present with **neonatal jaundice** (especially with Greek and Chinese ancestry) -Less common: **chronic nonspherocytic hemolytic anemia** (Northern European, Mediterranean, Asian males with neonatal jaundice)

(continued on next page)

Table 21.5: RBC Enzyme Defects *(cont.)*

	Pyruvate Kinase Deficiency	G6PD Deficiency
Laboratory findings	-Normochromic, normocytic, Coombs-negative anemia with **reticulocytosis and increased RDW** -Increased bilirubin -Bone marrow: **erythroid hyperplasia and active marrow** -Enzyme assay: decreased PK (not always), so **definitive diagnosis is with PCR**	-Increased bilirubin, LDH, ↓ Hgb, decreased haptoglobin -**Normal MVC, increased RDW, reticulocytosis** -Smear: fragmented RBCs (bite cells), polychromasia, microspherocytes, and normoblasts; **supravital stain: Heinz bodies** -Various screening tests available (dye, fluorescent); if positive, perform **quantitative enzyme assay**
Management	**Exchange transfusion** and phototherapy in newborn; transfusions for symptomatic anemia; **splenectomy** for moderate to severe disease	**Supportive treatment** for acute hemolysis; **transfusion** as needed; **splenectomy** in moderate to severe cases, mostly with chronic hemolysis

Abbreviations: *N-acetyl-p-aminophenol, APAP; acetylsalicylic acid, ASA; adenosine triphosphate, ATP; glucose-6 phosphate dehydrogenase, G6PD; hemoglobin, Hgb; lactate dehydrogenase, LDH; mean corpuscular volume, MVC; nicotinamide adenine dinucleotide phosphate–dependent oxidase, NADPH; polymerase chain reaction, PCR; protein kinase, PK; red blood cell, RBC; red blood-cell distribution width, RDW*

Autoimmune hemolytic anemia

Background/etiology

- Red blood cell (RBC) destruction due to **antibodies against RBC antigens; IgG against Rh complex** is most common
- **IgM (cold) antibodies** less common; usually occurs with certain **infections** (Epstein-Barr virus [EBV], HIV, cytomegalovirus [CMV], mycoplasma pneumonia) and less commonly with **inflammatory conditions** (systemic lupus erythematosus [SLE], inflammatory bowel disease), **immune deficiency**, and **malignancy**.

Physiology—IgG is a **warm antibody** (maximally active at 37.5°C [99.5°F]) → antibody-complement complex ingested by macrophages in the spleen and liver → **RBC is lysed**; IgM (cold antibody) → complement activation → generation of C3b and moderate **intravascular hemolysis**.

Clinical presentation—**Acute** pallor, jaundice, dark urine, fatigue, fever, tachypnea, tachycardia, hepatosplenomegaly plus signs and symptoms of the underlying disease

Laboratory findings—**Direct Coombs-positive** acute anemia with **reticulocytosis**, normal to increased white blood cells (WBCs) with normal platelets, microspherocytes, polychromatophilia, RBC clumping with cold antibodies (**high cold agglutinin titers**)

Treatment—No treatment for mild, self-limited disease; **transfuse with units negative for any alloantibodies identified** with severe symptomatic anemia; **corticosteroids** for moderately severe IgG disease (usually no response if IgM); **intravenous Ig (IVIG)** if poor response to at least 2 weeks of steroids; **splenectomy** for lack of response or continued need for large doses of steroids; immunosuppressives with chronic disease.

Hemoglobinopathies
Sickle-cell disease
Background/etiology
- Any genotype that contains **at least one sickle gene** (**Hgb S** making up at least 50% of the Hgb)
- Hgb S results from a substitution of valine for glutamic acid at the number 6 position of the β-globin chain
- In homozygous disease (**autosomal recessive**), only Hgb S is produced
- **Compound heterozygotes**: Hgb S/Hgb C, Hgb S/Hgb D, Hgb S/β-thalassemia, and Hgb S/Hgb E (and others)
- **Sickle-cell trait** (Hgb AS), the amount of Hgb S is <50%, with rare complications and normal life span; high prevalence in Africa and India because of **heterozygous survival advantage in areas of endemic malaria**
- Hgb S in the United States is prevalent in **African Americans**.

Physiology—Hgb S carries oxygen normally but **once oxygen is unloaded, RBC becomes distorted** and after multiple deoxygenation cycles, permanent damage occurs → **Hgb S polymerization and RBC sickling with low oxygen conditions**; the **abnormal RBC interacts with the vascular endothelium** → **inflammatory activation** → **vaso-occlusion**. Irreversible RBC damage → **hemolysis**; the bone marrow increases production, but cannot compensate → **moderate to severe anemia**.

Diagnosis—**Newborn diagnosis** (liquid chromatography): test all abnormal screens again at first visit and 6 months, and **Hgb electrophoresis of both parents** (if not known); will have Hgb screen with **Hgb F in the greatest quantity**, then Hgb S; compound heterozygotes with other patterns: Hgb S/β^0 (clinical course like Hgb S), Hgb SC (same symptoms but with less frequency); others are much less common. Smear: **anemia, reticulocytes, nucleated RBCs, target cells, sickle cells**.

Clinical findings and management issues
- Well-compensated (increased heart rate and stroke volume) **baseline anemia** with decreased stamina; **acute hemolytic episodes**:
  - **Aplastic crisis (with any hemolytic anemia)**: infection with **parvovirus B19** → acute, significant (life-threatening) decreases in Hgb with large reticulocytosis (instead of mild transient decrease in healthy people); **transfusions** are necessary until marrow activity restored.

- **Acute splenic sequestration:** first 5 years with persistence of any splenic tissue: acute onset of life-threatening anemia with significant reticulocytosis and **abdominal distension due to blood pooling in the spleen** (unknown reason); need **emergent transfusions**; prophylactic splenectomy for recurrence (common).

- Early **functional and then anatomic asplenia** and other immune dysfunction → risk of bacterial infections, especially with **encapsulated organisms** (*Staph. pneumoniae, Haemophilus influenzae* type B, *Salmonella* spp.) including sepsis, pneumonia, meningitis, and **osteomyelitis (*Staph. aureus* and *Salmonella*)**; not possible to differentiate between bacterial and viral infections with febrile illness, so **admit to the hospital**, obtain blood and urine **cultures, chest x-ray**, and possible lumbar puncture and start **empiric parenteral broad-spectrum antibiotics** (third-generation cephalosporin) until cultures are negative.

- **Vaso-occlusive episodes with ischemia: pain** is the most common feature and involves bone with the most marrow activity; earliest involvement with **metacarpals and metatarsals, at 6 months through 2 years—acute dactylitis (hand-foot syndrome; symmetric swelling of hands and/or feet)**; with increasing age, involves the **long bones** (maintain marrow activity) then the **vertebrae** during adolescence. Precipitators of the ischemic event = **hypoxemia, dehydration, acidosis, hypothermia, infection, and stress**. Ischemic vaso-occlusive attacks occur more in central body areas (as opposed to the extremities) with increasing age and may occur in the absence of any obvious precipitating factors.

  - **Must control pain adequately** with acetaminophen, **nonsteroidal anti-inflammatory drugs (NSAIDs)**, and increased oral hydration; then **codeine or oral morphine derivatives** with moderate pain, and **admission to the hospital with IV opiates** for peak pain (continuous infusion with fentanyl or nalbuphine; also patient-controlled analgesia in older children). IV hydration and blood transfusions will not alleviate pain and should be used only with clinical dehydration and a hemodynamic decrease of Hgb.

  - **Hydroxyurea** (raises Hgb F and Hgb level) is the **only effective drug to reduce the frequency of painful episodes** if given daily; short-term adverse effect is **myelosuppression**, and long-term effects not yet known; currently used selectively in children **>5 years who have had multiple painful episodes**.

- **Acute chest syndrome: new density on chest x-ray with pain, fever, and respiratory distress**; most underlying causes not found, but felt to be **infection** (most common *S. pneumoniae*, *M. pneumoniae*, and *C. pneumoniae*); preceding painful episode with use of an oral morphine derivative is the most common associated increased risk. Other etiologies: pulmonary infarction, atelectasis, fat embolism (bone infarction).

  - Obtain **chest x-ray** if fever or other findings.
  - Administer **oxygen.**
  - **IV hydration**
  - Provide **analgesia** that does not suppress respiration.
  - **Empiric antibiotics with IV third-generation cephalosporin and oral macrolide** to cover most likely organism.

- **Blood transfusion** for hypoxemia, increasing respiratory distress, or a previous admission for acute chest syndrome; if lack of improvement within hours, perform **exchange transfusion**.

- **Priapism:** involuntary erection lasting >30 minutes; episodes **longer than 3–4 hours** can result in fibrosis and impotence; initial treatment with **oral analgesia and sitz baths**; if >4 hours, blood is **aspirated from the corpora cavernosa followed by injection of dilute epinephrine**; effectiveness of transfusion or exchange transfusion is not supported.
- **Neurological complications: focal neurological defect** (most common presentation is **hemiparesis**): any deficit >24 hours and/or an MRI lesion consistent with infarct and correlating with clinical deficit. Also headache, seizures, and cerebral venous thrombosis.
  - **Oxygen and blood transfusion within an hour to raise the Hgb to >11.0 g/dL; then exchange transfusion to decrease the Hgb S to 30%**
  - **Immediate CT** scan to exclude hemorrhage, followed by an MRI
  - For primary prevention: **transcranial Doppler ultrasound** (blood velocity) yearly beginning at age 2–3 years; **prophylactic blood transfusion to maintain Hgb S at <30%** if blood velocity exceeds 200 cm/sec.
- Other complications: pulmonary hypertension, cholelithiasis, cholecystitis, avascular necrosis of the femoral or humeral head, renal disease (nephrotic syndrome, infarct, papillary necrosis, renal medullary carcinoma), retinopathy, psychosocial problems, cognitive and developmental delays, poor growth and delayed puberty

Other general management issues—**Oral daily penicillin prophylaxis beginning at age 2–4 months;** in addition to routine immunization with the PCV-13, additional doses of **PPV-23** should be administered after age 2 years; **allogenic bone marrow transplantation**: must use HLA-compatible full sibling and patient younger than 16 years of age with Hgb SS or Hgb S/beta^0-thalassemia with a history of severe disease.

Other hemoglobinopathies
- **Hgb E:** high incidence in Southeast Asians; especially in California: **Hgb E/β-thalassemia** (second most common worldwide globin mutation)
- **Hgb C:** same as Hgb S except that lysine is substituted for glutamic acid (mostly in African Americans); Hgb AC is asymptomatic; homozygous Hgb C results in mild anemia, splenomegaly, and cholelithiasis; no sickling
- **Hereditary methemoglobinemia:** absence of nicotinamide adenine dinucleotide (NADH) cytochrome b5 reductase → increased methemoglobin in RBCs (formed from constant loss of electrons to oxygen from Fe^{2+} → Fe^{3+}, which combines with water to produce methemoglobin); **toxic (acquired) methemoglobinemia** is more common (aniline dyes, lidocaine, nitrates, sulfonamides, infection, metoclopramide, chloroquine, fume inhalation, pesticides); **15% methemoglobin is associated with visible cyanosis and 70% is lethal** (lower with anemia); **oxygen saturation is low but PaO$_2$ is normal**; the blood may appear **brown** in color; infants are more vulnerable

to Hgb oxidation. Daily oral ascorbate for hereditary disease reduces the methemoglobin; **IV methylene blue for the toxic form** and then oral maintenance.

Alpha-thalassemia

Background/etiology—Inherited disorders of Hgb synthesis; **abnormal formation of globin chains → imbalance with the other normally produced chain →** accumulates in the cell as an unstable product → **cell destruction**. In alpha-thalassemia, α-globin production is reduced to absent with **relative excess of β- and γ-globin chains**. In the fetus, **γ^4 tetramers are formed (Hgb Barts)**; and after birth, **β^4 tetramers are formed (Hgb H)**. There are **four α-globin genes** (gene duplication), and the majority of clinical presentations are the result of complete **deletional mutations** (few nondeletional mutations; contrast to beta-thalassemia).

Clinical findings, diagnosis, and management

- **Silent trait** = deletion of **one gene**; common in **African Americans**; no clinical expression; usually identified if a sibling has two- or three-gene deletion; not identified by Hgb electrophoresis, as there are no abnormal hemoglobins and no relative increase in any Hgb—need molecular analysis.
- **Alpha-thalassemia trait** = deletion of **two genes** (cis or trans, depending on the chromosome from which the genes are deleted); African Americans and Mediterranean descent; **mild hypochromic, microcytic anemia (normal RDW)** without clinical problems (often diagnosed as **iron deficiency**); not identified by Hgb electrophoresis, as there are no abnormal hemoglobins and no relative increase in any Hgb—need molecular analysis for diagnosis.
- **Hgb H disease** = **three-gene** deletions; **Hgb Barts >25% in the newborn** period and easily diagnosed with **Hgb electrophoresis; at least one parent has alpha-thalassemia trait**; later β-tetramers develop (Hgb H; interact with RBC membrane to produce Heinz bodies), which can be identified electrophoretically; microcytosis and hypochromia with mild to moderate anemia (Hgb 7–11 g/dL), **target cells**, mild splenomegaly, and jaundice and cholelithiasis; typically do not require transfusions or splenectomy. Common in Southeast Asian populations.
- **Alpha-thalassemia major** = four-gene deletions; severe **fetal anemia resulting in hydrops fetalis**; newborn has **predominantly Hgb Barts** with small amounts of other fetal hemoglobins; anisocytosis and poikilocytosis; **immediate exchange transfusions** needed for the possibility of survival; transfusion-dependent and only cure is **bone marrow transplant**.

Beta-thalassemia

Background/etiology—There are only **two beta globin genes** (one on each chromosome; no duplication) and variation in β-chain synthesis occurs mostly due to **single base changes leading to partial reductions (β^+-thalassemia)**; if there is a gene deletion then there is **complete absence of β-globin production (β^0-thalassemia; thalassemia major = Cooley anemia)**; >200 mutations with 20 common alleles representing most around the world; **excess alpha chains form tetramers,** precipitate in the cells, and cause destruction; in the most severe forms maturation of RBCs is disrupted, → **ineffective erythropoiesis**; is **increased production in γ-chains (increased Hgb F) and in δ-chains (increased Hgb A_2)**.

Clinical findings, diagnosis, and management

- **Beta-thalassemia silent trait:** genotype is Hgb A/β^+-thalassemia (normal with micro-cytosis and very slightly elevated Hgb A_2)
- **Beta-thalassemia trait:** either β^+/Hgb A or β^0/Hgb A; normal clinically with **variable microcytosis, Hgb 10–12 g/dL, normal or decreased reticulocytes, and a normal RDW;** often confused with **iron deficiency**; identified by electrophoresis with **elevated Hgb F and Hgb A_2**
- **Thalassemia minor:** heterozygotes with a more severe phenotype than thalassemia trait; may have iron accumulation
- **Thalassemia intermedia:** any combination of mutations that produces a microcytic anemia with Hgb of about 7 g/dL; variable increases in Hgb F and A_2 and increase in RDW; splenomegaly, some medullary hyperplasia, and excessive iron stores; may require splenectomy, repeated transfusions, and chelation therapy
- **Thalassemia major (Cooley anemia): progressive hemolytic anemia, hypersplenism, and poor growth in the first months of life** and depending on the amount of Hgb F (20–100%; low amount of Hgb A_2); **transfusions** required from age 2 months to 2 years
  - **Severe anemia (Hgb 2–7 g/dL), few reticulocytes (ineffective erythropoiesis), increased RDW, nucleated RBCs, microcytosis and no normal-appearing RBCs;** increased serum bilirubin, serum ferritin and transferrin saturation (iron accumulation even without transfusion; **nutritional hemosiderosis**)
  - Without transfusions: cardiac decomposition and **medullary hyperplasia** $\rightarrow$ maxillary hyperplasia, frontal bossing, expanded medullary space of the skull with massive widening of the diploic spaces (producing the "hair-on-end" pattern); **pathological fractures, hepatosplenomegaly**
  - **Chronic transfusions** necessary for health and prevention of the complications $\rightarrow$ **transfusional hemosiderosis** (mostly avoided with iron chelators); best method of determining Fe stores liver biopsy to guide the use of chelators (but does not correlate to cardiac overload); **deferoxamine** (major side effects bone dysplasia, ototoxicity, and retinal changes) chelates Fe; deferiprone is a new iron chelator (FDA-approved) for use in children >2 years of age that is better at removing cardiac iron (major side effect is neutropenia)
  - Major problems: **cardiac toxicity** (hemosiderosis) and **endocrinopathies** (decreased growth, delayed sexual maturation, diabetes mellitus, hypothyroidism, hypoparathyroidism)
  - Best cure rate with bone marrow transplant from HLA-matched sib in children <15 years of age without hepatomegaly or excessive Fe stores

WHITE BLOOD CELL DISORDERS

Leukocytosis

Etiology

- **Neutrophilia**
  - **Increased production:** most common cause from **bacterial infection** (with increased bands); may have early neutrophilia with viral infections; also from inflammation (connective tissue disorders, inflammatory bowel disease, vasculitis syndromes), malignancy/myeloproliferative disease (transient myeloproliferative disorder with Down syndrome, Hodgkin disease, some solid tumors)
  - **Decreased vascular space egress: corticosteroids**, splenectomy, leukocyte adhesion deficiency
  - Decreased neutrophil margination: corticosteroids, epinephrine, physiological stress
  - **Increased marrow release:** infection, stress, hypoxia, endotoxins, corticosteroids

- **Lymphocytosis** (>4,000/µL): lymphocytes physiologically increased in infants; most common pathological increase is **viral infections** (may be accompanied by neutropenia) and very high counts with **pertussis.**
- **Eosinophilia** (>500/µL): allergy, asthma, drug hypersensitivity, parasites, some malignancies, chlamydia infections, and others less commonly
- **Monocytosis** (>950/µL): certain bacterial infections (tuberculosis [TB], Brucella); other infections: syphilis, mononucleosis, protozoal infections, rickettsial infections, malignancies (chronic myelogenous leukemia [CML], Hodgkin), autoimmune disease, vasculitis, sarcoidosis, recovery from neutropenia
- Basophilia (>150/µL): very rare; chronic myologenous leukemia

Management—Most important—treat the underlying condition; with **hyperleukocytosis** (WBC >100,000): hydration, urine alkalinization, and allopurinol for **uric acid excretion**; may rapidly decrease the WBC with leukapheresis or exchange transfusion

Neutropenia

Physiology/etiology

- The **absolute neutrophil count (ANC)** is the percentage of neutrophils plus bands in the total WBC count; neutropenia in whites is <1,500/µL and in blacks <1,000/µL; **severe neutropenia (with a significant risk of life-threatening infections) is <500/µL**
- Mechanisms are either a decreased production, maturational arrest, decreased release from the bone marrow, accelerated utilization, decreased survival, or marginal pool shifts in the peripheral circulation.
- **Congenital neutropenia**
  - **Kostmann syndrome** (presents in the first month of life with recurrent fever, disseminated infections, and ANC <200/µL); granulocyte colony-stimulating factor (G-CSF) receptor mutation → maturational arrest and depletion of mature neutrophils. Treated with G-CSF.

- Fanconi anemia: see Table 21.3
- Shwachman-Diamond syndrome: see Chapter 13
- **Infections:** various; usually in the first 24–48 hours to a week; due to margination, increased utilization (especially with bacterial infections) and decreased production
- **Drug/toxin-induced:** heavy metals, benzene, chemotherapy, radiation, sulfonamides, chloramphenicol, and others
- **Autoimmune: chronic benign neutropenia; antineutrophil antibodies** (IgG); most occur between 3 and 30 months of age and as a primary condition; less commonly with other pathologies (other autoimmune disease, malignancy); usually spontaneous recovery by age 5 years. **Mild, self-limited infections** (adequate bone marrow reserve): stomatitis, gingivitis, upper respiratory infection (URI), otitis media, abscesses; decreased or normal total WBC count with **neutrophils <1,000/µL (often remains <500/µL)** and normal RBCs and platelets; bone marrow shows myeloid **hyperplasia with a decrease in mature neutrophils**; treat infections and, if frequent, trimethoprim-sulfamethoxazole for prophylaxis; if no good response, use G-CSF or IVIG.
- **Cyclic:** autosomal dominant early hematopoietic precursor defect; **decreased neutrophils every 21 days**; treat with G-CSF

Diagnosis—CBC, differential and ANC at least two to three times per week for at least 8 weeks to make the diagnosis of cyclic neutropenia plus bone marrow aspiration; check immune status with quantitative immunoglobulins and CD4/CD8, pancreatic function, chromosomes (if pancytopenia for Fanconi), autoantibodies, skeletal survey (for congenital syndromes).

Management
- Follow CBC, differential and ANC frequently
- Cultures and chest x-ray with severely low ANC
- **Fever and neutropenia** associated with chemotherapy and Kostmann syndrome, → **broad-spectrum parenteral antibiotics** (vancomycin plus ceftazidime, cefepime, or carbapenem; or if vancomycin not indicated, then cefepime, ceftazidime, or carbapenem or an aminoglycoside plus an antipseudomonal beta-lactam)
- If persistent for more than 5 days, add amphotericin
- Cyclic neutropenia and Kostmann syndrome without fever is treated with **G-CSF.**

PLATELET DISORDERS

Thrombocytosis

Physiology/etiology

Normal platelet count is 150,000–400,000/μL; increased release of cytokines and thrombo-poietin, interleukin (IL)-6 and others → **reactive thrombocytosis** = exaggerated response to a primary problem (infection, inflammation); most commonly occurs with **pneumonia**; in **primary thrombocytosis** (rare in childhood), there is platelet production unregulated by normal feedback (most caused by CML, acute myelogenous leukemia [AML], or myelo-proliferative disorders). Causes of reactive thrombocytosis:

- Severe bacterial infections
- Inflammatory states: connective tissue disease, vasculitis (Kawasaki), inflammatory bowel disease
- With hemolytic anemias
- Post-splenectomy
- Tissue damage: trauma, surgery, burns
- Rebound: iron deficiency, recovery idiopathic thrombocytopenic purpura (ITP), bleed-ing, chemotherapy
- Malignancies: especially of soft tissue
- Renal disease: nephritis, nephrotic syndrome

Clinical presentation—**Reactive:** preceding illness, then increased platelets with no adverse effects; **primary:** usually with mucocutaneous bleeding, excessive bruising, headache, thromboses, splenomegaly, hepatomegaly

Laboratory findings—Reactive; increased erythrocyte sedimentation rate (ESR), C-reactive protein (CRP), and other acute-phase reactants; **increased normal-appearing megakaryocytes with no other abnormalities; increased serum thrombopoietin;** bone marrow: **hypercellular with increased megakaryocytes with or without fibrosis**

Management—Treat underlying condition; low dose aspirin for significant platelet increases associated with vasculitic syndromes (Kawasaki)

Thrombocytopenia

Physiology/etiology/diagnosis and management

Platelets <150,000/μL; **acquired etiologies** much more common than congenital; decreased production (bone marrow dysfunction; decreased, abnormal megakaryocytes), increased destruction (normal to increased megakaryocytes) or splenic sequestration.

- **Decreased production:** aplastic anemia, Fanconi anemia, Wiskott-Aldrich syndrome, thrombocytopenia-absent radius (TAR) syndrome, other hereditary thrombocytopenia syndromes; **acquired disorders:** infiltrative disorders (leukemia, lymphoma, histiocy-tosis, storage disease), drugs (chloramphenicol, chemotherapy, valproic acid, phenytoin, sulfonamides), radiation, infection (neonatal TORCH infections, HIV, overwhelming sepsis), neonatal hypoxia, placental insufficiency, nutritional deficiency (iron, megalo-blastic anemias)

- **Increased destruction or sequestration**
  - **Neonatal alloimmune thrombocytopenia:** development of maternal antibodies against **antigens (most common is HPA-1a) shared with the father on fetal platelets** (same pathophysiology as Rh disease); first pregnancy affected; neonate develops petecchiae and purpura (and at times significant bleeding; intracranial hemorrhage) in the first days of life with **normal platelets in the mother**; diagnosis with the presence of **maternal alloantibodies against the father's platelets**; treatment: **IVIG** starting in the second trimester to the mother (if the diagnosis is known from a previous pregnancy); otherwise, treat the infant with **washed maternal platelets** (most share the maternal alloantigens); usually complete resolution within 2–4 months.
  - **Nonimmune platelet destruction:** disseminated intravascular coagulation (DIC), hemolytic-uremic syndrome, thrombotic thrombocytopenic purpura (usually in adults, less so in adolescents); thrombotic **microangiopathy** with RBC destruction and consumptive thrombocytopenia; also with **Kasabach-Merritt syndrome:** platelet-trapping and activation of coagulation within a hemangioma
  - **Sequestration:** splenomegaly (most with some degree of anemia and leukopenia)
  - **Immune thrombocytopenia purpura (ITP): postviral** (1–4 weeks) **acquired immune-mediated platelet destruction** (antibody-coated platelets are recognized by the Fc-receptor of splenic macrophages and are removed); young child with **sudden onset of petechiae and purpura** and possible mucocutaneous bleeding with very low platelets; the physical exam is otherwise normal (**no hepatosplenomegaly or lymphadenopathy**); most resolve within 6 months and 20% go on to have **chronic ITP.** Very few have **intracranial hemorrhage.**
    - Laboratory findings: platelet counts are usually **<20,000/μL** and **platelet size is normal or increased**; normal Hgb (unless significant bleeding), indices, and WBC count and differential; bone marrow is normal except for **increased megakaryocytes** (with immature forms); bone marrow aspiration performed only if another cell line is affected or evidence of lymphoproliferative disease on physical exam; adolescents should be tested for SLE, and HIV should be considered in the sexually active adolescent.
    - Treatment: **mild to moderate illness** (platelets >20,000 with no bleeding) should just be followed; families provided with education and counseling; **IVIG** for more severely affected or ongoing bleeding for 1–2 days: will increase the platelet count to >20,000 in most; if unresponsive, **corticosteroids** used until platelet counts are >20,000 and then rapidly tapered. **Platelet transfusion contraindicated** (antibodies bind to autologous platelets) unless life-threatening bleeding.
    - **Chronic ITP:** continued thrombocytopenia for >6 months; evaluate for autoimmune disease, HIV, and nonimmune causes of chronic thrombocytopenia; **splenectomy** is usually successful in inducing complete remission.
- Qualitative platelet disorders
  - **Acquired:** liver disease, uremia, diseases with fibrin degradation products; **prolonged bleeding time** plus other coagulation abnormalities; treat the underlying

condition and/or infuse platelets, cryoprecipitate, or treat with **desmopressin** (helps to correct bleeding time). Also seen with drugs: acetylsalicylic acid (ASA) and NSAIDs, valproic acid, and high-dose penicillin.

- **Congenital** (life-threatening bleeding treated with platelet transfusion; chronic treatment with desmopressin)
  - **Glanzmann thrombasthenia** (autosomal recessive: partial or complete absence of glycoprotein IIb/IIIa from platelet membrane; platelets do not aggregate with adenosine diphosphate (ADP), collagen, epinephrine, and thrombin but do aggregate with ristocetin and von Willebrand factor (vWF). May have life-threatening hemorrhages.
  - **Bernard-Soulier syndrome:** absence of glycoprotein Ib (inability to bind ristocetin or vWF), V, and IX from the platelet surface; platelets are large and have an unusual shape; they do not aggregate with ristocetin but do with ADP, collagen, epinephrine, and thrombin. Often have severe hemorrhage.

COAGULATION DISORDERS
Hemophilia A and B

Etiology—Of all of the congenital coagulation disorders, 85% are **factor VIII deficiency (hemophilia A)**, 14% are **factor IX deficiency (hemophilia B)**, and all others are 1%. All racial groups affected, and most are **X-linked** (females can be affected if they are homozygous or with extreme lyonization).

Physiology—Factors IXa and VIIIa (**intrinsic pathway**) are required to accelerate the activation of factor X, with VIIa/tissue factor in the presence of Ca^{2+} and phospholipids, which is necessary for effective thrombin formation → platelet aggregation, clot retraction, and factor VIII activation; the abnormality in hemophilia is **slow clot formation** (platelet plug forms but not reinforced by fibrin clot); vWF binds to platelet GP Ib and brings factor VIII to the area of injury. Severity of disease is dependent upon a **wide variety of genetic defects** with coagulation factor levels at ≥5% (**mild**), 1–5% (**moderate**), or ≤1% (**severe**). Carriers are not symptomatic with factor VIII deficiency, but there may be increased bleeding with factor IX deficiency with significant trauma.

Clinical findings—The more severe the abnormality, the earlier and more severe is the bleeding. Bleeding may occur after birth (with **circumcision**) and a small number develop an **intracranial hemorrhage**; the major types of bleeding are **hemarthrosis and deep muscle hematomas**. Mild cases may not be diagnosed until there is a major trauma. Repeated bleeding leads to **joint destruction**, muscle weakness, compression damage, and atrophy. May be gastrointestinal (GI) and genitourinary (GU) bleeding, bleeding with tooth eruption or dental extraction, or intracranial hemorrhage resulting in death.

Laboratory studies—**Normal bleeding time, increased activated partial thromboplastin time (aPTT), normal prothrombin time (PT), and normal thrombin time; each factor may then be specifically assayed; inhibitors** are tested for by incubating the patient's plasma with normal plasma and determining whether there is neutralization of the factor tested for. Carriers have a factor VIII activity/vWF antigen ratio of less than 1 (normal is 1:1). Fetal testing can also be performed if the mutation is known (restriction fragment length polymorphism; RFLP) or with gene sequencing if unknown.

Management—**Recombinant factor VIII** products for mild to moderate bleeding; factor levels must be raised to 35–50%; and with major bleeding, to near 100%; there are specific protocols for all types of bleeding specifying dose per kg, frequency, and length of time that it should be administered. **Desmopressin acetate** (intranasal) is used for mild disease (releases the person's endogenous factor VIII). It is **not effective for factor IX deficiency**. With severe hemophilia, **prophylaxis** with the first hemorrhage (factor VIII via a central venous catheter; administered every 2–3 days to keep a minimum factor level) is now the standard of care; it has been very effective in preventing chronic joint disease. If a bleeding episode has not responded to replacement therapy, **inhibitors** have probably developed (less common with IX); these patients need to go through a **desensitization** process and if this fails, bleeding is treated with high-dose factor VIIa or activated prothrombin complex concentrates.

von Willebrand Disease (VWD)

Etiology—**Most common hereditary bleeding disorder;** different variants depending on mutations coding for different functional domains of the **vWF** (chromosome 12). Autosomal inheritance, but more girls are affected.

Physiology—**vWF** adheres to the subendothelium after vascular damage, and platelets then adhere through the glycoprotein Ib receptor. Platelets become activated, additional platelets are recruited, and **factor VIII** is brought in (**carried with vWF**). Phosphatidylserine is exposed, which aids in regulation of factor V- and VIII-dependent steps in the cascade.

Clinical findings—Hallmark is **mucocutaneous bleeding** (bruising, epistaxis, menorrhagia). There are seven types of VWD: **type 1 disease** is the most common (also types 2A, 2B, 2N, 2M, and type III; there is also a platelet-type called pseudo-VWD). They differ in general regarding whether the **protein is reduced but not absent** (type 1), **qualitatively normal** (type 2), or **absent** (type 3; similar to hemophilia).

Laboratory findings—**Type 1 VWD** often has normal bleeding time (normal to increased to significantly increased) and aPTT (abnormal in severe cases); no single assay can rule out the disease, so testing should include quantitative assay for vWF antigen (decreased, normal, or absent), vWF ristocetin cofactor activity (normal, decreased, or absent), factor VIII activity (normal or decreased), determination of vWF multimers (normal, normal but decreased, abnormal, or absent), ristocetin-induced platelet aggregation (normal, reduced, or absent), and platelet count (normal or decreased in type 2B). Diagnosis based on finding at least one low level of these.

Management—Elevating the level of vWF permits normal recovery and survival of factor VIII (because its gene is normal). In type 1 and some of type 2, **desamino-8-D-arginine vasopressin (DDAVP)** releases vWF from endothelial cells. Cells may not respond, however, in most of type 2 and all of type 3 disease, or if there is accelerated clearance of released vWF. If this is the case, **replacement therapy is with plasma-derived vWF concentrates** (which also contain factor VIII); minor bleeding may be managed with a combination of DDAVP and an antifibrinolytic (ε-aminocaproic acid).

Thrombotic Disorders

Etiology—Due to **prothrombotic states or hereditary thrombotic disorders**; in children, most common in sick neonates and then again in the second decade of life (but not in the first decade)

Most common acquired causes—Immobilization (trauma, surgery, burns), dehydration, polycythemia, **indwelling catheters**, pregnancy, inflammation (infection, inflammatory bowel disease, vasculitis), medications (oral **contraceptives**, L-asparaginase), nephrotic syndrome, liver disease, **malignancy, antiphospholipid syndrome**, vascular grafts, paroxysmal nocturnal hemoglobinuria, severe thrombocytosis, **DIC, hemolytic uremic syndrome (HUS), thrombotic thrombocytopenic purpura (TTP)**

Congenital disorders

- Deficiencies of the anticoagulant proteins: **antithrombin III, protein C, and protein S**; autosomal dominant; **venous thromboembolism** (deep venous thrombosis, renal vein thrombosis, cerebral venous thrombosis) early in life from antithrombin deficiency and protein C deficiency; **venous and arterial thromboembolism** (cerebrovascular and renal artery thrombosis) from protein S deficiency. Homozygous protein C deficiency → **neonatal purpura fulminans** (necrotic purpura of the skin and major vessel thromboses). Diagnosis through specific clotting assays of each individual protein. **Fresh frozen plasma** is the only source of protein C. After the neonatal period, **warfarin** is used. Thromboses treated with **anticoagulant therapy**.

- Resistance to activated protein C: mutation of **factor V Leiden** (not inactivated by activated protein C → unregulated active factor V); increased frequency of **venous thrombosis, especially in young women during pregnancy or on oral contraceptives**; increased risk of **recurrent abortions; most common mutation resulting in thrombosis in young adults**. Diagnosis is through molecular testing for factor V Leiden.

ONCOLOGY

Leukemias

Acute lymphoblastic leukemia (ALL)

Background

- Almost 80% of all childhood leukemia, with peak at 2–6 years and male predominance. Most from B-cell progenitors (most common: early pre-B cell), then T cells, then B cells
- More common in children with chromosomal abnormalities (**Down syndrome**, Turner), **ataxia-telangiectasia, Fanconi** syndrome, Diamond-Blackfan syndrome, Shwachman-Diamond syndrome, and neurofibromatosis type I
- Genetic and environmental factors (**radiation**, geographic clusters, and possible viruses) may be involved. Most have **chromosomal abnormalities**, which relate to prognosis; **t(9;22) = poor prognosis**

Clinical presentation

- Initial **nonspecific constitutional symptoms with intermittent low-grade fever**; often with **bone and/or joint pain**, which may be severe
- Then evidence of bone marrow failure: clinical evidence of **anemia and thrombocytopenia**
- Exam: pallor, petechiae, purpura, mucocutaneous bleeding, **lymphadenopathy, splenomegaly**, hepatomegaly (less often), **bone tenderness, and joint swelling**; if there is central nervous system (CNS) involvement (uncommon initially), it usually manifests as increased intracranial pressure (ICP); also may present with testicular or ovarian involvement.

Diagnosis

- CBC initially—**anemia and thrombocytopenia**; WBC counts most commonly <10,000 and no blasts are usually seen (may be seen as atypical lymphocytes).
- Next, **bone marrow aspiration is required and is diagnostic**; large homogeneous population of **lymphoblasts**
- **Lumbar puncture** for cerebrospinal fluid (CSF) examination (for staging); if blasts are present, there is CNS leukemia (worse).

Treatment

- **Remission induction:** eradicate leukemic cells from bone marrow with chemotherapy and corticosteroids; usually also **intrathecal chemotherapy**; almost all in **remission in 4–5 weeks**; patients with very poor prognosis may have a bone marrow transplant after first remission.
- **CNS therapy:** prevent later CNS relapse; **intrathecal and intensive systemic chemotherapy; patients having or who have had radiation are** in the highest risk group.
- 14 to 28 weeks of multiagent chemotherapy after remission
- **Maintenance phase:** daily mercaptopurine and weekly methotrexate for 2–3 years

Major complications

- **Tumor lysis syndrome** with start of treatment; major problem is with severe hyperuricemia which may precipitate renal failure; also hyperkalemia and hyperphosphatemia
- **Myelosuppression:** may need transfusions, erythropoietin, G-CSF; cultures and broad-spectrum antibiotics for fever and neutropenia (see previous discussion); prophylactic treatment of *Pneumocystis carinii*
- **Relapse**
  - **Bone marrow relapse** is a poor prognostic finding (up to 20%); intensive chemotherapy with agents not previously used, then best outcome with **allogenic stem cell transplant** (still, only few patients with long-term survival)
  - **CNS relapse: increased ICP or isolated cranial nerve palsies**; intrathecal chemotherapy plus irradiation plus systemic chemotherapy; good prognosis if just confined to CNS
  - **Testicular:** painless swelling of one or both testicles; systemic chemotherapy and local irradiation; good prognosis

Prognosis

Overall 5-year survival is 80%; average risk if presentation is at 1–10 years of age with <50,000 WBC and good initial response to treatment; **high risk of relapse and poor prognosis:** presentation at <1 year or >10 years of age plus WBC >50,000 (worse with >100,000), specific chromosomal anomalies, and poor initial response to treatment

Acute myelogenous leukemia (AML)

- Bone marrow cells are of the **myeloid/monocyte/megakaryocytes lines**
- No predisposing factors or environmental/genetic factors in most; some with identified chromosomal anomalies. Increased risk with exposure to **radiation, previous chemotherapy**, organic solvents, paroxysmal nocturnal hemoglobinuria, and other conditions (similar to those for acute lymphoblastic leukemia [ALL] risk)
- Marrow failure findings like in ALL plus **"blueberry muffin" spots** (extramedullary hematopoiesis), **gingival infiltration**, DIC, more common CNS symptoms, and discrete masses
- Bone marrow aspiration: **hypercellular with predominance of myeloid, monocyte precursors, and megakaryocytes**; special staining identifies as myeloperoxidase (myeloid)-containing cells.
- Multiagent chemotherapy leads to 80% remission rate (treatment is targeted to specific markers); long-term cure (up to 70%) with **stem cell transplant after remission.**

Chronic myelogenous leukemia (CML)

- Almost all with the **Philadelphia chromosome** [t(9;22)(q34;11)]
- **Initial chronic phase for 3–4 years** with nonspecific constitutional findings, plus increased WBC (mostly mature forms) but with an increased amount of immature forms, plus mild anemia and thrombocytosis; significant **splenic enlargement**, then

accelerated blast crisis with a large increase in WBCs → hyperviscosity (neurological signs and symptoms) and severe hyperuricemia
- Diagnosis—bone marrow and of the Philadelphia chromosome
- **Hydroxyurea** during the chronic phase gradually decreases the WBC count, then **bone marrow transplant or allogenic stem cell transplant** leads to an 80% cure.

Lymphomas

Hodgkin disease

Background
- Highest in pediatrics at **15–19 years of age** (but peaks at late 20s and then in the 50s); more in males. Familial clusters; associated with specific HLA types; EBV antigens demonstrated in some cases. Increased risk with **congenital and acquired immunodeficiencies**.
- Hallmark is the **Reed-Sternberg cell** (from germinal center B cells); disease arises in **lymphoid tissue** to adjacent lymph node areas with hematogenous spread to **liver, spleen, bone, bone marrow, and CNS**
- Standard (older) classification (newer classification more complex with additional types)
  - **Nodular sclerosing:** most common
  - **Mixed cellularity:** next most common; usually in younger patients with advanced disease and extranodal extension
  - **Lymphocytic predominance:** more common in younger males with localized disease
  - **Lymphocyte-depleted:** rare; seen more with HIV infection

Clinical presentation
- Most common: **nontender, firm, cervical or supraclavicular lymph nodes, often with some degree of mediastinal involvement (mass)**; rare hepatosplenomegaly; rare presentation below the diaphragm
- Other findings depend on location and extent of masses (compression or obstruction) or organ dysfunction (liver, bone marrow infiltration, pleural or pericardial effusion).
- May have **systemic symptoms (called B symptoms**; important for staging and prognosis): fever >39°C (102.2°F), weight loss 10% over 3 months, and drenching night sweats

Diagnosis
- Perform **chest x-ray for any mediastinal mass**
- **Nodal biopsy (excisional biopsy)**
- Tests for **staging** (I: single node or extralymphatic site, to IV: disseminated): CBC (marrow involvement); serum chemistries; liver function tests; **CT chest, abdomen and pelvis; gallium scan; PET scan**; then, if advanced or B symptoms, **bone marrow aspirate and biopsy**; bone scan if bone pain or increased alkaline phosphatase

Treatment—**Chemotherapy with or without low-dose radiation**; various regimens, depending on stage, patient age, B symptoms, presence of hilar nodes or bulky masses; **cycles of chemotherapy → cumulative toxicity** (second malignancy, sterility, pulmonary and cardiac dysfunction). Most relapses are in the first 3 years.

Prognosis—Poor prognosis with **bulky masses, stage III, or stage IV at diagnosis and the presence of any B symptoms**; if no remission within 12 months, myeloablative chemotherapy and **autologous stem cell transplant** with or without radiation; if good prognostic features and stage I–II, 5-year survival of 90%

Non-Hodgkin lymphoma (NHL)

Background

- Most present with new onset disease; small number secondary to **inherited or acquired immune deficiencies**, infections (HIV, EBV), or genetic syndromes (ataxia-telangiectasia)
- Derived from germinal center abnormalities; most in children are **high-grade and aggressive** (rapid growth and invasive); most present with **advanced disease, including bone marrow, CNS, and GI involvement**
- Four histological types
  - **Burkitt:** most common; B cell; **sporadic type (abdominal presentation**; more common in the United States) or endemic type (head and neck tumors; most in equatorial Africa; related to presence of EBV genome); disseminates to bone marrow and CNS
  - **Lymphoblastic:** next most common; most are T cell, smaller number B cell; **intrathoracic or mediastinal mass**; disseminates to bone marrow and CNS
  - **Diffuse large B cell:** third most common; primary mass is **abdominal or mediastinal**; rare dissemination to bone marrow and CNS
  - **Anaplastic large cell:** uncommon; most T cell, then null, then smallest number are B cell; primary is a **skin lesion and systemic findings** (fever, weight loss); disseminates easily to other areas of the skin, liver, spleen, lung, mediastinum

Clinical presentation—Painless, rapid increase in one or more lymph nodes; if mediastinal mass: respiratory symptoms, superior vena cava syndrome; if abdominal mass: ascites or intestinal obstruction, pain, and/or bone pain with dissemination

Diagnosis

- **Biopsy any nodes** and test for cell of origin, karyotype, and specialized genetic studies.
- Chest x-ray; CT scan chest, neck, abdomen, head, and pelvis; PET scan and bone scan
- Lumbar puncture with CSF cytology
- Bone marrow aspiration and biopsy
- CBC, chemistries, uric acid, calcium phosphorus, renal function, liver enzymes

Treatment

- **Multiagent systemic and intrathecal chemotherapy; surgery only for diagnosis, not debulking; radiation only in special circumstances**
- Hydration and allopurinol or recombinant urate oxidase (tumor lysis)
- If progressive or relapse, re-induction and then allogenic or autologous stem cell transplant; most have a good prognosis

Histiocytic Syndromes

Clonal proliferation and accumulation of cells of the **monocyte-macrophage system**

Table 21.6: Histiocytic Syndromes

	Class I = Langerhans' Cell Histiocytosis	**Class II**	**Class III**
Diseases	• **Eosinophilic granuloma, Hand-Schüller-Christian disease, Letterer-Siwe disease**	• Hemophagocytic lymphohistiocytosis, familial hemophagocytic lymphohistiocytosis, and infection-associated hemophagocytic syndrome	• Malignancies of cells of the monocyte-macrophage lines: **acute monocytic leukemia and malignant histiocytosis**
Cytology	• Clonal proliferation of cells of **monocyte line** with electron-microscopic findings of a **Langerhans cell** (antigen-presenting cell of the skin) • Lesions contain various proportions of Langerhans cells plus lymphocytes, granulocytes, monocytes, and eosinophils.	• Nonmalignant proliferative accumulation of macrophages • Uncontrolled hemophagocytosis and activation of inflammatory cytokines → **disseminated lesions of many organs**: infiltration with activated phagocytic macrophages and lymphocytes	
Signs and symptoms	• Most present as **single or multiple asymptomatic or painful (with swelling) skeletal lesions (skull mostly); half have skin findings** (similar to seborrhea) with local adenopathy and hepatosplenomegaly. • Other signs and symptoms depend on site of lesions (e.g., vertebral: cord collapse; hearing loss, otitis, and draining ears with middle ear destruction; osteolytic lesions with pathological fractures of long bones). • Also **CNS, bone marrow, and liver involvement**	• Generalized disease process with rash, fever, weight loss, hepatosplenomegaly, adenopathy, CNS signs and symptoms, and respiratory distress • Familial form also with **severe immune deficiency**	
Diagnosis	• **Tissue biopsy of skin or bone lesions;** detailed study of any organ involved on physical exam; chest x-ray, skeletal survey, CBC, chemistries, liver function tests	• Characteristic pathology in **skin and bone marrow biopsy;** increased liver enzymes and lipids with decreased fibrinogen; pancytopenia	

(continued on next page)

Table 21.6: Histiocytic Syndromes *(cont.)* — Note: No Class III for the categories on this page

	Class I = Langerhans' Cell Histiocytosis	Class II
Treatment	• **Single-system disease usually benign with spontaneous remission:** arrest bone lesion with curettage or low-dose radiation • With multisystem disease: multiagent chemotherapy; good response rate if early diagnosis	• Treat any underlying infection with supportive care; **secondary disease with identified infection and treatment has good outcome.** • Chemotherapy and immunosuppression protocols • **Familial form is ultimately fatal:** allogenic stem cell transplant will cure up to 60%.

Abbreviations: central nervous system, CNS

Neuroblastoma and Wilms Tumor

Table 21.7: Comparison of Neuroblastoma and Wilms Tumor

	Neuroblastoma	Wilms Tumor
Characteristics	Embryonal cell carcinoma of **peripheral sympathetic nervous system:** from undifferentiated small round cells to mature ganglion cells (ganglioneuroblastoma); **most common neoplasm in neonates; mean age 2 years; most by age 5 years**	**Nephroblastoma:** mixed embryonal neoplasm of the kidney; most are sporadic, small number with positive family history (autosomal dominant; one gene isolated); age **2–5 years**; most common with no ectopia or anaplasia (**with anaplasia: higher rates of relapse and death**)
Risks	Related to genetic (prognostic importance; risk-based treatment) and environmental factors (parental exposures); some may be familial	**WAGR, Beckwith-Wiedemann syndrome,** Sotos syndrome, neurofibromatosis-1, and isolated **hemihypertrophy and GU anomalies**
Location	Can occur at **any site along the sympathetic chain; most are adrenal or retroperitoneal;** the rest from any other ganglia	One or both kidneys (**7% bilateral**)

(continued)

	Neuroblastoma	Wilms Tumor
Presentation	• Most present with **firm, nodular, painful flank or midline mass; may be calcified or hemorrhagic** • May also present with **metastatic disease** (long bones, **skull**, lymph nodes, liver, and **skin**): bone pain, **bluish subcutaneous nodules**, proptosis, **periorbital ecchymoses** • Primary chest or abdominal tumors may present as an autoimmune paraneoplastic syndrome with **ataxia and opsomyoclonus** • **Catecholamine secretion** (sweating, tachycardia, hypertension) or **vasoactive intestinal polypeptide** (with secretory diarrhea) • Disease in infants <1 year of age (stage 4s): **subcutaneous nodes, massive hepatomegaly, no bone involvement, and a small primary tumor**	• **Asymptomatic abdominal mass noticed by a parent or MD** at a well-child visit; smooth and firm, of various sizes • Fewer with pain, vomiting, and hematuria; if there is renal ischemia: hypertension • Tumor can invade **renal veins or inferior vena cava** and embolize to heart or lungs
Diagnosis	• Almost all have increased **urinary metabolites: HVA and VMA**, which helps to confirm diagnosis prior to biopsy. • **Biopsy of tumor** • Diagnosis can be made with **neuroblasts in bone marrow with VMA or HVA in urine without a primary tumor biopsy.** • Staging (I, confined to origin; to IV, disseminated): plain films, CT, MRI, bone scan, PET scan, bone marrow aspirate and biopsy	• Abdominal flatplate and ultrasound; CT or MRI for confirmation of origin, extent, involvement of contralateral kidney, and invasion of vessels; may need **MRA or angiography** • Chest x-ray, CBC, liver function tests, chemistries, renal function tests • Staging correlates with prognosis (I, confined to kidney and excised completely; to IV, metastases; to **V, bilateral renal**).

(continued on next page)

Table 21.7: Comparison of Neuroblastoma and Wilms Tumor *(cont.)*

	Neuroblastoma	**Wilms Tumor**
Treatment	• Low risk: surgery and observation (**4s usually regresses spontaneously;** if recurrence (uncommon): chemotherapy and radiation almost always result in a cure • Intermediate risk: **surgery and chemotherapy** with or without radiation • High risk: induction chemotherapy, then surgery and radiation, then high-dose chemotherapy and **autologous stem cell transplant**	• **Surgical removal**; inspection of contralateral kidney, liver, retroperitoneal nodes with biopsies • First, establish patency of IVC: **if not patent, need preoperative chemotherapy.** • Chemotherapy with or without radiation, depending on stage • Bilateral: chemotherapy first, then either **unilateral nephrectomy and partial of the other kidney or bilateral partial nephrectomies,** depending on tumor extent; then postoperative chemotherapy and radiation • Worse with anaplasia, large tumor, advanced stage; **stage I and II with 90% cure rate**

Abbreviations: genitourinary, GU; homovanillic acid, HVA; inferior vena cava, IVC; vanillylmandelic acid, VMA; Wilms tumor, aniridia, GU abnormalities, and mental retardation, WAGR

Rhabdomyosarcoma

Background—**Most common soft-tissue sarcoma** (small, round cell tumor like Hodgkin, Ewing, neuroblastoma) in children; most are of the **head and neck**, then GU, then extremities (older children), then retroperitoneal and other sites (very uncommon); increased incidence with neurofibromatosis-1 and familial cancer syndrome

Pathology—Four histological types:

- **Embryonal:** most common; intermediate prognosis
- **Botryoid:** next most common; projects into a body cavity like a bunch of grapes (vagina, uterus, bladder, nasopharynx, middle ear)
- **Alveolar:** third most common; chromosomal translocations; trunk and extremities; poorest prognosis
- **Pleomorphic:** adult type; rare in children

Clinical presentation—Presence of a **painful mass**; specific symptoms dependent on **displacement or obstruction of adjacent tissue and location** (e.g. nasal obstruction, cranial nerve palsies, proptosis); **sarcoma botryoides**: projecting out from vagina; early dissemination to lungs and bone

Diagnosis—Biopsy with microscopic examination, immunochemical staining, cytogenetic and molecular genetic analysis; CT or MRI of area involved; plain films, ultrasound, chest CT, bone scan, bone marrow aspirate and biopsy

Treatment and prognosis—Pre- and postoperative chemotherapy with or without radiation; up to 90% survive with **complete resection** and 70% long-term with incomplete resection; <50% survive with **dissemination**; younger children do better than older

Gonadal and Germ Cell Tumors

Background—Most in children are **germ cell tumors** (GCTs; most in females are sacrococcygeal tumors in infants; ovarian tumors uncommon; testicular tumors more common <4 years of age and after puberty). Increased risks: Klinefelter syndrome (mediastinal tumors); Down syndrome, cryptorchidism, infertility, testicular atrophy, and inguinal hernias (testicular tumors); gonadal dysgenesis (gonadoblastomas).

Types
Primordial GCTs—May have benign and malignant elements in different areas of the tumor; characteristic chromosomal anomalies; teratomas, germinomas (seminomas, ovarian dysgerminoma), endodermal sinus tumor, embryonal cell carcinoma, choriocarcinomas,x yolk-sac tumors, and gonadoblastomas

Non-GCTs
From coelomic epithelium; ovarian: epithelial and sex cord/stromal tumors (granulosa cell tumor); testicular: Leydig cell, Sertoli cell tumors

Clinical presentation
- **Teratomas** present with masses in many locations; most **are sacrococcygeal** and are diagnosed in utero, or at or shortly after birth
- **Germinomas** may present in the gonads or are intracranial or mediastinal (extragonadal tumors tend to be midline)
- **Non-GCTs are very uncommon**; most are **ovarian** (granulosa cell), then **Sertoli and Leydig cell tumors** of the testes; often associated with virilization, feminization, or precocious puberty.

Diagnosis—Increased alpha-fetoprotein (AFP) with endodermal sinus tumors and minimally with teratomas; increased beta-human chorionic gonadotropin (beta-hCG) with choriocarcinomas and germinomas; increased lactate dehydrogenase (LDH) with any; evaluate with chest x-ray, abdominal ultrasound, CT, MRI, CT chest, and bone scan.

Treatment—Resection of anything that can be resected (not CNS tumors); radiation and chemotherapy for any non-resectable and CNS lesions; overall survival 80% (worse for adolescents and extragonadal tumors)

Liver Tumors

- Rare in childhood; most are **malignant**; tumors in first 6 months of life; more commonly benign vascular tumors or hamartomas
- **Hepatoblastoma**
  - Most common <3 years old; associated with **Beckwith-Wiedemann syndrome** and adenomatous polyposis
  - Presents with **large asymptomatic abdominal mass** (most from right lobe) then weight loss, anorexia and vomiting, and anemia; metastases to **regional nodes and lungs**
  - Diagnosis: **increased AFP**; ultrasound, then CT or MRI plus CT of chest and bone scan
  - Treatment: outcome depends on **complete resection** plus chemotherapy; poor survival if unresectable with metastases; long-term survival with **liver transplant**

- **Hepatocellular carcinoma**
  - Mostly in **adolescents**; associated with **hepatitis B or C**; also increased with certain inborn errors and liver abnormalities
  - **Hepatic mass, abdominal distension with pain**; may rupture with hemoperitoneum
  - Diagnosis: **increased AFP**; same diagnostic studies as hepatoblastoma
  - Treatment: up to 40% can have complete resection but **only 30% long-term survival**; chemotherapy; **liver transplant**

Brain Tumors

- Represent second most frequent malignancy in childhood; higher incidence **<7 years of age**; highest morbidities and mortality among all malignancies; some familial hereditary syndromes; previous exposure to radiation
  - **Early infancy:** most are **supratentorial**, especially **teratomas and choroid plexus tumors**; may present with CSF obstruction and evidence of increased intracranial pressure (vomiting, lethargy, bulging fontanels)
  - **Late infancy, preschool to middle childhood:** most **infratentorial**, especially **juvenile pilocytic astrocytoma and medulloblastoma**; common presentation with headache, nausea, vomiting, and papilledema; also problems with equilibrium, gait, coordination, and visual changes
  - **Late childhood and adolescence:** most **supratentorial**, especially **diffuse astrocytoma**; presentation with motor weakness and abnormal reflexes, sensory changes, focal deficits, seizures, speech problems

- The majority are from: **juvenile pilocytic astrocytoma, medulloblastoma, ependymoma, and craniopharyngioma**. Presentation dependent on location, type, and patient age; often initial subtle changes; head circumference may increase in an infant with open sutures.

- Diagnosis: thorough **neurological and ophthalmological** evaluation; best imaging test is **MRI; lumbar puncture** for CSF cytology except with new-onset hydrocephalus or an infratentorial lesion

Astrocytomas

- **Juvenile pilocytic astrocytoma:** most common; anywhere, but most in the **cerebellum; low-grade, rarely invasive with low potential for metastases**
- **Fibrillary astrocytoma** is next most common; diffusely infiltrating; **low-grade astrocytoma, anaplastic astrocytoma, and glioblastoma multiforme**; oligodendrogliomas are uncommon; originate in white matter and spread to cortex (infiltrating)

Ependymal tumors

- **Ependymomas:** most common; noninvasive tumor arising from **lining of ventricle**; almost all **posterior fossa**; anaplasia is rare; average age is 6 years (younger children with poorer outcome)
- **Choroid plexus tumors: most common tumor <1 year of age**; arise from **choroid plexus in lateral ventricles**; papillomatous is most common (surgical resection → cure), then carcinomatous (poor prognosis); may present with **obstruction and increased ICP.**

Embryonal tumors (primary neuroectodermal tumors; PNET)

- **Most common group of malignant CNS tumors;** metastases to the neuraxis
- **Medulloblastoma:** most common; **cerebellar**, most in the midline vermis; causes **4th ventricular obstruction and hydrocephalus with increased ICP and cerebellar dysfunction**; younger children present with **dissemination on diagnosis** and have a poor prognosis; treated with **surgical resection** (better prognosis with gross total resection) **and chemotherapy**; radiation (with many complications) is used based on more advanced staging.

Craniopharyngioma

- **Suprasellar** solid tumor with cystic components; **minimally invasive**; may be **calcified**; presentations: **decreased visual acuity, nystagmus, visual field defects, neuroendocrine findings (panhypopituitarism, deceased growth velocity)**
- **Gross total resection is curative with or without radiation; no role for chemotherapy**

Brain-stem tumors

- Types: **focal, dorsally exophytic, cervicomedullary, and diffuse intrinsic**
- Presentation: gaze palsy, cranial nerve palsies, upper motor neuron defects
- **Surgery for focal and dorsally exophytic tumors** (low-grade gliomas); have a favorable outcome; cervicomedullary tumors are sensitive to **radiation; diffuse infiltrative pontine gliomas have a very poor outcome**—no surgical resection is possible; with radiation, survival is about 12 months.

NEUROLOGICAL DISORDERS

SPECIFIC SIGNS AND SYMPTOMS OF NEUROLOGIC DYSFUNCTION

Headache

The following classifications follow the 2004 International Classification of Headache Disorders, Classification Subcommittee of the International Headache Society.

Migraine headache

Migraine without aura

- **Strong family history**; migraine in one or both parents
- **Monophasic** headache (i.e., just the headache phase)
- Pain **gradually increases in intensity.**
- Child **looks sick and wants to lie down in a dark, quiet place.**
- Moderate to intense pain, **unilateral, throbbing/pulsating**, worse with physical activity
- Associated with **nausea and vomiting, photophobia, and phonophobia** (of sound) during the headache
- Lasts from several hours to a few days

Migraine with aura

- **Strong family history**
- **Biphasic** headache: **decreased cerebral blood flow** and transient neurological abnormalities (**aura**), then **increased blood flow** (headache symptoms)
- **Aura types:** visual (less common in children; almost any visual pattern), **sensory symptoms** (paresthesias), **body image distortion** ("Alice in Wonderland" syndrome), **hemiplegia** (familial or sporadic hemiplegic migraine), or **brain-stem** signs (vasoconstriction of basilar and posterior cerebral arteries; occipital headache, ataxia, vertigo, brief loss of consciousness). May be followed by a typical migraine headache (as above), non-migraine headache, or without headache.

Childhood periodic symptoms (precursors to migraine)

- **Cyclic vomiting:** episodes of **vomiting multiple times over at least an hour with complete resolution followed by deep sleep and return to normal**

- **Abdominal migraine:** recurrent episodes of **dull, moderate to severe mid-abdominal pain** (periumbilical or poorly localized) **for at least an hour to a few days**; nausea, vomiting, and/or pallor at the time of the pain

Diagnosis—History and physical with careful **neurologic and funduscopic examination**; neuroimaging should be used only with:

- **Abnormal neurological signs**, **focal** neurological signs and symptoms during the headache or aura (except those classic for aura), **persisting/recurring** during the headache, or visual signs and symptoms during the **peak** of the headache (rather than the aura)
- Migraine with **seizure**
- Headache on **awakening from sleep** and/or **occurring early in the morning with increase in frequency and severity**
- Recent worsening of school performance and/or behavioral changes
- Headache occurring as a result of a cough
- Cluster headaches in a preadolescent
- Child <6 years of age with main complaint of headache

Management
- Avoid exacerbating stimuli.
- Treat acute attack with rest in a quiet and dark place, **acetaminophen, or nonsteroidal anti-inflammatory drug (NSAID)** if mild, brief, and infrequent.
- If nausea and vomiting: **antiemetic** (dimenhydrinate rectal suppository).
- Triptans not FDA-approved in children, but have been shown to be safe and effective; best to use **intranasal Sumatriptan** (can repeat one time in at least 2 hours; **not** for basilar or hemiplegic migraines).
- With frequent headaches or when child is missing school, **consider prophylaxis**; safest drug is **propranolol** (≥7 years old). Others: **calcium channel blockers, anticonvulsants** (valproate, topiramate, gabapentin), **antihistamines** (cyproheptadine), and **antidepressants** (amitriptyline). **Biofeedback and self-hypnosis** are very effective in children >8 years of age.

Cluster headaches
- **Clusters of headaches** (30–90-minute episodes; multiple per day) **occurring over weeks to months, separated by periods of 1–2 years**
- Always **unilateral** (same side during each attack), starting **around/behind an eye** → **ipsilateral hemicranium**
- **Severe, throbbing, or constant**
- **Child cannot lie still (contrast to migraine)**
- Often associated with autonomic dysfunction (unilateral Horner syndrome, sweating, flushing, tearing)
- **Very uncommon in children**, especially <10 years of age
- Usually no family history

- Obtain **head CT** if occurs prior to adolescence
- Treat attack with **oxygen** with or without sumatriptan (suppress recurrences with **prednisone** over 2–3 weeks).

Organic headaches

- Sporadic headaches **early in the morning** or after arising, then become **diffuse and generalized, more frontal and occipital**. Increased intensity with anything that **increases intracranial pressure (ICP)**, e.g., cough, sneeze; irritability, lethargy, and **morning vomiting**; headache may become constant.
- **Causes with increased ICP:** infection, tumors, hydrocephalus, subdural hematoma, lead poisoning, pseudotumor cerebri
- **Causes without increased ICP:** acute subarachnoid hemorrhage, aneurysm, arteriovenous malformation, thromboembolism, severe hypertension, collagen vascular disease affecting the central nervous system (CNS)
- Diagnosis: careful history and physical, **neurological and funduscopic exams, blood pressure, and neuroimaging** (CT or MRI)

Tension/stress headaches

Anxiety → contraction of scalp and neck muscles → dull ache; more **during the day**, particularly in **school; does not throb, and no nausea and vomiting**; increases and decreases in intensity; mostly **frontal** (but can be occipital or both); **very common in children; underlying emotional or stressful factors and/or psychosocial problems**; may also be associated with caffeine excess/withdrawal. Treatment: **remove provoking factors** when possible; may need psychological counseling; **mild analgesics** for pain; **biofeedback and self-hypnosis**.

Altered Consciousness

Definitions/pathophysiology

- **Lethargy:** difficulty in maintaining arousal (but can be aroused to communicate)
- **Obtundation:** severe decrease in alertness, but alerts to stimuli other than pain
- **Stupor:** unresponsive except to painful stimuli
- **Coma:** unresponsive to any stimuli, including pain
  - Stupor and coma: from primary dysfunction of the ascending reticular activating system and/or both cerebral cortices, or from secondary problems affecting both cerebral cortices, e.g., increased ICP
- **Delirium:** an agitated confusional state (agitation, confusion, delusions, hallucinations); may alternate with drowsiness and have motor abnormalities; assumed to be an organic encephalopathy until proven otherwise
- **Encephalopathy:** diffuse brain disorder with altered states of consciousness, altered cognition/personality and/or seizures; visual hallucinations almost always represent an organic encephalopathy

Etiology

- **Toxic:** toxins, illicit drugs, medications, carbon monoxide
- **Hypoxic-ischemic encephalopathy:** cardiac arrest, drowning, perinatal, hemorrhage
- **Infections:** meningitis, encephalitis, postinfectious encephalitis, abscess, empyema
- **Metabolic:** decreased osmolality (hypoglycemia, hyponatremia, hypernatremia), inborn errors of metabolism, endocrine disorders (thyroid, adrenal, parathyroid), hepatic encephalopathy, uremic encephalopathy, hypertensive encephalopathy, Reye syndrome, lead encephalopathy
- **Cardiovascular:** vasculitis, subarachnoid hemorrhage, severe congestive heart failure, thromboembolism
- **Increased intracranial pressure:** hemorrhage, cerebral edema, tumors, hydrocephalus
- **Trauma:** concussion, contusion, epidermal or subdural hematoma, intracranial hemorrhage
- **Vasculitis**
- **Seizures** and postictal states
- **Psychological and psychogenic:** schizophrenia, panic disorder, conversion reaction, catatonia
- **Metabolic:** diabetic ketoacidosis (DKA), hypoglycemia, hyponatremia, hypernatremia, hypomagnesemia, endocrine (as above), uremia, hepatic encephalopathy, hypertensive encephalopathy, inborn errors of metabolism

Diagnosis—History: initial **rapid assessment**: events leading up to current state, recent illnesses, ongoing/known illnesses, use of medications, possibility of ingestions/exposures, history of migraines or seizures, family history of neurological disorders

Exam

- Vital signs and general findings: evidence of trauma, skin perfusion, rashes
- Respiratory pattern
  - **Cheyne-Stokes breathing:** periods of hyperpnea alternating with apnea; **bilateral damage anywhere along the descending path from forebrain to upper pons**; sign of **impending uncal or transtentorial herniation**
  - **Kussmaul breathing:** fast, deep breathing: compensation for **metabolic acidosis**
  - **Central neurogenic hyperventilation:** sustained, rapid, deep hyperventilation; lesions just **ventral to the aqueduct or 4th ventricle**
  - **Medullary and pontine lesions: apneustic breathing** (pause with full inspiration) or irregular breathing with pauses (no pattern)
- **Eyes and pupils**
  - Funduscopic exam: hemorrhages, papilledema
  - **Light reflex:** present in most metabolic causes; **absent usually with structural lesions, some drugs, and asphyxia**
    - **Unilateral pupil constriction plus Horner syndrome:** hypothalamic lesion; impending uncal herniation

- ◦ **Mid-position fixed pupils:** midbrain; impending transtentorial herniation; massive barbiturates
- ◦ **Dilated, fixed pupils:** unilaterally dilated—uncal herniation; bilateral—anoxia, bilaterally compressed 3rd cranial nerves, large dose of an anticholinergic
- ◦ **Small, reactive pupils:** organophosphates, sedative-hypnotics, phenothiazines, clonidine
- ◦ **Pinpoint, reactive pupils:** pontine lesion, narcotics
- ◦ **Dilated, reactive pupils:** anticholinergics, amphetamines, cocaine, carbamazepine, postictal

- **Tonic lateral eye deviation** (both eyes): seizures originating in the hemisphere opposite the direction of gaze, or a destructive lesion in the hemisphere of the direction of gaze
- **Oculocephalic reflex** ("doll's eyes"): a positive response with an intact brain stem is conjugate deviation of the eyes opposite to the direction of head-turning; random eye movements occur with a pons or midbrain lesion; sign of impending uncal/ transtentorial herniation
- **Oculovestibular reflex:** instill ice water in alternate ears 15 minutes apart; normal response with an intact brain stem: eyes deviate toward the irrigated ear and slowly return to the midline; if the ipsilateral eye abducts and the opposite does not, lesion of the medial longitudinal fasciculus; presence of slow movement indicates unilateral hemispheric function (corticopontine pathway must be intact); presence of skew deviation (hypertropic; one eye above the other) or no response indicates a brainstem lesion

- **Trunk and limb position** at rest and with painful stimulus
  - Spontaneous movements of all limbs: mild hemispheric depression without a structural abnormality
  - **Hemiplegia or monoplegia:** abnormality in contralateral hemisphere
  - **Flaccid paralysis:** dysfunction of lower pons or medulla
  - **Extensor response to pain (decerebrate rigidity):** brain-stem compression (midbrain or upper pons); most severe form is **opisthotonus**; sign of impending uncal/ transtentorial herniation
  - **Flexor arm and extensor leg response to pain = decorticate rigidity:** hemispheric dysfunction with intact brain stem; uncommon in children, but seen after head trauma; sign of impending uncal/transtentorial herniation

Management

- **ABCDE** of initial management: **a**irway and cervical spine protection, **b**reathing and ventilation, **c**irculation and control of bleeding, **d**isability (exam, as above), **e**xposure and environmental control (undress patient for complete visualization, and prevent hypothermia)
- Obtain **Dextrostix** first and **give IV D25/W**, 2–4 mL/kg push; continue infusion with D10 if positive response.

- **Other labs:** CBC, erythrocyte sedimentation rate (ESR), electrolytes, glucose, BUN, creatinine, Ca, P, Mg, liver enzymes and liver function tests (including ammonia), arterial blood gas (ABG) and carboxyhemoglobin, toxicology screen urinalysis, cultures, chest x-ray, cervical spine x-ray, and pelvic x-ray (if any evidence of trauma).
- **CT head** as soon as stable, then lumbar puncture if not contraindicated by CT; consider **EEG.**
- Give **naloxone** with any hypoventilation or CNS depression; if no response to 10 mg, opiates are not the cause.
- Mild **initial hyperventilation with 100% oxygen** for evidence of increased ICP, 25% **mannitol** IV, **restrict fluids, and ICP monitoring with neurosurgical consult**
- Correct electrolyte, acid-base abnormalities, empiric antibiotics for likely infection, specific therapies for toxidromes, control seizures; admit to pediatric intensive care unit (PICU) when stable.

Closed Minor Head Trauma in Children

Definition—A 2–20-year-old patient seen within 24 hours of head injury who appears normal at exam

Management

- **No initial loss of consciousness:** thorough history and physical; + neurological; observe at clinic, office, Emergency Room (ER), or home under a competent caregiver
- **Brief loss of consciousness** (<1 minute), but not for suspected child abuse, previously known neurological problems, or cerebrospinal fluid (CSF) shunts: history and physical, including neurological exam with observation; consider CT scan; CT better than MRI for acute head trauma); discharge if normal with observation or has a normal CT scan.

Movement Disorders

Ataxia

Definition—Inability to make smooth, accurate, and coordinated movements; problem with **cerebellum and/or posterior column sensory pathways** (fine control of posture and movement); may be generalized or involve just gait or the hands and arms; acute or chronic onset

Most common etiologies
Acute/recurrent:

- **Drugs:** alcohol, anticonvulsants
- **Postinfectious:** acute cerebellar ataxia: autoimmune response 2–3 weeks after a viral infection in a young child (adenovirus, enteroviruses, varicella); sudden onset of severe truncal ataxia with vomiting, horizontal nystagmus, and dysarthria; also acute brainstem encephalitis and other uncommon immune-mediated disorders in children (e.g., multiple sclerosis)

- Migraine: basilar
- Benign paroxysmal vertigo
- Neuroblastoma (see Chapter 21), frontal lobe (association fibers to cerebellum), and cerebellar tumors
- **Trauma:** hemorrhage, vascular occlusion, postconcussion
- **Vasculitis**
- Hereditary disorders: certain **inborn errors** and **hereditary ataxia** disorders with episodic or recurrent ataxia

Chronic/progressive:

- **Congenital malformations:** posterior fossa, e.g., Chiari, Dandy-Walker malformation, cerebellar aplasia/hypoplasia
- **Brain tumors**
- **Metabolic disorders:** abetalipoproteinemia (see Chapter 13), Hartnup disease (defect in transport of neutral amino acids by intestinal mucosa and renal tubules), maple syrup urine disease (see Chapter 2), pyruvate dehydrogenase deficiency, respiratory chain disorders, and others
- **Hereditary degenerative disease**
  - Ataxia-telangiectasia (see Chapter 9)
  - Adrenoleukodystrophy
  - **Friedreich ataxia:** autosomal recessive abnormality of gene coding for mitochondrial protein **frataxin** → oxidative injury due to **excessive mitochondrial iron deposits**; affects spinocerebellar tracts, dorsal columns, pyramidal tracts, cerebellum, and medulla; **slowly progressive ataxia before age 10 years**, initial involvement of primarily lower extremities, then weakness of hands and feet, dysarthria, loss of deep tendon reflexes (DTRs), loss of vibratory and position sense, nystagmus, and extensor plantar response; **progressive kyphoscoliosis and other skeletal problems**; **progressive hypertrophic cardiomyopathy** usual cause of death. Symptomatic treatment and antioxidants (slow progression somewhat).
  - Others: extremely rare

Chorea and Athetosis

- **Chorea:** rapid, irregular, uncontrolled movements of the hands and feet with an abnormal gait
- **Athetosis:** distal writhing movements of the extremities with or without chorea
- **Rigidity** through range of motion in flexors and extensors

Most common etiologies

- **Infections:** encephalitis (various viruses, including HIV), bacterial endocarditis, scarlet fever, diphtheria, toxoplasmosis
- **Postinfectious:** postviral encephalitis, **Sydenham chorea** (sole neurological manifestation of rheumatic fever, see Chapter 12);

- **Autoimmune disorders:** especially **SLE** (may be the presenting sign), often with antiphospholipid antibodies
- **Metabolic/toxic:** carbon monoxide, organophosphates, heavy-metal poisoning; liver/renal failure, hypoparathyroidism, hyperthyroidism, hypo- or hypernatremia
- **Basal ganglia lesions** (vascular, masses, multiple sclerosis)
- **Drugs:** stimulants (cocaine, amphetamines), dopamine agonists and receptor blockers, anticholinergics, anticonvulsants, calcium channel blockers, tricyclic antidepressants (TCAs), oral contraceptives, lithium, and others
- **Hereditary: Huntington disease:** mutation in huntingtin protein → formation of abnormal inclusions within nuclei of neurons → decreased transcriptional activations; rare to start in children (<1% begin under age 10 years; much more rapid with average age from diagnosis to death of 8 years); neuropsychiatric findings in **Wilson disease** include chorea; other rare genetic causes
- Most common causes of athetosis: **extrapyramidal cerebral palsy** (kernicterus, asphyxia, certain metabolic disorders), cerebral palsy in former premature infants, dopamine-blocking drugs, and after circulatory arrest for complex cardiac surgery

Dystonia

- **Sustained muscle contractions with abnormal posture**, twisting, and repetitive movements
- **Generalized primary dystonia:** due to a number of genetic disorders (many gene loci); initially intermittent (stress-aggravated), then involvement of extremities, axial muscles, face, and tongue → impaired swallowing and speech
- **Secondary dystonia: perinatal asphyxia, kernicterus,** drugs (phenytoin, carbamazepine, phenothiazines); **Wilson disease** (particularly basal ganglia involvement: often progressive dystonia, tremors, rigidity, choreoathetosis, and dysarthria); may respond to large doses of trihexyphenidyl; many other drugs and procedures may be beneficial (intrathecal baclofen, stereotaxic surgery)

Tremor

Involuntary rhythmic oscillations of part of the body

- **Familial essential tremor:** autosomal dominant trait; slowly progressive; mostly upper extremities; disappears with rest; severe cases may respond to propranolol or primidone
- **Myoclonic tremors:** sudden, brief, jerky, involuntary movements with a tremor; mostly after hypoxic cerebellar injury or certain neurodegenerative disease
- **Jitteriness:** mostly in **healthy term infants while crying or being examined; rhythmic tremors of equal amplitude around a fixed axis; abnormal if occurs while awake and alert or persists after first 2 weeks of life**; also many possible organic causes: hypoglycemia, hypocalcemia, hypomagnesemia, anemia, infection, maternal drugs
- Drug-induced (amphetamines, valproate, TCAs, caffeine, theophylline, neuroleptics) or initial manifestation of a metabolic disorder

Tics

- **Involuntary**, **repetitive**, **nonrhythmic**, spasmodic movements of any muscle group, exacerbated by stress
- **Transient tic disorder:** most common movement disorder of childhood; more common in boys and with a family history; typical behaviors: eye-blinking, facial movements, throat-clearing; lasts weeks to <1 year; no treatment needed
- **Chronic motor tic disorder:** tics in up to three muscle groups at a time; may continue into adulthood
- **Gilles de la Tourette syndrome:** most are probably autosomal dominant but no gene locus has been identified; lifelong condition beginning age 2–21 years; **multiple motor tics in different parts of the body and at least one vocal tic prior to the age of 21** (echolalia, obscene words, barking, and others; uncontrollable) **with increase and decrease of findings over a year**. May also have concomitant attention deficit hyperactivity disorder (ADHD) and obsessive-compulsive disorder (OCD); ultimate severity is determined by severity during adolescence. Treatment is for those with significant social and academic problems: behavior management, biofeedback, **haloperidol** (dopamine blocker; adverse effects: restlessness, acute dystonic reaction, drug-induced parkinsonism, tardive dyskinesia, depression), clonidine, and other drugs.

CNS INFECTION
Acute Bacterial Meningitis

Background

Most occur from **hematogenous dissemination** from a distant site (less commonly from a contiguous source of infection); usually with **rapid invasion from recent bacterial colonization of the nasopharynx**; often previous/ongoing **viral infection** → enhances entry into CNS via the **choroid plexus and the meninges** → circulates through the CSF and subarachnoid space and multiplies rapidly; **polymorphonuclear cell (PMN) invasion and chemotactic factors** → a significant **inflammatory response** → **cytokine** production.

Etiology

- Most common cause in children is *Neisseria meningitidis* (sporadic: equal distribution between types B, C, and Y in the United States; vs. epidemic: usually type A)
- Increased risk with **close contact and recent colonization**; highest rate <5 years of age with second peak at age 15–24 years
- Since immunization, there has been a significant decline in incidence of *Haemophilus influenzae* type B (HiB; under-vaccinated, especially in underdeveloped) and *Strep. pneumoniae* (invasive disease peaks in first 2 years)
  - Seen more with incomplete immunizations or abnormal immune status, including **functional/anatomic asplenia**
  - Also seen with **CSF leaks, cochlear implants**, and from contiguous infections, e.g., otitis media, sinusitis, and pneumonia

- Other organisms less common and associated with specific circumstances/ abnormalities.

Clinical presentation

- Most common—**insidious over days** with **viral symptoms** then **nonspecific findings of CNS infection** (lethargy, irritability, fever, headache, photophobia, hypotension, and tachycardia).
- Then with or without evidence of **meningeal irritation**: nuchal rigidity, back pain, positive Brudzinski (supine passive flexion of neck → flexion of knees and hips) and Kernig (pain with extension of legs after 90-degree flexion of hips) signs; **not consistent findings at 12–18 months of age (absence does not rule out diagnosis)**
- **Increased ICP:** persistent headache, bulging fontanel, split sutures, 3rd- and 6th-nerve palsies, hypertension with decreased heart rate, apnea, abnormal posturing, stupor, coma (papilledema usually suggests a more chronic cause)
- May present with **focal neurological signs and seizures** (cerebritis, infarction, electrolyte abnormalities, subdural effusion)
- Alteration in mental status; **coma** → poor prognosis

Table 22.1: CSF Results for Various Etiologies of Meningitis

	WBCs, mm3 (NL = <5, 75% lymphs)	Glucose, mg/dL (NL = >50 or 75% serum glucose)	Protein, mg/dL (NL = 20–45)	Opening pressure, mm H$_2$O (NL = 50–80)	Gram stain
Bacterial	Elevated in the hundreds to thousands (usually not <100–200); mostly PMNs	Decreased (<50% serum)	Elevated into the hundreds	Elevated usually in the hundreds	Causative organism seen
Partially treated	Widely variable depending on the time of pretreatment, but usually elevated to at least a slight degree (to many thousands); may see mostly mononuclear cells	May be normal to decreased	Elevated into the hundreds	May be normal to variably elevated	Antibiotics may sterilize CSF and Gram stain may be negative; possible diagnosis with antigen detection
Viral (or meningo-encephalitis)	Usually elevated into the hundreds (not thousands); mostly mononuclear cells (but may see early PMNs); some viruses are associated with significant elevations of WBCs	For most viruses, is usually in the normal range	May be slightly to moderately elevated (<200)	Normal to slightly elevated (100–200)	Negative; need viral culture, PCR, EEG, CT/MRI
TB	Variably increased but usually <500; PMNs may be seen early but lymphocytes are prominent through rest of course	Decreased similar to bacterial; will continue to decrease until treatment	Usually quite high; often into the thousands	Elevated to variable degrees	Not seen; usually not seen with acid-fast smear; best way to detect is PCR of CSF
Fungal	Variably increased similar to TB (<500) with PMNs early and then mononuclear cells	Decreased similar to bacterial (and TB); will continue to decrease until treatment	May be normal to moderately elevated (<500)	Elevated to variable degrees	May see fungal elements; can culture organisms

Abbreviations: cerebrospinal fluid, CSF; normal limits, NL; polymerase chain reaction, PCR; polymorphonuclear cells, PMN; tuberculosis, TB; white blood cell, WBC

Diagnosis—Obtain **blood culture** and perform lumbar puncture, but not immediately if: **increased ICP** (other than a bulging fontanel), **severe cardiopulmonary compromise, infection of the skin over the site, and thrombocytopenia with bleeding**; if there is a delay in diagnosis (because of the need to perform a CT scan), then **do not delay antibiotics**; perform lumbar puncture (LP) after excluding brain abscess or after treating ICP.

Management

- **Start antibiotics as soon as possible** (and if LP has to be delayed); treat shock, increased ICP, and any organ failure.
- **Initial empiric antibiotics** (prior to culture and sensitivities) per susceptibilities to *Strep. pneumoniae*; most strains plus HiB plus *N. meningitidis* will be sensitive to the combination of **vancomycin with either cefotaxime or ceftriaxone**.
  - If allergic to penicillin/cephalosporins and at least 1 month of age, may use **IV chloramphenicol**.
- 10–14-day course with IV penicillin or a third-generation cephalosporin if *Strep. pneumoniae* is sensitive to penicillin and there are no complications; if resistant, complete with vancomycin
- 5–7-day course with IV penicillin for uncomplicated *N. meningitidis*
- 7–10-day course IV with the antibiotic with the best sensitivity for uncomplicated **HiB**
- **Partially treated** meningitis and no positive culture: use a third-generation antibiotic IV for 7–10 days; if no improvement or with focal signs, obtain CT or MRI.
- For **gram-negative meningitis**, use a third-generation cephalosporin (cefotaxime or ceftriaxone for most; ceftazidime for *Pseudomonas aeruginosa*) for 3 weeks, or for at least 2 weeks after cultures are negative.
- CSF should be sterile 24–48 hours after the appropriate dosing of a sensitive antibiotic; **no routine repeat LP** except for gram-negative meningitis or with beta-lactamase–resistant *Strep. pneumoniae*.
- **Dexamethasone** just prior to (or concurrently with) the antibiotics with **HiB** (at least **6 weeks** of age) **reduces the incidence of sensorineural hearing loss**; studies have not shown an advantage for the use of corticosteroids with the other organisms (except for tuberculosis [TB] meningitis).
- Fluids (IV; nothing-by-mouth [NPO]) should initially be **restricted to one-half to two-thirds maintenance** due to **increased ICP and syndrome of inappropriate antidiuretic hormone secretion (SIADH**; which is very common); fluids should not be restricted with dehydration and/or shock

Complications and outcome

- Up to one-third have a **subdural effusion**: increased head circumference (in infants), **seizures**, and **prolonged or recurrent fever**; head CT or MRI is diagnostic; symptomatic effusions in infants may be aspirated through the anterior fontanel.
- SIADH may exacerbate cerebral edema.
- **Prolonged fever** (>10 days) in a small number; most from intercurrent viral illness, then nosocomial or secondary bacterial infection, drug reaction, or thrombophlebitis
- **Secondary fever** (fever after an afebrile period): most due to a nosocomial infection

- Seizures, increased ICP, cranial nerve palsies, stroke, herniation, venous sinus thrombosis
- Most common outcome morbidity is **sensorineural hearing loss** (highest with *Strep. pneumoniae* then *N. meningitidis* and HiB); due to labyrinthitis and/or direct damage to the 8th nerve; all need hearing test.
- Other morbidities: recurrent seizures, mental retardation, developmental delay, visual abnormalities, behavioral problems
- Mortality highest with ***Strep. pneumoniae***; severe abnormalities occur in up to 20%—especially if <6 months old; also increased with seizures after the **fourth day**, focal presentation, and coma.

Prophylaxis of contacts—All close contacts to the index case diagnosed with **N. meningitidis** should be given **rifampin** every 12 hours for 2 days as soon as possible; household contacts of the index case diagnosed with **HiB** should be given rifampin once per day for 4 days; there is no prophylaxis with *Strep. pneumoniae*.

Meningoencephalitis

Background—Infection of the **meninges and brain tissue** is due to most common **enteroviruses**; spread by person-to-person contact; most cases are self-limited

Etiology

- **Viruses:** enterovirus, arboviruses, herpes simplex virus (HSV), varicella zoster virus (VZV), cytomegalovirus (CMV), Epstein-Barr virus (EBV), measles, adenovirus, and many others
- **Bacteria:** TB, *Rickettsia* spp., *Chlamydia* spp., *Bartonella* spp., *Brucella* spp., and many others
- **Fungi:** *Candida* spp., *Cryptococcus neoformans*, *Coccidioides immitis*, and many others
- **Parasites:** *Schistosoma* spp., *Trichinella spiralis*, *Toxocara canis*, and many others
- **Noninfectious etiologies** (vaccines, systemic disease, immune-mediated disease, malignancy, drugs, toxins, CSF shunts, and others less commonly)

Clinical presentation—From **mild to severe and focal to diffuse, onset is usually acute** with a few days of fever and at times a rash, then headache (frontal, generalized, retrobulbar) in older children and irritability and lethargy in infants; then nausea, vomiting, photophobia, and neck, back, and leg pain are common; altered consciousness, abnormal movements, seizures, focal neurological signs, flaccid paralysis (anterior horn cell involvement), nuchal rigidity

Diagnosis—Clinical presentation plus CSF fluid → mild mononuclear predominance (see Table 22.1); isolation of the virus more likely early in the course and most common with enteroviruses (can increase yield with nasopharyngeal, fecal, and urine cultures); **PCR** is better for enteroviruses and HSV; may also obtain acute and convalescent serum titers, especially for non-enteroviral infections.

Management—Supportive treatment, except for etiologies for which there is a specific anti-infective drug (e.g., acyclovir with HSV), and treat complications; most children recover completely but, depending on the organism, there may be sequelae (motor, seizures, deafness, visual, behavioral, auditory).

Brain Abscess

Background—Most common in **neonates and at 4–8 years of age**; from **heart emboli** (right-to-left shunts), immune disorders, meningitis, contiguous infection (mastoiditis, sinusitis, orbital cellulitis), other soft-tissue infection of the face or scalp, dental infection, penetrating trauma, CSF shunt infections; most in frontal, parietal, and temporal lobes of either hemisphere; most are single but may be multiple and involve more than one lobe

Etiology—Various **streptococcal species**, **anaerobes**, **gram-negative aerobes**; **Citrobacter** most common in neonate; most have one cultured organism, but two or more may be present

Clinical presentation—Nonspecific early findings such as **low-grade fever, headache, and lethargy**; then with progression of inflammation: worsening headache, vomiting, seizures, focal signs, papilledema, coma; if the cerebellum is involved: ataxia, nystagmus, headache, and vomiting

Diagnosis—Blood culture is positive in only a small number; peripheral white blood cell (WBC) count is normal to increased; CSF is variable: WBCs and protein normal to minimally increased and glucose may be normal to low; culture is rarely positive (if the diagnosis is suspected, and LP should not be performed because of the possibility of herniation); **diagnostic study of choice is MRI.**

Management

- If **etiology is not known** or suspected, start vancomycin plus third-generation cephalosporin plus metronidazole; otherwise, antibiotic selection is based on most likely etiology from the history and physical and if the patient is immunocompromised.
- **Antibiotics alone** if abscess diameter <2 cm, of short duration (<2 weeks), and with no evidence of increased ICP and intact neurological exam, but need weekly neuroimaging
- **Antibiotics and aspiration** if symptomatic and encapsulated
- **Surgery** (rare): >2.5 cm, gas-containing, multiloculated, posterior fossa, fungal; mortality is higher (usually <10%) if <1 year old, multiple abscesses, coma, or no CT done; long-term sequelae at >50%

NEURODEGENERATIVE DISEASE

- **Progressive deterioration** of neurological function with **loss of speech, vision, hearing, intellect, feeding ability, and/or ambulation with or without seizures** affecting either the white or gray matter. Outcome is **fatal** but diagnosis is important for genetic counseling and future prevention.

- Etiology:
  - Sphingolipidoses (see Chapter 2)
  - **Neuronal ceroid lipofuscinoses:** most common class; autosomal recessive; storage of autofluorescent substances within lysosomes of neurons and other tissues; all with some combination of cerebellar ataxia, myoclonic seizures, cognitive deterioration, blindness (optic atrophy; brown macular discoloration; consistent finding in all), dementia, microcephaly, dystonic posturing
  - **Adrenoleukodystrophies** (ALDs): X-linked recessive; accumulation of **very long-chain fatty acids in neural tissue and adrenals (adrenal cortical insufficiency)**; classic ALD begins at age 5–15 years; early findings: decreased school performance, behavioral changes, and gait disturbance, then generalized seizures, upper motor signs, ataxia, and pseudobulbar palsy; adrenal insufficiency may precede neurological findings in about half. MRI shows **periventricular demyelination progressing anteriorly.** Death usually within 10 years of onset unless bone marrow transplant done or if given a mixture of glyceryl trioleate and glyceryl trierucate (**Lorenzo's oil**) prior to age 6 with any MRI changes.
  - Sialidosis: autosomal recessive; accumulation of sialic acid-oligosaccharide complexes secondary to deficiency in lysosomal enzyme neuraminidase. Slow decrease in visual function and a retinal cherry-red spot plus progressive myoclonus (lack of ambulation) and generalized seizures or multiorgan disease (coarse facial features, skeletal anomalies, lymphocytes with cytoplasmic vacuoles).
  - Others: Menkes disease (Chapter 2), Rett disorder (Chapter 5), subacute sclerosing panencephalitis, and others rarely.

CEREBRAL PALSY

Background

Most common **chronic motor disability that begins in childhood**—from any of a number of disorders of **early brain development**; the features can change over time; may be abnormalities of cognition, speech, hearing, vision, feeding, and behavior; some may also have a seizure disorder. In many cases, **antenatal factors resulting in abnormal brain development** can be identified, however **<10% are associated with perinatal asphyxia. Most are born at term without problems during labor and delivery.** Increased risk with **low birth weight** (especially very low birth weight) and **antenatal/intrapartum maternal infection.** Most occurring in infants born prematurely are due to **intraventricular hemorrhage and/or periventricular leukomalacia** (white-matter necrosis; see Chapter 1). **MRI with white-matter abnormalities at 40 weeks postconceptional age predictive of cerebral palsy at age 2 years.**

Classification and Features

- **Spastic hemiplegia**
  - Most common cause—**in-utero or neonatal stroke due to thrombophilic disorders.**
  - Decreased movements on **one side; upper extremity** > lower: **early hand preference; difficulty with hand use; growth arrest, especially of the hand (more than the foot)**
  - Delayed walking and then abnormal gait; **spasticity** with toe-walking; some with seizures, some with cognitive dysfunction, including mental retardation
  - **Increased DTRs, clonus, extensor plantar response**
  - MRI shows **atrophy of a cerebral hemisphere with hydrocephalus ex vacuo** (due to expansion of the lateral ventricle into space previously occupied by brain tissues)

- **Spastic diplegia**
  - Most common cause—periventricular leukomalacia (**PVL**) (leg fibers in periventricular white matter affected primarily).
  - Bilateral spasticity of **legs** > **arms**
  - Early detection—use of **arms for crawling, while dragging legs**; legs with **scissoring** when held in suspension under axillae; may also be excessive hip adduction and the paraspinal muscles may be affected (**unable to sit**); walking delayed (**toe-walking**) and impaired growth of the lower extremities with disuse atrophy. Intelligence is usually normal and there are no or minimal seizures.

- **Spastic quadriplegia**
  - Causes: **multicystic cortical encephalomalacia, PVL, malformations**
  - **All extremities** with **hypertonicity and spasticity** and decreased movement and athetosis; increased DTRs, clonus, extensor plantar response; **most severe form; flexion contractures occur**
  - High association with **mental retardation, seizures, supranuclear bulbar palsies (swallowing, speech), and visual problems**

- **Extrapyramidal (choreoathetoid)**
  - Most likely associated with **asphyxia, kernicterus, mitochondrial disorders, and other genetic problems**
  - Initial hypotonia, poor head control with persistent head lag; then variable increase in tone with rigidity and dystonia over years; generally no upper motor signs or seizures, and most do not have cognitive problems
  - Feeding difficulties, drooling, speech problems

Diagnosis

History and physical, including thorough neurological and ophthalmological exams to preclude neurodegenerative disease, metabolic disorders, spinal cord abnormalities, or muscular dystrophies; blood chemistries, acid-base analysis, glucose, hepatic and renal function, and urinalysis; **MRI of brain and spinal cord** for structural lesions, effects of hypoxia-ischemia; **test hearing and vision; genetic evaluation and counseling**

Management

Multidisciplinary team involving neurology, orthopedics, physiatry, psychology, and dental; **therapists**: physical, occupational, speech, feeding, and developmental; educator, social worker, nutritionist. Teach **daily activities** and how to function and play (**therapy only optimizes function**); use of **adaptive equipment**, **prevention of contractures**, improvement of **communication skills with special equipment**; management of **eye and hearing problems**, **behavior management**, management of **learning and cognitive disorders**; surgical procedures to decrease muscle spasms; **spasticity drugs** (baclofen, dantrolene, levodopa, carbamazepine, benzodiazepines, trihexyphenidyl, selected muscle injection of **botulinum toxin**)

CEREBROVASCULAR DISEASE

Arterial Thromboembolism

Presentations

- **Stroke:** abrupt change in neurological function from either interrupted blood supply → **ischemia and infarction** identified on CT after 24 hours (area of increased lucency that enhances with contrast)
- **Hemorrhage** → tissue disruption, compression, and vasospasm (area of increased density on non-enhanced CT scan)
- Many secondary events leading to neuronal injury and death; if neurological exam normalizes within 24 hours, it may be due to a **transient ischemic attack** (no permanent brain damage).
  - Major cerebral arteries: **internal carotid artery** occlusion (shedding of emboli from a thrombus): progressive flaccid hemiplegia and lethargy and aphasia if dominant hemisphere involvement; may have focal seizures; **vertebral basilar circulation** (most common with neck trauma, especially at C1-C2): acute headache and brainstem dysfunction; multiple infarcts = **embolization or vasculitis**; infarction of the **middle cerebral artery or one of its branches** (anterior or posterior cerebral arteries): sudden hemiplegia plus hemiparesis, hemianopia, and aphasia (dominant hemisphere). Seizures may precede the hemiplegia.
  - **Occlusion of small arteries:** unilateral neurological signs with complete recovery due to small area of involvement (except in few cases with bilateral findings, progressive deterioration, and poor outcome)

Most common causes

- **Trauma** (head, neck, intraoral)
- **Infection** (local infections of the head and neck, meningitis, encephalitis)
- **Cerebrovascular malformations**
- **Vasculitis and autoimmune disease**, **drugs** (amphetamines, cocaine)
- **Heart disease** (arrhythmias, myxoma, prosthetic heart valves, cyanotic defects, bacterial endocarditis, acute rheumatic fever)
- **Hemoglobinopathies** (sickle cell)

- **Coagulation disorders**, certain **metabolic diseases** associated with stroke (homocystinuria)
- **Vasculopathies** (moyamoya disease)

Venous Thrombosis

Causes and presentations—Slow-evolving diffuse neurological signs and symptoms with seizures in neonates and focal neurological signs (hemiplegia) in older children; both may have signs of **increased intracranial pressure.**

- **Septic causes:** meningitis (superficial cortical and deep penetrating veins), encephalitis, otitis media, mastoiditis, sinusitis and orbital cellulitis (cavernous sinus thrombosis)
- **Aseptic causes:** vascular malformations (impaired venous drainage), trauma (head, sinus, jugular vein), **inherited prothrombotic disorders,** acquired prothrombotic states (pregnancy, nephrotic syndrome, antiphospholipid syndrome), inflammation (rheumatic disease, inflammatory bowel disease), drugs (oral contraceptives), dehydration, malignancy, polycythemia

Intracranial Hemorrhage

Causes and presentations

- **Intraparenchymal hemorrhage:** loss of consciousness, seizures and hemiplegia; large collections of blood can shift midline structures and increase ICP; **subarachnoid hemorrhage:** severe headache, nuchal rigidity, and progressive loss of consciousness
- **Intraventricular/periventricular hemorrhage in preterm newborns** (see Chapter 1)
- **Intraventricular hemorrhage at term:** from choroid plexus and/or germinal matrix; most have problems from delivery with some degree of hypoxia; most common presentation is seizures on the second day of life or apnea, cyanosis, and seizures in 1st hours of life; both may have posthemorrhagic hydrocephalus
- Hemorrhage secondary to **congenital or acquired bleeding disorders**
- **Traumatic hemorrhage**
- **Aneurysms:** most are at the bifurcation of major arteries at the base of the brain; rarely rupture during childhood; associations with polycystic kidney disease and coarctation; initial rupture → **subarachnoid hemorrhage** and may be progressive; may be gaze and pupillary abnormalities (pressure on the oculomotor nerve). Lumbar puncture will be **grossly bloody and centrifuged fluid is xanthochromic.**
- **Arteriovenous malformations (AVMs):** relatively small number symptomatic in childhood; may be an abnormal communication between choroidal arteries and veins → vein of Galen malformation, choroid plexus malformation, and shunts between the cerebellar arteries and straight sinus; usually present with **high-output congestive heart failure or progressive hydrocephalus and increased ICP (CSF obstruction);** difficult to treat and are associated with a poor outcome. Also between superficial arteries and veins → result in AVM within the cerebral hemispheres; vast majority are **supratentorial.**

Pseudotumor Cerebri

✓ Increased ICP with normal CSF analysis, normal brain, and normal ventricles on imaging

✓ Headache, vomiting, diplopia in most; then neck stiffness, tinnitus, ataxia, paresthesias; not acutely ill and normal mental state; no focal signs observed except for abducens nerve palsy; also papilledema present (may have optic atrophy if untreated)

✓ Normal imaging and CSF; must assess baseline visual fields

✓ Causes: Most are idiopathic if >11 years old; most causes found <6 years of age; drugs (steroid withdrawal, vitamin A, tetracycline), head trauma, infections (otitis, sinusitis), systemic disorders (iron deficiency, systemic lupus erythematosus, vitamin A and D deficiencies, leukemia), metabolic (adrenal insufficiency, treatment of diabetic ketoacidosis, hyperthyroidism, hypoparathyroidism) and pregnancy

✓ Many can be reversed with withdrawal of CSF to reduce the opening pressure to half (sometimes need serial); then acetazolamide; if progressive optic atrophy: ventriculoperitoneal shunt

---

Diagnostic studies—Initial screen may be with a CT scan, (will only detect large area of infarction); better test should be **perfusion MRI imaging, MR angiography, and MR venography** (detect early cerebral ischemia and allow assessment of cerebral vessels); a **four-vessel angiogram** is indicted to detect sites of intracranial hemorrhage or vasculitis. Other tests include ECG and echocardiography for heart disease, infection evaluation, evaluation of connective tissue disease and vasculitis (ESR, antinuclear antibodies [ANA], rheumatoid factor [RF], C3, C4), lipid disorders (lipid profile), coagulation disorders (lupus anticoagulant, factor V Leiden, proteins C and S, antithrombin III, antiphospholipid antibodies), metabolic disorders (homocystinuria), and drugs (urine, blood toxicology screen).

Management—**No antithrombolytic agent** if significant intracerebral hemorrhage and hypertension; supportive care; surgical evacuation of large hematoma; after a stroke, long-term therapy with **low-dose aspirin; low molecular-weight heparin or warfarin** for several months with cardiac emboli, aneurysm dissection, high-grade cerebral artery stenosis, and severe prothrombotic conditions.

CONGENITAL CNS ANOMALIES
Neural Tube and Neuronal Migration Defects

Background—Failure of neural tube SP-closure between the third and fourth weeks of gestation; affected by many periconceptional factors; prenatal screening with **alpha-fetoprotein** levels at 16–18 weeks (increased)

Spina bifida occulta—Midline opening of posterior rami of vertebrae **without any protrusion of neural tissues**; usually at L5-S1; most are **asymptomatic** unless they are associated with more serious defects; clue to diagnosis with any **lumbosacral midline cutaneous defect**: in general, the more severe the defect, the more severe the underlying anomaly

Meningocele—**Meninges protrude through posterior vertebral defect with a normal cord**; usually **covered by skin (fluid-filled fluctuant mass)**—need an **MRI** to evaluate for the presence of any neural tissue, **head CT scan for the possibility of hydrocephalus** (see below), urological evaluation for bladder dysfunction (also bowel dysfunction)

Meningomyelocele

- **Protrusion of neural tissue through posterior midline vertebral defects anywhere along the neuraxis (most are lumbosacral)**; with **low sacral lesions**, bowel and bladder involvement is the major problem; with **midlumbar lesions**, also flaccid paralysis, areflexia, various sensory deficits, and deformations of the lower extremities; **increasing neurological deficits with lesions that are more cephalad** (until upper thorax to cervical where there are minimal deficits)
- Genetic predisposition
- Decreased incidence with **maternal periconceptional use of folic acid through 12 weeks' gestation** (end of neurulation)
- Most associated with **obstructive hydrocephalus = type II Chiari malformation** due to (downward displacement of the hindbrain through the foramen magnum with proximal obstruction and ventricular enlargement); if not treated, → **hindbrain dysfunction** (apnea, vocal cord paralysis, stridor, upper extremity spasticity)
- Diagnosis: evaluate for other anomalies and urological function; need **MRI of the area involved and CT of the head for hydrocephalus**
- Treatment: both meningocele and meningomyelocele need to be repaired with **ventriculoperitoneal (VP) shunt** for hydrocephalus; bladder needs to be catheterized regularly (and repeat evaluations of renal and urological function), and enemas or suppositories for bowel dysfunction. Most will have **functional ambulation** with lower lesions (from midlumbar), and about half with higher lesions with the use of **orthotic devices**. Higher incidence of **seizures and learning problems.**

Encephalocele—Protrusion of just **meninges** (good prognosis) or **brain tissue through the skull** (may or may not be covered with skin); mostly in the **occiput** (but also frontal); many are associated with **other anomalies** that result in hydrocephalus; a higher incidence of **visual abnormalities, microcephaly, mental retardation, and seizures**; perform initial plain films of the skull and cervical spine, then examine contents of sac with ultrasound, and finally complete brain **MRI** prior to surgery.

Anencephaly—Primary defect is the failure of closure of the rostral neuropore (the last part of the neural tube to close) → a **large skull defect associated with a poorly formed, small to absent brain; other anomalies** such as congenital heart disease; recurrence risk is about 4%; most that are born alive die within a few days

Lissencephaly—**Absence of cerebral convolutions with a poorly formed sylvian fissure** due to early abnormal neuroblasts migration; isolated or as part of a syndrome; includes **lateral ventriculomegaly and white-matter heterotropias;** seizures, microcephaly, developmental delay, and optic nerve hypoplasia with microphthalmia. Poor outcome.

Schizencephaly—**Unilateral or bilateral clefts in the cerebral hemispheres** (secondary to abnormalities of morphogenesis) with surrounding abnormal brain tissue; may be fused or unfused; unilateral may present with neonatal hemiparesis; bilateral (and with a greater extent) with severe **mental retardation, seizures, microcephaly, spastic quadriplegia** (bilateral); CT scan can usually define the lesions; MRI may be added for more detail if needed.

Porencephaly—**Intracerebral cysts** resulting from developmental defects or acquired disease (e.g., infarction); most near the sylvian fissure **and communicate with the subarachnoid space or ventricular system;** abnormal adjacent gyri and an encephalocele; microcephaly, mental retardation, spasticity, seizures, optic atrophy, and other anomalies; **acquired lesions are generally unilateral without communication.**

Holoprosencephaly—**Defective cleavage of the prosencephalon and failure of induction of the forebrain** (noncleaved midline structures on CT or MRI are diagnostic; may be diagnosed with prenatal ultrasound) with varying degrees of severity usually **associated facial anomalies** (cyclopia and others); in the lobar form, there is a **single ventricle, absent falx, and fused basal ganglia;** more than half associated with **chromosomal abnormalities (trisomy 13, 18)** and there is a high mortality rate

Agenesis of the corpus callosum—**X-linked recessive or autosomal dominant;** may be associated with **syndromes and specific chromosomal anomalies;** wide range of intelligence and neurological deficits (usually associated with other brain abnormalities). CT or MRI is diagnostic.

Hydrocephalus
- **Obstructive/noncommunicating**: congenital or acquired lesion within the ventricular system → impaired circulation of CSF with proximal ventricular enlargement
  - Most common; mostly at **aqueduct or 4th ventricle**
  - **Aqueductal stenosis:** may be inherited as an X-linked trait or occur from a gliosis (meningitis, subarachnoid hemorrhage, intrauterine viral infection); intraventricular hemorrhage in a premature infant; may also occur with neurofibromatosis type 1 (NF-1)

- **Posterior fossa: brain tumors, Chiari type I** (adolescent or adult with headache and progressive lower extremity spasticity, usually without hydrocephalus) **and II malformation, Dandy-Walker malformation**
  - ◦ **Dandy-Walker malformation:** cystic expansion of 4th ventricle due to lack of formation of its roof; almost all with **hydrocephalus, cerebellar hypoplasia, agenesis of the cerebellar vermis**; infant with large head, **prominent occiput** + transillumination; **cerebellar signs**, long-tract signs, delay in motor and cognitive development; the cystic cavity and lateral ventricle (if hydrocephalus) need to be shunted
- **Nonobstructive/communicating:** obliteration of subarachnoid cisterns or malfunction of arachnoid villi → impaired absorption of CSF; most common after subarachnoid hemorrhage, leukemic infiltrates, intrauterine infection, TB, or pneumococcal meningitis
  - Increased production of CSF due to a **choroid plexus papilloma** (rare)
  - Clinical findings: infants with **rapidly increasing head circumference, bulging anterior fontanel, distended scalp veins, broad forehead, and the setting-sun sign** (eyes drift downward); increased DTRs, clonus, positive Babinski reflex, and spasticity; diagnosis more difficult in older children due to fused sutures: irritability, lethargy, vomiting, headache, personality changes, decreased school performance; **papilledema, pyramidal tract signs, 3rd- and 6th-nerve palsies**
  - Diagnosis initially with **ultrasound** through the anterior fontanel of an infant (serial ultrasounds to follow progress in preterm infant with intraventricular hemorrhage [IVH]; see Chapter 1); better anatomical diagnosis of brain and related problems with CT or MRI
  - Treatment: **VP shunt** (problems with occlusion and infection, especially from coagulase-negative *Staph. aureus*) with increasing/symptomatic hydrocephalus; increased incidence of developmental delay, decreased cognitive development, poor memory skills, visual and behavioral problems

Hydranencephaly—**Absent cerebral hemispheres or remnants present within a sac** and intact midbrain and brain stem; caused by early bilateral internal carotid artery occlusion; **rapid increase in head size postnatally with positive transillumination**; seizures, spastic quadriplegia, and no cognitive development; usually treated with VP shunt for palliation

Other Spinal Cord Disorders

Tethered cord

- Occult spinal dysraphism often indicated by **overlying cutaneous defect** (see above); the highest risk is with a **caudal appendage (tail), dermal sinus above the gluteal folds and lipomas**; if these are present, lower spine should be evaluated with **MRI**
- **Tethered cord:** persistence of a thick, ropelike filum terminale—anchors the conus at or below L2; abnormal tension then leads to decreased blood supply; other anomalies may also be present
- Infants present with **asymmetric lower-extremity growth** (seen as asymmetry of the gluteal folds), deformations, muscle wasting, **delay in walking**, then toe-walking and

regression of lower-extremity function; also bowel and bladder dysfunction; if missed (or in milder cases), older children will have diffuse lower-extremity pain.

- **MRI** will show the defect; **surgical transection**; physical therapy may be needed.

Diastematomyelia—**Division of the spinal cord into two halves by a fibrocartilaginous or bony septum from the posterior vertebral bodies** (half are at L1-L3) secondary to an abnormality of tube fusion; **movement of the cord produces more trauma**; asymptomatic or with motor and sensory abnormalities of the lower extremities (usually unilateral) and may include urinary incontinence; diagnosis is with **CT or MRI**; treatment is excision

Syringomyelia—**Cystic structure within the spinal cord** (may be localized or may communicate with CSF) felt to form due to constriction of the central canal at the level of the foramen magnum during development → CSF cannot flow cephalad; the ones that are communicating with CSF are usually **associated with a Chiari type I malformation,** and the **noncommunicating ones are acquired** (tumors, infection, trauma, infarction); symptoms rare, but if present involve the **lateral spinothalamic tracts** (asymmetric loss of pain and temperature sensation in the upper extremities with preservation of light touch); with progression, there is involvement of the **corticospinal tracts** → wasting of hand muscles with no DTRs in the upper extremities and upper motor neuron signs in the lower extremities; diagnosis is with **MRI**; treatment is **surgical**

NEUROCUTANEOUS SYNDROMES
Neurofibromatosis type 1 (von Recklinghausen disease)
Background
Autosomal dominant disorder (half as new mutations) **high penetrance rate so there are carriers with clinical findings**; mutation at 17q11.2—wide range of mutations resulting in decreased function of **neurofibromin**; genetic testing may be performed; prenatal diagnosis may be made if one parent has been diagnosed with the disease; some features may be present at birth, others later

Note: NF-2 is diagnosed with either bilateral 8th-nerve acoustic neuromas on CT or MRI, or a parent or sibling with the diagnosis, and either unilateral 8th-nerve masses or two of the following findings: subcapsular lens opacities, neurofibroma, meningioma, glioma, or schwannoma; most distinctive feature is bilateral acoustic neuromas (hearing loss).

Diagnostic features—Diagnosis is clinical (no routine neuroimaging for diagnosis); need at least two of the following:

- **Café-au-lait spots:** usually the first feature; at birth or in infancy; increase in size and number through childhood

- **Pathological feature: neurofibromas:** can be present in all organ systems; appear on the skin prior to puberty and to some degree in all by adulthood; nodules/tags in the skin, deeper tissue, or subcutaneous tissues; increase in size and number with puberty and pregnancy but are intermittent throughout life; **plexiform neurofibromas** are usually congenital: soft-tissue enlargement or patch of hyperpigmentation with or without hyperkeratosis.
- **Osseous abnormality:** most common is scoliosis but this is not diagnostic; **tibial dysplasia** (is diagnostic; **cortical thinning of long bones**), when present, occurs at birth (anterolateral bowing of the lower leg) → increased risk of fractures; also diagnostic is **sphenoid dysplasia**
- **Axillary/inguinal freckling:** freckles (similar to facial freckles); most commonly seen at ages 3–5 years in the majority of patients and is usually the second noted feature
- **Optic glioma:** in about 15% of patients; **most common CNS tumor**; develops in children <6 years; may be visual loss, proptosis, and precocious puberty (if in the optic chiasm); symptomatic lesions are treated with carboplatin and vincristine before surgery. A routine yearly eye exam should be performed in every patient.
- **Lisch nodules: iris hamartomas**; occur beginning in early adolescence; do not cause clinical problems

Complications—About one-third develop serious complications; extreme degree of variability within each family

- Most mildly affected; cannot predict significant complications in childhood
- Increased risk of **lifelong malignancy**; most are **peripheral malignant sheath tumors** (pain and increased growth of a plexiform or deep nodular neurofibroma); others: **pheochromocytoma, rhabdomyosarcoma, Wilms tumor, leukemia, vascular tumors, brain tumors**
- **Gastrointestinal (GI) neurofibromas** → bleeding, anemia, malabsorption, and obstruction
- **Seizures** occur in <10%, most not related to any specific etiology
- **Non-ossifying fibromas of long bones**, especially distal femur and proximal tibia; more common during adolescence
- **Progressive kyphoscoliosis with pulmonary function deterioration**
- **Hypertension: essential is most common**; also renovascular hypertension, secondary to tumors and coarctation
- Increased incidence of mental retardation; **most have average to low-average intelligence; specific learning disabilities in more than half**
- Poor fine motor coordination; decreased tone, balance, and gait abnormalities; speech problems
- Increased incidence of ADHD

Diagnostic and management issues
General
- Evaluate clinically **for new neurofibromas and progression of lesions; no routine diagnostic imaging without signs and symptoms**
- Yearly **blood-pressure check**
- Careful **neurodevelopmental evaluation at each visit**
- Yearly **ophthalmological exam**
- Evaluate any **skeletal changes**

Specific
- Prenatal visit: if known diagnosis in a parent, **refer for genetic counseling**
- **Neonates:** negative findings do not rule out diagnosis; examine all first-degree relatives, including slit-lamp exam (>90% of affected adults will have Lisch nodules)
- **First year:** follow growth and development (most are shorter than average and have increased head size due to increased brain volume); careful exam for neurofibromas, proptosis, rapid increase in head size, focal neurological signs, skeletal abnormalities, and development
- **First 5 years:** follow speech and motor skills carefully; if evidence of persistent headaches, seizures, marked increase in head size, or plexiform neurofibromas of the head, obtain MRI.
- **Childhood:** refer for surgery for any disfigurement; evaluate for learning problems, ADHD, and social adjustment; follow for onset and development of puberty; refer to psychiatrist/psychologist as needed for specific problems.
- **Adolescence:** endocrine studies and possible MRI if abnormal pubertal development; discuss issues regarding transitioning to adulthood.

Tuberous Sclerosis

Background—**Autosomal dominant with spontaneous mutations; wide variations within the same family;** the younger the presentation, the greater risk of mental retardation

Diagnostic features
- **Major features**
  - **Characteristic skin lesions**
    - **Ash-leaf macule:** must have at least three; occur on trunk and extremities; better visualized with Woods UV lamp
    - **Sebaceous adenoma:** typically will develop between ages 4–6 years; small, red nodules over nose and cheeks that later coalesce and enlarge
    - **Shagreen patch:** rough, raised lesion that looks like orange peel, especially on the lumbosacral skin
  - **Brain lesions**
    - Pathological lesion is the **tuber** (decreased neurons with astrocytes and multinucleated giant neurons; increased number correlates to increased neurological

impairment); occur in **cerebral convolutions and project into the ventricular system; may become calcified and cause obstructive hydrocephalus**; brain tumors are less common than in NF-1.

◦ Most common neurological problem is **seizure disorder** (also cognitive impairment, behavioral abnormalities, autism): presenting seizure in infancy is the **infantile spasm**; difficult to control; may develop into myoclonic seizures with severe cognitive and neurobehavioral impairment; most common seizures when disease presents in **older children, are generalized**

- **Eye lesions:** mulberry tumors from the nerve head in the retina, disc lesions, hamartomas, or pigmented areas
- Tumors in the **heart, kidneys, or lungs**
  ◦ Half have a **rhabdomyoma of the heart**; tend to resolve slowly; may cause arrhythmias or heart failure. Kidneys are affected in most after age 10 years; angiomyolipomas and/or renal cysts. Pulmonary: lymphangiomyomatosis

Initial diagnostic studies—With clinical diagnosis (based on above criteria), obtain head CT or MRI, renal ultrasound, cardiac echocardiogram, and chest x-ray; repeat studies are done only with specific signs and symptoms (as is the case with NF-1); any evidence of increased ICP requires immediate investigation for possible surgery due to CSF obstruction or mass lesion

Management—Issues are the same as with NF-1; most important treatment issue is **control of seizures** (which may be difficult).

Sturge-Weber Syndrome

Background—Sporadic presentation; **abnormal development of the primordial vascular bed** in early stages of cerebral vascularization; brain becomes **calcified and atrophic**

Clinical features—The **nevus (port wine stain)** is present at birth; it is **unilateral** (on the side of the abnormal brain development) and always involves **the forehead and upper eyelid** (not all congenital port wine stains are due to Sturge-Weber); **ipsilateral glaucoma; seizures occur in the first year of life (focal tonic-clonic and contralateral to the side of the nevus)** and become **refractory, and hemiparesis slowly develops; severe learning disorders and mental retardation**

Diagnosis—A **skull film** will show occipito-parietal intracranial calcifications (**"railroad track" appearance**); CT: calcifications, and shows **unilateral atrophy and hydrocephalus ex vacuo**; MRI for exact size and location of vascular malformation and any white-matter lesions

Treatment—Most important management issue is **seizure control**; manage behavioral and learning problems (special education); surveillance of complications—no routine studies unless signs and symptoms, except for routine evaluations of intraocular pressure; if seizures become refractory in the first 2 years, treatment of choice is **hemispherectomy; pulsed dye laser** for port wine stain

NEUROMUSCULAR DISEASE

Spinal Muscular Atrophies (SMAs)

Background—**Progressive denervation of muscle with subsequent atrophy** due to continuation of the normal process of **programmed neuronal cell death through the perinatal and postnatal period**; normally, the **survivor motor neuron (SMN) gene** arrests the process—it is mutated in the SMAs. Most are autosomal recessive, and is seen in all ethnic groups.

Types and findings

- **SMA-1: Werdnig-Hoffman disease; severe infantile type**; severe hypotonia, weakness, and decreased muscle mass in the first months of life; no DTRs; fasciculations seen most easily in the tongue, face, and jaw; eventual involvement of the diaphragm; presents with decreased feeding, decreased movement, lack of head control, increased flaccidity, and then respiratory weakness and distress; vast majority die in the first 2 years
- **SMA 2: late infantile; most common**; progressive weakness and scoliosis through early school years and often later; wheelchair-dependent
- **SMA 3: juvenile type = Kugelberg-Welander disease**; progressive weakness in proximal muscles, especially shoulders; remain ambulatory for most of their life, (middle adulthood)

Diagnostic findings—**Best test is to obtain blood for genetic evaluation of the SMN gene**; muscle biopsy (which usually is not necessary) shows nonspecific findings of denervation atrophy; EMG: nonspecific signs of denervation and fibrillation potentials

Management—There is **no cure**, and nothing will delay the progression; treatment is symptomatic.

Myasthenia Gravis

Background—**Rapid fatigue of striated muscles from immune-mediated neuromuscular blockade** → decreased acetylcholine receptors (circulating receptor-binding antibodies) → decreased responsiveness of the motor endplate. Most are **not hereditary**, but there are familial, non-immune forms, associations with Hashimoto thyroiditis and collagen vascular disease.

Clinical findings

- **Juvenile form:** ptosis and some degree of extraocular muscle weakness is the first sign; also possibly poor head control, dysphagia, and facial weakness → feeding problems; most will have involvement of the limb girdle and distal muscles of the hands; fatigue occurs late in the day or when tired (rapid fatigue of muscles with repetitive or sustained contractions). If untreated, may lead to respiratory failure.
- **Transient neonatal myasthenia:** infants born to mothers with myasthenia due to **transplacental antibodies**; infants may have decreased suck and swallow, generalized hypotonia, decreased motor activity, and weakness and respiratory insufficiency for days to weeks. May require nasogastric (NG) feeds and ventilation; strength returns as antibodies wane; no increased risk for myasthenia at a later age
- **Congenital myasthenia:** no maternal disease; permanent, severe disease without spontaneous remission; rare

Diagnosis—**EMG is specific for the diagnosis; decreased response to repetitive stimuli until the muscle is refractory**; process is **reversed after a cholinesterase inhibitor is given**; NCV is normal; **anti-acetylcholine antibodies** are an inconsistent finding. Administer **edrophonium** (**Tensilon test**; short-acting cholinesterase inhibitor); ptosis, ophthalmoplegia, and fatigability of other muscles improves improve within a few seconds.

Management

- Mild disease may require **no therapy**
- Otherwise, **cholinesterase inhibitors** are the primary therapy: **neostigmine methylsulfate IM or oral neostigmine bromide or pyridostigmine** (greater dose but slightly longer-acting)
- No response (large antibody titers), **prednisone, intravenous Ig (IVIG), or plasmapheresis**
- Potential complication—**do not tolerate neuromuscular blockade during anesthesia** (may have paralysis for weeks)
- **Aminoglycosides also potentiate the blockade** and should be avoided.
- Disease may undergo spontaneous remission or persist into adulthood.

Hereditary Motor-Sensory Neuropathies (HMSN)

Background—Number of identified types, but **type 1 (Charcot-Marie-Tooth disease)** is by far the most common; leads to **peroneal muscular atrophy**; is the **most common genetic neuropathy**; most are **autosomal dominant** with high degree of expressivity

Clinical presentation—Most are asymptomatic until **late childhood to adolescence; peroneal and tibial nerves are involved first** → **gradual wasting of muscles of the anterior compartment of the lower leg (clumsy due to frequent falls); muscle wasting is progressive** and eventually develops a **storklike appearance**; also **foot drop and foot arch abnormalities**; most require assistance from orthotic devices; **forearms may also be involved:** atrophy of the muscles of the forearms and hands may lead to a **claw-hand deformity.**

Laboratory diagnosis—The most important initial step is **NCV test—slowing**; there is no need for an EMG or muscle biopsy; **sural nerve biopsy** is diagnostic and shows interstitial hypertrophic neuropathy; definitive diagnosis may be made with molecular genetics.

Management—Ankle stabilization, orthotic devices, physical therapy, splinting, protect legs and knees from trauma, surgical ankle fusion; burning paresthesias treated with phenytoin or carbamazepine; no treatment delays the progression.

Guillain-Barré Syndrome

Background—Mostly motor **postinfectious polyneuropathy**; usually occurs after a **nonspecific viral illness** by about 10 days (especially associated with *Campylobacter jejuni and Helicobacter pylori*); may also occur after rabies vaccine, influenza vaccine, and oral polio vaccine (no longer available in the United States)

Clinical findings—Begins with **lower-extremity weakness, progresses cephalad to the trunk, upper extremities, and bulbar muscles (Landry ascending paralysis); may be initial sensory involvement**: tenderness and paresthesias on palpation of the muscles; eventually (over days to weeks) **flaccid paralysis of all four extremities. Bulbar involvement is a sign of impending respiratory failure; DTRs are lost early**; involvement of the **autonomic nervous system** (lability in blood pressure, cardiac rate, and possibly asystole). A small number suffer an acute relapse during the recovery phase, and some have a chronic relapsing form for months to years.

Laboratory diagnosis—Most important test (and usually the only one needed) is **LP**: CSF shows a dissociation of protein and cells, i.e., **there is an increase in CSF protein with a normal glucose and no pleocytosis (and culture is negative)**; there is greatly reduced motor, and sometimes sensory NCVs; there may be positive **antiganglioside antibodies.**

Management—**Admit all** in the early stages for observation (for respiratory compromise); slowly progressive disease is just observed (symptomatic treatment); **rapidly progressive disease is treated with IVIG**; if ineffective → **plasmapheresis and/or immunosuppressive drugs** (steroids are not effective); some centers use **IVIG plus interferon**; chronic neuropathic pain may be treated with gabapentin. Most recover completely within 2–3 weeks (muscle function recovered in inverse direction, with DTRs last to recover); some have various degrees of residual defects or a chronic neuropathy (permanent axonal loss); poor outcome with cranial nerve involvement and respiratory failure.

Muscular Dystrophies
Duchenne and Becker

Background—Becker is essentially the same disease as Duchenne, but in a milder, more protracted form; most common **hereditary primary myopathy** (all races and ethnic groups around the world); most cases are **X-linked recessive**; up to one-third are new mutations without female carriers. There is significantly decreased **muscle dystrophin**.

Clinical presentation
- Infants may be mildly hypotonic with poor head control and delay in motor skills.
- Possible hip-girdle weakness at age 2 years and lordosis may be prominent by age 3 years
- By 3–6 years, **hip-waddle and Gower sign** are evident (hands on ground and legs in a progressive climb to standing).
- **Calf pseudohypertrophy** (muscle replaced with fat and collagen)
- Most will walk without orthotics up to age 10 years, with orthotics until age 12, and then are wheelchair-dependent with a **rapid progression of scoliosis, thoracic deformities, and contractures**; then progressive weakness and respiratory muscle weakness → **increased infections and progressive decrease in pulmonary function**; gradual loss of DTRs
- **Cardiomyopathy** is present in almost all
- **Intellectual impairment** in all; most have some form of **learning disability.**
- Death usually occurs by age 18–20 years (respiratory failure, infection, aspiration, heart failure).

Laboratory diagnosis—**First screen with a serum CK**—will be 15,000–35,000 IU (normal is up to 160 IU, and a normal value is not consistent with the diagnosis); specific diagnosis may be obtained **first with a PCR of blood sample for the dystrophin gene** mutation, however one-third are falsely negative (due to several reasons with respect to the genome and testing methods); the **most accurate study needs to be performed—muscle biopsy** (more invasive; not done initially) with specific immunochemical studies of the **abnormal dystrophin protein**.

Management—**No cure or slowing of progressive deterioration**; treatment is **supportive with a multidisciplinary team**: physiotherapy (delays contractures), orthotic devices, good nutritional counseling (avoid obesity), calcium supplementation (decrease incidence of osteoporosis), digoxin, manage psychobehavioral and adjustment issues; some studies show that early use of corticosteroids improves long-term prognosis as well as short-term improvements.

Myotonic dystrophy

Background—Second most common muscular dystrophy in North America; **autosomal dominant**; due to a trinucleotide expansion on chromosome 19 of a gene coding for a protein kinase; each successive affected generation tends to be more severely involved.

Clinical findings

- Infants are either normal at birth or have facial wasting (with a number of characteristic findings) and **hypotonia**
- **Mild weakness develops over years and is then progressive (wasting of the distal muscles, especially the hand, forearm, and anterior compartment of the lower leg);** then tongue atrophy and wasting of the neck and proximal muscles (may also develop a Gower sign).
- Condition is **slowly progressive through adolescence and adulthood.**
- **Myotonia not evident until after age 5 years—very slow relaxation of a muscle group after contraction** (can see this if the patient makes tight fists and tries to open them quickly); speech becomes slurred; there may be problems swallowing and with ophthalmoplegia.
- In the **severe congenital form,** infants are **born to mothers with myotonic dystrophy;** there are **congenital contractures, generalized hypotonia, and weakness at birth; infants are flaccid with muscle wasting and usually need NG feedings and possibly ventilation** (poor prognosis).

Laboratory findings—**EMG shows a myotonic pattern**; CK is normal to slightly increased; specific diagnosis and prenatal diagnosis can be made with **molecular genetic analysis**; muscle biopsy is not needed for diagnosis and may show variable findings.

Management—There is **no specific treatment**; treat individual problems; physiotherapy and orthopedics as necessary; certain drugs raise the depolarization threshold of muscle and may decrease myotonia and improve function (phenytoin, carbamazepine, procainamide).

SEIZURES

Simple febrile seizures

Definition

- **Generalized seizure lasting <15 minutes occurring once in a 24-hour period** (complex = longer than 15 minutes, focal, >1 in a 24-hour period)
- Prior to onset, child has a **normal history and no evidence of CNS infection or metabolic disturbance**
- Typical age is **6 months–5 years**
- **High rate of recurrence**, especially if **first seizure occurs <12 months of age.**
- **No long-term risk for any problems.**
- **Simple febrile seizures are benign events, and almost all have a good prognosis.**

Increased risk of afebrile seizures and treatment issues

- With positive family history of epilepsy, <12 months of age with first seizure, or multiple febrile seizures; there is no evidence that treatment prevents the later development of epilepsy

- Some anticonvulsants may prevent the recurrence of repeated febrile seizures. If significant parental anxiety with non-treatment, then intermittent **oral diazepam at the onset of a fever** may prevent a seizure.

Evaluation—**Consider LP with the first febrile seizure in a child <12 months of age**, where clinical signs and symptoms of meningitis are less obvious. There is increased likelihood of CNS infection as a cause of the fever and the seizure if the child is still seizing on arrival at the ER, with a focal seizure, or with abnormal neurological findings on examination. Consider LP if the first seizure occurs between age 12 and 18 months, and it should not be routine if the child is >18 months of age (only if signs and symptoms suggest the diagnosis). **EEG is not predictive and should not be performed. No benefit to obtaining routine blood studies. No routine neuroimaging.**

Neonatal Seizures

Background—Do not commonly have generalized tonic-clonic seizures (decreased arborization and myelination). Typical seizures include focal (especially extremities and face), multifocal clonic (many muscle groups involved), tonic (extremity and trunk rigidity with fixed eye deviation), myoclonic (distal muscle jerks), and **subtle** (chewing, salivation, apnea, blinking, color changes, "bicycling"); subtle seizures may be associated with autonomic changes, lack of suppression with gentle restraint and no effect of sensory stimuli on the activity.

Classification—Either a **clinical seizure with a consistent EEG event** (these are epileptic and generally respond to treatment with anticonvulsants), a **clinical seizure with an inconsistent EEG event** (usually neurologically depressed to comatose and usually due to hypoxic-ischemic encephalopathy; they are likely to be non-epileptic and may or may not respond to therapy), or **electrical seizures without clinical seizures** (generally due to an abnormal background EEG in a coma and not on anticonvulsants).

Most causes—Most important is **hypoxic-ischemic encephalopathy**; consider also infection (sepsis, meningitis), metabolic causes (electrolyte abnormalities, acid-base disorders, inborn errors of metabolism), birth trauma and hemorrhage, structural abnormalities, and maternal conditions (illness, drugs, medications) or treatments (accidental injection of lidocaine into the fetus).

Other neonatal seizures

- **Benign familial neonatal seizures**: autosomal dominant, occurring on **the second to third day of life** with multiple daily seizures and normality between seizures; stop at age 1–6 months with good prognosis
- **Fifth-day fits**: days 4–6 with normal infants; multifocal seizures occurring <24 hours
- **Pyridoxine deficiency**: rare; generalized clonic seizures shortly after birth are resistant to anticonvulsants; pyridoxine is required for the synthesis of glutamic acid decarboxylase, needed to make gamma aminobutyric acid (GABA); if suspected, give pyridoxine

IV during EEG monitoring and seizures stop immediately in most cases; still need a 6-week trial before discontinuing due to lack of effect.

Management—Most seizures in the neonate are treated with phenobarbital and/or phenytoin.

Unprovoked Seizures Beyond the Neonatal Period

Partial seizures

Simple partial seizures

Description: relatively short, **focal, asymmetric tonic or clonic seizure without loss of consciousness**; some with a vague aura; remain awake and can talk during seizure; no postictal period

EEG: unilateral, bilateral, or multifocal spikes or sharp waves

Principal treatment: carbamazepine, phenytoin; adjuncts: leviractam, oxcarbazepine, zonisamide

Complex partial seizures

Description: focal seizure that may begin as a simple partial seizure, but some degree of loss of consciousness at some point (or from the beginning); automatisms are common after loss of consciousness (lip-smacking, salivation, walking, running, others); can become **secondarily generalized**; usually somewhat longer than simple partial seizures; there is a postictal period.

EEG: anterior **temporal lobe** sharp waves or focal/multifocal spikes; may see this on the interictal EEG, but may be normal and other specialized EEG methods may be needed to demonstrate abnormal electrical activity. **CT/MRI** for temporal lobe pathology.

Principal treatment: carbamazepine, phenytoin; clobazam, lamotrigine, tiagabine as an adjunct; gabapentin as an add-on for refractory seizures (age 12 years and older); topiramate for refractory seizures

Benign partial epilepsy

Description: onset from **rolandic (centrotemporal gyri)** without a pathological lesion; focal, tonic-clonic with paresthesias mostly involving the **face**, and most commonly during sleep; brief loss of consciousness and the seizure may secondarily generalize; onset from toddler to mid-adolescence with **peak at age 9–10 years**; often a positive family history of seizures; child is otherwise normal; good prognosis

EEG: repetitive spikes from **rolandic gyri with normal background**

Principal treatment: if seizures are frequent, the drug of choice is carbamazepine (continued for 2 years or between ages 14–16 years with spontaneous remission).

Generalized seizures

Absence (petit mal) seizures

Description: sudden cessation of motor activity or speech with blank facial expression and eyelid-flickering; most common in girls >5 years of age; total duration is short with resumption of pre-seizure activity; no aura or postictal state, but may have automatisms; may be multiple in a 24-hour period.

EEG: 3/second spike and generalized wave discharge

Principal management: ethosuximide, valproic acid; lamotrigine as single therapy for complex form

Generalized tonic-clonic seizures

Description: may present from the outset or follow a partial seizure; activity may be **preceded by an aura** (which represents the focal site of origin of the seizure); **sudden loss of consciousness** with eyes rolling back; then **tonic contractions**, cyanosis, and apnea, followed by **rhythmic clonic contractions**; then gradual slowing; may bite tongue, but vomiting is rare; also loss of sphincter tone (mostly bladder); **significant postictal period**, then deep sleep with subsequent vomiting and bifrontal headache

EEG: variable findings

Principal management: phenobarbital, primidone, phenytoin, carbamazepine, valproic acid; lamotrigine as an adjunct; gabapentin, topiramate as an add-on medication for secondarily generalized seizures

Myoclonic seizures

Benign myoclonus of infancy

Description: clusters of myotonic movements (brief, symmetric muscle contractions) mostly of the neck, trunk, and extremities; **typically stop by age 2 years; normal infant with normal development**

EEG: normal

Principal management: none

Myoclonic epilepsy of early childhood

Description: repetitive myoclonic movements that may occur multiple times in a day; may be preceded by tonic-clonic seizures; onset usually in first years of life; some have positive family history of seizures; **good prognosis in most** (learning problems; small number with mental retardation)

EEG: fast spike waves of >2.5 Hz with a normal background

Principal management: valproic acid, nitrazepam, lamotrigine

Complex myoclonic seizures

Description: often begins as many seizures in the first year of life; up to about one-third have delayed development; less common family history; more common with **hypoxic-ischemic encephalopathy**; **poor prognosis**

- **Lennox-Gastaut syndrome:** intractable myoclonic plus tonic seizures with interictal awake slow spike-and-wave pattern on EEG; may be refractory to treatment; significant increase in behavioral problems and mental retardation; may respond to a ketogenic diet (mechanism of action unknown); also clonazepam, nitrazepam, lamotrigine (also for complex myoclonic seizures)

Juvenile myoclonic epilepsy

Description: genetic locus for frequent myoclonic jerks on awakening, abating in late afternoon; then, after a few years, early morning tonic-clonic seizures with myoclonus; **typical onset age 12–16 years; normal exam**

EEG: 4–6/sec irregular spike-and-wave pattern

Principal management: valproic acid for life (usually a good response)

Infantile spasms

Description: brief, symmetric contraction of the neck, trunk, and extremities—usually clusters over minutes; usually starts at **age 4–8 months**; most with specific problems (prenatal, perinatal, postnatal) and have **poor prognosis** (mental retardation and neurological dysfunction); major association with **tuberous sclerosis** (see previous section); the few that have no previous problems have good prognosis; felt to be due to overproduction of corticotrophin-releasing hormone → neuronal hyperexcitability

EEG: hypsarrhythmia (chaotic, high-voltage, bilaterally asynchronous slow-wave activity)

Principal management: adrenocorticotropic hormone (ACTH), vigabatrin (especially with tuberous sclerosis)

Management of a first unprovoked seizure

- Careful history, physical, neurological, ophthalmological exams and family history; ask parent to demonstrate (rather than describe) seizure
- Always check serum **glucose**, but other labs only as warranted per the history and physical.
- Perform **EEG:** useful for seizure type, prediction of recurrence risk, focal abnormalities, or epileptic syndromes
- **No neuroimaging** unless focal deficits found on the physical exam
- **No treatment—watchful waiting** (<50% will go on to have another seizure)
- BUT . . . **≥2 seizures in an interval of >24 hours is suggestive of a seizure disorder**; again, history, family history, and physical exam are the most important in terms of diagnosis; no routine labs; **consider LP; obtain EEG in all; MRI for newly**

diagnosed epilepsy (especially if neurological deficits, partial seizure, or focal EEG abnormalities)

- Goal is to use the most appropriate **single anticonvulsant with the least side effects**, with increase in the dose until seizure control; serum levels are monitored at first but not routinely thereafter (unless there is a specific reason to do so); look for drug reaction mostly in first 3 months and monitor labs (no routine labs thereafter); use drug(s) for at least **2 seizure-free years** prior to discontinuation.

Management of status epilepticus

Definition: continuous seizure activity lasting **>30 minutes**, or serial seizures between **which there is no return to consciousness**; most are **generalized tonic-clonic seizures**; may be an initial manifestation of encephalitis or meningitis; the more the seizure is prolonged, the greater chance of neuronal injury.

Management:

- Airway (oral airway; intubate if necessary; suction), breathing (provide oxygen), circulation
- Check vital signs; **Dextrostix or bedside glucose**
- Place **NG tube**
- IV fluids: give **5 mL/kg 10% dextrose IV push** if low glucose.
- Draw blood for electrolytes, Ca, Mg, **ABG** (and others as needed based on information obtained); consider LP only when patient is stabilized.
- Quick exam for evidence of trauma, increased ICP, infection, retinal hemorrhage, dehydration, breathing pattern; more comprehensive exam when seizures are controlled
- **IV anticonvulsant** (not IM): administer short-acting benzodiazepine (**lorazepam preferred**; greater duration with decreased risk of hypotension and respiratory arrest) directly into a vein; if no IV: may give **rectal gel diazepam or buccal/nasal midazolam**
- Follow with **loading dose of phenytoin (fosphenytoin)**; follow ECG with loading; if not effective, give **phenobarbital**; if not effective, consider **diazepam infusion, barbiturate coma, paraldehyde, or general anesthesia.**
- If seizures do not recur, begin maintenance 12–24 hours later.

Index

REFERENCES

1. Alter, BP, Lipton, JM. Fanconi Anemia, *eMedicine* (2007).

2. Altman, LC, Becker, JW, Williams, PV, eds., *Allergy in Primary Care*. Philadelphia: Saunders, 2000.

3. Ambalavanan, N. Fluid, electrolyte, and nutrition management of the newborn. *eMedicine* (2008).

4. American Academy of Allergy, Asthma and Immunology. *The Allergy Report, Volumes 1, 2, and 3*. Milwaukee: American Academy of Allergy, Asthma and Immunology, 2000.

5. American Academy of Child and Adolescent Psychiatry. Practice parameter for the assessment and treatment of children and adolescents with suicidal behavior. *J Am Acad Child Adolesc. Psychiatry* (2001) 40 (Suppl): 24S–51S.

6. American Academy of Child and Adolescent Psychiatry. Practice parameters for the assessment and treatment of children, adolescents and adults with autism and other pervasive developmental disorders. *J Am Acad Child Adolesc. Psychiatry* (1999) 38 (Suppl): 32S–54S.

7. American Academy of Pediatrics. Dietary recommendations for children and adolescents: A guide for practitioners. *Pediatrics* (2006) 117: 544–59.

8. American Academy of Pediatrics. Guidance for effective discipline. *Pediatrics* (1998) 101: 723–28.

9. American Academy of Pediatrics. Management of hyperbilirubinemia in the newborn infant 35 or more weeks of gestation. *Pediatrics* (2004) 114: 297–316.

10. American Academy of Pediatrics Policy Statement. Breastfeeding and the use of human milk. *Pediatrics* (2005) 115: 496–506.

11. American Academy of Pediatrics Task Force on Infant Sleep Position and Sudden Infant Death Syndrome. The changing concept of sudden infant death syndrome: Diagnostic coding shifts, controversies regarding the sleeping environment, and new variables to consider in reducing risk. *Pediatrics* (2005) 116: 1245–55.

12. American Academy of Pediatrics, Committee on Bioethics. Appropriate boundaries in the pediatrician-family-patient relationship. *Pediatrics* (1999) 104(2): 334–36.

13. American Academy of Pediatrics, Committee on Bioethics. Professionalism in pediatrics: Statement of principles. Policy Statement. *Pediatrics* (2007) 120(4): 895–97.

14. American Academy of Pediatrics, Committee on Nutrition. Prevention of pediatric overweight and obesity. *Pediatrics* (2003) 112: 424–30.

15. American Academy of Pediatrics, Committee on Public Education. Media violence. *Pediatrics* (2001) 108: 1222–26.

16. American Psychiatric Association. *Diagnostic and Statistical Manual of Mental Disorders, 4th Edition, Text Revision.* Washington, DC: American Psychiatric Publishing, Inc., 2000.

17. Arnon, S, and Litmanovitz, I. Diagnostic tests in neonatal sepsis. *Curr Opin Infect Dis.* (June 2008) 21(3): 223–37.

18. Badawy, M, and Conners, GP. Lead toxicity. *eMedicine* (2008).

19. Baddour, LM, Wilson, WR, et al. Infective endocarditis: Diagnosis, antimicrobial therapy and management of complications: A statement for healthcare professionals from the Committee on Rheumatic Fever, Endocarditis and Kawasaki Disease, Council on Cardiovascular Disease. *Circulation* (June 14, 2005) 111 (23): e394–434.

20. Baraitser, M, and Winter, RM. *Color Atlas of Congenital Malformation Syndromes.* London: Mosby-Wolfe, 1996.

21. Barclay, L. Guidelines issue for treating atopic eczema in children. *Medscape Medical News* (2008).

22. Barclay, L. Guidelines revised on use of 7-valent pneumococcal conjugate vaccine in children. *Medscape Medical News* (2008).

23. Barlow, J, and Stewart-Brown, S. Child abuse and neglect. *Lancet* (2005) 365: 1750–52.

24. Basco, WT. Teens at risk: A focus on adolescent suicide. *Medscape Pediatrics* (2006).

25. Benseler, SM, Silverman, ER. Systemic lupus erythematosis. *Pediatric Clinics of North America* (2005) 52: 443–67.

26. Bhagwagar, Z. Bipolar disorder. *Medscape CME,* 2007.

27. Boyer, SG, and Boyer, KM. Update on TORCH infections in the newborn infant. *NBIN* (2004) 4(1).

28. Boyle, JS, and Holstege, CP. Plant poisoning, caladium, dieffenbachia, and philodendron. *Medscape* (2008).

29. Cardoso, F, Seppi, K, et al. Seminar on choreas. *Lancet* (2006) 5: 589–602.

30. Centers for Disease Control. *Childhood and Adolescent Immunization Schedule,* 2009.

31. Centers for Disease Control. Parasitic Diseases page. Recreational water-associated illnesses (accessed 2009).

32. Chan, JCM, Williams, DM, and Roth, KS. Kidney failure in infants and children. *Pediatr Rev* (2002) 23: 47–59.

33. Chen, LH, and Keystone, JS. New strategies for the prevention of malaria in travelers. *Infect Dis Clin N Am.* (2005) 19: 185–210.

34. Chin, TK, Chin, EM, et al. Rheumatic heart disease. *eMedicine* (2008).

35. Clark, BJ III. Treatment of heart failure in infants and children. *Heart Dis* (2000) 2: 354–61.

36. Committee on Infectious Diseases, American Academy of Pediatrics. *Red Book: 2009 Report of the Committee on Infectious Diseases.* Elk Grove Village: American Academy of Pediatrics, 2009.

37. Defendi, GL, and Tucker, JR. Acetaminophen toxicity. *eMedicine* (2008).

38. Department of Health and Human Services, Centers for Disease Control and Prevention. Diagnosis and management of foodborne illnesses. *MMWR* (2004) 53: 11–12.

39. Dias, PJ. Adolescent substance abuse: Assessment in the office. *Pediatr Clin N Am* (2002) 49: 269–300.

40. Dixon, SD, and Stein, MT, eds. *Encounters with Children: Pediatric Behavior and Development.* St. Louis: Mosby, 2000.

41. Emslie, GJ, Hamrin, V, and Gibbons, R. A multidisciplinary approach to treating major depressive disorder in the adolescent patient. *Medscape CME,* 2009.

42. Fanaroff, AA, and Martin, RJ, eds. *Neonatal-Perinatal Medicine: Diseases of the Fetus and Infant, 8th Edition.* St. Louis: Mosby, 2006.

43. Feldman, HM. Evaluation and management of language and speech disorders in preschool children. *Pediatr Rev* (2005) 26: 131–41.

44. Fenichel, GM. *Clinical Pediatric Neurology, 4th Edition.* Philadelphia: WB Saunders, 2001.

45. Finberg, L, ed. *Saunders Manual of Pediatric Practice.* Philadelphia: WB Saunders, 2002.

46. Freudenthal, W, Ralston, M. Organophosphate toxicity. *eMedicine* (2008).

47. Friedman, AL. Pediatric hydration therapy: Historical review and a new approach. *Kidney Int* (2005) 67: 380–88.

48. Garges, HP, Moody, MA, and Cotton, CM. Neonatal meningitis: What is the correlation among cerebrospinal fluid cultures, blood cultures and cerebrospinal fluid parameters? *Pediatrics* (Apr 2006) 117(4): 1094–1100.

49. Gillberg, C, and Soderstrom, H. Learning disability. *Lancet* (2003) 362: 811–21.

50. Goldstein, RJ. Hydrocarbon toxicity. *eMedicine* (2008).

51. Graham, JM. *Smith's Recognizable Patterns of Human Deformation, 3rd Edition.* Philadelphia: Saunders, 2007.

52. Green, M. *Pediatric Diagnosis: Interpretation of Symptoms and Signs in Children and Adolescents, 6th Edition.* Philadelphia: WB Saunders, 1998.

53. Grosse, SD, and Dezateaux, C. Newborn screening for inherited metabolic disease. *Lancet* (2007) 396: 5–6.

54. Guarino, A, Albano, F, et al. Oral rehydration: Toward a real solution. *J Pediatr Gastroenterol Nutr* (2001) 33: S2–S12.

55. Hagan, JF, Shaw, JS, Duncan, PM, eds. *Bright Futures: Guidelines for Health Supervision of Infants, Children and Adolescents, 3rd Edition.* Elk Grove Village: American Academy of Pediatrics, 2008.

56. Harper, J. Megaloblastic anemia. *eMedicine* (2007).

57. Haycook, GB. Hypernatremia: Diagnosis and management. *Arch Dis Child Educ Pract Ed* (2006) 91: ep8–ep13.

58. Hazinski, MF et al., eds. *PALS Provider Manual.* Dallas: American Heart Association, 2007.

59. Headache Classification Subcommittee of the International Headache Society. *The International Classification of Headache Disorders, 2nd Edition. Cephalagia* (2004) 24 (Suppl 1): 9–160.

60. Hendricks, KM, Duggan, C, and Walker, WA. *Manual of Pediatric Nutrition, 3rd Edition.* Hamilton: BC Decker, 2000.

61. Horenstein, MS, and Hamilton, RM. Syncope. *eMedicine* (2008).

62. Huang, LH, Portwine, C, and Miller, R. Transient erythroblastopenia of childhood. *eMedicine* (2007).

63. Ilowite, NT. Current treatment of juvenile rheumatoid arthritis. *Pediatrics* (Jan 2002) 109(1): 109–15.

64. Inoue, S. Autoimmune and chronic benign neutropenia. *eMedicine* (2007).

65. Inoue, S. Leukocytosis. *eMedicine* (2008).

66. Inoue, S. Thrombocytosis. *eMedicine* (2007).

67. Joffe, A, and Blythe, M, eds. *Handbook of Adolescent Medicine. State of the Art Reviews. Adolescent Medicine* (2003) 14: 231–62.

68. Johnson, CF. Child sexual abuse. *Lancet* (2004) 364: 462–70.

69. Jolley, CD. Failure to thrive. *Curr Probl Pediatr Adolesc Health Care* (2003) 33: 183–206.

70. Jones, KL. *Smith's Recognizable Patterns of Human Malformation, 6th Edition.* Philadelphia: Saunders, 2005.

71. Kaultman, H, and Shah, M. Evaluation of the child with an arrhythmia. *Pediatr Clin N Am* (2004) 51: 1537–51.

72. Kavey, RE, Daniels, SR, Lauer, RM, et al. American Heart Association guidelines for primary prevention of atherosclerotic cardiovascular disease beginning in childhood. *Circulation* (March 2003) 107 (11): 1562–66.

73. Kazdin, AE. Treatment of antisocial behavior in children and adolescents. *Eye on Psi Chi* (2009) vol. 12, issue 3.

74. Kelly, WF, Oppenheimer, JJ, and Argyros, GJ. Allergic and environmental asthma. *eMedicine* (2009).

75. Kliegman, RM, Behrman, RE, Jenson, HB, Stanton, BF, eds. *Nelson Textbook of Pediatrics, 18th Edition.* Philadelphia: Saunders Elsevier Inc, 2007.

76. Kliegman, RM, Greenbaum, LA, and Lye PS, eds. *Practical Strategies in Pediatric Diagnosis and Therapies, 2nd Edition.* Philadelphia: Elsevier, 2004.

77. Kliegman, RM, Marcdante, KJ, et al., eds. *Nelson Essentials of Pediatrics, 5th Edition.* Philadelphia: Elsevier, 2006.

78. Krawczyk, J, Gharahbaghian, L, and Rutkowski, A. Cough and cold preparation toxicity. *eMedicine* (2006).

79. Lappa, S, and Moscicki, A. The pediatrician and the sexually active adolescent: A primer for sexually transmitted diseases. *Pediatr Clin N Am* (1997) 44: 1430.

80. Larcombe, J. Urinary tract infection in children. *Clin Evid* (2004) Jun (11): 509–23.

81. Lawrence, DT, Holstege, CP, and Emery, KC. Iron toxicity. *eMedicine* (2006).

82. Lee, MT. Acute anemia. *eMedicine* (2009).

83. Levine, MD, Carey, WB, Crocker, AC, eds. *Developmental-Behavioral Pediatrics, 3rd Edition.* Philadelphia: WB Saunders Company, 1999.

84. Lie, D. Guidelines address proper screening and treatment of lead-related disease in children. *Medscape CME*, 2007.

85. Lie, D. New guidelines issued for evaluating physical abuse in children. Medscape.com: Medscape LLC, 2007.

86. Liu, A. Comprehensive management of pediatric asthma: Using the guidelines to develop effective, long-term plans. *Medscape CME*, 2008.

87. Long, WA, ed. *Fetal and Neonatal Cardiology*. Philadelphia: WB Saunders, 1990.

88. Marshall, SA, Landau, ME et al. Conversion disorders. *eMedicine* (2008).

89. Matsui, H, Adachi, I et al. Anatomy of coarctation, hypoplastic and interrupted aortic arch: Relevance to interventional/surgical treatment. *Expert Rev Cardiovasc Ther.* (2007) 5(5): 871–80.

90. Murata, P. New guidelines for antiviral therapy and prophylaxis for influenza in children. *Medscape Medical News* (2007).

91. Murata, P. Pediatric guidelines updated for influenza vaccination in 2008–2009. *Medscape Medical News* (2008).

92. National Institutes of Health. *National Asthma Education Prevention Program (NAEPP)*. www.nhlbi.nih.gov, 2007.

93. Newburger, JW, Takahasi, M, Gerber, MA et al. Diagnosis, treatment and long-term management of Kawasaki disease. *Pediatrics* (2004) 114: 1708–33.

94. Nicholls, D, and Viner, R. Eating disorders and weight problems. *BMJ* (2005) 330: 950–53.

95. Perkin, RM, Swift, JD et al., eds. *Pediatric Hospital Medicine: Textbook of Inpatient Management*. Philadelphia: Lippincott Williams and Wilkins, 2007.

96. Pliszka, SR, and Burkstein, OG. *Attention-Deficit/Hyperactivity Disorder*. Guidelines Pocketcard, Version 3.0. Baltimore: International Guidelines Center, 2007.

97. Pomeranz, AJ, Busey, SL et al., eds. *Pediatric Decision-Making Strategies*. Philadelphia: WB Saunders, 2002.

98. Raj, A, and Bertolone, S. Sickle cell anemia. *eMedicine* (2006).

99. Robertson, J, Shilkofski, N, eds. *The Harriet Lane Handbook, 17th Edition*. Philadelphia: Mosby, Inc, 2005.

100. Rodbard, Helena, and Vega, Charles. Diabetes screening, diagnosis and therapy in pediatric patients with type 2 diabetes. *Medscape J Med* (2008) 10(8): 184.

101. Rodriguez-Cruz, E, and Ettinger, LM. Hypertension. *eMedicine* (2008).

102. Rogers, MC, ed. *Textbook of Pediatric Intensive Care, 4th Edition*. Baltimore: Williams and Wilkins, 2008.

103. Saiman, L, and Siegel, J. Infection control recommendations for patients with cystic fibrosis: Microbiology, important pathogens and infection control practices to prevent patient-to-patient transmission. *Am J Infect Control.* (2003) 31 (3 Suppl): S1–62.

104. Sankar, R. Initial treatment of epilepsy with antiepileptic drugs: Pediatric issues. *Neurology* (2004) 63 (10 Suppl 4): S30–39.

105. Satou, G, Herzberg, G, and Erickson, LC. Congestive heart failure. *eMedicine* (2006).

106. Sawaf, H, and Lorenzana, A. Hemophilia A and B. *eMedicine* (2008).

107. Schilsky, ML, and Oikonomou, I. Inherited Metabolic Liver Disease. *Curr Opin Gastroenterol.* (2005) 21(3): 275–82.

108. Schwaderer, AL, and Schwartz, GJ. Back to basics: Acidosis and alkalosis. *Pediatr Rev* (2004) 25: 350–57.

109. Schwarz, SM. Biliary atresia. *eMedicine* (2007).

110. Scrivner, CR, Beaudet, AL et al., eds. *The Metabolic and Molecular Basis of Inherited Disease, 8th Edition.* New York: McGraw-Hill, 2001.

111. Sheldon, SH. *Evaluating Sleep in Infants and Children.* Philadelphia: Lippincott-Raven, 1996.

112. Silberstein, SD. Migraine. *Lancet* (2004) 363: 381–91.

113. Sills, RH, and Meck, M. Hereditary elliptocytosis and related disorders. *eMedicine* (2008).

114. Slap, GB. Menstrual disorders in adolescence. *Best Pract Res Clin Obstet Gynecol* (2003) 17: 75–92.

115. Snyder, CL, Splide, TL, and Rice, H. Fluid management for the pediatric surgical patient. *eMedicine* (2008).

116. Soghoian, S, Doty, CI et al. Carbon monoxide toxicity. *eMedicine* (2008).

117. Soghoian, S, Doty, CI et al. Tricyclic antidepressant toxicity. *eMedicine* (2008).

118. Springer, Shelley C. et al. Bowel obstruction in the newborn. *eMedicine* (2004).

119. Stam, J. Thrombosis of cerebral veins and sinuses. *New Engl J Med* (2005) 352: 1791–98.

120. Steering Committee on Quality Improvement and Management, American Academy of Pediatrics. *Pediatric Clinical Practice Guidelines and Policies: A Compendium of Evidence-based Research for Pediatric Practice, 9th Edition.* Elk Grove: American Academy of Pediatrics, 2009.

121. Steiner, MJ, DeWalt, DE, and Byerley, JS. Is the child dehydrated? *JAMA* (2004) 291: 2746–54.

122. Stiehm, ER, Ochs, HD, and Winkelstein, JA. *Immunologic Disorders of Infants and Children, 5th Edition.* Philadelphia: Elsevier, 2004.

123. Sun, SS. National estimates of the timing of sexual maturation and racial differences among US children. *Pediatrics* (2002) 110(5): 911–19.

124. Suresh, GK, and Soll, RF. Overview of surfactant replacement trials. *J Perinatol* (May 2005) 25 Suppl 2: S40–44.

125. Taeusch, HW, Ballard, RA, Gleason, CA, eds. *Avery's Diseases of the Newborn, 8th Edition.* Philadelphia: WB Saunders, 2004.

126. Tanner, JM. *Growth at Adolescence, 2nd Edition.* Oxford: Blackwell Scientific Publications, 1962.

127. Taussig, LM, Landau, LI, eds. *Pediatric Respiratory Medicine.* St. Louis: Mosby, 2008.

128. Volpe, JJ, ed. *Neurology of the Newborn, 5th Edition.* Philadelphia: WB Saunders, 2008.

129. Waseem, M, Aslam, M, and Gersheimer, JR. Salicylate toxicity. *eMedicine* (2008).

130. Wheeler, D, Vimalachandra, D et al. Antibiotics and surgery for vesicoureteral reflux: A meta-analysis of randomized controlled trials. *Arch Dis Child* (2003) 88: 688–94.

131. Wilson, W, Taubert, KA et al. Prevention of infective endocarditis: Guidelines from the American Heart Association: Rheumatic fever, endocarditis and Kawasaki Disease Committee. *Circulation* (October 9, 2007) 116 (15): 1736–54.

132. Yaish, HM. Pyruvate kinase deficiency. *eMedicine* (2007).

133. Yaish, HM. Thalassemia. *eMedicine* (2007).